IARC MONOGRAPHS

ON THE

EVALUATION OF THE
CARCINOGENIC RISK
OF CHEMICALS TO HUMANS

Sex Hormones (II)

VOLUME 21

This publication represents the views and expert opinions
of an IARC Working Group on the
Evaluation of the Carcinogenic Risk of Chemicals to Humans
which met in Lyon,
21-27 November 1978

December 1979

INTERNATIONAL AGENCY FOR RESEARCH ON CANCER

IARC MONOGRAPHS

In 1971, the International Agency for Research on Cancer (IARC) initiated a programme on the evaluation of the carcinogenic risk of chemicals to humans involving the production of critically evaluated monographs on individual chemicals.

The objective of the programme is to elaborate and publish in the form of monographs critical reviews of data on carcinogenicity for groups of chemicals to which humans are known to be exposed, to evaluate these data in terms of human risk with the help of international working groups of experts in chemical carcinogenesis and related fields, and to indicate where additional research efforts are needed.

International Agency for Research on Cancer 1979

PRINTED IN SWITZERLAND

ISBN 92 832 1221 5

CONTENTS

SEX HORMONES (II)

Lyon, 21-27 November 1978

Members

H.A. Bern, Professor of Zoology, Cancer Research Laboratory, University
of California, 230 Warren Hall, Berkeley, California 94720,
USA *(Chairman)*

H.M. Bolt, Institut für Toxikologie der Universität Tübingen, Lothar
Meyer-Bau, Wilhelmstrasse 56, 7400 Tübingen 1, Federal Republic
of Germany

U.H. Ehling, Gesellschaft für Strahlen- und Umweltforschung MBH München,
Institut für Biologie, Abteilung für Genetik, Ingolstädter
Landstrasse 1, Post Oberschleissheim, 8042 Neuherberg, Federal
Republic of Germany

L. Elbling, Institut für Krebsforschung der Universität Wien, IX,
Borschkegasse 8a, 1090 Vienna, Austria

A.L. Herbst, Chairman, Department of Obstetrics and Gynecology,
The University of Chicago, The Chicago Lying-In Hospital, 5841
Maryland Avenue, Chicago, Illinois 60637, USA

R.N. Hoover, Head, Environmental Studies Section, Environmental
Epidemiology Branch, Division of Cancer Cause and Prevention,
National Cancer Institute, Bethesda, Maryland 20014, USA

R. Kroes, Deputy Director, Central Institute for Nutrition and Food
Research (TNO), Utrechtseweg 48, Zeist, The Netherlands *(Vice-Chairman)*

H. Nagasawa, Head, Carcinogenesis Section, Pharmacology Division,
National Cancer Center Research Institute, Tsukiji 5-chome,
Chuo-ku, Tokyo, Japan

M.A. Quinn, Department of Obstetrics and Gynaecology, University of
Melbourne, Parkville, Victoria 3052, Australia

E. Stern, Professor of Epidemiology, University of California,
School of Public Health, Los Angeles, California 90024, USA

H. Tuchmann-Duplessis, Université René Descartes, UER Biomédicale,
Laboratoire d'Embryologie, 45 rue des Saints-Pères, 75270 Paris
Cedex 06, France

S.D. Vesselinovitch, The University of Chicago, Department of Radiology, Section of Radiation Biology and Experimental Oncology, 950 East 59th Street, Chicago, Illinois 60637, USA

M.P. Vessey, Professor, Department of Social and Community Medicine, University of Oxford, 8 Keble Road, Oxford OX1 3QN, UK

Representative from the National Cancer Institute

J.I. Munn, Assistant to the Scientific Coordinator for Environmental Cancer, Landow Building, Room 8C25, Division of Cancer Cause and Prevention, National Cancer Institute, Bethesda, Maryland 20014, USA

Representative from SRI International

J.G.T. Johansson, Medicinal Chemist, Bio-Organic Chemistry Department, Life Sciences Division, SRI International, 333 Ravenswood Avenue, Menlo Park, California 94025, USA

Representative from the Commission of the European Communities

M.-T. van der Venne, Commission of the European Communities, Health and Safety Directorate, Bâtiment Jean Monnet, Plateau du Kirchberg, Luxembourg, Great Duchy of Luxembourg

Representative from the World Health Organization

D.B. Thomas, Special Programme of Research in Human Reproduction, World Health Organization, 1211 Geneva 27, Switzerland

Representative from the US Pharmaceutical Manufacturers' Association

R. Dorfman, Syntex Laboratories, Inc., 3401 Hillview Avenue, Palo Alto, California 94304, USA

Observers

P.A. Desaulles, Director of Metabolic and Endocrine Research, Biological Department, Pharmaceutical Division, Ciba-Geigy Ltd, 4002 Basel, Switzerland

R. Hess, Director of Toxicology, Ciba-Geigy Ltd, 4022 Basel, Switzerland

Secretariat

R. Althouse[1], Unit of Chemical Carcinogenesis

H. Bartsch, Unit of Chemical Carcinogenesis *(Rapporteur section 3.2)*

---

[1]Present address: University of Oxford, Department of the Regius Professor of Medicine, Radcliffe Infirmary, Oxford OX2 6HE, UK

M. Castegnaro, Unit of Environmental Carcinogens

J.A. Cooper[1], Unit of Epidemiology and Biostatistics *(Co-rapporteur section 3.3)*

L. Griciute, Chief, Unit of Environmental Carcinogens

J.E. Huff[2], Unit of Chemical Carcinogenesis *(Co-secretary)*

D. Mietton, Unit of Chemical Carcinogenesis *(Library assistant)*

R. Montesano, Unit of Chemical Carcinogenesis *(Rapporteur section 3.1)*

C. Partensky, Unit of Chemical Carcinogenesis *(Technical editor)*

I. Peterschmitt, Unit of Chemical Carcinogenesis, WHO, Geneva *(Bibliographic researcher)*

V. Ponomarkov[3], Unit of Chemical Carcinogenesis

R. Saracci, Unit of Epidemiology and Biostatistics *(Co-rapporteur section 3.3)*

L. Tomatis, Chief, Unit of Chemical Carcinogenesis *(Head of the Programme)*

E.A. Walker, Unit of Environmental Carcinogens *(Rapporteur sections 1 and 2.3)*

E. Ward, Montignac, France *(Editor)*

J.D. Wilbourn, Unit of Chemical Carcinogenesis *(Co-secretary)*

Secretarial assistance

    A.V. Anderson
    M.J. Ghess
    R.B. Johnson
    J.A. Smith

---

[1] Present address: Deputy Associate Director, Carcinogenesis Program, Division of Cancer Cause & Treatment, National Cancer Institute, Bethesda, MD 20014, USA

[2] Present address: National Institute of Environmental Health Sciences, P.O. Box 12233, Research Triangle Park, North Carolina 27709, USA

[3] Present address: Laboratory of Comparative Oncology, Cancer Research Center, USSR Academy of Medical Sciences, Kashirskoye Shosse 6, Moscow 115478, USSR

The term 'carcinogenic risk' in the *IARC Monograph* series is taken to mean the probability that exposure to the chemical will lead to cancer in humans.

Inclusion of a chemical in the monographs does not imply that it is a carcinogen, only that the published data have been examined. Equally, the fact that a chemical has not yet been evaluated in a monograph does not mean that it is not carcinogenic.

Anyone who is aware of published data that may alter the evaluation of the carcinogenic risk of a chemical for humans is encouraged to make this information available to the Unit of Chemical Carcinogenesis, International Agency for Research on Cancer, Lyon, France, in order that the chemical may be considered for re-evaluation by a future Working Group.

Although every effort is made to prepare the monographs as accurately as possible, mistakes may occur. Readers are requested to communicate any errors to the Unit of Chemical Carcinogenesis, so that corrections can be reported in future volumes.

IARC MONOGRAPH PROGRAMME ON THE EVALUATION OF THE

CARCINOGENIC RISK OF CHEMICALS TO HUMANS

PREAMBLE

BACKGROUND

In 1971, the International Agency for Research on Cancer (IARC) initiated a programme on the evaluation of the carcinogenic risk of chemicals to humans with the object of producing monographs on individual chemicals*. The criteria established at that time to evaluate carcinogenic risk to humans were adopted by all the working groups whose deliberations resulted in the first 16 volumes of the *IARC Monograph* series. In October 1977, a joint IARC/WHO *ad hoc* Working Group met to re-evaluate these guiding criteria; this preamble reflects the results of their deliberations(1) and those of a subsequent IARC *ad hoc* Working Group which met in April 1978(2).

OBJECTIVE AND SCOPE

The objective of the programme is to elaborate and publish in the form of monographs critical reviews of data on carcinogenicity for groups of chemicals to which humans are known to be exposed, to evaluate these data in terms of human risk with the help of international working groups of experts in chemical carcinogenesis and related fields, and to indicate where additional research efforts are needed.

The monographs summarize the evidence for the carcinogenicity of individual chemicals and other relevant information. The critical analyses of the data are intended to assist national and international authorities in formulating decisions concerning preventive measures. No recommendations are given concerning legislation, since this depends on risk-benefit evaluations, which seem best made by individual governments and/or international agencies. In this connection, WHO recommendations on food additives(3), drugs(4), pesticides and contaminants(5) and occupational carcinogens(6) are particularly informative.

---

*Since 1972, the programme has undergone considerable expansion, primarily with the scientific collaboration and financial support of the US National Cancer Institute.

The *IARC Monographs* are recognized as an authoritative source of information on the carcinogenicity of environmental chemicals. The first users' survey, made in 1976, indicates that the monographs are consulted routinely by various agencies in 24 countries.

Since the programme began in 1971, 21 volumes have been published(7) in the *IARC Monograph* series, and 449 separate chemical substances have been evaluated (see also cumulative index to the monographs, p. 565). Each volume is printed in 4000 copies and distributed *via* the WHO publications service (see inside covers for a listing of IARC publications and back outside cover for distribution and sales services).

SELECTION OF CHEMICALS FOR MONOGRAPHS

The chemicals (natural and synthetic, including those which occur as mixtures and in manufacturing processes) are selected for evaluation on the basis of two main criteria: (a) there is evidence of human exposure, and (b) there is some experimental evidence of carcinogenicity and/or there is some evidence or suspicion of a risk to humans. In certain instances, chemical analogues were also considered.

Inclusion of a chemical in a volume does not imply that it is carcinogenic, only that the published data have been examined. The evaluations must be consulted to ascertain the conclusions of the Working Group. Equally, the fact that a chemical has not appeared in a monograph does not mean that it is without carcinogenic hazard.

The scientific literature is surveyed for published data relevant to the monograph programme. In addition, the IARC Survey of Chemicals Being Tested for Carcinogenicity(8) often indicates those chemicals that are to be scheduled for future meetings. The major aims of the survey are to prevent unnecessary duplication of research, to increase communication among scientists, and to make a census of chemicals that are being tested and of available research facilities.

As new data on chemicals for which monographs have already been prepared and new principles for evaluating carcinogenic risk receive acceptance, re-evaluations will be made at subsequent meetings, and revised monographs will be published as necessary.

WORKING PROCEDURES

Approximately one year in advance of a meeting of a working group, a list of the substances to be considered is prepared by IARC staff in consultation with other experts. Subsequently, all relevant biological data are collected by IARC; in addition to the published literature, US Public Health Service Publication No. 149(9) has been particularly

valuable and has been used in conjunction with other recognized sources
of information on chemical carcinogenesis and systems such as CANCERLINE,
MEDLINE and TOXILINE. The major collection of data and the preparation
of first drafts for the sections on chemical and physical properties, on
production, use, occurrence and on analysis are carried out by SRI
International under a separate contract with the US National Cancer
Institute. Most of the data so obtained on production, use and occurrence
refer to the United States and Japan; SRI International and IARC supplement this information with that from other sources in Europe. Biblio-
graphical sources for data on mutagenicity and teratogenicity are the
Environmental Mutagen Information Center and the Environmental Teratology
Information Center, both located at the Oak Ridge National Laboratory,
USA.

Six to nine months before the meeting, reprints of articles containing relevant biological data are sent to an expert(s), or are used by the
IARC staff, for the preparation of first drafts of the monographs. These
drafts are edited by IARC staff and are sent prior to the meeting to all
participants of the Working Group for their comments. The Working Group
then meets in Lyon for seven to eight days to discuss and finalize the
texts of the monographs and to formulate the evaluations. After the
meeting, the master copy of each monograph is verified by consulting the
original literature, then edited and prepared for reproduction. The
monographs are usually published within six months after the Working Group
meeting.

DATA FOR EVALUATIONS

With regard to biological data, only reports that have been published
or accepted for publication are reviewed by the working groups, although
a few exceptions have been made. The monographs do not cite all of the
literature on a particular chemical: only those data considered by the
Working Group to be relevant to the evaluation of the carcinogenic risk
of the chemical to humans are included.

Anyone who is aware of data that have been published or are in press
which are relevant to the evaluations of the carcinogenic risk to humans
of chemicals for which monographs have appeared is urged to make them
available to the Unit of Chemical Carcinogenesis, International Agency
for Research on Cancer, Lyon, France.

THE WORKING GROUP

The tasks of the Working Group are five-fold: (a) to ascertain that
all data have been collected; (b) to select the data relevant for the
evaluation; (c) to ensure that the summaries of the data enable the reader
to follow the reasoning of the committee; (d) to judge the significance

of the results of experimental and epidemiological studies; and (e) to
make an evaluation of the carcinogenic risk of the chemical.

Working Group participants who contributed to the consideration and
evaluation of chemicals within a particular volume are listed, with their
addresses, at the beginning of each publication (see p. 5). Each member
serves as an individual scientist and not as a representative of any
organization or government. In addition, observers are often invited
from national and international agencies, organizations and industries.

GENERAL PRINCIPLES FOR EVALUATING THE CARCINOGENIC RISK OF CHEMICALS

The widely accepted meaning of the term 'chemical carcinogenesis',
and that used in these monographs, is the induction by chemicals of
neoplasms that are not usually observed, the earlier induction by chemicals
of neoplasms that are usually observed, and/or the induction by chemicals
of more neoplasms than are usually found - although fundamentally different
mechanisms may be involved in these three situations. Etymologically, the
term 'carcinogenesis' means the induction of cancer, that is, of malignant
neoplasms; however, the commonly accepted meaning is the induction of
various types of neoplasms or of a combination of malignant and benign
tumours. In the monographs, the words 'tumour' and neoplasm' are used
interchangeably (In scientific literature the terms 'tumourigen', 'oncogen'
and 'blastomogen' have all been used synonymously with 'carcinogen',
although occasionally 'tumourigen' has been used specifically to denote
the induction of benign tumours).

Experimental Evidence

Qualitative aspects

Both the interpretation and evaluation of a particular study as well
as the overall assessment of the carcinogenic activity of a chemical
involve several qualitatively important considerations, including:
(a) the experimental parameters under which the chemical was tested,
including route of administration and exposure, species, strain, sex, age,
etc.; (b) the consistency with which the chemical has been shown to be
carcinogenic, e.g., in how many species and at which target organ(s);
(c) the spectrum of neoplastic response, from benign neoplasia to multiple
malignant tumours; (d) the stage of tumour formation in which a chemical
may be involved: some chemicals act as complete carcinogens and have
initiating and promoting activity, while others are promoters only; and
(e) the possible role of modifying factors.

There are problems not only of differential survival but of differential toxicity, which may be manifested by unequal growth and weight gain
in treated and control animals. These complexities should also be considered in the interpretation of data, or, better, in the experimental design.

Many chemicals induce both benign and malignant tumours; few instances are recorded in which only benign neoplasms are induced by chemicals that have been studied extensively. Benign tumours may represent a stage in the evolution of a mqlignant neoplasm or they may be 'end-points' that do not readily undergo transition to malignancy. If a substance is found to induce only benign tumours in experimental animals, the chemical should be suspected of being a carcinogen and requires further investigation.

Hormonal carcinogenesis

Hormonal carcinogenesis presents certain distinctive features: the chemicals involved occur both endogenously and exogenously; in many instances, long exposure is required; tumours occur in the target tissue in association with a stimulation of non-neoplastic growth, but in some cases, hormones promote the proliferation of tumour cells in a target organ. Hormones that occur in excessive amounts, hormone-mimetic agents and agents that cause hyperactivity or imbalance in the endocrine system may require evaluative methods comparable with those used to identify chemical carcinogens; particular emphasis must be laid on quantitative aspects and duration of exposure. Some chemical carcinogens have significant side effects on the endocrine system, which may also result in hormonal carcinogenesis. Synthetic hormones and anti-hormones can be expected to possess other pharmacological and toxicological actions in addition to those on the endocrine system, and in this respect they must be treated like any other chemical with regard to intrinsic carcinogenic potential.

Quantitative aspects

Dose-response studies are important in the evaluation of carcinogenesis: the confidence with which a carcinogenic effect can be established is strengthened by the observation of an increasing incidence of neoplasms with increasing exposure.

The assessment of carcinogenicity in animals is frequently complicated by recognized differences among the test animals (species, strain, sex, age), in route(s) of administration and in dose/duration of exposure; often, target organs at which a cancer occurs and its histological type may vary with these parameters. Nevertheless, indices of carcinogenic potency in particular experimental systems (for instance, the dose-rate required under continuous exposure to halve the probability of the animals remaining tumourless(10)) have been formulated in the hope that, at least among categories of fairly similar agents, such indices may be of some predictive value in other systems, including humans.

Chemical carcinogens differ widely in the dose required to produce a given level of tumour induction, although many of them share common biological properties which include metabolism to reactive (electrophilic (11-13)) intermediates capable of interacting with DNA. The reason for this variation in dose-response is not understood but may be due either to

differences within a common metabolic process or to the operation of
qualitatively distinct mechanisms.

Statistical analysis of animal studies

Tumours which would have arisen had an animal lived longer may not
be observed because of the death of the animal from unrelated causes, and
this possibility must be allowed for. Various analytical techniques have
been developed which use the assumption of independence of competing risks
to allow for the effects of intercurrent mortality on the final numbers
of tumour-bearing animals in particular treatment groups.

For externally visible tumours and for neoplasms that cause death,
methods such as Kaplan-Meier (i.e., 'life-table', 'product-limit' or
'actuarial') estimates(10), with associated significance tests(14,15),
are recommended.

For internal neoplasms which are discovered 'incidentally'(14) at
autopsy but which did not cause the death of the host, different estimates
(16) and significance tests(14,15) may be necessary for the unbiased study
of the numbers of tumour-bearing animals.

All of these methods(10,14-16) can be used to analyse the numbers of
animals bearing particular tumour types, but they do not distinguish
between animals with one or many such tumours. In experiments which end
at a particular fixed time, with the simultaneous sacrifice of many
animals, analysis of the total numbers of internal neoplasms per animal
found at autopsy at the end of the experiment is straightforward. However,
there are no adequate statistical methods for analysing the numbers of
particular neoplasms that kill an animal host.

Evidence of Carcinogenicity in Humans
====

Evidence of carcinogenicity in humans can be derived from three
types of study, the first two of which usually provide only suggestive
evidence: (1) reports concerning individual cancer patients (case reports),
including a history of exposure to the supposed carcinogenic agent; (2)
descriptive epidemiological studies in which the incidence of cancer in
human populations is found to vary (spatially or temporally) with exposure
to the agent; and (3) analytical epidemiological studies (e.g., case-
control or cohort studies) in which individual exposure to the agent is
found to be associated with an increased risk of cancer.

An analytical study that shows a positive association between an
agent and a cancer may be interpreted as implying causality to a greater
or lesser extent, if the following criteria are met: (a) there is no
identifiable positive bias (By 'positive bias' is meant the operation of
factors in study design or execution which lead erroneously to a more
strongly positive association between an agent and disease than in fact
exists. Examples of positive bias include, in case-control studies,

better documentation of exposure to the agent for cases than for controls,
and, in cohort studies, the use of better means of detecting cancer
in individuals exposed to the agent than in individuals not exposed);
(b) the possibility of positive confounding has been considered (By 'positive confounding' is meant a situation in which the relationship between
an agent and a disease is rendered more strongly positive than it truly
is as a result of an association between that agent and another agent
which either causes or prevents the disease. An example of positive
confounding is the association between coffee consumption and lung cancer,
which results from their joint association with cigarette smoking); (c)
the association is unlikely to be due to chance alone; (d) the association
is strong; and (e) there is a dose-response relationship.

In some instances, a single epidemiological study may be strongly
indicative of a cause-effect relationship; however, the most convincing
evidence of causality comes when several independent studies done under
different circumstances result in 'positive' findings.

Analytical epidemiological studies that show no association between
an agent and a cancer ('negative' studies) should be interpreted according
to criteria analogous to those listed above: (a) there is no identifiable
negative bias; (b) the possibility of negative confounding has been
considered; and (c) the possible effects of misclassification of exposure
or outcome have been weighed.

In addition, it must be recognized that in any study there are
confidence limits around the estimate of association or relative risk.
In a study regarded as 'negative', the upper confidence limit may indicate
a relative risk substantially greater than unity; in that case, the study
excludes only relative risks that are above this upper limit. This usually
means that a 'negative' study must be large to be convincing. Confidence
in a 'negative' result is increased when several independent studies
carried out under different circumstances are in agreement.

Finally, a 'negative' study may be considered to be relevant only to
dose levels within or below the range of those observed in the study and
is pertinent only if sufficient time has elapsed since first human exposure
to the agent. Experience with human cancers of known etiology suggests
that the period from first exposure to a chemical carcinogen to development
of clinically observed cancer is usually measured in decades and may be in
excess of 30 years.

Experimental Data Relevant to the Evaluation of Carcinogenic Risk to Humans

No adequate criteria are presently available to interpret experimental
carcinogenicity data directly in terms of carcinogenic potential for humans.
Nonetheless, utilizing data collected from appropriate tests in animals,
positive extrapolations to possible human risk can be approximated.

Information compiled from the first 17 volumes of the *IARC Monographs*
(17-19) shows that of about 26 chemicals or manufacturing processes now
generally accepted to cause cancer in humans, all but possibly two (arsenic
and benzene) of those which have been tested appropriately produce cancer
in at least one animal species. For several (aflatoxins, 4-aminobiphenyl,
diethylstilboestrol, melphalan, mustard gas and vinyl chloride), evidence
of carcinogenicity in experimental animals preceded evidence obtained from
epidemiological studies or case reports.

In general, the evidence that a chemical produces tumours in experimental animals is of two degrees: (a) *sufficient evidence* of carcinogenicity is provided by the production of malignant tumours;   and (b)
limited evidence of carcinogenicity reflects qualitative and/or quantitative
limitations of the experimental results.

For many of the chemicals evaluated in the first 20 volumes of the
IARC Monographs for which there is *sufficient evidence* of carcinogenicity
in animals, data relating to carcinogenicity for humans are either insufficient or nonexistent.   In the absence of adequate data on humans, it is
reasonable, for practical purposes, to regard such chemicals as if they
presented a carcinogenic risk to humans.

Sufficient evidence of carcinogenicity is provided by experimental
studies that show an increased incidence of malignant tumours: (i) in
multiple species or strains, and/or (ii) in multiple experiments (routes
and/or doses), and/or (iii) to an unusual degree (with regard to incidence,
site, type and/or preocity of onset).   Additional evidence may be provided
by data concerning dose-response, mutagenicity or structure.

In the present state of knowledge, it would be difficult to define a
predictable relationship between the dose (mg/kg bw/day) of a particular
chemical required to produce cancer in test animals and the dose which would
produce a similar incidence of cancer in humans.   The available data suggest,
however, that such a relationship may exist (20,21), at least for certain
classes of carcinogenic chemicals.   Data that provide *sufficient evidence* of
carcinogenicity in test animals may therefore be used in an approximate
quantitative evaluation of the human risk at some given exposure level, provided that the nature of the chemical concerned and the physiological,
pharmacological and toxicological differences between the test animals and
humans are taken into account.   However, no acceptable methods are currently
available for quantifying the possible errors in such a procedure, whether
it is used to generalize between species or to extrapolate from high to low
doses.   The methodology for such quantitative extrapolation to humans
requires further development.

Evidence for the carcinogenicity of some chemicals in experimental
animals may be limited for two reasons.   Firstly, experimental data may
be restricted to such a point that it is not possible to determine a causal
relationship between administration of a chemical and the development of a

particular lesion in the animals. Secondly, there are certain neoplasms, including lung tumours and hepatomas in mice, which have been considered of lesser significance than neoplasms occurring at other sites for the purpose of evaluating the carcinogenicity of chemicals. Such tumours occur spontaneously in high incidence in these animals, and their malignancy is often difficult to establish. An evaluation of the significance of these tumours following administration of a chemical is the responsibility of particular Working Groups preparing individual monographs, and it has not been possible to set down rigid guidelines; the relevance of these tumours must be determined by considerations which include experimental design completeness of reporting.

Some chemicals for which there is *limited evidence* of carcinogenicity in animals have also been studied in humans with, in general, inconclusive results. While such chemicals may indeed be carcinogenic to humans, more experimental and epidemiological investigation is required.

Hence, '*sufficient evidence*' of carcinogenicity and '*limited evidence*' of carcinogenicity do not indicate categories of chemicals: the inherent definitions of those terms indicate varying degrees of experimental evidence, which may change if and when new data on the chemicals become available. The main drawback to any rigid classification of chemicals with regard to their carcinogenic capacity is the as yet incomplete knowledge of the mechanism(s) of carcinogenesis.

In recent years, several short-term tests for the detection of potential carcinogens have been developed. When only inadequate experimental data are available, positive results in validated short-term tests (see p. 23) are an indication that the compound is a potential carcinogen and that it should be tested in animals for an assessment of its carcinogenicity. Negative results from short-term tests cannot be considered sufficient evidence to rule out carcinogenicity. Whether short-term tests will eventually be as reliable as long-term tests in predicting carcinogenicity in humans will depend on further demonstrations of consistency with long-term experiments and with data from humans.

EXPLANATORY NOTES ON THE MONOGRAPH CONTENTS

Chemical and Physical Data (Section 1)

The Chemical Abstracts Service Registry Number and the latest Chemical Abstracts Primary Name (9th Collective Index)(22) are recorded in section 1. Other synonyms and trade names are given, but no comprehensive list is provided. Further, some of the trade names are those of mixtures in which the compound being evaluated is only one of the ingredients.

The structural and molecular formulae, molecular weight and chemical and physical properties are given. The properties listed refer to the

pure substance, unless otherwise specified, and include, in particular,
data that might be relevant to carcinogenicity (e.g., lipid solubility) and
those that concern identification. A separate description of the composition of technical products includes available information on impurities and
formulated products.

Production, Use, Occurrence and Analysis (Section 2)

The purpose of section 2 is to provide indications of the extent of
past and present human exposure to this chemical.

Synthesis

Since cancer is a delayed toxic effect, the dates of first synthesis
and of first commercial production of the chemical are provided. In
addition, methods of synthesis used in past and present commercial production are described. This information allows a reasonable estimate to be
made of the date before which no human exposure could have occurred.

Production

Since Europe, Japan and the United States are reasonably representative industrialized areas of the world, most data on production, foreign
trade and uses are obtained from those countries. It should not, however,
be inferred that those nations are the sole or even the major sources or
users of any individual chemical.

Production and foreign trade data are obtained from both governmental
and trade publications by chemical economists in the three geographical
areas. In some cases, separate production data on organic chemicals manufactured in the United States are not available because their publication
could disclose confidential information. In such cases, an indication of
the minimum quantity produced can be inferred from the number of companies
reporting commercial production. Each company is required to report on
individual chemicals if the sales value or the weight of the annual production exceeds a specified minimum level. These levels vary for chemicals
classified for different uses, e.g., medicinals and plastics; in fact,
the minimal annual sales value is between $1000 and $50 000 and the minimal
annual weight of production is between 450 and 22 700 kg. Data on production
in some European countries are obtained by means of general questionnaires
sent to companies thought to produce the compounds being evaluated. Information from the completed questionnaires is compiled by country, and the
resulting estimates of production are included in the individual monographs.

Use

Information on uses is meant to serve as a guide only and is not
complete. It is usually obtained from published data but is often complemented by direct contact with manufacturers of the chemical. In the case

of drugs, mention of their therapeutic uses does not necessarily represent
current practice nor does it imply judgement as to their clinical efficacy.

Statements concerning regulations and standards (e.g., pesticide
registrations, maximum levels permitted in foods, occupational standards
and allowable limits) in specific countries are mentioned as examples only.
They may not reflect the most recent situation, since such legislation is
in a constant state of change; nor should it be taken to imply that other
countries do not have similar regulations.

Occurrence

Information on the occurrence of a chemical in the environment is
obtained from published data, including that derived from the monitoring
and surveillance of levels of the chemical in occupational environments,
air, water, soil, foods and tissues of animals and humans. When available,
data on the generation, persistence and bioaccumulation of a chemical are
also included.

Analysis

The purpose of the section on analysis is to give the reader an indication, rather than a complete review, of methods cited in the literature.
No attempt is made to evaluate critically or to recommend any of the methods.

Biological Data Relevant to the Evaluation of Carcinogenic Risk to Humans (Section 3)

In general, the data recorded in section 3 are summarized as given
by the author; however, comments made by the Working Group on certain
shortcomings of reporting, of statistical analysis or of experimental
design are given in square brackets. The nature and extent of impurities/
contaminants in the chemicals being tested are given when available.

Carcinogenicity studies in animals

The monographs are not intended to cover all reported studies. Some
studies are purposely omitted (a) because they are inadequate, as judged
from previously described criteria(23-26) (e.g., too short a duration, too
few animals, poor survival); (b) because they only confirm findings that
have already been fully described; or (c) because they are judged irrele-
vant for the purpose of the evaluation. In certain cases, however, such
studies are mentioned briefly, particularly when the information is considered to be a useful supplement to other reports or when it is the only
data available. Their inclusion does not, however, imply acceptance of
the adequacy of their experimental design and/or of the analysis and
interpretation of their results.

Mention is made of all routes of administration by which the compound
has been adequately tested and of all species in which relevant tests have

been done(5,26). In most cases, animal strains are given (General characteristics of mouse strains have been reviewed(27). Quantitative data are
given to indicate the order of magnitude of the effective carcinogenic
doses. In general, the doses and schedules are indicated as they appear
in the original paper; sometimes units have been converted for easier
comparison. Experiments on the carcinogenicity of known metabolites,
chemical precursors, analogues and derivatives, and experiments on factors
that modify the carcinogenic effect are also reported.

Other relevant biological data

Lethality data are given when available, and other data on toxicity
are included when considered relevant. The metabolic data are restricted
to studies that show the metabolic fate of the chemical in animals and
humans, and comparisons of data from animals and humans are made when
possible. Information is also given on absorption, distribution, excretion
and placental transfer.

Embryotoxicity and teratogenicity

Data on teratogenicity from studies in experimental animals and from
observations in humans are also included. There appears to be no causal
relationship between teratogenicity(28) and carcinogenicity, but chemicals
often have both properties. Evidence of teratogenicity suggests transplacental transfer, which is a prerequisite for transplacental carcinogenesis.

Indirect tests (mutagenicity and other short-term tests)

Data from indirect tests are also included. Since most of these tests
have the advantage of taking less time and being less expensive than mammalian carcinogenicity studies, they are generally known as 'short-term'
tests. They comprise assay procedures which rely on the induction of
biological and biochemical effects in *in vivo* and/or *in vitro* systems.
The end-point of the majority of these tests is the production not of
neoplasms in animals but of changes at the molecular, cellular or multi-
cellular level: these include the induction of DNA damage and repair,
mutagenesis in bacteria and other organisms, transformation of mammalian
cells in culture, and other systems.

The short-term tests are proposed for use (a) in predicting potential
carcinogenicity in the absence of carcinogenicity data in animals, (b) as
a contribution in deciding which chemicals should be tested in animals,
(c) in identifying active fractions of complex mixtures containing carcinogens, (d) for recognizing active metabolites of known carcinogens in human
and/or animal body fluids and (e) to help elucidate mechanisms of carcinogenesis.

Although the theory that cancer is induced as a result of somatic
mutation suggests that agents which damage DNA *in vivo* may be carcinogens,

the precise relevance of short-term tests to the mechanism by which cancer
is induced is not known. Predictions of potential carcinogenicity are
currently based on correlations between responses in short-term tests and
data from animal carcinogenicity and/or human epidemiological studies.
This approach is limited because the number of chemicals known to be
carcinogenic in humans is insufficient to provide a basis for validation,
and most validation studies involve chemicals that have been evaluated
for carcinogenicity only in animals. The selection of chemicals is in
turn limited to those classes for which data on carcinogenicity are
available. The results of validation studies could be strongly influenced
by such selection of chemicals and by the proportion of carcinogens in the
series of chemicals tested; this should be kept in mind when evaluating
the predictivity of a particular test. The usefulness of any test is
reflected by its ability to classify carcinogens and noncarcinogens, using
the animal data as a standard; however, animal tests may not always
provide a perfect standard. The attainable level of correlation between
short-term tests and animal bioassays is still under investigation.

Since many chemicals require metabolism to an active form, tests
that do not take this into account may fail to detect certain potential
carcinogens. The metabolic activation systems used in short-term tests
(e.g., the cell-free systems used in bacterial tests) are meant to approximate the metabolic capacity of the whole organism. Each test has its
advantages and limitations; thus, more confidence can be placed in the
conclusions when negative or positive results for a chemical are confirmed
in several such test systems. Deficiencies in metabolic competence may
lead to misclassification of chemicals, which means that not all tests
are suitable for assessing the potential carcinogenicity of all classes of
compounds.

The present state of knowledge does not permit the selection of a
specific test(s) as the most appropriate for identifying potential carcinogenicity. Before the results of a particular test can be considered to be
fully acceptable for predicting potential carcinogenicity, certain criteria
should be met: (a) the test should have been validated with respect to
known animal carcinogens and found to have a high capacity for discrimin-
ating between carcinogens and noncarcinogens, and (b), when possible, a
structurally related carcinogen(s) and noncarcinogen(s) should have been
tested simultaneously with the chemical in question. The results should
have been reproduced in different laboratories, and a prediction of carcinogenicity should have been confirmed in additional test systems. Confidence
in positive results is increased if a mechanism of action can be deduced
and if appropriate dose-response data are available. For optimum usefulness,
data on purity must be given.

The short-term tests in current use that have been the most extensively
validated are the *Salmonella typhimurium* plate-incorporation assay(29-33),
the X-linked recessive lethal test in *Drosophila melanogaster*(34), unscheduled DNA synthesis(35) and *in vitro* transformation(33,36). Each is compatible with current concepts of the possible mechanism(s) of carcinogenesis.

An adequate assessment of the genetic activity of a chemical depends
on data from a wide range of test systems. The monographs include, therefore, data not only from those already mentioned, but also on the induction
of point mutations in other systems(37-42), on structural(43) and numerical
chromosome aberrations, including dominant lethal effects(44), on mitotic
recombination in fungi(37) and on sister chromatid exchanges(45-46).

The existence of a correlation between quantitative aspects of mutagenic and carcinogenic activity has been suggested(5,44-50), but it is not
sufficiently well established to allow general use.

Further information about mutagenicity and other short-term tests
is given in references 45-53.

Case reports and epidemiological studies

Observations in humans are summarized in this section.

Summary of Data Reported and Evaluation (Section 4)

Section 4 summarizes the relevant data from animals and humans and
gives the critical views of the Working Group on those data.

Experimental data

Data relevant to the evaluation of the carcinogenicity of a chemical
in animals are summarized in this section. Results from validated mutagenicity and other short-term tests are reported if the Working Group
considered the data to be relevant. Dose-response data are given when
available. An assessment of the carcinogenicity of the chemical in animals
is made on the basis of all of the available data.

The animal species mentioned are those in which the carcinogenicity
of the substance was clearly demonstrated. The route of administration
used in experimental animals that is similar to the possible human exposure
is given particular mention. Tumour sites are also indicated. If the
substance has produced tumours after prenatal exposure or in single-dose
experiments, this is indicated.

Human data

Case reports and epidemiological studies that are considered to be
pertinent to an assessment of human carcinogenicity are described. Human
exposure to the chemical is summarized on the basis of data on production,
use and occurrence. Other biological data which are considered to be
relevant are also mentioned. An assessment of the carcinogenicity of the
chemical in humans is made on the basis of all of the available evidence.

Evaluation

This section comprises the overall evaluation by the Working Group of the carcinogenic risk of the chemical to humans. All of the data in the monograph, and particularly the summarized information on experimental and human data, are considered in order to make this evaluation.

References

1. IARC (1977) IARC Monograph Programme on the Evaluation of the
    Carcinogenic Risk of Chemicals to Humans. Preamble.
    IARC intern. tech. Rep. No. 77/002

2. IARC (1978) Chemicals with *sufficient evidence* of carcinogenicity
    in experimental animals - *IARC Monographs* volumes 1-17.
    IARC intern. tech. Rep. No. 78/003

3. WHO (1961) Fifth Report of the Joint FAO/WHO Expert Committee on
    Food Additives. Evaluation of carcinogenic hazard of food addi-
    tives. WHO tech. Rep. Ser., No. 220, pp. 5, 18, 19

4. WHO (1969) Report of a WHO Scientific Group. Principles for the
    testing and evaluation of drugs for carcinogenicity. WHO tech.
    Rep. Ser., No. 426, pp. 19, 21, 22

5. WHO (1974) Report of a WHO Scientific Group. Assessment of the
    carcinogenicity and mutagenicity of chemicals. WHO tech. Rep.
    Ser., No. 546

6. WHO (1964) Report of a WHO Expert Committee. Prevention of cancer.
    WHO tech. Rep. Ser., No. 276, pp. 29, 30

7. IARC (1972-1978) IARC Monographs on the Evaluation of the
    Carcinogenic Risk of Chemicals to Humans, Volumes 1-18, Lyon,
    France

    Volume 1 (1972) Some Inorganic Substances, Chlorinated Hydrocarbons,
    Aromatic Amines, *N*-Nitroso Compounds and Natural Products
    (19 monographs), 184 pages

    Volume 2 (1973) Some Inorganic and Organometallic Compounds
    (7 monographs), 181 pages

    Volume 3 (1973) Certain Polycyclic Aromatic Hydrocarbons and
    Heterocyclic Compounds (17 monographs), 271 pages

    Volume 4 (1974) Some Aromatic Amines, Hydrazine and Related
    Substances, *N*-Nitroso Compounds and Miscellaneous Alkylating
    Agents (28 monographs), 286 pages

    Volume 5 (1974) Some Organochlorine Pesticides (12 monographs),
    241 pages

    Volume 6 (1974) Sex Hormones (15 monographs), 243 pages

Volume 7 (1974)   Some Anti-thyroid and Related Substances,
    Nitrofurans and Industrial Chemicals (23 monographs), 326 pages

Volume 8 (1975)   Some Aromatic Azo Compounds (32 monographs),
    357 pages

Volume 9 (1975)   Some Aziridines, *N-*, *S-* and *O*-Mustards and
    Selenium (24 monographs), 268 pages

Volume 10 (1976)   Some Naturally Occurring Substances (32 monographs),
    353 pages

Volume 11 (1976)   Cadmium, Nickel, Some Epoxides, Miscellaneous
    Industrial Chemicals and General Considerations on Volatile
    Anaesthetics (24 monographs), 306 pages

Volume 12 (1976)   Some Carbamates, Thiocarbamates and Carbazides
    (24 monographs), 282 pages

Volume 13 (1977)   Some Miscellaneous Pharmaceutical Substances
    (17 monographs), 255 pages

Volume 14 (1977)   Asbestos (1 monograph), 106 pages

Volume 15 (1977)   Some Fumigants, the Herbicides 2,4-D and
    2,4,5-T, Chlorinated Dibenzodioxins and Miscellaneous
    Industrial Chemicals (18 monographs), 354 pages

Volume 16 (1978)   Some Aromatic Amines and Related Nitro Compounds –
    Hair Dyes, Colouring Agents and Miscellaneous Industrial
    Chemicals (32 monographs), 400 pages

Volume 17 (1978)   Some *N*-Nitroso Compounds (17 monographs),
    365 pages

Volume 18 (1978)   Polychlorinated biphenyls and Polybrominated
    biphenyls (2 monographs), 140 pages

Volume 19 (1979)   Some Monomers, Plastics and Synthetic Elastomers,
    and Acrolein (17 monographs), 513 pages

Volume 20 (1979)   Some Halogenated Hydrocarbons (25 monographs),
    609 pages

Volume 21 (1979)   Sex Hormones (II)   (22 monographs), 583 pages

8. IARC (1973-1978)   Information Bulletin on the Survey of Chemicals
    Being Tested for Carcinogenicity, Numbers 1-7, Lyon, France

        Number 1 (1973) 52 pages
        Number 2 (1973) 77 pages
        Number 3 (1974) 67 pages
        Number 4 (1974) 97 pages
        Number 5 (1975) 88 pages
        Number 6 (1976) 360 pages
        Number 7 (1978) 460 pages
        Number 8 (1979) 604 pages

9. PHS 149 (1951-1976)   Public Health Service Publication No. 149,
    Survey of Compounds which have been Tested for Carcinogenic
    Activity, Washington DC, US Government Printing Office

        1951 Hartwell, J.L., 2nd ed., Literature for the years through
              1947 on 1329 compounds, 583 pages

        1957 Shubik, P. & Hartwell, J.L., Supplement 1, Literature for
              the years 1948-1953 on 981 compounds, 388 pages

        1969 Shubik, P. & Hartwell, J.L., edited by Peters, J.A.,
              Supplement 2, Literature for the years 1954-1960 on 1048
              compounds, 655 pages

        1971 National Cancer Institute, Literature for the years
              1968-1969 on 882 compounds, 653 pages

        1973 National Cancer Institute, Literature for the years
              1961-1967 on 1632 compounds, 2343 pages

        1974 National Cancer Institute, Literature for the years
              1970-1971 on 750 compounds, 1667 pages

        1976 National Cancer Institute, Literature for the years
              1972-1973 on 966 compounds, 1638 pages

10. Pike, M.C. & Roe, F.J.C. (1963)   An actuarial method of analysis
    of an experiment in two-stage carcinogenesis. Br. J. Cancer,
    17, 605-610

11. Miller, E.C. & Miller, J.A. (1966) Mechanisms of chemical carcino-
    genesis: nature of proximate carcinogens and interactions with
    macromolecules. Pharmacol. Rev., 18, 805-838

12. Miller, J.A. (1970)   Carcinogenesis by chemicals: an overview -
    G.H.A. Clowes Memorial Lecture. Cancer Res., 30, 559-576

13. Miller, J.A. & Miller, E.C. (1976) The metabolic activation of
     chemical carcinogens to reactive electrophiles. In:
     Yuhas, J.M., Tennant, R.W. & Reagon, J.D., eds, Biology of
     Radiation Carcinogenesis, New York, Raven Press

14. Peto, R. (1974) Guidelines on the analysis of tumours rates and
     death rates in experimental animals. Br. J. Cancer, 29, 101-105

15. Peto, R. (1975) Letter to the editor. Br. J. Cancer, 31, 697-699

16. Hoel, D.G. & Walburg, H.E., Jr (1972) Statistical analysis of
     survival experiments. J. natl Cancer Inst., 49, 361-372

17. Tomatis, L. (1977) The value of long-term testing for the implen-
     tation of primary prevention. In: Hiatt, H.H., Watson, J.D.
     & Winsten, J.A., eds, Origins of Human Cancer, Book C, Cold
     Spring Harbor, N.Y., Cold Spring Harbor Laboratory, pp. 1339-
     1357

18. IARC (1977) Annual Report 1977, Lyon, International Agency for
     Research on Cancer, p. 94

19. Tomatis, L., Agthe, C., Bartsch, H., Huff, J., Montesano, R.,
     Saracci, R., Walker, E. & Wilbourn, J. (1978) Evaluation of
     the carcinogenicity of chemicals: a review of the IARC Monograph
     Programme, 1971-1977. Cancer Res., 38, 877-885

20. Rall, D.P. (1977) Species differences in carcinogenesis testing.
     In: Hiatt, H.H., Watson, J.D. & Winsten, J.A., eds, Origins
     of Human Cancer, Book C, Cold Spring Harbor, N.Y., Cold Spring
     Harbor Laboratory, pp. 1383-1390

21. National Academy of Sciences (NAS) (1975) Contemporary Pest Control
     Practices and Prospects: the Report of the Executive Committee,
     Washington DC

22. Chemical Abstracts Service (1978) Chemical Abstracts Ninth Collective
     Index (9CI), 1972-1976, Vols 76-85, Columbus, Ohio

23. WHO (1958) Second Report of the Joint FAO/WHO Expert Committee on
     Food Additives. Procedures for the testing of intentional food
     additives to establish their safety and use. WHO tech. Rep.
     Ser., No. 144

24. WHO (1967) Scientific Group. Procedures for investigating intentional
     and unintentional food additives. WHO tech. Rep. Ser., No. 348

25. Berenblum, I., ed. (1969) Carcinogenicity testing. UICC tech Rep.
     Ser., 2

26. Sontag, J.M., Page, N.P. & Saffiotti, U. (1976) Guidelines for
     carcinogen bioassay in small rodents. Natl Cancer Inst.
     Carcinog. tech. Rep. Ser., No. 1

27. Committee on Standardized Genetic Nomenclature for Mice (1972)
     Standardized nomenclature for inbred strains of mice. Fifth
     listing. Cancer Res., 32, 1609-1646

28. Wilson, J.G. & Fraser, F.C. (1977) Handbook of Teratology, New York,
     Plenum Press

29. Ames, B.N., Durston, W.E., Yamasaki, E. & Lee, F.D. (1973) Carcino-
     gens are mutagens: a simple test system combining liver homo-
     genates for activation and bacteria for detection. Proc. natl
     Acad. Sci. (Wash.), 70, 2281-2285

30. McCann, J., Choi, E., Yamasaki, E. & Ames, B.N. (1975) Detection
     of carcinogens as mutagens in the Salmonella/microsome test:
     assay of 300 chemicals. Proc. natl Acad. Sci. (Wash.), 72,
     5135-5139

31. McCann, J. & Ames, B.N. (1976) Detection of carcinogens as mutagens
     in the Salmonella/microsome test: assay of 300 chemicals:
     discussion. Proc. natl Acad. Sci. (Wash.), 73, 950-954

32. Sugimura, T., Sato, S., Nagao, M., Yahagi, T., Matsushima, T.,
     Seino, Y., Takeuchi, M. & Kawachi, T. (1977) Overlapping of
     carcinogens and mutagens. In: Magee, P.N., Takayama, S.,
     Sugimura, T. & Matsushima, T., eds, Fundamentals in Cancer
     Prevention, Baltimore, University Park Press, pp. 191-215

33. Purchase, I.F.M., Longstaff, E., Ashby, J., Styles, J.A.,
     Anderson, D., Lefevre, P.A. & Westwood, F.R. (1976) Evaluation
     of six short term tests for detecting organic chemical carcino-
     gens and recommendations for their use. Nature (Lond.), 264,
     624-627

34. Vogel, E. & Sobels, F.H. (1976) The function of Drosophila in
     genetic toxicology testing. In: Hollaender, A., ed.,
     Chemical Mutagens: Principles and Methods for Their Detection,
     Vol. 4, New York, Plenum Press, pp. 93-142

35. San, R.H.C. & Stich, H.F. (1975) DNA repair synthesis of cultured
     human cells as a rapid bioassay for chemical carcinogens.
     Int. J. Cancer, 16, 284-291

36. Pienta, R.J., Poiley, J.A. & Lebherz, W.B. (1977) Morphological
     transformation of early passage golden Syrian hamster embryo
     cells derived from cryopreserved primary cultures as a reliable
     in vitro bioassay for identifying diverse carcinogens. Int. J.
     Cancer, 19, 642-655

37. Zimmermann, F.K. (1975) Procedures used in the induction of mitotic recombination and mutation in the yeast *Saccharomyces cerevisiae*. Mutat. Res., 31, 71-86

38. Ong, T.-M. & de Serres, F.J. (1972) Mutagenicity of chemical carcinogens in *Neurospora crassa*. Cancer Res., 32, 1890-1893

39. Huberman, E. & Sachs, L. (1976) Mutability of different genetic loci in mammalian cells by metabolically activated carcinogenic polycyclic hydrocarbons. Proc. natl Acad. Sci. (Wash.), 73, 188-192

40. Krahn, D.F. & Heidelburger, C. (1977) Liver homogenate-mediated mutagenesis in Chinese hamster V79 cells by polycyclic aromatic hydrocarbons and aflatoxins. Mutat. Res., 46, 27-44

41. Kuroki, T., Drevon, C. & Montesano, R. (1977) Microsome-mediated mutagenesis in V79 Chinese hamster cells by various nitrosamines. Cancer Res., 37, 1044-1050

42. Searle, A.G. (1975) The specific locus test in the mouse. Mutat. Res., 31, 277-290

43. Evans, H.J. & O'Riordan, M.L. (1975) Human peripheral blood lymphocytes for the analysis of chromosome aberrations in mutagen tests. Mutat. Res., 31, 135-148

44. Epstein, S.S., Arnold, E., Andrea, J., Bass, W. & Bishop, Y. (1972) Detection of chemical mutagens by the dominant lethal assay in the mouse. Toxicol. appl. Pharmacol., 23, 288-325

45. Perry, P. & Evans, H.J. (1975) Cytological detection of mutagen-carcinogen exposure by sister chromatid exchanges. Nature (Lond.), 258, 121-125

46. Stetka, D.G. & Wolff, S. (1976) Sister chromatid exchanges as an assay for genetic damage induced by mutagen-carcinogens. I. *In vivo* test for compounds requiring metabolic activation. Mutat. Res., 41, 333-342

47. Bartsch, H. & Grover, P.L. (1976) Chemical carcinogenesis and mutagenesis. In: Symington, T. & Carter, R.L., eds, Scientific Foundations of Oncology, Vol. IX, Chemical Carcinogenesis, London, Heinemann Medical Books Ltd, pp. 334-342

48. Hollaender, A., ed. (1971a,b, 1973, 1976) Chemical Mutagens: Principles and Methods for Their Detection, Vols 1-4, New York, Plenum Press

49. Montesano, R. & Tomatis, L., eds (1974) Chemical Carcinogenesis Essays, Lyon (IARC Scientific Publications No. 10)

50. Ramel, C., ed. (1973) Evaluation of genetic risk of environmental chemicals: report of a symposium held at Skokloster, Sweden, 1972. Ambio Spec. Rep., No. 3

51. Stoltz, D.R., Poirier, L.A., Irving, C.C., Stich, H.F., Weisburger, J.H. & Grice, H.C. (1974) Evaluation of short-term tests for carcinogenicity. Toxicol. appl. Pharmacol., 29, 157–180

52. Montesano, R., Bartsch, H. & Tomatis, L., eds (1976) Screening Tests in Chemical Carcinogenesis, Lyon (IARC Scientific Publications No. 12)

53. Committee 17 (1976) Environmental mutagenic hazards. Science, 187, 503–514

INTRODUCTION

    Effects of oestrogens
    Effects of progestins
    Effects of androgens

BIOLOGICAL ACTIVITIES OF STEROID HORMONE PREPARATIONS

PHYSIOLOGICAL PRODUCTION AND ACTION OF SEX HORMONES IN HUMANS

    Childhood
    The normal menstrual cycle
    Anovulatory menstrual cycles
    Postmenopausal and ovariectomized women
    Pregnant women
    Men
    Mechanisms of action of sex hormones
    The interpretation of hormone values in females

PHARMACOLOGY OF SYNTHETIC OESTROGENS AND PROGESTINS

    Mode of action of hormonal contraceptives in women

METABOLISM OF THE SEX HORMONES

    Humans
    Experimental mammals

ANALYTICAL METHODS

HORMONES AND CARCINOGENICITY

HORMONES AND MUTAGENICITY

HORMONES AND EMBRYOTOXICITY AND TERATOGENICITY

    Diethylstilboestrol
    Progestins and androgens
    Oestrogens, progestins and oral contraceptives
    Clomiphene and clomiphene citrate

REFERENCES

INTRODUCTION

The compounds considered in this volume are listed in Table 1.
With the exception of chlorotrianisene, clomiphene, dienoestrol and
diethylstilboestrol, they are steroid derivatives; in order to avoid
semantic complications, all of the compounds dealt with are referred to
as 'sex hormones', even though most of them do not occur naturally.
They have all been used in some form of therapy in humans, and many have
found widespread use in oral hormonal contraceptive agents.

The Working Group also considered methallenoestril, quinoestradol
and quinoestrol; however, monographs on these compounds were not prepared
because of the scarcity of available data, particularly on carcinogenicity.

In considering the carcinogenic activity of the sex hormones, it is
necessary to relate their pathogenic activities to their varying physiological properties. The naturally occurring oestrogens, oestradiol-17β,
oestriol and oestrone, the androgen testosterone and the progestin
progesterone are present in all vertebrate species as secretions of the
ovaries, testes and/or adrenal glands or as products of the mammalian
placenta. As such, they form part of the total endocrine environment,
the interrelations and control of which are complex. For background
information see Hafez & Evans (1973), Turner & Bagnara (1976) and Williams
(1974); for more detailed accounts of the steroid hormones, see Applezweig
(1962, 1964), Azarnoff (1975), Briggs & Brotherton (1970), Briggs &
Christie (1976), Brotherton (1976), Crosignani & James (1974), Fuchs &
Klopper (1977), Johns (1976) and Schulster *et al*. (1976).

Basically, the compounds considered are oestrogens, androgens or
progestins; the general activities of these three classes of compounds
are outlined below in relation to growth, differentiation and development.
Classification of hormones with regard to these types of biological
activity cannot be rigid, because it is based on a number of physiological
effects, which individual compounds may cause to varying degrees. In
addition, activity often varies according to the route of administration,
the vehicle used and the species, sex and strain.

The sex hormones are used widely in human medicine for a large
variety of conditions, apart from their use as oral contraceptive agents:
in the treatment of dysmenorrhoea, endometriosis and dysfunctional
uterine bleeding, and as replacement therapy in patients with gonadal
dysgenesis and in women with symptoms of the climacteric. Their use in
the prevention of postmenopausal osteoporosis is currently being assessed,
as is their role in the treatment of advanced breast and endometrial
carcinoma. In obstetric practice, progestins have been used in the
management of threatened abortion and to prevent premature labour, and
local oestrogens have been used successfully to 'prime' the unripe
cervix to induction of labour.

TABLE 1

List of compounds reviewed

Compound	CAS[a] No.	CAS[a] preferred nomenclature
Oestrogens		
Chlorotrianisene	569-57-3	1,1',1''-(1-Chloro-1-ethenyl-2-ylidene)tris(4-methoxy-benzene)
Conjugated oestrogens	–	A mixture of compounds, mainly sodium oestrone sulphate
Dienoestrol	84-17-3	4,4'-(1,2-Diethylidene-1,2-ethanediyl)bisphenol
Diethylstilboestrol	56-53-1	4,4'-(1,2-Diethyl-1,2-ethenediyl)bisphenol
Diethylstilboestrol dipropionate	130-80-3	4,4'-(1,2-Diethyl-1,2-ethenediyl)bisphenol dipropionate
Ethinyloestradiol[b]	57-63-7	(17α)-19-Norpregna-1,3,5(10)-trien-20-yne-3,17-diol
Mestranol[b]	72-33-3	(17α)-3-Methoxy-19-norpregna-1,3,5(10)-trien-20-yn-17-ol
Methallenoestril[c]	517-18-0	β-Ethyl-6-methoxy-α,α-dimethyl-2-naphthalene propanoic acid
Oestradiol-17β	50-28-2	(17β)-Estra-1,3,5(10)-triene-3,17-diol
Oestradiol 3-benzoate	50-50-0	Estra-1,3,5(10)-triene-3,17-diol(17β)-3-benzoate
Oestradiol dipropionate	113-38-2	Estra-1,3,5(10)-triene-3,17-diol(17β)-dipropionate
Oestradiol-17β-valerate	979-32-8	(17β)-Estra-1,3,5(10)-triene-3,17-diol 17-pentanoate
Polyoestradiol phosphate	28014-46-2	(17β)-Estra-1,3,5(10)-triene-3,17-diol polymer with phosphoric acid
Oestriol	50-27-1	(16α,17β)-Estra-1,3,5(10)-triene-3,16,17-triol

Compound	CAS[a] No.	CAS[a] preferred nomenclature
Oestrone	53-16-7	3-Hydroxyestra-1,3,5(10)-trien-17-one
Oestrone benzoate	2393-53-5	3-(Benzoyloxy)estra-1,3,5(10)-trien-17-one
Quinoestradol[c]	1169-79-5	(16α,17β)-3-(Cyclopentyloxy)-estra-1,3,5(10)-triene-16,17-diol
Quinoestrol[c]	152-43-2	(17α)-3-(Cyclopentyloxy)-19-norpregna-1,3,5(10)-trien-20-yn-17-ol
Progestins		
Chlormadinone acetate[b]	302-22-7	17-(Acetyloxy)-6-chloro-pregna-4,6-diene-3,20-dione
Dimethisterone[b]	79-64-1	(6α,17β)-17-Hydroxy-6-methyl-17-(1-propynyl)-androst-4-en-3-one
Ethynodiol diacetate[b]	297-76-7	(3β,17α)-19-Norpregn-4-en-20-yne-3,17-diol diacetate
17α-Hydroxyprogesterone caproate	630-56-8	17-[(1-Oxohexyl)oxy]pregn-4-ene-3,20-dione
Lynoestrenol[b]	52-76-6	(17α)-19-Norpregn-4-en-20-yn-17-ol
Medroxyprogesterone acetate	71-58-9	(6α)-17(Acetyloxy)-6-methyl-pregn-4-ene-3,20-dione
Megestrol acetate	595-33-5	17-(Acetyloxy)-6-methylpregna-4,6-diene-3,20-dione
Norethisterone[b]	68-22-4	(17α)-17-hydroxy-19-norpregn-4-en-20-yn-3-one
Norethisterone acetate[b]	51-98-9	(17α)-17-(Acetyloxy)-19-norpregn-4-en-20-yn-3-one acetate
Norethynodrel[b]	68-23-5	(17α)-17-Hydroxy-19-norpregn-5(10)-en-20-yn-3-one
Norgestrel[b]	797-63-7	(17α)-13-Ethyl-17-hydroxy-18,19-dinorpregn-4-en-20-yn-3-one
Progesterone	57-83-0	Pregn-4-ene-3,20-dione
Androgens		
Testosterone	58-22-0	(17β)-17-Hydroxyandrost-4-en-3-one

Compound	CAS^a No.	CAS^a preferred nomenclature
Testosterone enanthate	315-37-7	(17β)-17-[(1-Oxoheptyl)oxy]androst-4-en-3-one
Testosterone propionate	57-85-2	(17β)-17-(1-Oxopropoxy)androst-4-en-3-one
Others		
Clomiphene	911-45-5	2-[4-(2-Chloro-1,2-diphenylethenyl)phenoxy]-N,N,-diethylethanamine
Clomiphene citrate	50-41-9	2-[4-(2-Chloro-1,2-diphenylethenyl)phenoxy]-N,N-diethylethanamine 2-hydroxy-1,2,3-propanetricarboxylate (1:1)

^{a}Chemical Abstracts Service

^{b}Used in oestrogen-progestin oral contraceptive preparations

^{c}Considered by the Working Group, but no monograph prepared (see p. 35)

In males, metastatic carcinoma of the prostate is treated with diethylstilboestrol and other oestrogenic compounds. Oestrogens are also used to develop secondary female sex characteristics in transsexual males, and androgens to suppress these characteristics in transsexual females. Androgens have been used in the treatment of male hypogonadism, in the treatment of symptoms of the climacteric and in advanced mammary tumours in women. Clomiphene citrate now has established usage in the induction of ovulation in anovulatory women; its use in oligospermic males is currently being assessed. Sex hormones are also used in veterinary medicine and as supplements to feedstuffs to promote growth of food animals.

In 1972, an estimated 250.6 million monthly cycles of oral contraceptives (the percent based on the 'minipill' is unknown) were purchased by retail pharmacies in the following countries (percent of total): US (35.6), Federal Republic of Germany (17.1), UK (7.6), Canada (6.8), France (6.1), Brazil (4.1), The Netherlands (4.0), Australia (3.6), Argentina (1.6), Belgium (1.6), Italy (1.5), Mexico (1.4), Austria (1.3), Spain (1.1), Yugoslavia (1.0), New Zealand (0.78), Finland (0.75), Greece (0.12), Colombia (0.65), Central America (0.4), Venezuela (0.33), Peru (0.27), Puerto Rico (0.17), Turkey (0.6), the Philippines (0.25), Iran (0.24) and Lebanon (0.1) (Piotrow & Lee, 1974). In 1977, an estimated 325 million cycles were bought by pharmacies (Anon., 1979).

In 1973, the US, Sweden and UNICEF provided about 54 million monthly cycles of oral contraceptives to various areas of the world. In 1978, it was estimated that over 80 million women around the world use oral contraceptives (WHO, 1978).

Effects of oestrogens

Oestrogens are responsible, together with other hormones, for the development and maintenance of the female sex organs and for the regulation of the menstrual cycle in primates and of the oestrus cycle in other mammals.

Oestrogens produce marked proliferative effects in all tissues derived from the Mullerian duct system. In the uterus, oestrogens initially induce fluid retention and stimulation of epithelial multiplication. The endometrium becomes thickened and highly vascularized. In menstruating species, the glands elongate, but they do not secrete. The secretion of cervical mucus is stimulated, and in the absence of progestin this constitutes a most sensitive indicator of oestrogenic activity. The multiplication of vaginal epithelial cells is stimulated, the infiltration of leucocytes is inhibited and, in rodents, there is keratinization.

In the secondary sex tissues, oestrogens are responsible for proliferation of the ducts in the mammary gland (the human breast) and for an increase in the size and pigmentation of the nipples. In the human female, oestrogens are responsible for the typical distribution of fat in the breasts and hips and for the regulation of characteristic hair growth.

Oestrogens have marked effects on the hypothalamus. This part of the brain regulates the release of a hormone (luteinizing hormone releasing hormone: LHRH), which is responsible for the episodic secretion of follicle-stimulating hormone (FSH) and luteinizing hormone (LH). There are two functional pools of LH, one an acutely releasable pool and the other a reserve pool; the activities of these two pools at any given point in the ovulatory cycle are determined by the pattern of secretion of LHRH, the action of which is amplified or impeded by oestrogens (Hoff *et al.*, 1977).

It is now believed that androgens exert their effects within the central nervous system by initial conversion to oestrogens, although they have a biological action of their own elsewhere (Naftolin *et al.*, 1975). Aromatase, the enzyme which converts androgens to oestrogens, is present in particularly high concentrations in the central neuroendocrine tissue of the foetus. Other enzymes associated with steroid metabolism have also been demonstrated in the brain: these include C-2 oestrogen hydroxylase, the concentration of which is particularly high in the hypothalamus of the human foetus (Fishman *et al.*, 1976), and 17β-oxidore-ductase (Naftolin *et al.*, 1975). Thus, the local production of oestrogens in the brain by the aromatizing system is closely associated with systems for the formation of oestrogen metabolites, including the catechol oestrogens (2-hydroxyoestrogens). In addition, the recent finding that 2-hydroxyoestrone binds to hypothalamic and uterine cytosol receptors and can elevate serum LH levels in immature male rats indicates that these oestrogen metabolites could play a role in the regulation of the reproductive processes (Fishman *et al.*, 1976). In another area, it has been shown that production of some of the androgens, notably androstenedione, dehydroepiandrosterone and its sulphate, decreases after the menopause. Before the menopause, oestrogen of ovarian origin potentiates the effect of adrenocorticotrophic hormone (ACTH) on the zona reticularis; this effect is lost after the menopause but can be regained by the administration of oestrogens (Abraham & Maroulis, 1975). Oestrogens also increase the levels of transcortin in plasma, thus increasing the proportion of protein-bound cortisol; this results in an increased secretion of corticotrophin and a rise in the levels of total plasma cortisol. Oestrogens also cause an increase in plasma sex hormone binding globulin, which binds testosterone and oestradiol. Prolactin release by the pituitary has been shown to be under the control of an inhibitory factor released by the hypothalamus. Release of prolactin is also influenced, both directly and indirectly, by circulating oestrogens: it is markedly increased by oestrogen administration.

Thus, it can be concluded that oestrogens have a much wider range of functions than was first appreciated, and it is likely that many more are yet to be discovered.

Oestrogens have a wide variety of effects in other systems, including plasma protein synthesis, blood coagulation and carbohydrate and lipid metabolism. A discussion of these effects and of the indications and contraindications for their use is clearly beyond the scope of the present monograph. It must be stressed, however, that there is concern with regard to the side effects of oestrogens, which has given rise to a considerable volume of literature (see Boston Collaborative Drug Surveillance Program, 1973; Richardson & MacLaughlin, 1978; Royal College of General Practitioners, 1974; Vessey & Doll, 1976; WHO, 1971, 1973).

Effects of progestins

Progesterone is the only important natural progestin, but many synthetic steroids have similar biological properties. The normal role of progesterone is to prepare the uterus for implantation and to maintain pregnancy. To achieve this normal response, prior stimulation with oestrogen is essential. The action of progesterone on the oestrogen-primed uterus is to induce further development of the endometrial glands and the secretion of glycogen into the uterine cavity; further action leads to the decidual changes. The maintenance of pregnancy is dependent on the continuing production of sufficient amounts of progesterone.

Progesterone acts as a potent antioestrogen on endocervical secretion and rapidly inhibits both the quantity and quality of the fertile-type mucus induced at the oestrogen peak at mid-cycle. Progesterone causes proliferation of acini in the oestrogen-stimulated ducts of the breast; it may also inhibit prolactin release from the pituitary and thus inhibit lactation. Raised progestin levels inhibit the release of LH at mid-cycle, and higher levels inhibit FSH production.

Bioassays for progestins are less satisfactory than those for the other hormones. They are conducted on oestrogen-primed animals, and the end-point may be either glandular endometrial proliferation, deciduoma formation or the maintenance of pregnancy.

Effects of androgens

Testosterone is the most potent natural androgen, although many of its derivatives have varying degrees of androgenic activity. Androgens are necessary for the maintenance of germinal tissue in the testis and for the differentiation and growth of the secondary sex organs in males. Vestigial remnants of the male accessory tissues in the female are stimulated by androgens, and it is probable that low levels of androgenic activity are an essential component of the normal female hormonal environment. Development of the prostate and seminal vesicles and of their secretions is stimulated by androgens. Secretion by the sebaceous glands is also increased, and pigmentation of the skin is stimulated. The characteristic distribution and growth of hair in the male are determined by androgenic activity.

Androgens have a marked anabolic effect: increased protein synthesis, particularly in muscle and bone, results in an increased rate of body growth in the presence of a functioning pituitary. There is retention of nitrogen, phosphorus and potassium and an increased use of body fat for protein synthesis.

In females, androgens have activities comparable with those of the progestins on the breast, uterus and vagina. In addition, they stimulate hypertrophy of the clitoris.

BIOLOGICAL ACTIVITIES OF STEROID HORMONE PREPARATIONS

The compounds considered have varying degrees of oestrogenic, androgenic or progestational activity. The degrees of activity depend on the route of administration and on the animal used. Furthermore, metabolites of the administered compounds may themselves have important physiological effects, depending on the animal used. Because of these factors, it is practically impossible to calculate exactly the potencies of sex hormones in humans from animal data. An acceptable approximation for comparing potencies of these compounds in humans may be to establish minimally effective doses, e.g., the amounts required in oral contraception to inhibit ovulation. Data relating potencies of the various hormone preparations are given in Tables 2, 3 and 4.

PHYSIOLOGICAL PRODUCTION AND ACTION OF SEX HORMONES IN HUMANS

Childhood

The sequence of changes seen in girls as they pass from childhood to adulthood is, first, the beginning of breast development (thelarche) followed closely by growth of pubic hair (puberty), both of which usually commence between the ages of 9 and 13 yrs; then uterine bleeding (menarche), which usually occurs between the ages of $11\frac{1}{2}$ and $15\frac{1}{2}$ yrs (Marshall & Tanner, 1969); and, finally, full reproductive function (ovulation). The age of onset of these events is very variable and seems to depend partly on body weight (Frisch, 1974a,b).

Little information is available on the levels and sources of the oestrogen production which accompanies these events. Using a very sensitive assay method, urinary oestrogen excretion was measured in 38 girls and 24 boys aged between 2 and 13 yrs; serial assays were performed in 8 girls for periods of up to 5 yrs, as they passed through thelarche, puberty, menarche and first ovulation. Up till the age of 8 yrs, the total urinary oestrogen values were within the very low range of 0.09-0.5 µg/24 hrs, with no differences seen between the sexes (Brown et al., 1978). Assuming that the metabolic clearance rate of oestrogens in children is not greatly different from that in adults, these urinary

TABLE 2

Relative oestrogenic potencies ^{a} in mice^b and rats^c

| | Vaginal keratinization | | Uterine weight | |
| | S.c. administration | Oral administration | S.c. administration | |
	(mice)	(mice)	(mice)	(rats)
Oestradiol-l7β	1	1	1	1-1.2
Oestrone	0.3	0.4-0.5	1-1.1	1-1.3
Oestriol	0.015	1	0.3-0.35	0.30-0.32
Ethinyloestradiol	1.2	≥ 10	1.2-1.3	1.3-1.5
Mestranol	0.6	≥ 7.5	0.6-0.7	-
Conjugated oestrogens	0.4-0.5	≥ 1	0.5-0.6	-
Oestrone piperazine sulphate	0.3-0.4	0.4-0.6	0.5	-
Diethylstilboestrol	0.3	3	≥ 1	1.14-1.28
Chlorotrianisene	0.001-0.005	0.3-0.6	0.1-0.15	-
Dienoestrol	-	-	0.9-1.0	1-1.15

^{a}Based either on induction of vaginal keratinization (Allen Doisy test) or on increase in uterine weight (Rubin's test) in immature or ovariectomized rats or mice

^{b}From Brotherton (1976) and Emmeus & Martin (1962)

^{c}From Morgan (1963)

TABLE 3

Relative progestational activity in rabbits and rats

	METHOD I[a]		METHOD II[b]
	S.c. administration	Oral administration	S.c. administration
Progesterone	1	1	1
17α-Hydroxyprogesterone caproate	-	-	< 0.1
Chlormadinone acetate	75	330	4-6
Medroxyprogesterone acetate	30	300	50-100
Megestrol acetate	25-30	250	10-15
Ethynodiol diacetate	2-5	100	5-7
Lynoestrenol	1-2.5	150	3-5
Norethisterone	1.5	100	6-10
Norethisterone acetate	2.5	200	20-30
Norethynodrel	1-2.5	30-50	2-3
dl-Norgestrel	10	300	50-150
Dimethisterone	1-2.5	50-100	1-3

[a]Method I: The end-point was the degree of glandular proliferation in the endometrium of oestrogen-primed, immature, castrated rabbits (Clauberg, 1930; Desaulles & Krähenbühl, 1960, 1962; McPhail, 1935; Neumann, 1968).

[b] Method II: The end-point was the capacity to block spontaneous ovulation in normal cycling female rats (Desaulles & Krähenbühl, 1964; Neumann, 1968; Tausk & de Visser, 1972).

TABLE 4

Approximate relative potencies of progestins in humans[a]

	Oral potency	Antigonadotrophic potency[b]	Oestrogenic activity	Androgenic activity
Progesterone	1	1	0	-
17α-Hydroxyprogesterone caproate	1[c]	< 0.1	0	-
Chlormadinone acetate	60	3-6	0	-
Medroxyprogesterone acetate	50	50-100	0	++
Megestrol acetate	70	-	0	-
Ethynodiol diacetate	3	10	+	0
Lynoestrenol	8	2-3	++	0
Norethisterone	20	30-100	+	+++
Norethisterone acetate	10	30-100	+	++
Norethynodrel	5	10-20	+++	0
dl-Norgestrel	60	-	0	+++
Dimethisterone	5	1-3	0	-

[a] From Brotherton (1976). Norethynodrel and to a lesser degree lynoestrenol enhance the levels of plasma corticoid binding globulin.

[b] Inhibition of ovulation

[c] S.c. administration

oestrogen values would be equivalent to serum oestradiol-17β and oestrone concentrations of approximately 0.2-1.0 pg/ml and 0.5-2.5 pg/ml, respectively and to total production rates of these two oestrogens of 0.4-2.0 μg per day. Such serum values are below the sensitivity of current radioimmunoassays, but values of this order have been obtained in young children using a highly sensitive mass-spectrometric method. Brown *et al.* (1978) noted that serial estimations performed over an 8-month period in a girl at the age of 3 and 4 yrs gave values which fluctuated over a 4.5-fold range (0.08-0.34 μg/24 hrs). Expressed on a logarithmic scale, these fluctuations were almost as great as those seen in follicular activity during the menstrual cycle.

Between the ages of 8-11 yrs, the oestrogen values began to increase above 0.5 μg/24 hrs, the increase being more rapid in girls than in boys. Breast development was first noted in the girls as the urinary oestrogen values rose to between 0.6-1.0 μg/24 hrs: thus, a level of urinary oestrogen excretion of approximately 1.0 μg/24 hrs represents the level of oestrogen production required to initiate breast development. This would be equivalent to a production rate of approximately 4 μg per day. At this time, the oestrogen values were showing cyclical variations of irregular periodicities. The oestrogen values continued to rise, and uterine bleeding (menarche) occurred as the peak urinary values exceeded 15 μg/24 hrs. This level would be equivalent to a production rate of approximately 60 μg per day. Thus, the oestrogen level required for menarche was approximately 10-15 times that required for thelarche. In all the subjects studied, the first cycles were anovulatory. Establishment of ovulation was a variable event, occurring within 3 months of menarche in 1 subject and more than 1 yr after menarche in another. The change from anovulatory to ovulatory cycles was a gradual process and was accompanied by an increasing and more prolonged production of progesterone premenstrually, until the full pattern of the ovulatory cycle emerged (Brown *et al.*, 1978).

While the fluctuating oestrogen levels seen at menarche were clearly mainly of ovarian (follicular) origin and consisted, therefore, of oestradiol-17β, the sources and identity of the oestrogen secreted before menarche were unclear. The low oestrogen values encountered before 8 yrs of age (0.09-0.5 μg/24 hrs) were similar to those seen in postmenopausal women after bilateral adrenalectomy and oophorectomy (0.12-0.75 μg/24 hrs), using the same assay method (Brown *et al.*, 1978); in the ablated patients these values presumably represented peripheral production of oestrogens from extraglandular androgen precursors (Brown & Matthew, 1962). The values are also similar to those seen in women with primary amenorrhoea associated with absent breast development and delayed puberty due to ovarian agenesis.

Boon *et al.* (1972) measured androstenedione, testosterone, dehydro-epiandrosterone and its sulphate and androsterone sulphate in the plasma of children aged between 1 day and 20 yrs. In the younger children, the assay methods were operating at the limits of their sensitivities, and many levels were undetectable. However, these workers concluded from their results, and from those recorded in the literature, that 50% of the plasma values for children aged 1-8 yrs fell within the following ranges: androstenedione, boys = 160-550 (mean, 580), girls = 20-970 (mean, 690) pg/ml; testosterone, boys = 0-160 (mean, 250), girls = 0-150 (mean, 110) pg/ml; dehydroepiandrosterone, boys = 0-160 (mean, 640), girls = 0-1060 (mean, 540) pg/ml; dehydroepiandrosterone sulphate, boys = 0-180 (mean, 110), girls = 0-270 (mean, 200) pg/ml; and androsterone sulphate, boys = 0-40 (mean, 20), girls = 0-20 (mean, 50) pg/ml. The values were practically the same for the two sexes. Thus, compared with adults, all of the androgen values in this age group were low; this was particularly true of dehydroepiandrosterone and its sulphate, which are considered to be almost entirely of adrenal origin. In children over the age of 8 yrs, the plasma concentrations of all the androgens increased, the most marked being a 10-fold increase in testosterone values in the boys.

A possible sequence of oestrogen production in girls is, therefore, as follows: between the ages of 1-8 yrs, small amounts of oestrone are produced by peripheral conversion of androstenedione, which is synthesized in small amounts by the adrenals and perhaps by extraglandular sites and the ovaries. After the age of 8 yrs, the ovaries start producing increasing amounts of oestradiol-17β, which eventually reach the level required for the initiation of breast development; this oestrogen production also provides the stimulus for increased androgen secretion by the adrenal cortex and thus initiates puberty. This adrenal androgen provides additional precursor for increased peripheral oestrone production. The change is accompanied by increasing rhythmical follicular activity within the ovary, which eventually produces sufficient oestradiol-17β to initiate endometrial growth and uterine bleeeding (menarche). Finally, ovulation is established, followed by the additional participation of progesterone in the oestrogen cycle.

The normal menstrual cycle

A characteristic pattern of interdependent fluctuating hormone levels is found during the fertile ovarian cycle. This is illustrated in Figure 1. The cycle commences with a small rise in FSH production, which reaches 10-30% above threshold level. This causes follicles within the ovary to develop and to secrete increasing amounts of oestrogen, which then depress the FSH production to below the threshold level. The oestrogen secretion reaches a peak and then falls. During this time, the dominant follicle is acquiring increasing sensitivity to LH. The elevated oestrogen levels act on the hypothalamus to produce LHRH, which triggers the massive release of LH that induces ovulation. This LH peak is accompanied by a smaller peak in FSH. After ovulation, the developing corpus luteum produces increasing amounts of oestrogen and progesterone, which rise to a maximum and then fall before the onset of menstruation.

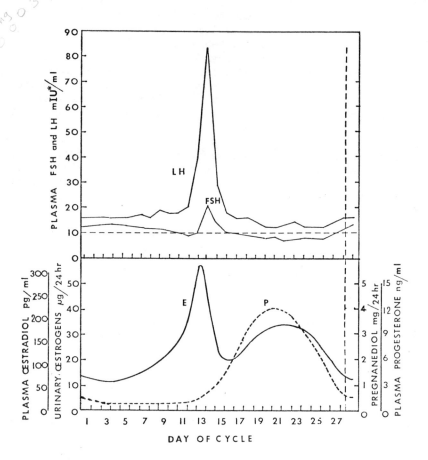

Figure 1.   The natural sequence of FSH, LH, oestradiol (E) and pro-
             gesterone (P) during the ovulatory cycle in women, expressed
             as plasma concentrations. Urine concentrations of the
             steroid metabolites are also given.

    Horizontal broken line = threshold level of FSH below which no folli-
cular development occurs

    Vertical broken line = onset of menstruation

    Data on FSH and LH are from Ross *et al.* (1970), and the plasma and
urine concentrations are means from the literature.

    *
     milli-International Units

The concentrations of oestradiol-17β, oestrone, progesterone and testosterone in the plasma and of their metabolites in the urine at various stages of the cycle are shown in Tables 5 and 6. 17β-Oestradiol is the major oestrogen secreted by the ovaries: the concentrations in ovarian blood are 10-20 times those in peripheral blood (Lloyd *et al.*, 1971). Its circulatory level shows substantial fluctuations throughout the cycle, reflecting the development and involution of the ovarian follicle and corpus luteum. Most of the circulating oestradiol (94%) is derived from secreted oestradiol, and the remainder by conversion from oestrone and, to a lesser extent, testosterone (Baird *et al.*, 1969).

The source of circulating oestrone is more complex. It has been shown that 1.3% of circulating androstenedione is converted to oestrone, accounting for approximately 40 μg/24 hrs of oestrone production (Siiteri & MacDonald, 1973). This contribution varies minimally during the cycle and so makes up 10-50% of total oestrone production, depending on the amount of oestrone being secreted directly. Another 20-34% of oestrone is derived from oestradiol-17β (Longcope & Williams, 1974).

Only a small amount of progesterone is secreted by the ovaries during the follicular phase, but during the luteal phase levels rise, and the concentration of progesterone in ovarian blood is 10-20 times that in peripheral blood. Secretion of oestradiol and progesterone by the ovaries occurs episodically, and definite fluctuations in plasma levels occur over short periods of time (Korenman & Sherman, 1973; West *et al.*, 1973).

The total production of oestradiol-17β during a 28-day cycle amounts to 5.0 mg, of which 0.9 mg is produced during the first 9 days, 1.6 mg are produced during the 6 days of the mid-cycle peak and 2.5 mg are produced during the 13 days of the luteal phase. The total ovarian production of progesterone during the luteal phase amounts to 230 mg. These calculations are based on the population means shown in Figure 1. For corresponding days of the cycle, the steroid values found in a female population vary over a 3- to 4-fold range, so that the upper limits of normal levels can be calculated approximately by multiplying the mean values by 2 and the lower limits by dividing them by 2.

In young women, the principal ovarian androgen is androstenedione (see Table 6), with a mean plasma concentration of 1800 pg/ml. During the cycle, its concentration remains relatively stable; it has a mid-cycle peak that is 15% higher than the level seen early or late in the cycle (Abraham, 1974; Judd & Yen, 1973). About 50% of androstenedione is derived from the ovaries, adrenal secretion being responsible for the remainder (Judd *et al.*, 1974a).

In contrast, the circulating level of testosterone is much lower, averaging 300 pg/ml. It has a mean concentration about 20% higher at mid-cycle (Abraham, 1974; Judd & Yen, 1973). Only 10% of circulating

TABLE 5

Plasma concentrations and blood production rates (BPR) of oestradiol-17β, oestrone, progesterone and testosterone and urine excretions of 'total' oestrogens and pregnanediol in women and men[a]

	Oestradiol-17β		Oestrone		Progesterone		Testosterone		'Total' urine	
	Plasma pg/ml	BPR μg/24hr	Plasma ng/ml	BPR μg/24hr	Plasma ng/ml	BPR mg/24hr	Plasma ng/100ml	BPR mg/24hr	Oestrogens μg/24hr[b]	Pregnanediol mg/24hr[c]
Women										
Early follicular phase	65	85	60	130	0.6	1.2	40	0.3	15	0.4
Mid-cycle peak E	260	340	100	220					60	0.7
Luteal maximum	150	200	100	220	13	26			45	4.0
Post-meno-pause	5	5	17	30	0.3	0.6			7	0.2
Late pregnancy	18,000	80,000[d]	6,000	80,000[d]	100	200			30,000	45
Men	20	50	30	55	0.4	0.8	660	6.6	15	0.5

[a]Values for plasma concentrations are means from the literature, and the BPRs were calculated from the data of Baird *et al.* (1969)

[b]Values from Brown *et al.* (1968)

[c]Values from Barrett & Brown (1970)

[d]Total oestriol, oestrone and oestradiol-17β

TABLE 6

Metabolic clearance rates (MCR), blood production rates (BPR) and peripheral plasma or serum concentration of relevant oestrogens and androgens in premenopausal women, postmenopausal women and in men (means and ranges are given)[a]

Steroid	MCR (1/day)	BPR (µg/day)	Plasma or serum concentrations		
			basal (pg/ml)	after oophorectomy (pg/ml)	ovarian vein (pg/ml)
Oestradiol					
Premenopausal	1170 (900-1500)	80 (40-500)	170 (30-400)	14 (5-30)	8000 (70-40,000)
Postmenopausal	910 (600-1000)	11 (5-20)	12 (5-25)	14 (6-25)	31 (14-54)
Oestrone					
Premenopausal	1870 (1470-2500)	101 (80-400)	120 (40-200)		880 (90-3800)
Postmenopausal	1600 (1200-1850)	48 (30-80)	30 (18-50)	39 (17-60)	72 (40-120)
Androstenedione					
Premenopausal	1800 (1200-2500)	3250 (200-4500)	1800 (1100-2500)	900 (300-2200)	70,000 (1000-300,000)
Postmenopausal	1800 (1000-2700)	1600 (700-2300)	900 (400-1300)	700 (200-1200)	3450 (450-13,000)
Men	2300 (1700-3300)	2000 (1500-3000)	890 (650-1300)		

Table 6 (continued)

Steroid	MCR (l/day)	BPR (µg/day)	Plasma or serum concentrations		
			basal (pg/ml)	after oophorectomy (pg/ml)	ovarian vein (pg/ml)
Testosterone					
Premenopausal	600 (450-1000)	180 (110-300)	300 (180-500)	130 (40-270)	3950 (740-20,000)
Postmenopausal	600 (510-780)	140 (40-240)	230 (70-400)	100 (40-200)	3030 (600-8700)
Men	1000 (800-1400)	6000 (3000-10,000)	6000 (3000-10,000)		

Plasma or serum concentrations (pg/ml ± SD)

Steroid	Premenopausal	Postmenopausal	Oophorectomized
Dihydrotestosterone	250 ± 60	120 ± 30	50
Dehydroepiandrosterone	5000 ± 1500	1600 ± 500	1260 ± 360
Dehydroepiandrosterone sulphate	2000 ± 500 x 10³	400 ± 100 x 10³	

[a] From Abraham et al., 1969; Baird & Guevara, 1969; Barberia & Thorneycroft, 1974; Benjamin & Deutsch, 1976; Calanog et al., 1976; Greenblatt et al., 1976; Grodin et al., 1973; Judd et al., 1974a,b, 1976; Longcope, 1971; Longcope & Williams, 1974; Maroulis & Abraham, 1976; Poortman et al., 1973; Rader et al., 1973; Tulchinsky & Korenman, 1970; Vermeulen, 1976; Yen et al., 1975

testosterone is due to direct ovarian secretion, the bulk being derived
from peripheral conversion of androstenedione (Bardin & Lipsett, 1967;
Horton & Tait, 1966).

Anovulatory menstrual cycles

Anovulatory cycles are characterized by absence of the normal
increases in progesterone production during the luteal phase. Two main
patterns of oestrogen production have been described (Brown & Matthew,
1962): one shows constantly elevated oestrogen values and bleeding,
usually irregularly, as a break-through phenomenon; the other shows a
single peak of oestrogen production, with maximum values which sometimes
exceed those of the normal cycle, and oestrogen withdrawal bleeding
occurs as the values fall after the peak. There are, however, many
variants of this pattern: a small transient increase in progesterone
production may sometimes be observed after the oestrogen peak; but all
gradations occur, from this small increase, through an inadequate luteal
phase to the full pattern of the ovulatory cycle. In the intermediate
patterns it may be difficult to decide whether ovulation has occurred or
not. The gonadotrophin patterns are variable: the early rise in FSH
may be delayed or absent, or the mid-cycle peaks of LH and FSH may be
reduced or absent (Faiman & Ryan, 1967). The total oestrogen production
throughout an ovulatory cycle does not exceed that of the upper range of
the ovulatory cycle, even in those with temporary high values; thus,
the condition is not associated with excessive oestrogen production but
with the absence of progesterone production.

Postmenopausal and ovariectomized women

With the approach of the menopause, there is a striking increase in
the variability of cycle length, due either to irregular maturation of
residual follicles with diminished responsiveness to gonadotrophin
stimulation, or to anovulatory bleeding following oestrogen withdrawal
without evidence of corpus luteum function. Elevation of FSH levels in
the presence of normal LH values has been observed (Sherman *et al.*,
1976).

Although the normal ovary practically ceases to produce oestrogens
following the menopause, it is still capable of androgen secretion;
furthermore, ultrastructural studies have shown that the postmenopausal
ovary still contains small numbers of apparently normal oocytes within
primordial follicles (Costoff & Mahesh, 1975).

Metabolic clearance rates, blood production rates and peripheral
plasma and ovarian concentrations of oestrogens and androgens in pre-
and postmenopausal women and in men are shown in Table 6.

The relative contributions of the ovaries and adrenals to the
overall production of oestradiol-17β, oestrone, androstenedione and
testosterone have been assessed. Current evidence suggests that the

postmenopausal ovaries secrete only minimal amounts of oestrone and
oestradiol-17β but are responsible for about 30% of the production of
androstenedione, and at least 50% of the production of testosterone.
Most, if not all, of the circulating oestrogen in postmenopausal women
is derived from extraglandular conversion of androgen precursors. There
is a close correlation between the peripheral and ovarian vein concentrations of tesosterone but not of the other steroids, confirming that the
ovaries are the main site of production of testosterone only. Similar
conclusions have been reached using experiments involving either adrenal
stimulation with ACTH or suppression with dexamethasone (Barberia &
Thorneycroft, 1974; Judd *et al.*, 1974a,b; Vermeulen, 1976).

Pregnant women

Pregnancy is characterized by the production of relatively enormous
amounts of oestrogens and progesterone. Thus, at term, the total daily
productions of oestrogens and progesterone are of the order of 100 and
200 mg, respectively (Brown, 1957; Lin *et al.*, 1972). In very early
pregnancy, the luteal phase levels of oestrogens and progesterone are
maintained. However, the growing placenta produces increasing amounts
of these steroids, and also of oestriol, and by the 7th week after
ovulation becomes the major site of hormone production. The proportion
of oestriol to total oestrogens increases as pregnancy advances, and at
term oestriol accounts for 70% of the total production (Brown, 1957).
Placental oestradiol-17β and oestrone are derived by aromatization
of dehydroepiandrosterone secreted by the foetal adrenals, and the
oestriol is produced from the same compound after being 16-hydroxylated
by the foetal liver [the 'foeto-placental unit (Diczfalusy, 1969)].
The mean plasma concentrations of unconjugated oestradiol-17β, oestrone
and oestriol in the maternal circulation at term are 18, 6 and 12 ng/ml,
respectively, and 99, 97 and 82% of these are bound to protein. Concentrations of the unbound unconjugated oestrogens are 3-6 times higher in the
foetal than in the maternal circulation, indicating that the foetus is
exposed to high plasma concentrations of these oestrogens (Tulchinsky,
1973).

Pregnancy is also characterized by the production by the placenta
of large amounts of human chorionic gonadotrophin (HCG) and of human
placental lactogen. The production of HCG can be detected as early as
10 days after ovulation and thus forms the basis for pregnancy tests
(Thomas *et al.*, 1973).

Men

Plasma concentrations of oestradiol-17β, oestrone, progesterone and
testosterone in men are given in Table 5. The high plasma testosterone
values are derived almost entirely from the secretion of testosterone by
the testes (Baird *et al.*, 1969). In the absence of chromosomal abnormalities,
the testes of the normal male secrete only small amounts of oestradiol-
17β, and by far the majority of daily oestradiol-17β production is

accounted for by conversion from testosterone. Likewise, the major part
of daily oestrone production can be accounted for by conversion of
adrenal androstenedione (Kelch *et al.*, 1972; Siiteri & MacDonald, 1973).

Mechanisms of action of sex hormones

Considerable progress has been made in elucidation of the mechanisms
of action of the sex steroid hormones at tissue level, and this has made
possible an understanding of the effects of various agents used in the
treatment of breast and endometrial cancer. Steroid hormones appear to
enter all cells by passive or facilitated diffusion, but they are retained
only in their target organs, due to the presence of specific cytoplasmic
receptors. Oestrogen is first bound with high affinity (dissociation
constant about 10^{-10}M) to cytoplasmic 8S receptor proteins, which dissociate
into a 4S-5S form with the oestrogen attached. This oestrogen receptor
complex is then transferred to the target-cell nucleus where it binds to
a non-histone complex, leading to increased synthesis of messenger RNA
and resultant specific proteins. A more general increase in the synthesis
of various types of RNA and proteins becomes obvious a few hours later;
stimulation of DNA synthesis occurs even later. The length of time the
oestrogen-receptor complex occupies the nucleus appears to be crucial to
its biological effect. The number of oestrogen receptors within the
cytoplasm of the endometrial cell reflects the endogenous concentration
of oestrogen throughout the cycle, increasing during the follicular
phase to a peak at the time of ovulation and then decreasing again.
Similar mechanisms of action pertain to both progesterone and dihydrotestosterone. For more detailed information, the reader is referred to
Chan & O'Malley (1976) and Jensen & deSombre (1972). Alternative mechanisms
of action have been proposed: see, for example, Szego (1965, 1974).

The interpretation of hormone values in females

The wide ranges of oestrogen values found in ovulating women are
the result of different stages in normal cyclical ovarian activity. The
plasma concentrations and daily production rates of oestradiol-17β and
oestrone in postmenopausal women are much lower and show practically no
overlap with those of premenopausal women. The metabolic clearance
rates of many steroids are influenced by a number of factors, including
oophorectomy and decrease with age (Longcope, 1971; Vermeulen, 1976),
and their plasma concentrations show circadian and day-to-day variations,
even in postmenopausal women. In one study, 8 steroids, including
oestradiol-17β, oestrone, androstenedione, testosterone, dihydrotestosterone
and dehydroepiandrosterone, were measured every 4 hrs for 24 hrs in the
plasma of postmenopausal women (Vermeulen, 1976): all except oestradiol-
17β showed significant daily variations (1.4- to 2.6-fold), with higher
values occurring between 8 a.m. and 10 a.m. and the lowest values between
8 p.m. and midnight. The plasma concentrations of the steroids also
showed marked short-term fluctuations. In another study, serum concentrations of oestradiol-17β, oestrone, androstenedione and testosterone were

measured in 6-12 serial samples taken over a 3-day period between 8 and
9 a.m. The mean coefficients of variation of the serial values in any
one individual were between 20% and 40% for all four steroids, with some
values differing by a factor of 4 or more (Judd *et al.*, 1974b, 1976).
These large variations were observed in pre- and postmenopausal women,
with and without endometrial cancer, and before and after oophorectomy.
The variations were as great between serial samples from the same individual
as they were between individuals. This phenomenon resembles that reported
for cortisol and dehydroisoandrosterone, two steroids that are secreted
episodically by the adrenals in the same circadian pattern (Rosenfeld *et
al.*, 1975). Finally, it is now firmly established that the conversion
of androstenedione to oestrone is affected by such variables as obesity
and age (Edman & MacDonald, 1978; Edman *et al.*, 1978; Hemsell *et al.*,
1974; Rizkallah *et al.*, 1975).

These considerable variations and different factors create serious
difficulties for obtaining representative values of blood concentrations
of hormones, especially from women in the postmenopausal years.

PHARMACOLOGY OF SYNTHETIC OESTROGENS AND PROGESTINS

The doses of the synthetic oestrogens and progestins that are
commonly used in combinations for hormonal contraception or in gynaecological or other treatment are listed in Table 7. It can be assumed that
contraceptive doses are near the minimum required for suppression of
ovulation and, therefore, have the same order of biological activity as
the maximum levels found during the normal cycle and early pregnancy.
It is difficult to obtain more precise information on relative potencies
in humans.

Mode of action of hormonal contraceptives in women

Most hormonal contraceptives act by suppressing ovulation through
the natural feed-back mechanisms which operate between the ovaries,
hypothalamus and pituitary during the menstrual cycle. The doses shown
in Table 7 generally achieve this effect. Although, under certain
conditions, oestrogens may stimulate pituitary gonadotrophin production,
under other conditions they are the most powerful inhibitors of pituitary
function known. Given alone to suppress ovulation, they cause irregular
uterine bleeding, and when the medication is stopped, ovulation may
occur at the time expected for withdrawal bleeding. Progestins alone
are weaker and less complete inhibitors of pituitary function, and
approximately 50 times the dose is required to obtain equivalent inhibition.
Consequently, the two hormones are usually given in combination.

Treatment starts on day 5 of the cycle and continues through to day
25; withdrawal bleeding occurs on day 28. Additional contraceptive
action is provided by the abnormal responses of the female genital tract
to progestin given early in the cycle. For example, progestin inhibits
the production of fertile-type cervical mucus and prevents sperm penetration.
In the sequential 'pill', first oestrogen alone is given, followed by a
combination of oestrogen and progestin; this produces a more normal

TABLE 7

Examples of doses and combinations of synthetic oestrogens and progestins

Use	Oestrogen	Progestin	Regime	Examples
Sequential contraception	Ethinyl oestradiol 0.1 mg	Dimethisterone 25 mg	16 + 5	Oracon[a]; Ovin
	Mestranol 0.08 mg	Chlormadinone acetate 2 mg	15 + 5	C-Quens[a]; Sequens
Combination contraception	Ethinyl oestradiol 0.05 mg	Norethisterone acetate 2.5 mg	21	Norlestrin; Prolestrin
	Ethinyl oestradiol 0.05 mg	Norethisterone acetate 1.0 mg	21	Minovlar; Anovlar 1 mg
	Ethinyl oestradiol 0.05 mg	dl-Norgestrel 0.5 mg	21	Ovral; Eugynon
	Ethinyl oestradiol 0.05 mg	Ethynodiol diacetate 1.0 mg	21	Ovulen 50; Demulen
	Ethinyl oestradiol 0.03 mg	d-Norgestrel 0.15 mg	21	Microgynon 21; Ovranette
	Ethinyl oestradiol 0.02 mg	Norethisterone acetate 1.5 mg	21	Loestrin 1/20; Zorane 1/20
	Mestranol 0.08 mg	Norethisterone 1.0 mg	21	Ortho-Novin 1/80; Norinyl 1/80
	Mestranol 0.075 mg	Norethynodrel 5.0 mg	20	Conovid; Enavid 5
	Mestranol 0.06 mg	Norethisterone 10.0 mg	20	Ortho Novum 10 mg
Oral progestin-only contraception		Norethisterone 0.35 mg	Continuous	Micronor; Noriday
		dl-Norgestrel 0.075 mg	Continuous	Neogest; Ovrette
		d-Norgestrel 0.03 mg	Continuous	Microlut; Microval
Injectable progestin contraception		Medroxyprogesterone acetate 150 mg	I.m. every 3 months	Depo-Provera; Depo-Clinovir 150

Table 7 (continued)

Use	Oestrogen	Progestin	Regime	Examples
Climacteric symptoms	Oestradiol-17β 1.0 mg 2.0 mg		21	Estrace
	Conjugated oestrogens 0.3 mg 0.625 mg 1.25 mg 2.5 mg		21	Premarin
	Oestradiol valerate 2.0 mg	dl-Norgestrel 0.5 mg	11 + 10[b]	Cyclo-progynova
	Conjugated oestrogens 0.625 mg 1.25 mg	dl-Norgestrel 0.5 mg	21 + 7	Prempak
Endometriosis	Ethinyl oestradiol 0.05 mg	dl-Norgestrel 0.5 mg	Daily for 6 months	Duoluton
		Norethisterone 5.0 mg	Daily for 6 months	Primolut N
Prostatic, mammary carcinoma	Diethylstilboestrol 25 mg 100 mg		1-4, three times daily	
	Fosfestrol[e] 250 mg		1-2, three times daily	Honvan
Endometrial carcinoma		Medroxyprogesterone acetate 100 mg	3-4 tablets daily	Provera
Mammary carcinoma		17α-Hydroxyprogesterone caproate	250 mg i.m. weekly	Primolut Depot

[a] Withdrawn; 15/16 days oestrogen followed by 5 days oestrogen plus progestin

[b] 11 tablets containing 2.0 mg oestradiol valerate; 10 tablets containing 2.0 mg oestradiol valerate plus 0.5 mg dl-norgestrel

[e] Diethylstilboestrol diphosphate

preparation of the female genital tract, but the effectiveness appears to be lower. In the 'mini-pill', progestin alone is given continuously in small doses, which do not usually inhibit ovulation; contraception is achieved by the abnormal effect of continuous progestin action on the genital tract; 'spotting', or irregular vaginal bleeding, is a common complication.

The combination type of oral contraception abolishes the early rise in FSH and the later peaks of LH and FSH. The sequential pill abolishes both the early and mid-cycle rises in FSH, but aberrant peaks of LH occur during both the administration of oestrogen and of progestin (Swerdloff & Odell, 1969). In the absence of stimulation by FSH, follicles do not develop in the ovaries, and oestrogen and progesterone productions remain at uniformly low levels.

METABOLISM OF THE SEX HORMONES

Humans

The natural steroid hormones are rapidly metabolized and eliminated: oestradiol-17β and progesterone have half-lives of 20 minutes and testosterone one of 11 minutes (Sandberg & Slaunwhite, 1956, 1957, 1958). Some conversions occur peripherally, but the major site of metabolism is in the liver. Elimination of glucuronide and/or sulphate conjugates of metabolites occurs *via* the urine or *via* the bile. Conjugates thus secreted into the gut are partly split by enzymes of the intestinal microflora. The resulting products may be reabsorbed (enterohepatic circulation) and reconjugated. Ultimately, the steroids are excreted in the urine, although a certain amount is excreted in the faeces. The main urinary metabolites of oestradiol-17β and oestrone are the conjugates of oestriol, 2-hydroxyoestrone, oestrone, 16α-hydroxyoestrone and oestradiol, given in order of decreasing quantitative importance; approximately 20 other metabolites are eliminated by this route. The main urinary metabolite of progesterone is the fully reduced compound, pregnanediol, which accounts for 15% of the progesterone produced (Klopper & Michie, 1956); other products include the partly reduced compound, pregnanolone, and various stereo-isomers of pregnanediol. The main metabolites of testosterone are the two stereo-isomeric oxidation-reduction products, androsterone (5α-androstane-3α-ol-17-one) and aetiocholanolone (5β-androstane-3α-ol-17one). The relative proportions of the various metabolites formed from oestradiol-17β and testosterone are influenced by the level of thyroid activity (Fishman *et al.*, 1965; Gallagher *et al.*, 1960). A minor route for the metabolism of testosterone involves aromatization to oestrogens, and this forms an important source of the oestrogens found in men and in postmenopausal women (see p. 54).

Synthetic steroids may be metabolized in humans by the same mechanisms as are the natural compounds. For example, the main metabolites of norethynodrel, ethynodiol diacetate and norgestrel are the 3α- and 3β-alcohols derived from reduction of the unsaturated structures in ring A, the ethinyl group at position 17 being retained (Cook *et al.*, 1972, 1973; DeJongh *et al.*, 1968). The products are eliminated as the glucuronides and sulphates (Layne *et al.*, 1963).

Experimental mammals

The problem of species differences, which is fundamental to the interpretation of toxicological data, is closely related to differences in metabolism of the compounds investigated. Present knowledge about the metabolism of sex steroids and related hormonally-active compounds indicates that not one of the species used for toxicological testing truly mimics human behaviour in this respect (see Table 8). Hence, metabolic differences must be taken into account in evaluating species-related toxicological effects of sex steroids.

Oestrogens are converted, both *in vivo* and *in vitro*, by oxidative enzymes in the liver to reactive metabolites that attach irreversibly to proteins (Bolt & Kappus, 1974; Horning *et al.*, 1978; Kappus *et al.*, 1973; Marks & Hecker, 1969) or to nucleic acids (Blackburn *et al.*, 1977). Progestins also bind irreversibly to proteins to varying degrees (Chen & Lee, 1975; Kappus & Remmer, 1975). Additional information is needed before a definite statement can be made about the involvement of reactive metabolites of natural and synthetic sex hormones in carcinogenesis, although this has been suggested (Horning *et al.*, 1978). All animal species in which hormone metabolism has been studied have shown certain differences when compared with humans. Further information regarding these differences would facilitate both the design and evaluation of toxicological and carcinogenicity studies in different species, and the need for more research is emphasized.

For a review of the metabolism of natural and synthetic oestrogens, see Bolt (1979).

ANALYTICAL METHODS

Analytical methods have been developed for the analysis of hormones in (1) pharmaceutical products (bulk chemicals, tablets, creams, etc.); (2) biological samples (plasma, urine, tissues, etc.); and (3) environmental samples (meat for human consumption, air from industrial environments, drinking-water, etc.). The choice of analytical method thus depends on the sample matrix in which the hormone occurs.

For pharmaceutical products, which are generally relatively pure materials, no extensive clean-up procedures are necessary, and a simple extraction, followed by a titrimetric, spectrophotometric or chromatographic assay is usually adequate.

In biological samples, hormones usually occur as conjugates, at low levels, in a complicated matrix. A more sensitive clean-up procedure, involving hydrolysis, extraction, chromatographic separation or derivatization, is usually required. A number of chromatographic methods have been developed for the final separation and detection: these include thin-layer chromatography, high-pressure liquid chromatography and various gas chromatographic techniques, in conjunction with flame-ionization

TABLE 8

Some species differences in the metabolism of sex hormones by experimental mammals in relation to man

Mammal	Metabolic process	Reference
Mouse	High faecal excretion of diethylstilboestrol	Helton et al. (1978a,b)
Rat	Faecal excretion of oestrogens predominates	Bolt & Remmer (1972a,b)
Guinea-pig	Negligible transformation of oestrone to oestradiol	Yoshizawa et al. (1977)
Rabbit	Ring-D-homoannulation of ethinyloestradiol is a major pathway	Abdel-Aziz & Williams (1969)
	Occurrence of oestradiol-17α	Breuer & Knuppen (1969)
Dog	Low conversion of oestradiol to oestriol	Beling et al. (1975)
	Major differences in pharmacokinetics and metabolism of 17α-hydroxyprogesterone progestins and of oestrogens	Forchielli & Murthy (1970) Kirdani & Sandberg (1974)
Non-human primates	Mostly quantitative differences in steroid metabolite patterns	Goldzieher & Kraemer (1972)

detection, electron-capture detection or mass-spectrometric detection of one or several characteristic ions. In view of the time-consuming nature of many of these clean-up procedures, increasing use is being made of radioimmunoassay, which requires little preliminary sample purification and is highly sensitive and specific. Methods similar to those employed for biological samples are used for environmental samples.

Analytical methods for the individual sex hormones are tabulated in the respective monographs.

HORMONES AND CARCINOGENICITY

The mechanism(s) by which hormones result in cancer development is not understood. Although many carcinogens show a mutagenic action, none of the hormones (including diethylstilboestrol) nor any of their metabolic products has so far been shown convincingly to be mutagenic; however, there have been reports of covalent binding of diethylstilboestrol metabolites to DNA and of results in short-term tests that indicate interactions with DNA (see monograph on diethylstilboestrol, p. 173).

Hormones may be essential to carcinogenesis by preparing the background on which tumours may ultimately arise. Thus, mammary tumours arise from mammary tissue that is in an appropriate developmental state: hormones that directly stimulate mammary gland development provide the necessary substrate. In laboratory rodents, these hormones include those of the ovary, the adrenal cortex and the pituitary. The hormones of these endocrine glands can be viewed as essential factors for the development of mammary cancer, although this does not mean that they should be considered as having a direct carcinogenic action.

In laboratory mice, both oestrogen and prolactin increase the incidence of mammary tumours by their actions on the mammary gland. In virgin mice of a strain in which the milk-borne mammary tumour virus (MTV)[1] is unexpressed, continuous exposure to prolactin may cause tumours to appear. The role of oestrogen is even more complex, since it can also stimulate prolactin secretion. Oestrogen and prolactin, and probably progesterone, all contribute to the development of mammary tumours in carcinogen-exposed rats.

When investigating carcinogenesis with female animal models, it is important to take into account essential differences in reproductive physiology; animals with spontaneous oestrus cycles, with functional corpora lutea (dog) and without (mouse and rat), and with reflex ovulation

---

[1]In this volume, MTV$^+$ indicates the presence of a virus able to express its biological activity, whereas MTV$^-$ refers to a virus in an occult or biologically inactive form.

(rabbit) may respond differently to exogenous hormones. The differences which occur in the basic endocrine relationships in a range of laboratory animal species as compared with those in man have been discussed at length by Neumann & Elger (1972). The importance of species differences in the metabolism of sex hormones is outlined on p. 60.

Another important consideration in interpreting the relevance of various animal models to the human experience is the epizoology of the cancer being investigated, compared with its corresponding epidemiology. For example, while pregnancy confers relative protection against breast cancer in humans and in rats, it increases the breast cancer risk in mice. Additionally, although the reproductive physiology of dogs is different from that of humans, the protective effects of early age at first pregnancy and of oophorectomy at a young age against the development of breast cancer appear to be the same in both species.

Hormones may stimulate carcinogenesis by providing a background – normal (permissive) or abnormal (teratogenic, see pp. 64-67) - for subsequent tumorigenesis by chemical, physical or viral agents or by promoting the growth and metastasis of tumours once they have been initiated, or in a variety of other ways. The following list of possible mechanisms is undoubtedly incomplete and in part speculative:

1. Hormones may increase the binding of chemical carcinogens to cellular constituents, e.g., by influencing metabolic activation systems.

2. Hormones may activate oncogenic virus production (e.g., mammary tumour virus in mice).

3. Hormones may be immunosuppressive and could thus influence tumour occurrence and growth.

4. Exposure to hormones may result in lesions (preneoplastic) which provide an environment for the survival of cells with abnormal growth potentials.

5. Hormones may influence the rate of progression of preneoplastic cells to neoplastic cells.

6. Hormones may preferentially stimulate proliferation of abnormal cell populations.

7. Hormones may stimulate the DNA synthesis and mitosis essential for fixation of the transformed state.

8. Hormones, by stimulating the proliferation of normal cells with a definite number of cell divisions, may exhaust the normal cell population and thus eliminate their inhibitory influence over the proliferation of abnormal cells (Nandi, 1978).

9. As a result of hormonal imbalance in a target organ, proliferation may be favoured over functional differentiation; conversely, certain hormonal milieux in target organs may favour specific synthetic and secretory activities and hence reduce tumorigenic potential.

HORMONES AND MUTAGENICITY

The majority of mutagenicity studies on the sex hormones considered in this volume were carried out before the statistical concepts for mutagenicity testing were developed (Vollmar, 1977); therefore, many results, especially those from cytogenetic studies, are inconclusive.

The Working Group also noted the scarcity of mutagenicity studies on sex hormones, particularly of those using mammalian germ cells, such as cytogenetic studies on oocytes, spermatocytes and spermatogonia. Only two dominant lethal tests have been reported, one on a combination of mestranol and lynoestrenol and the other on norethisterone acetate; the authors considered these to be positive, although confirmation is required.

Before a definite statement about the possible mutagenicity of sex hormones can be made, therefore, additional studies are required.

HORMONES AND EMBRYOTOXICITY AND TERATOGENICITY

Many steroidal sex hormones cause antifertility, embryotoxicity and foetotoxicity in several species, and such effects are usually dose-related. Some oestrogens also produce teratogenic effects and impaired fertility in exposed offspring. Certain progestins, testosterone and testosterone derivatives have a virilizing effect on the foetus.

In humans, birth defects have been observed in foetuses after maternal ingestion of various drugs. However, only in a limited number of cases is it possible to ascribe a particular defect to a specific drug. If an adverse effect is to be produced, exposure must occur during the relevant susceptible period of embryogenesis; and in interpreting the results of a study, the influence of the drug must be distinguished from any effects of the condition for which the drug was administered.

Diethylstilboestrol

Non-neoplastic alterations in the genital tract are commonly found in female children born to women who received diethylstilboestrol during pregnancy. These changes include vaginal adenosis, cervical ectropion and transverse fibrous ridges on the cervix or in the vagina. In addition, there is some evidence of alterations in the structure of the fundus of the uterus. Changes in the male genital tract include epididymal cysts, testicular abnormalities and alterations in the seminal fluid. Many of these changes appear to be related to disturbances in the development of the Mullerian tract in females and of the Wolffian duct in males. They are considered in greater detail in the monograph on diethylstilboestrol (see p. 173).

Neonatal mice provide a useful model for studying the long-term effects of prenatal exposure of humans to diethylstilboestrol and sex steroids (Bern, 1979; Bern *et al.*, 1975, 1976; Forsberg, 1972, 1975, 1976; Kohrman, 1978). Both mice and rats are born with incompletely developed genital tracts, in a stage similar to that in the first trimester in humans. In mice, the first few days after birth constitute a critical period during which injection of sex steroids or diethylstilboestrol may induce irreversible changes in the genital tract. Although hormones injected into neonatal mice are not metabolized by the placenta (as may occur in humans exposed prenatally), the responses observed are similar to those that occur in mice exposed prenatally, either transplacentally or directly (Kimura, 1975; McLachlan, 1977; McLachlan *et al.*, 1975). Some of these responses, such as vaginal adenosis (Forsberg, 1976, 1979) and epididymal cysts (McLachlan *et al.*, 1975), resemble those seen in humans after transplacental exposure to diethylstilboestrol (Gill *et al.*, 1976, 1977; Herbst, 1978; Herbst *et al.*, 1975a,b). Even when the animal model system involves transplacental administration, however, it should be remembered that the placenta of different species may handle steroids and diethylstilboestrol in different ways.

Progestins and androgens

Masculinization of the external genitalia in female foetuses has been observed after their exposure *in utero* to large doses of progestational agents, especially 19-nor steroids, which also have some androgenic activity. The changes include clitoral hypertrophy, labio-scrotal fusion, and occasionally the occurrence of penile urethra. Similar changes have been reported after exposure to combinations of these compounds with oestrogens. Advancement of skeletal maturation has also been noted (Breibart *et al.*, 1963). Milder degrees of masculinization have been reported with progestational compounds that have a lesser degree of androgenic activity, such as medroxyprogesterone acetate (Burstein & Wasserman, 1964). Androgens themselves produce similar masculinizing effects on the foetus, but drugs such as methyltestosterone, testosterone, 19-normethyltestosterone and methylandrostenediol, have apparently been less widely used than progestins during pregnancy (Grumbach & Ducharme, 1960).

Oestrogens, progestins and oral contraceptives

There is no evidence that children born to women who used oral contra-ceptives at times prior to pregnancy have an increased frequency of birth defects (Peterson, 1969; Robinson, 1971; Rothman & Louik, 1978; Royal College of General Practitioners, 1976).

Chromosome abnormalities (principally triploidy and tetraploidy) in foetuses have been reported to be more common following the use of oral contraceptives by their mothers (Alberman *et al.*, 1976; Carr, 1970; Harlap *et al.*, 1979), but these findings have not been confirmed (Bishun, 1976; Klinger *et al.*, 1976; Lauritsen, 1975).

It has been suggested that more congenital abnormalities occur in infants born to women who became pregnant while actually taking oral contraceptives. The defects described include the VACTERL syndrome (a pattern of multiple anomalies: vertebral, anal, cardiac, tracheal, esophageal, renal, limb) (Nora & Nora, 1973, 1975; Nora *et al.*, 1978), cardiovascular abnormalities (Heinonen *et al.*, 1977; Janerich *et al.*, 1977; Levy *et al.*, 1973; Rothman *et al.*, 1979) and limb reduction defects (Janerich *et al.*, 1974). A VACTERL syndrome was seen in a child of a mother given hormone therapy at the beginning of pregnancy (Kaufman, 1973). Other authors have found no evidence of such abnormalities (Mulvihill *et al.*, 1974; Vessey *et al.*, 1976).

The evidence relating the use of hormonal pregnancy tests to congenital malformations is stronger, but not conclusive (Gal *et al.*, 1967; Greenberg *et al.*, 1975; Janerich *et al.*, 1977; Laurence *et al.*, 1971; Oakley *et al.*, 1973). Studies that implicate hormones used to support pregnancy are difficult to interpret, since the indication for which the drug was given might itself be expected to be associated with an increased risk of birth defects.

Clomiphene and clomiphene citrate

Clomiphene citrate alone or in combination with gonadotrophic hormones stimulates the synthesis of sex hormones in the gonads and induces germ-cell maturation. It is thus used to induce ovulation. Higher risks of multiple births and abortions, among other side effects accompanying use of this agent, are well documented.

A slight increase of chromosomal anomalies has been reported in early embryos of mice and rabbits after superovulation (Fujimoto *et al.*, 1974; Maudlin & Fraser, 1977; Takagi & Sasaki, 1976); however, negative effects have also been reported (Fechheimer & Beatty, 1974). After superovulation induced by conjugated oestrogens and gonadotrophic hormones, an inheritable limb defect in connection with neural tube defects and a shifted sex ratio favouring females to males (2:1) can occur in the F1 generation of Swiss albino mice, which is transmitted over several generations. The highly increased steroid hormone levels

may be the origin of these inheritable lesions (Elbling, 1973, 1975a,b,c).
Smith & Chrisman (1975) could not confirm these effects in other mouse
strains.

In humans, neural tube defects have been reported in the 11 children
of 10 women given clomiphene to induce ovulation [Barrett & Hakim
(1973) (1 case), Dyson & Kohler (1973) (2 cases), Field & Kerr (1974) (2
cases), Nevin & Harley (1976) (4 women, 5 children) and Sandler (1973)
(1 case)]. Other authors have reported no increase in congenital defects
following clomiphene usage (Hack *et al.*, 1972).

It has been suggested that subfertility in women may be associated
with an increased prevalence of congenital defects (Ahlgren *et al.*,
1976). Additionally, a high proportion of early spontaneous abortuses
have been shown to be chromosomally abnormal (Boué & Boué, 1973; Dhadial
et al., 1970); however, no information is available on the karyotypes
of abortuses from subfertile women or of those from women given clomiphene
to induce superovulation. Chromosome analyses may help to clarify the
problem. At present, no definite association has been demonstrated
between clomiphene administration and congenital defects in humans.

References

Abdel-Aziz, M.T. & Williams, K.I.H. (1969) Metabolism of 17α-ethynyl-
    estradiol and its 3-methyl ether by the rabbit; an *in vivo* D-
    homoannulation. Steroids, 13, 809-820

Abraham, G. (1974) Ovarian and adrenal contribution to peripheral
    androgens during the menstrual cycle. J. clin. Endocrinol. Metab.,
    39, 340-346

Abraham, G.E. & Maroulis, G.B. (1975) Effect of exogenous estrogen on
    serum pregnenolone, cortisol and androgens in postmenopausal women.
    Obstet. Gynecol., 45, 271-274

Abraham, G.E., Lobotsky, J. & Lloyd, C.W. (1969) Metabolism of
    testosterone and androstenedione in normal and ovariectomised women.
    J. clin. Invest., 48, 696-703

Ahlgren, M., Källén, B. & Rannevik, G. (1976) Outcome of pregnancy
    after clomiphene therapy. Acta obstet. gynecol. scand., 55, 371-375

Alberman, E., Creasy, M., Elliott, M. & Spicer, C. (1976) Maternal
    factors associated with fetal chromosomal anomalies in spontaneous
    abortions. Br. J. Obstet. Gynaecol., 83, 621-627

Anon. (1979) OCs - Update on usage, safety, and side effects.
    Population Reports, Series A, No. 5, Washington DC, George Washington
    University Medical Center, Department of Medical & Public Affairs,
    pp. A-133-186

Applezweig, N. (1962) Steroid Drugs, New York, McGraw-Hill

Applezweig, N. (1964) Steroid Drugs, Vol. 2, San Francisco, Holden-Day

Azarnoff, D.L. (1975) Steroid Therapy, Philadelphia, Saunders

Baird, D.T. & Guevara, A. (1969) Concentration of unconjugated estrone
    and estradiol in peripheral plasma in nonpregnant women throughout
    the menstrual cycle, castrate and postmenopausal women and in men.
    J. clin. Endocrinol. Metab., 29, 149-156

Baird, D.T., Horton, R., Longcope, C. & Tait, J.F. (1969) Steroid dynamics under steady-state conditions. Recent Prog. Horm. Res., 25, 611-664

Barberia, J.M. & Thorneycroft, I.H. (1974) Simultaneous radioimmunoassay of testosterone and dihydrotestosterone. Steroids, 23, 757-766

Bardin, C.W. & Lipsett, M.B. (1967) Testosterone and androstenedione blood production rates in normal women and women with idiopathic hirsutism or polycystic ovaries. J. clin. Invest., 46, 891-902

Barrett, S.A. & Brown, J.B. (1970) An evaluation of the method of Cox for the rapid analysis of pregnanediol in urine by gas-liquid chromatography. J. Endocrinol., 47, 471-480

Barrett, S. & Hakim, C. (1973) Anencephaly, ovulation stimulation, subfertility and illegitimacy. Lancet, ii, 916-917

Beling, C.G., Gustafsson, P.-O. & Kasström, H. (1975) Metabolism of estradiol in greyhounds and German shepherd dogs. Acta radiol., Suppl. 344, 109-120

Benjamin, F. & Deutsch, S. (1976) Plasma levels of fractionated estrogens and pituitary hormones in endometrial carcinoma. Am. J. Obstet. Gynecol., 126, 638-647

Bern, H.A. (1979) The neonatal mouse - tumorigenesis after short-term exposure to hormones and its possible relevance to human syndromes. In: Proceedings, Symposium on Endocrine-Induced Neoplasia, Omaha, NA, Eppley Institute for Research in Cancer (in press)

Bern, H.A., Jones, L.A., Mori, T. & Young, P.N. (1975) Exposure of neonatal mice to steroids: longterm effects on the mammary gland and other reproductive structures. J. Steroid Biochem., 6, 673-676

Bern, H.A., Jones, L.A., Mills, K.T., Kohrman, A. & Mori, T. (1976) Use of the neonatal mouse in studying long-term effects of early exposure to hormones and other agents. J. Toxicol. environ. Health, Suppl. 1, 103-116

Bishun, N.P. (1976) Chromosomes and oral contraceptives. Proc. R. Soc. Med., 69, 353-356

Blackburn, G.M., Orgee, L. & Williams, G.M. (1977) Oxidative bonding of natural oestrogens to DNA by chemical and metabolic means. J. chem. Soc. chem. Commun., 11, 386-387

Bolt, H.M. (1979) Metabolism of estrogens - natural and synthetic. Pharm. Ther , 4, 155-181

Bolt, H.M. & Kappus, H. (1974)   Irreversible binding of ethynyl-estradiol metabolites to protein and nucleic acids as catalyzed by rat liver microsomes and mushroom tyrosinase. J. Steroid Biochem., 5, 179-184

Bolt, H.M. & Remmer, H. (1972a)   Retention, metabolsm and elimination of 17α-ethynyl-estradiol-3-methyl ether (mestranol). Xenobiotica, 2, 77-88

Bolt, H.M. & Remmer, H. (1972b)   The accumulation of mestranol and ethynylestradiol metabolites in the organism. Xenobiotica, 2, 489-498

Boon, D.A., Keenan, R.E., Slaunwhite, W.R., Jr & Aceto, T., Jr (1972) Conjugated and unconjugated plasma androgens in normal children. Pediatr. Res., 6, 111-118

Boston Collaborative Drug Surveillance Program (1973)   Oral contraceptives and venous thromboembolic disease, surgically confirmed gall bladder disease and breast tumours. Lancet, i, 1399-1404

Boué, J.C. & Boué, A. (1973)   Increased frequency of chromosomal anomalies in abortions after induced ovulation. Lancet, i, 679-680

Breibart, S., Bongiovanni, A.M. & Eberlein, W.R. (1963)   Progestins and skeletal maturation. New Engl. J. Med., 268, 255

Breuer, H. & Knuppen, R. (1969)   Comparative studies on the metabolism of estrogens in the rabbit under various experimental conditions: in vivo, during perfusion, in vitro. Adv. Biosci., 3, 71-79

Briggs, M.H. & Brotherton, J. (1970)   Steroid Biochemistry and Pharmacology, London, Academic Press

Briggs, M.H. & Christie, G.A. (1976)   Advances in Steroid Biochemistry and Pharmacology, Vol. 4, London, Academic Press

Brotherton, J. (1976)   Sex Hormone Pharmacology, London, Academic Press

Brown, J.B. (1957)   The relationship between urinary oestrogens and oestrogens produced in the body. J. Endocrinol., 16, 202-212

Brown, J.B. & Matthew, G.D. (1962)   The application of urinary estrogen measurements to problems in gynecology. Recent Prog. Horm. Res., 18, 337-373

Brown, J.B., MacLeod, S.C., MacNaughtan, C., Smith, M.A. & Smith B. (1968) A rapid method for estimating oestrogens in urine using a semi-automatic extractor. J. Endocrinol., 42, 5-15

Brown, J.B., Harrisson, P. & Smith, M.A. (1978) Oestrogen and pregnanediol excretion through childhood, menarche and first ovulation. J. biosoc. Sci., Suppl. 5, 45-64

Burstein, R. & Wasserman, H.C. (1964) The effect of Provera on the fetus. Obstet. Gynecol., 23, 931-934

Calanog, A., Sall, S., Gordon, G.G., Olivo, J. & Southern, A.L. (1976) Testosterone metabolism in endometrial cancer. Am. J. Obstet. Gynecol., 124, 60-63

Carr, D.H. (1970) Chromosome studies in selected spontaneous abortions. I. Conception after oral contraceptives. Can. med. Assoc. J., 103, 343-348

Chan, L. & O'Malley, B.W. (1976) Mechanism of action of the sex steroid hormones. New Engl. J. Med., 294, 1322-1328

Chen, C. & Lee, S.-G. (1975) Covalent binding of norethynodrel to proteins and glutathione initiated by rat liver oxygenase. Mol. Pharmacol., 11, 409-420

Clauberg, C. (1930) Physiology and pathology of sex hormones, in particular of the hormones of the corpus luteum. I. Biological test for luteinizing hormone (the specific hormone of the corpus luteum) in young rabbits (Ger.). Zbol. Gynäkol., 2757-2770

Cook, C.E., Twine, M.E., Tallent, C.R., Wall, M.E. & Bressler, R.C. (1972) Norethynodrel metabolites in human plasma and urine. J. Pharmacol. exp. Ther., 183, 197-205

Cook, C.E., Karim, A., Forth, J., Wall, M.E., Ranney, R.E. & Bressler, R.C. (1973) Ethynodiol diacetate metabolites in human plasma. J. Pharmacol. exp. Ther., 185, 696-702

Costoff, A. & Mahesh, V.B. (1975) Primordial follicles with normal oocytes in the ovaries of postmenopausal women. J. Am. Geriatr. Soc., 23, 193-196

Crosignani, P.G. & James, V.H.T., eds (1974) Recent Progress in Reproductive Endocrinology, London, Academic Press

DeJongh, D.C., Hribar, J.D., Littleton, P., Fotherby, K., Rees, R.W.A., Shrader, S., Foell, T.J. & Smith, H. (1968) The identification of some human metabolites of norgestrel, a new progestational agent. Steroids, 11, 649-664

Desaulles, P.A. & Krähenbühl, C. (1960) Modern developments in the
    field of gestagen therapy (Ger.). In: Nowakowski, H., ed.,
    Moderne Entwicklungen auf dem Gestagengebiel. Hormone in der
    Veterinär-medizin, Berlin, Springer, pp. 1-10

Desaulles, P.A. & Krähenbühl, C. (1962) Comparison of activities of certain
    synthetic gestagens (Fr.). Acta endocrinol., 40, 217-231

Desaulles, P.A. & Krähenbühl, C. (1964) Comparison of the anti-fertility
    and sex hormonal activities of sex hormones and their derivatives.
    Acta endocrinol., 47, 444-456

Dhadial, R.K., Machin, A.M. & Tait, S.M. (1970) Chromosomal anomalies in
    spontaneously aborted human fetuses. Lancet, ii, 20-21

Diczfalusy, E. (1969) Steroid metabolism in the human foeto-placental
    unit. Acta endocrinol. (KbH.), 61, 649-664

Dyson, J.L. & Kohler, H.G. (1973) Anencephaly and ovulation stimulation.
    Lancet, i, 1256-1257

Edman, C.D. & MacDonald, P.C. (1978) Effect of obesity on conversion of
    plasma androstenedione to estrone in ovulatory and anovulatory young
    women. Am. J. Obstet. Gynecol., 130, 456-461

Edman, C.D., Aiman, E.J., Porter, J.C. & MacDonald, P.C. (1978)
    Identification of the estrogen product of extraglandular aromatization
    of plasma androstenedione. Am. J. Obstet. Gynecol., 130, 439-447

Elbling, L. (1973) Does gonadotrophin-induced ovulation in mice cause
    malformations in the offspring? Nature, 246, 37-39

Elbling, L. (1975a) Malformations and abnormality of the sex ratio after
    hormone treatment of mice (Ger.). Wien. klin. Wschr., 87, 68-71

Elbling, L. (1975b) Congenital malformations in mice after gonado-
    trophin-induced ovulation. Proc. Soc. exp. Biol. (N.Y.), 149, 376-379

Elbling, L. (1975c) Malformations induced by hormones in mice and their
    transmission to the offspring. Exp. Pathol., 11, 115-122

Emmeus, C.W. & Martin, L. (1962) Estrogens. In: Dorfman, R.I., ed.,
    Methods in Hormone Research, Vol. III, London, Academic Press,
    pp. 1-75

Faiman, C. & Ryan, R.J. (1967) Serum follicle-stimulating hormone and
    luteinizing hormone concentrations during the menstrual cycle as
    determined by radioimmunoassays. J. clin. Endocrinol. Metab., 27,
    1711-1716

Fechheimer, N.S. & Beatty, R.A. (1974) Chromosomal abnormalities and sex ratio in rabbit blastocysts. J. Reprod. Fertil., 37, 331-341

Field, B. & Kerr, C. (1974) Ovulation stimulation and defects of neural-tube closure. Lancet, ii, 1511

Fishman, J., Hellman, L., Zumoff, B. & Gallagher, T.F. (1965) Effect of thyroid on hydroxylation of estrogen in man. J. clin. Endocrinol. Metab., 25, 365-368

Fishman, J., Naftolin, F., Davies, I.J., Ryan, K.J. & Petro, Z. (1976) Catechol estrogen formation by the human fetal brain and pituitary. J. clin. Endocrinol. Metab., 42, 177-180

Forchielli, E. & Murthy, D.V.K. (1970) Metabolism of chlormadinone acetate in the human and in laboratory animals (Abstract no. 123). Exerpta Medica Internatl Congr. Ser., 210, 64-65

Forsberg, J.-G. (1972) Estrogen, vaginal cancer, and vaginal development. Am. J. Obstet. Gynecol., 113, 83-87

Forsberg, J.-G. (1975) Late effects in the vaginal and cervical epithelia after injections of diethylstilboestrol into neonatal mice. Am. J. Obstet. Gynecol., 121, 101-104

Forsberg, J.-G. (1976) Animal model: estrogen-induced adenosis of vagina and cervix in mice. Am. J. Path., 84, 669-672

Forsberg, J.-G. (1979) Developmental mechanism of estrogen-induced irreversible changes in the mouse cervicovaginal epithelium. Natl Cancer Inst. Monogr., 51, 41-56

Frisch, R.E. (1974a) A method of prediction of age of menarche from height and weight at ages 9 through 13 years. Pediatrics, 53, 384-390

Frisch, R.E. (1974b) Critical weight at menarche, initiation of the adolescent growth spurt, and control of puberty. In: Grumbach, M.M., Grave, G.D. & Mayer, F.E., eds, Control of the Onset of Puberty, New York, John Wiley & Sons, pp. 403-423

Fuchs, F. & Klopper, A., eds (1977) Endocrinology of Pregnancy, 2nd ed., New York, Harper & Row

Fujimoto, S., Pahlavan, N. & Dukelow, W.R. (1974) Chromosomal abnormalities in rabbit preimplantaiton blastocysts induced by superovulation. J. Reprod. Fertil., 40, 177-181

Gal, I., Kilman, B. & Stern, J. (1967) Hormonal pregnancy tests and congenital malformation. Nature, 216, 83

Gallagher, T.F., Hellman, L., Bradlow, H.L., Zurnoff, B. & Fukushima, D.K.
    (1960) The effects of thyroid hormones on the metabolism of steroids.
    Ann. N.Y. Acad. Sci., 86, 605-611

Gill, W.B., Schumacher, G.F.B. & Bibbo, M. (1976) Structural and
    functional abnormalities in the sex organs of male offspring of mothers
    treated with diethylstilbestrol (DES). J. reprod. Med., 16, 147-153

Gill, W.B., Schumacher, G.F.B. & Bibbo, M. (1977) Pathological semen and
    anatomical abnormalities of the genital tract in human male
    subjects exposed to diethylstilbestrol in utero. J. Urol., 117,
    477-480

Goldzieher, J.W. & Kraemer, D.C. (1972) The metabolism and effects of
    contraceptive steroids in primates. Acta endocrinol., Suppl. 166,
    389-421

Greenberg, G., Inman, W.H.W., Weatherall, J.A.C. & Adelstein, A.M.
    (1975) Hormonal pregnancy tests and congenital malformations.
    Br. med. J., ii, 191-192

Greenblatt, R.B., Colle, M.L. & Mahesh, V.B. (1976) Ovarian and adrenal
    steroid production in the postmenopausal woman. Obstet. Gynecol.,
    47, 383-387

Grodin, J.M., Siiteri, P.K. & MacDonald, P.C. (1973) Source of estrogen
    production in postmenopausal women. J. clin. Endocrinol. Metab., 36,
    207-214

Grumbach, M.M. & Ducharme, J.R. (1960) The effects of androgens on fetal
    sexual development. Androgen induced female pseudohermophrodism.
    Fertil. Steril., 11, 157-180

Hack, M., Brish, M., Serr, D.M., Insler, V., Salomy, M. & Lunenfeld, B.
    (1972) Outcome of pregnancy after induced ovulation. Follow-up of
    pregnancies and children born after clomiphene therapy. J. Am. med.
    Assoc., 220, 1329-1333

Hafez, E.S.E. & Evans, T.N. (1973) Human Reproduction. Conception and
    Contraception, Hagerstown, MD, Harper & Row

Harlap, S., Shiono, P., Pellegrin, F., Golbus, M., Bachman, R., Mann, J.,
    Schmidt, L. & Lewis, J.P. (1979) Chromosome abnormalities in oral
    contraceptive breakthrough pregnancies. Lancet, i, 1342-1343

Heinonen, O.P., Slone, D., Monson, R.R., Hook, E.B. & Shapiro, S. (1977)
    Cardiovascular birth defects and antenatal exposure to female sex
    hormones. New Engl. J. Med., 296, 67-70

Helton, E.D., Gough, B.J., King, J.W., Jr, Thenot, J.P. & Horning, E.C. (1978a) Metabolism of diethylstilbestrol in the C3H mouse: chromatographic systems for the quantitative analysis of DES metabolic products. Steroids, 31, 471-484

Helton, E.D., Hill, D.E., Gough, B.J., Lipe, G.W., King, J.W., Jr, Horning, E.C. & Thenot, J.P. (1978b) Comparative metabolism of diethylstilbestrol in the mouse, rhesus monkey, and chimpanzee. J. Toxicol. environ. Health, 4, 482-483

Hemsell, D.L., Grodin, J.M., Brenner, P.F., Siiteri, P.K. & MacDonald, P.C. (1974) Plasma precursors of estrogen. II. Correlation of the extent of conversion of plasma androstenedione to estrone with age. J. clin. Endocrinol. Metab., 38, 476-479

Herbst, A.L., ed. (1978) Intrauterine Exposure to Diethylstilbestrol in the Human, Chicago, IL, American College of Obstetricians & Gynecologists

Herbst, A.L., Poskanzer, D.C., Robboy, S.J., Friedlander, L. & Scully, R.E. (1975a) Prenatal exposure to stilbestrol. A prospective comparison of exposed female offspring with unexposed controls. New Engl. J. Med., 292, 334-339

Herbst, A.L., Scully, R.E. & Robboy, S.J. (1975b) Vaginal adenosis and other diethylstilbestrol related abnormalities. Clin. Obstet. Gynecol., 18, 185-194

Hoff, J.D., Lasley, B.L., Wang, C.F. & Yen, S.S.C. (1977) The two pools of pituitary gonadotropin: regulation during the menstrual cycle. J. clin. Endocrinol. Metab., 44, 302-312

Horning, E.C., Thenot, J.-P. & Helton, E.D. (1978) Toxic agents resulting from the oxidative metabolism of steroid hormones and drugs. J. Toxicol. environ. Health, 4, 341-361

Horton, R. & Tait, J.F. (1966) Androstenedione production and inter-conversion rates measured in peripheral blood and studies on the possible site of its conversion to testosterone. J. clin. Invest., 45, 301-313

Janerich, D.T., Piper, J.M. & Glebatis, D.M. (1974) Oral contraceptives and congenital limb-reduction defects. New Engl. J. Med., 291, 697-700

Janerich, D.T., Dugan, M.J., Standfast, S.J. & Strite, L. (1977) Congenital heart disease and prenatal exposure to exogenous sex hormones. Br. med. J., i, 1058-1060

Jensen, E.V. & deSombre, E.R. (1972) Mechanism of action of the female
    sex hormones. Ann. Rev. Biochem., 41, 203-230

Johns, W.F. (1976) Steroids (Organic Chemistry Series 2), Vol. 8, London,
    Butterworths

Judd, H.L. & Yen, S.S.C. (1973) Serum androstenedione and testosterone
    levels during the menstrual cycle. J. clin. Endocrinol. Metab., 36,
    475-481

Judd, H.L., Lucas, W.E. & Yen, S.S.C. (1974a) Effect of oophorectomy on
    circulating testosterone and androstenedione levels in patients with
    endometrial cancer. Am. J. Obstet. Gynecol., 118, 793-798

Judd, H.L., Judd, G.E., Lucas, W.E. & Yen, S.S.C. (1974b) Endocrine
    function of the postmenopausal ovary: concentration of androgens
    and estrogens in ovarian and peripheral vein blood. J. clin.
    Endocrinol. Metab., 39, 1020-1024

Judd, H.L., Lucas, W.E. & Yen, S.S.C. (1976) Serum 17β-estradiol and
    estrone levels in postmenopausal women with and without endometrial
    cancer. J. clin. Endocrinol. Metab., 43, 272-278

Kappus, H. & Remmer, H. (1975) Metabolic activation of norethisterone
    (norethindrone) to an irreversibly protein-bound derivative by rat
    liver microsomes. Drug Metab. Disposition, 3, 338-344

Kappus, H., Bolt, H.M. & Remmer, H. (1973) Irreversible protein binding
    of metabolites of ethynylestradiol in vivo and in vitro. Steroids,
    22, 203-225

Kaufman, R.L. (1973) Birth defects and oral contraceptives. Lancet, i,
    1396

Kelch, R.P., Jenner, M.R., Weinstein, R., Kaplan, S.L. & Grumbach, M.M.
    (1972) Estradiol and testosterone secretion by human, simian and
    canine testes, in males with hypogonadism and in male pseudoherma-
    phrodites with the feminizing testes syndrome. J. clin. Invest.,
    51, 824-830

Kimura, T. (1975) Persistent vaginal cornification in mice treated with
    estrogen prenatally. Endocrinol. jpn., 22, 497-502

Kirdani, R.Y. & Sandberg, A.A. (1974) The fate of estriol in dogs.
    Steroids, 23, 667-686

Klinger, H.P., Glasser, M. & Kava, H.W. (1976) Contraceptives and the
    conceptus. I. Chromosome abnormalities of the fetus and the
    neonate related to maternal contraceptive history. Obstet. Gynecol.,
    48, 40-48

Klopper, A. & Michie, E.A. (1956) The excretion of urinary pregnanediol
    after the administration of progesterone. J. Endocrinol., 13,
    360-364

Kohrman, A.K. (1978) The newborn mouse as a model for study of the effects
    of hormonal steroids in the young. Pediatrics, 62, Suppl., 1143-1150

Korenman, S.G. & Sherman, B.M. (1973) Further studies on gonadotrophin
    and estradiol secretion during the preovulatory phase of the human
    menstrual cycle. J. clin. Endocrinol. Metab., 36, 1205-1209

Laurence, M., Miller, M., Vowles, M., Evans, K. & Carter, C. (1971)
    Hormonal pregnancy tests and neural tube malformations. Nature,
    233, 495-496

Lauritsen, J.G. (1975) The significance of oral contraceptives in causing
    chromosome anomalies in spontaneous abortions. Acta obstet. gynecol.
    scand., 54, 261-264

Layne, D.S., Golab, T., Arai, K. & Pincus, G. (1963) The metabolic fate
    of orally administered ^{3}H-norethynodrel and ^{3}H-norethindrone in
    humans. Biochem. Pharmacol., 12, 905-911

Levy, E.P., Cohen, A. & Fraser, F.C. (1973) Hormone treatment during
    pregnancy and congenital heart defects. Lancet, i, 611

Lin, T.J., Lin, S.C., Erlenmeyer, F., Kline, I.T., Underwood, R.,
    Billiar, R.B. & Little, B. (1972) Progesterone production rates
    during the third trimester of pregnancy in normal women, diabetic
    women, and women with abnormal glucose tolerance. J. clin. Endocrinol.
    Metab., 34, 287-297

Lloyd, C.W., Lobotsky, J., Baird, D.T., McCracken, J.A., Weisz, J., Pupkin,
    M., Zanartu, J. & Puga, J. (1971) Concentration of unconjugated
    estrogens, androgens and gestagens in ovarian and peripheral venous
    plasma of women: the normal menstrual cycle. J. clin. Endocrinol.
    Metab., 32, 155-166

Longcope, C. (1971) Metabolic clearance and blood production rates of
    estrogens in postmenopausal women. Am. J. Obstet. Gynecol., 111,
    778-781

Longcope, C. & Williams, K.I.H. (1974) The metabolism of estrogens in
    normal women after pulse injections of ^{3}H-estradiol and ^{3}H-estrone.
    J. clin. Endocrinol. Metab., 38, 602-607

Marks, F. & Hecker, E. (1969) Metabolism and mechanism of action of
    oestrogens. XII. Structure and mechanism of formation of water-
    soluble and protein-bound metabolites of oestrone in rat-liver
    microsomes in vitro and in vivo. Biochim. biophys. Acta, 187, 250-265

Maroulis, G.B. & Abraham, G.E. (1976) Ovarian and adrenal contributions to peripheral steroid levels in postmenopausal women. Obstet. Gynecol., 48, 150-154

Marshall, W.A. & Tanner, J.M. (1969) Variations in pattern of pubertal changes in girls. Arch. Dis. Child., 44, 291-303

Maudlin, I. & Fraser, L.R. (1977) The effect of PMSG dose on the incidence of chromosomal anomalies in mouse embryos fertilized in vitro. J. Reprod. Fertil., 50, 275-280

McLachlan, J.A. (1977) Prenatal exposure to diethylstilbestrol in mice: toxicological studies. J. Toxicol. environ. Health, 2, 527-537

McLachlan, J.A., Newbold, R.R. & Bullock, B. (1975) Reproductive tract lesions in male mice exposed prenatally to diethylstilbestrol. Science, 190, 91-992

McPhail, M.K. (1935) The assay of progestin. J. Physiol., 83, 145-156

Morgan, C.F. (1963) A comparison of topical and subcutaneous methods of administration of sixteen oestrogens. J. Endocrinol., 26, 317-329

Mulvihill, J.J., Mulvihill, C.G. & Neill, C.A. (1974) Congenital heart defects and prenatal sex hormones. Lancet, i, 1168

Naftolin, F., Ryan, K.J., Davies, I.J., Reddy, V.V., Flores, F., Petro, Z., Kuhn, M., White, R.J., Takaoka, Y. & Wolin, L. (1975) The formation of estrogens by central neuroendocrine tissues. Recent Prog. Horm. Res., 31, 295-319

Nandi, S. (1978) Hormonal carcinogenesis: a novel hypothesis for the role of hormones. J. environ. Pathol. Toxicol., 2, 13-20

Nandi, S. (1978) Role of hormones in mammary neoplasia. Cancer Res., 38, 4046-4049

Neumann, F. (1968) Chemical constitution and pharmacologic action (Ger.). In: Langecker, H., ed., Handbuch der experimenteller Pharmakologie, Vol. 22, Die Gestagene, Berlin, Springer, pp. 680-1025

Neumann, F. & Elger, W. (1972) Critical considerations of the biological basis of toxicity studies with steroid sex hormones (Ger.). In: Plotz, E.J. & Haller, J., eds, Methods in Steroid Toxicology for Research and Clinical Application of Steroids, Los Altos, CA, Geron-X, pp. 10-81

Nevin, N.C. & Harley, J.M.G. (1976) Clomiphene and neural tube defects. Ulster med. J., 45, 59-64

Nora, A.H. & Nora, J.J. (1975) A syndrome of multiple congenital
    anomalies associated with teratogenic exposure. Arch. environ.
    Health, 30, 17-21

Nora, J.J. & Nora, A.H. (1973) Birth defects and oral contraceptives.
    Lancet, i, 941-942

Nora, J.J., Nora, A.H., Blu, J., Ingram, J., Fountain, A., Peterson, M.,
    Lortscher, R.H. & Kimberling, W.J. (1978) Exogenous progestogen and
    oestrogen implicated in birth defects. J. Am. med. Assoc., 240,
    837-843

Oakley, G.P., Jr, Flynt, J.W., Jr & Falek, H. (1973) Hormonal pregnancy
    tests and congenital malformations. Lancet, ii, 256-257

Peterson, W.F. (1969) Pregnancy following oral contraceptive therapy.
    Obstet. Gynecol., 34, 363-367

Piotrow, P.T. & Lee, C.M. (1974) Oral contraceptives - 50 million users.
    Population Reports, Series A, No. 1, Washington DC, George Washington
    University Medical Center, Department of Medical & Public Affairs,
    pp. A-1-A-26

Poortman, J., Thijssen, J.H.H. & Schwarz, F. (1973) Androgen production
    and conversion to estrogens in normal postmenopausal women and in
    selected breast cancer patients. J. clin. Endocrinol. Metab., 37,
    101-109

Rader, M.D., Flickinger, G.L., deVilla, G.O., Jr, Mikuta, J.J. & Mikhail,
    G. (1973) Plasma estrogens in postmenopausal women. Am. J. Obstet.
    Gynecol., 116, 1069-1073

Richardson, G.S. & MacLaughlin, D.T., eds (1978) Hormonal biology of
    endometrial cancer. A series of workshops on the biology of human
    cancer. Report no. 8. UICC Tech. Rep. Ser., Vol. 42, Geneva,
    International Union Against Cancer

Rizkallah, T.H., Tovell, H.M.M. & Kelly, W.G. (1975) Production of estrone
    and fractional conversion of circulating androstenedione to estrone
    in women with endometrial cancer. J. clin. Endocrinol. Metab., 40,
    1045-1056

Robinson, S.C. (1971) Pregnancy outcome following oral contraceptives.
    Am. J. Obstet. Gynecol., 109, 354-358

Rosenfeld, R.S., Rosenberg, B.J., Fukushima, D.K. & Hellman, L. (1975)
    24-Hour secretory pattern of dehydroisoandrosterone and dehydro-
    isoandrosterone sulfate. J. clin. Endocrinol. Metab., 40, 850-855

Ross, G.T., Cargille, C.M., Lipsett, M.B., Rayford, P.L., Marshall, J.R., Strott, C.A. & Rodbard, D. (1970) Pituitary and gonadal hormones in women during spontaneous and induced ovulatory cycles. Recent Prog. Horm. Res., 26, 1-62

Rothman, K.J. & Louik, C. (1978) Oral contraceptives and birth defects. New Engl. J. Med., 299, 522-524

Rothman, K.J., Fyler, D.C., Goldblatt, A. & Kreidberg, M.B. (1979) Exogenous hormones and other drug exposures of children with congenital heart disease. Am. J. Epidemiol., 109, 433-439

Royal College of General Practitioners (1974) Oral Contraceptives and Health, London, Pitman Medical

Royal College of General Practitioners (1976) The outcome of pregnancy in oral contraceptive users. Br. J. Obstet. Gynaecol., 83, 608-616

Sandberg, A.A. & Slaunwhite, W.R., Jr (1956) Metabolism of 4-C^{14}-testosterone in human subjects. I. Distribution in bile, blood, feces and urine. J. clin. Invest., 35, 1331-1339

Sandberg, A.A. & Slaunwhite, W.R., Jr (1957) Studies of phenolic steroids in human subjects. II. The metabolic fate and hepato-biliary-enteric circulation of C^{14}-estrone and C^{14}-estradiol in women. J. clin. Invest., 36, 1266-1278

Sandberg, A.A. & Slaunwhite, W.R., Jr (1958) The metabolic fate of C^{14}-progesterone in human subjects. J. clin. Endocrinol. Metab., 18, 253-265

Sandler, B. (1973) Anencephaly and ovulation stimulation. Lancet, ii, 379

Schulster, D., Burstein, S. & Corbe, A. (1976) Molecular Endocrinology of Steroid Hormones, New York, John Wiley & Sons

Sherman, B.M., West, J.H. & Korenman, S.G. (1976) The menopausal transition: analysis of LH, FSH, estradiol, and progesterone concentrations during menstrual cycles of older women. J. clin. Endocrinol. Metab., 42, 629-636

Siiteri, P.K. & MacDonald, P.C. (1973) Role of extraglandular estrogen in human endocrinology. In: Greep, R.O. & Astwood, E.B., eds, Handbook of Physiology, Vol. 2, Bethesda, MD, American Physiological Society, pp. 615-629

Smith, C.M. & Chrisman, C.L. (1975) Failure of exogenous gonadotrophin controlled ovulation to cause digit abnormalities in mice. Nature, 253, 631

Swerdloff, R.S. & Odell, W.D. (1969) Serum luteinizing and follicle stimulating hormone levels during sequential and nonsequential contraceptive treatment of eugonadal women. J. clin. Endocrinol. Metab., 29, 157-163

Szego, C.M. (1974) The lysosome as a mediator of hormone action. Recent Prog. Horm. Res., 30, 171-233

Szego, C.M. (1965) Role of histamine in mediation of hormone action. Fed. Proc., 24, 1343-1352

Takagi, N. & Sasaki, M. (1976) Digynic triploidy after superovulation in mice. Nature, 264, 278-281

Tausk, M. & De Visser, J. (1972) International Encyclopedia of Pharmacology and Therapeutics, Section 48, Vol. II, Elmsford, N.Y., Pergamon Press, pp. 35-194

Thomas, K., De Hertogh, R., Pizarro, M., Van Exter, C. & Ferin, J. (1973) Plasma LH-HCG, 17β-estradiol, estrone and progesterone monitoring around ovulation and subsequent nidation. Int. J. Fertil., 18, 65-73

Tulchinsky, D. (1973) Placental secretion of unconjugated estrone, estradiol and estriol in the maternal and the fetal circulation. J. clin. Endocrinol. Metab., 36, 1079-1087

Tulchinsky, D. & Korenman, S.G. (1970) A radio-ligand assay for plasma estrone; normal values and variations during the menstrual cycle. J. clin. Endocrinol. Metab., 31, 76-80

Turner, C.D. & Bagnara, J.T. (1976) General Endocrinology, 6th ed., Philadelphia, Saunders

Vermeulen, A. (1976) The hormonal activity of the postmenopausal ovary. J. clin. Endocrinol. Metab., 42, 247-253

Vessey, M.P. & Doll, R. (1976) Ovulation of existing techniques. Is 'the pill' safe enough to continue using? Proc. R. Soc. (Lond.), 195, 69-80

Vessey, M., Doll, R., Peto, R., Johnson, B. & Wiggins, P. (1976) A long-term follow-up study of women using different methods of contraception - an interim report. J. biosoc. Sci., 8, 373-427

Vollmar, J. (1977) Statistical problems in mutagenicity tests. Arch. Toxicol., 38, 13-25

West, C.D., Mahafan, D.K., Chavré, V.J., Nabors, C.J. & Tyler, F.H. (1973)
   Simultaneous measurement of multiple plasma steroids by radio-
   immunoassay demonstrating episodic secretion. J. clin. Endocrinol.
   Metab., 36, 1230-1236

WHO (1971) Methods of fertility regulation: advances in research and
   clinical experience. World Health Org. tech. Rep. Ser., No. 473

WHO (1973) Advances in methods of fertility regulation. World Health
   Org. tech. Rep. Ser., No. 527

WHO (1978) Steroid contraception and the risk of neoplasia. Report of
   a WHO Scientific Group. World Health Org. tech. Rep. Ser., No. 619

Williams, R.H. (1974) Textbook of Endocrinology, 5th ed., Philadelphia,
   Saunders

Yen, S.S.C., Martin, P.L., Burner, A.M., Czekala, N.M., Greaney, M.O.,
   Jr & Callantine, M.R. (1975) Circulating estradiol, estrone and
   gonadotropin levels following the administration of orally active
   17β-estradiol in postmenopausal women. J. clin. Endocrinol. Metab.,
   40, 518-521

Yoshizawa, I., Ohuchi, R., Nakagawa, A. & Kimura, M. (1977) Metabolism
   of estrone-6,7-^{3}H in guinea pigs. Yakugaku Zasshi, 97, 197-201

OESTROGENS AND PROGESTINS IN RELATION TO HUMAN CANCER

ENDOGENOUS SEX HORMONES AND HUMAN CANCER

Factors which affect the extraglandular conversion of androgens to oestrogens and their relation to endometrial cancer

Measurement of conversion rates
Sites of extraglandular aromatization
Conversion rates in various clinical conditions

Measurement of endogenous oestrogen values in blood and urine of postmenopausal women with and without endometrial cancer

Evidence that oestrone produced by the extraglandular route may not be as biologically active as ovarian oestradiol

The modulating effects of oestriol on the response of the breast and endometrium to oestradiol and oestrone

The modulating effects of progesterone on the carcinogenic action of oestrogens

The modulating effects of androgens on the development of breast cancer

Summing-up

EXOGENOUS SEX HORMONES AND HUMAN CANCER

Oestrogens used in treatment

Early studies
Recent studies

    (a)   Endometrial cancer
    (b)   Breast cancer
    (c)   Other cancers
    (d)   Benign breast disease

Androgens used in treatment

Hormonal contraception

Breast
    (a)   Gross and microscopic changes
    (b)   Benign breast disease
    (c)   Breast cancer

Uterus
    (a)   Non-neoplastic changes in the cervix
    (b)   Cervical neoplasia
    (c)   Endometrial cancer
    (d)   Trophoblastic tumours
    (e)   Uterine fibroids
Ovary
    (a)   Non-neoplastic and benign lesions
    (b)   Ovarian cancer
Pituitary
Malignant melanoma
Liver
    (a)   Benign neoplasms
    (b)   Malignant tumours

REFERENCES

ENDOGENOUS SEX HORMONES AND HUMAN CANCER

Factors which affect the extraglandular conversion of androgens to
oestrogens and their relation to endometrial cancer

Measurement of conversion rates

Rates of conversion of androstenedione to oestrone are measured in
women with endometrial cancer by administering a tracer dose, containing
^{3}H-oestrone and ^{14}C-androstenedione, as a single i.v. injection. The
fraction of plasma androstenedione that is converted to oestrone at the
aromatization sites in the tissues and which enters the blood can be
calculated by comparing the ^{3}H:^{14}C ratio in the oestrone and androstenedione
extracted from the blood with the ratio injected. Metabolic clearance
rates can also be calculated, and these, together with the endogenous
serum values, provide an estimate of daily production rates. Accurate
measurement of the isotope ratios in the plasma is difficult because
only very small amounts of radioactivity appear in these fractions;
therefore, conversion rates are often calculated from the isotope ratios
in the much more abundant urinary metabolites of oestrone. The model
depends on adequate mixing and equilibration of the administered tracers
in the various hormone pools of the body. Discrepancies between calculations
based on plasma hormones and those based on urinary metabolites have
provoked the challenge that these models may not be valid (Rizkallah *et
al.*, 1975). It has been shown recently that when ^{3}H-oestrone and ^{14}C-
androstenedione are given by i.v. infusion, the time taken to reach
steady-state conditions in plasma depends on the weight of the subject:
within 7 hrs for thin subjects and up to 48 hrs for the grossly obese.
Calculations of conversion rates based on urinary metabolites require
that all urine be collected until the tracer is completely eliminated;
this took 3 days for thin subjects and up to 7 days for the obese. When
these factors were controlled, the calculations based on blood and on
urine agreed, and it was concluded that the model was valid (Edman *et
al.*, 1978). Most of the studies reported, however, have utilized less-
than-ideal lengths of time for infusion and urine collection; these
deficiencies would exaggerate the differences due to obesity.

Sites of extraglandular aromatization

Human fat tissue can aromatize androgens to oestrogen *in vitro*
(Nimrod & Royan, 1975), and this was thought to be the main site *in vivo*
(MacDonald *et al.*, 1978). However, muscle is also involved; in men,
20-25% of extraglandular production of oestrone occurs in muscle and 10-
15% in adipose tissue, making a total of 30-40% in these two sites
(Longcope *et al.*, 1978). No information is available on the relative
contributions of other sites.

Conversion rates in various clinical conditions

Certain clinical conditions are associated with increased secretion of androstenedione, which then provides the substrate for increased peripheral production of oestrone. In 6 young anovulatory women with ovarian hyperthecosis, average daily production rates of androstenedione and testosterone were 3-8 times the normal; most of this excess androgen was produced by the ovaries. The daily production rates of oestrogen exceeded the average production rate seen in ovulating women; oestrone formed from plasma androstenedione accounted for most of the oestrogen produced (Aiman *et al.*, 1978). In normally ovulating women, practically all of the oestrogen is secreted as such by the ovaries. A postmenopausal patient with an ovarian tumour of the surface epithelium (a mucinous cystadenocarcinoma associated with hyperplastic stromal cells and endometrial hyperplasia) produced 5 times the normal amount of androstenedione; this was derived from the tumour, and it accounted for all of the raised oestrone production (5 times normal) (MacDonald *et al.*, 1976). A virilized postmenopausal woman with bilateral benign cystic teratomas associated with clusters of hyperplastic cells scattered within the stroma of the ovaries produced 10 times the normal amount of testosterone; this was derived from the ovaries, presumably from the hyperplastic stromal cells, and, together with the normal production of androstenedione, accounted for most of the oestrone produced and 75% of the oestradiol (Aiman *et al.*, 1977).

Other clinical states are also associated with increased extraglandular conversion of androstenedione to oestrone. Cirrhosis of the liver in men is accompanied by a general disturbance of androgen metabolism; this leads to an increase in the blood concentration of androstenedione, which is converted more efficiently to oestrone (Gordon *et al.*, 1975). Any reduction in the transhepatic clearance of androstenedione appears to be accompanied by its increased conversion to oestrone, and of oestrone to oestriol.

Age is an important factor in determining conversion rates of plasma androstenedione to oestrone. In a study of 23 women aged 19-73 years and of 26 males aged 12-82 years, with body weights selected to be within the range of 60-80 kg, significant correlations were found between conversion rates and age (correlation coefficient, r = 0.86 for the women and 0.62 for the men). The regression lines were linear and passed through 1% conversion at 20 years and 3% at 70 years of age for both sexes (Hemsell *et al.*, 1974).

Obesity is another very important factor. The conversion of plasma androstenedione to oestrone was measured in 24 ovulating and 31 anovulatory women aged 13-40 years with weights ranging from 41-159 kg. Highly significant correlations were found between conversion rates and body weights in the two groups (both r = 0.81). The regression lines were superimposable in the two groups; they curved exponentially and passed through 0.9% conversion at 45 kg, 1.8% at 90 kg and 3.6% at 135 kg body weight. Thus, the conversion rate approximately doubled for every increase of 45 kg in body weight over 45 kg (Edman & MacDonald, 1978).

Likewise, significant correlations were found between conversion rates of androstenedione to oestrone and body weights in 25 postmenopausal women with endometrial cancer aged 47-78 years with body weights of 61-195 kg and 25 controls aged 50-81 years with body weights of 47-165 kg (both r = 0.69). When body weight was expressed in terms of excess over ideal weight, the correlation coefficients were not altered. The regression lines were again superimposable in the two groups; they curved exponentially and passed through 2% conversion at 45 kg body weight, 4% at 100 kg and 8% at 160 kg, which represented a doubling in conversion for every 60 kg increase in body weight over 45 kg. Thus, in very obese postmenopausal women weighing between 110 and 195 kg, the efficiency of conversion of plasma androstenedione to oestrone was 2-4 times that in postmenopausal women of normal weight and 3-10 times that in non-obese premenopausal women. The similarity between the results obtained in the cancer patients and those in the controls showed that the conversion rates were entirely accounted for by weight and age and were independent of cancer status. Nevertheless, the authors emphasized that the conditions associated with increased extraglandular production of oestrone from androstenedione, whether by increased availability of androstenedione or by more efficient conversion, were all associated with increased rates of endometrial cancer (MacDonald *et al.*, 1978).

Measurement of endogenous oestrogen values in blood and urine of post-menopausal women with and without endometrial cancer

Serum oestradiol-17β and oestrone concentrations were measured in 16 postmenopausal patients with endometrial cancer and in 10 controls, with body weights matched as closely as possible. No significant differences were found between the mean serum levels of either oestradiol-17β or oestrone in the two groups, and no correlations were found between the oestrogen values and the subjects' ages, heights or years after the menopause. However, correlations (r = 0.62 for oestradiol-17β and 0.57 for oestrone) were found between body weight and oestrogen values in the cancer patients but not in the controls. This positive correlation could have been unduly influenced by the inclusion in the cancer group of a very obese patient who weighed 100 kg and had high oestrogen values. If high oestrogen values are defined as those above the 90th percentile for the control group, 19% of the cancer patients had high serum oestradiol-17β values (>17.3 pg/ml) and 44% had high oestrone values (>33.5 pg/ml), a distribution which did not reach signifance, probably because of the small numbers involved (Judd *et al.*, 1976).

In a well-controlled study, 20 postmenopausal patients with endometrial cancer and 30 controls were matched by age, weight and diabetic status, although the mean weight of the cancer group was greater than that of the controls (74 kg compared with 67 kg). Values for plasma oestradiol-17β and oestrone were significantly higher in the cancer patients than in the controls (P<0.02 for oestradiol-17β and P<0.001 for oestrone); and these differences were still significant after further adjustment for the difference in body weights. Thus, 50-55% of the cancer patients had values for oestradiol-17β and oestrone higher than the corresponding 90th percentiles for the control group. No correlations were found between the oestrogen values and the subjects' ages, heights or years since the menopause; however, correlations were found between body weights and oestrogen values in the cancer group (r = 0.47 for oestradiol-17β and 0.53 for oestrone), but not in the controls. This was probably due again to the high incidence of very obese subjects in the cancer group. Plasma FSH values were significantly lower in the cancer patients than in the controls, in keeping with the higher oestrogen values (Benjamin & Deutsch, 1976).

Urinary oestrogen excretion was measured in 36 postmenopausal women with endometrial cancer, in 11 postmenopausal women with atypical hyperplasia in 42 normal controls and in 18 oophorectomized women, using a rapid assay which measured 'total' urinary oestrogens and a specific assay which measured oestradiol, oestrone and oestriol, corrected to 100% recovery. The mean values in the control group were not significantly different from those in the oophorectomized patients; nevertheless, the highest total oestrogen value in the oophorectomized patients was 4.7 μg/24 hrs, whereas 11 of the 42 control women had values higher than this, the greatest being 8.6 μg/24 hrs. The mean values of all the oestrogen fractions in the cancer group were significantly higher than those of the controls, and this difference persisted after oophorectomy, suggesting that the oestrogen was not of ovarian origin. The patients with atypical hyperplasia had mean oestrogen values 3 times those of the cancer patients and 6 times those of the controls; these high values were reduced by oophorectomy to the oestrogen levels of the cancer patients, suggesting that it was mainly of ovarian origin. No correlations were found between the oestrogen values and the ages of the subjects or their body weights (Rome et al., 1977). Further analysis of the data shows that 40% of the cancer patients had oestrogen values which were above the 90th percentiles of the controls.

Urinary oestrogen excretion was also measured in 102 women with postmenopausal bleeding, and a weak correlation (r = 0.41) was found between oestrogen values and body weight in those patients who did not have ovarian pathology. The highest total urinary oestrogen value in this group was 21 μg/24 hrs, which was found in the most obese patient, who weighed 107 kg and had a hyperplastic endometrium (Reti et al., 1978).

Evidence that oestrone produced by the extraglandular route may not be as biologically active as ovarian oestradiol

Oestradiol-17β and oestrone are synthesized in body tissues by the extraglandular aromatization of androgens, which are secreted by the adrenals and ovaries and are perhaps produced in small amounts in the body tissues. Androstenedione and testosterone are the two main androgens involved in this process, and they are interconvertible. Androstenedione is present in the blood of pre- and postmenopausal women in approximately 4 times the concentration of testosterone, and it is converted peripherally to oestrone 4 times more efficiently than testosterone is converted to oestradiol-17β. The androstenedione-oestrone route is thus by far the more important and is the one that is usually measured. Oestradiol-17β and oestrone are also interconvertible and are further metabolized to the same urinary metabolites, irrespective of which oestrogen is produced or its source. For further details of these conversions and their significance, see reviews by Baird *et al.* (1968, 1969) and by Siiteri & MacDonald (1973).

Since many of the conditions in which increased extraglandular production of oestrone occurs are associated with an increased risk of endometrial and breast cancer, MacDonald and his coworkers have proposed that increased extraglandular production of oestrone is a causative factor in the development of these cancers, particularly in the endometrium (Siiteri *et al.*, 1974). This concept has been a most important advance; it is largely convincing, although not completely adequate.

A hirsute amenorrhoeic patient with ovarian hyperthecosis has been described who had persistently raised urinary oestrogen excretion, of 20-47 μg/24 hrs. Surprisingly, on curretage, no endometrium was obtained, despite the fact that this level of oestrogen excretion would normally be associated with gross stimulation of the endometrium and episodes of bleeding. It was suggested that either the excess androgen was antagonizing the effects of the oestrogen or the oestrogen being measured was not derived from the ovarian oestradiol but was a general metabolite of the excess androgen production (Brown & Matthew, 1962). It has now been established that the latter mechanism is a characteristic feature of ovarian hyperthecosis (Aiman *et al.*, 1978), but it is also likely that excess circulating androgens may interfere with the action of oestrogen on the endometrium.

In 38 postmenopausal women with ovarian tumours, raised urinary oestrogen excretion values were found in 4 of the 5 patients with sex-cord mesenchymal tumours (4 granulosa-theca-cell tumours and 1 thecoma), in 14 of the 30 patients with tumours of the surface epithelium and in both patients with metastatic tumours. The one patient with a benign cystic adult teratoma had normal values (Rome *et al.*, 1973). It was noted that the urinary oestrogen values correlated well with the clinical signs of oestrogenic activity in the patients with 'functional' mesenchymal tumours, but not in the patients with 'non-functional' tumours. It was

postulated that the former secreted oestradiol, in view of its evident
biological activity, whereas the latter probably secreted androgen which
was then converted peripherally to oestrogen (Laverty *et al.*, 1975).
The conclusion with regard to 'non-functional' ovarian tumours (non-
endocrine tumours) has now been confirmed; the excess steroid production
has its origin in the hyperplastic stroma associated with these tumours
(Aiman *et al.*, 1977; MacDonald *et al.*, 1976). This demonstrates that
the extraglandular route of oestrogen biosynthesis predominates in the
two notable exceptions to the rule that raised oestrogen excretion is
always associated with proliferation of the endometrium (provided a
functional endometrium is present); it provides evidence that oestrone
from this source is not as biologically active as an equivalent amount
of oestradiol-17β produced by the ovaries.

On the other hand, oestrone appears to be bound to the cytoplasmic
receptor of the target cell and to be translocated to the nucleus; it
differs from oestradiol-17β only in that it is bound about 25% less
efficiently (Siiteri *et al.*, 1974). Since the circulating level of
oestrone is 3-4.5 times higher than that of oestradiol in postmenopausal
women, oestrone may effectively compete with oestradiol-17β for binding
sites in the cytoplasm; and in view of its stable, high circulating
concentration, it may ultimately have the same proliferative activity as
oestradiol. It has been shown in rats that repeated doses of oestriol
(which binds to the cytoplasmic receptor with a similar affinity to that
of oestrone) have an effect similar to that of oestradiol-17β in eliciting
early uterotrophic response but that only oestradiol-17β can cause true
uterine growth (Anderson *et al.*, 1975).

It is possible that oestradiol-17β itself may be important in the
development of hyperplastic endometria in postmenopausal women, since
high urinary secretion of oestrogens in postmenopausal women with atypical
endometrial hyperplasia fell following oophorectomy to levels similar to
those seen in women with endometrial cancer (Rome *et al.*, 1977). It has
recently been observed that levels of serum sex-binding globulin are
markedly reduced in obese postmenopausal women, with and without endometrial
cancer, resulting in higher levels of free oestradiol (Siiteri, 1978).

Obviously, much research still needs to be done in this important
area to ascertain why high circulating oestrogen levels are associated
with excessive endometrial growth in some women and not in others with
similar constitutional backgrounds.

The modulating effects of oestriol on the response of the breast and
endometrium to oestradiol and oestrone

Oestriol can depress the growth-promoting action of oestradiol-17β
and oestrone on the uterus of rats (Hisaw *et al.*, 1954; Huggins &
Jensen, 1955); it competes with oestradiol-17β for receptor binding proteins
in rat uteri (Brecher & Wotiz, 1967); and it protects the rat mammary
gland against tumour induction by 7,12-dimethylbenzanthracene (Lemon,
1970; Terenius, 1971). These and similar findings have led to the

hypothesis (the 'oestriol hypothesis') that oestriol is an impeded or anti-oestrogen which can protect the breast and uterus against the carcinogenic action of the more potent oestradiol-17β and oestrone. Epidemiological observations have been interpreted as supporting this hypothesis (MacMahon et al., 1973). However, in humans, obesity increases the risk of endometrial and possibly breast carcinoma and also favours the conversion of oestradiol-17β to oestriol (Brown & Strong, 1965; Wynder et al., 1960, 1966).

Numerous investigations have been made to test indirectly the oestriol hypothesis, including the recent epidemiological endocrine studies of MacMahon and Cole and their colleagues. These workers postulate that an increased production of oestriol early in reproductive life explains many of the epidemiological characteristics of breast cancer. In studies of populations with different rates of breast cancer they showed that the ratio of oestriol:oestrone plus oestradiol excreted in the urine was inversely correlated with breast cancer risk. The ratio was significantly higher (P<0.001) in Japanese and Chinese women in Asia, with low rates of breast cancer, than in American and Canadian Caucasians, with high cancer rates (MacMahon et al., 1974). Intermediate values of the ratio were found in Asian migrants in Hawaii with intermediate breast cancer rates (Dickinson et al., 1974) and in American women who had had a pregnancy before the age of 24 years (low risk), compared with nulliparous women or women who had had a later first birth (double the risk) (Cole et al., 1976).

Nevertheless, recent work has shown that the oestriol hypothesis is untenable in its original form. Animal experiments have shown that the impeding effect of oestriol operates only when oestriol is present in approximately the same concentration as oestradiol and oestrone. It has now been shown that free oestriol is practically absent from the plasma of nonpregnant women, the concentrations being usually less than 4-30 pg/ml, compared with 100-400 pg/ml for oestradiol-17β and oestrone (Kim et al., 1974; Mishell et al., 1971; Raju et al., 1975; Rotti et al., 1975). Oestriol is apparently conjugated in the liver as rapidly as it is formed from oestrone and oestradiol-17β, and little or no free oestriol appears as such in the blood. Even the most generous calculations show that there is insufficient free oestriol in blood to have any modulating effect on the action of oestradiol and oestrone, the short-fall being a factor of 10 or more. Raju et al. (1977) have recently demonstrated that oestriol-3-glucuronide (oestriol-3-glucosiduronate) is the predominant form of oestriol in serum during the menstrual cycle (in contrast with pregnant women, in whom oestriol-3-sulphate-16-glucosiduronate is the predominant conjugate) and that high concentrations of oestriol-3-sulphate are present in human breast cyst fluid. It is thus possible that the effects noted are mediated by different conjugates of oestriol.

Oestriol is now prescribed for the relief of menopausal symptoms in the belief that it is a safe oestrogen. Recent work has shown, however, that, weight for weight, oestriol is as active as oestradiol in inducing uterotrophic responses in rats during the first 3 hrs after administration. Oestriol is a 'weak' oestrogen because it is not bound as strongly as oestradiol-17β to the nuclear oestrogen receptor and is rapidly lost from the system; but the uterotrophic effect of oestriol is greatly enhanced when it is given in repeated 3-hourly doses, a phenomenon well known to the early bioassayers (Anderson et al., 1975). Thus, oestriol may not be very different from oestradiol-17β in its carcinogenic potential for the endometrium, when doses with similar biological activities are used.

The modulating effects of progesterone on the carcinogenic action of oestrogens

Progesterone has a profound effect on the action of oestradiol-17β on human endometrium: it decreases the number of uterine receptors for oestradiol-17β and increases the ability of the endometrium to inactivate oestradiol-17β by increasing dehydrogenase activity (Tseng & Gurpide, 1974).

The list of conditions associated with high risk of endometrial carcinoma in humans comprises all circumstances in which excess oestrogen is produced without the possibility of ovulation. These include ovarian tumours, increased peripheral production of oestrone from androgens, polycystic ovarian disease and any situation in which oestrogen alone is administered over long periods of time. Two patients with Turner's syndrome due to a mosaic chromosomal constitution showed, on repeated endometrial biopsy, a progression from cystic glandular hyperplasia, through atypical hyperplasia to adenocarcinoma. Both excreted raised amounts of urinary oestrogens, one 36-48 μg/24 hrs and the other 13-20 μg/24 hrs, but no evidence of ovulation was detected during the 2-5-year study, even when clomiphene citrate was administered (Ostor et al., 1978). Furthermore, approximately 30% of women with endometrial cancer have a history of involuntary infertility, compared with a figure of 10% for the overall population; and infertility is also a risk factor in breast cancer. It is pertinent, therefore, to compare the hormone patterns found in ovulatory and anovulatory cycles and to assess the relative incidence of these two conditions in various age groups.

The average 28-day ovulatory menstrual cycle, with ovulation occurring on day 14, is characterized by low oestrogen and progesterone values early in the cycle. The oestrogen values begin to rise on about day 7 and rapidly reach a peak on day 13; they then fall, rise to a second maximum on day 21 and fall before onset of menstruation. Progesterone production begins to increase on the day of the preovulatory oestrogen peak, reaches a maximum on day 21 and falls before the onset of menstruation. The important feature is that, in the absence of functioning

ovarian tumours, raised progesterone values are found only following
ovulation; this provides the most reliable hormonal parameter that
ovulation has occurred. Furthermore, during the normal cycle, *raised*
oestrogen values in the presence of *low* progesterone output occur on
average for only the 5-6 days before ovulation. In other words, raised
oestrogen values unopposed by progesterone occur during only 20% of the
total duration of the normal cycle. Generally, an increase in the
length of the cycle is due merely to an increase in the number of
low-oestrogen days at the beginning of the cycle, although anovulatory
function may sometimes occur during this period.

Anovulatory cycles are characterized by persistently low progesterone
values. Two patterns of oestrogen production are observed. In one, the
oestrogen values are elevated and remain more or less constant, and
bleeding occurs as a breakthrough phenomenon. In the other pattern, the
oestrogen values rise to a peak, which resembles or exceeds that of the
normal cycle; but this is not followed by a rise in progesterone or by
a second rise in oestrogens, and bleeding occurs as a withdrawal phenomenon.
Variations in this second pattern include a small rise in progesterone
production after the oestrogen peak; and all gradations from a frankly
anovulatory cycle, through a deficient luteal phase to the full pattern
of the ovulatory cycle may be encountered (Brown & Matthew, 1962). An
important feature of the ovulatory cycle is that, providing a responsive
endometrium is present, bleeding always occurs with the fall in progesterone
production. Even in the unusual case of abnormal oestrogen production
during the luteal phase, the fall in progesterone output overrides the
effect of continuing or rising oestrogen production. In contrast, the
bleeding which occurs during or after an anovulatory cycle is an irregular
phenomenon and may not occur at all. Depending on the levels of oestrogen
production and their duration, the endometrium may be stimulated well
past the normal proliferative changes and reach severe hyperplasia, such
as cystic glandular hyperplasia. Furthermore, anovulatory cycles, which
are the most common cause of dysfunctional bleeding, are usually inter-
spersed with ovulatory cycles. It is only in exceptional circumstances,
such as in the conditions associated with high risk of endometrial
cancer, that anovulatory ovarian activity persists for long periods of
time. It would thus appear that the action of progesterone on the
oestrogen-primed endometrium and the subsequent progesterone withdrawal
bleeding may help to prevent the establishment of potentially malignant
areas of endometrium.

The modulating effects of androgens on the development of breast cancer

Differences in the excretion of androgen metabolites have been
documented in patients with breast cancer as compared with controls
(Bulbrook *et al.*, 1964; Marmorston *et al.*, 1965; Stern *et al.*, 1964);
and a prospective study has shown that in patients who went on to develop
breast cancer, the excretion of androgen metabolites (particularly of
aetiocholanolone) was, on the average, lower than that in those who did

not develop such a tumour (Hayward, 1970). This reduction in androgen
excretion may be due to a reduced production rate of dehydroepiandrosterone
and its sulphate (Poortman *et al.*, 1973). The exact relationship of
such findings to the development of breast cancer is as yet unclear.

Summing-up

The data reviewed are generally consistent, the discrepancies noted
being mainly due to inadequacies in the methods used and the populations
studied. Thus, the high correlation between age and conversion of
plasma androstenedione to oestrone found in infusion studies was not
reflected by endogenous oestrogen values in postmenopausal women. This
is explained by the different age ranges involved, the infusion studies
being performed on subjects aged 12-82 years, whereas the measurement of
the endogenous values was necessarily restricted to postmenopausal women
with half this age range. The correlations between peripheral oestrone
production and obesity were much less significant for the endogenous
values than in the infusion studies, and in some populations no correlation
was demonstrated. At least three factors account for this. Firstly, in
most of the conversion studies involving obese subjects, the tracers
were not infused long enough (48 hrs) to achieve complete steady-state
conditions, and the urine collections were incomplete (less than 7
days). These deficiencies would have amplified the effects of obesity
on the conversion rates. Secondly, if muscle and body fat contribute
only 40% of the overall conversion of androstenedione to oestrone,
factors affecting conversion at other sites could mask the effect of
body weight on the endogenous values. Thirdly, some very obese subjects,
weighing up to 195 kg, with very high conversion rates were included in
the infusion studies; these were not adequately matched in the studies
of endogenous oestrogen values.

MacDonald *et al.* (1978) frequently mention the occurrence of endometrial hyperplasia in patients with high conversion rates to oestrone.
However, insufficient data were presented to confirm or disprove the
finding from the endogenous values that the biological effects of this
oestrone were considerably less than the equivalent production of ovarian
oestradiol-17β. Furthermore, MacDonald *et al.* (1978) were unable to
demonstrate a specific effect of endometrial cancer on the extraglandular
conversion rates of androstenedione to oestrone, the effects noted being
entirely accounted for by weight and age. Their model may not have been
precise enough to show the small differences between the cancer cases
and controls that were demonstrated by assays of the endogenous hormones
in blood and urine, which themselves had well-recognized deficiencies.

All approaches point to a strong association between raised oestrogen
production in the persistent absence of ovulation and an increased risk
of endometrial cancer. Two routes seem to be involved in this process.
In the first, ovarian oestradiol-17β is secreted either continuously

over long periods of time or in fluctuations, so that the endometrium is stimulated through the stages of normal proliferation to hyperplasia, reaching adenomatous hyperplasia, atypical hyperplasia and eventually carcinoma in some cases. This would appear to be the most common route in premenopausal patients and may also be the route in those few postmenopausal women in whom progression through atypical hyperplasia to carcinoma takes place. The other route involves the production of oestrone by extraglandular conversion of androstenedione; this would appear to be the most common route in postmenopausal women. The oestrone may not have sufficient oestrogenic activity to cause proliferative changes in the endometrium, but it does provide facultative support for the development of cancer; and this would seem to be the situation in 50-60% of these patients. However, when the production of oestrone is increased by any process, the chances of developing cancer are very greatly increased; this would seem to be the situation in 40-50% of postmenopausal women who develop endometrial cancer. Further work is obviously required, using more precise methods and better controlled populations, before categorical statements can be made.

Although the above association between oestrogen production, anovulation and endometrial cancer appears to be well founded, a similar correlation has not yet been demonstrated for breast cancer. However, several of the risk factors associated with endometrial cancer are also risk factors for breast cancer: the two cancers themselves are associated, and the epidemiology of breast cancer clearly indicates that sex hormones play a central part.

EXOGENOUS SEX HORMONES AND HUMAN CANCER

The possible role of exogenous sex hormones in human cancer has been reviewed recently (Anon., 1977; Thomas, 1978; WHO, 1978).

In preparing sections 3.3 of the individual monographs, the Working Group excluded many reports because they did not clearly identify a specific substance to which the individuals were exposed, or because exposure was to multiple hormonal agents. When people were described, for example, as having received 'oestrogen replacement therapy', it was felt that it would be unjustified to attribute the observed effects to any specific compound, even though one compound may have been used preponderantly during the relevant period of time. When appropriate, however, such reports have been cited below.

Oestrogens used in treatment

Early studies

Until the mid- to late-1960s, only a small proportion of the general population had used oestrogens, and only a very small proportion had used them for a number of years. Thus, early case-control studies of

this exposure (Arthes *et al.*, 1971;   Jensen & Østergaard, 1954;   Wynder
et al., 1966) are inadequate.

Six cohort studies reported in the early literature
(Geist *et al.*, 1941;   Gordan, 1961;   Leis, 1966;   Schleyer-Saunders,
1960;   Wallach & Henneman, 1959;   Wilson, 1962) have been cited as
providing evidence that oestrogen replacement therapy is associated with
'protection' against virtually all forms of cancer, particularly those
of the breast and reproductive organs (Defares, 1971).   However, in each
of these studies, rather than identifying a group of exposed persons and
then following them up, information was simply extracted from existing
medical records.   In some instances, a group comprised only those patients
who were followed up to a certain date;   in others, patients were included
only up to the date they were last seen, with no additional follow-up
being attempted, and there was no common closing date.   These methods
may have resulted in underestimates of the number of cases of cancer.

In several of the studies, only a small number of patients and/or a
short follow-up period were involved.   This is critical, since most
carcinogenic effects manifest themselves only after long latent periods,
and the relevant follow-up period may be many years after initial exposure.
Indeed, endocrine phenomena associated with changes in breast cancer
risk (oophorectomy and early age at natural menopause) do not exert
their effect for about 10 years (Trichopoulos *et al.*, 1972).   In addition,
small cohorts and short follow-up make it likely that relatively small
increases in risk will be overlooked.   With this in mind, it is important
to note in the six studies cited above that: (a) in two, no women were
followed for more than 10 years (Geist *et al.*, 1941;   Gordan, 1961);
(b) in one, only 86/304 women were followed for more than 10 years
(Wilson, 1962);   (c) in one, the number followed for 10 years could not
be determined, but the longest follow-up was only 15 years (Schleyer-
Saunders, 1960);   (d) in one, although the longest follow-up was 25
years, the average for all 292 patients was 5 years, indicating that
very few women were followed up for more than 10 years (Wallach & Henneman,
1959);   (e) in one, the entire study group consisted of those that had
used the medication for at least 10 years, but the longest follow-up was
only 14 years after starting use (Leis, 1966).

These studies also suffer from flaws in some of the analyses.   When
an expected value was given, the manner of derivation was not given.   In
one (Leis, 1966), although the definition of the study group required 10
years of use, the 10 years preceding entry into the study appear to have
been included erroneously in the calculation of an expected value.   Five
of the 6 studies involved women who had had a hysterectomy and were thus
not at risk for certain tumours;   and only one study (Wilson, 1962) took
this into account when calculating the expected value for tumours of the
reproductive organs.   Finally, no adjustment was made for the protective
effect against breast cancer risk of oophorectomy or early age at natural
menopause, and no mention was made of risk in relation to parity, previous
history of benign disease, age at onset of oestrogen use, or risk by
interval from first use.

In summary, in the few case-control studies carried out prior to the early 1970s to evaluate the risk associated with menopausal oestrogen use, the population exposed, particularly to long-term use, was too small for an adequate evaluation. Each of the six follow-up studies was deficient either in conduct or in analysis, and they are thus inconclusive.

Recent studies

(a) Endometrial cancer

In 1975, two case-control studies were published that associated the use of oestrogens for symptoms of the climacteric with a relatively high risk of endometrial cancer (Smith *et al.*, 1975; Ziel & Finkle, 1975). In one study, a 4-8-fold excess risk of this cancer was reported among women who had used oestrogens, compared with women with ovarian cancer, cancer of the uterine cervix and other cancers of the reproductive organs, who were diagnosed at the same cancer clinic (Smith *et al.*, 1975). In the second study, an 8-fold increased risk of endometrial cancer was reported among oestrogen users, on the basis of records of members of a prepaid health plan, in comparison with a sample of all plan members of similar age, race, residence, duration of health plan membership and uterine status (intact). This study also indicated a dose-response relationship between risk and number of years of use, the risk progressing to a 14-fold excess among those who used oestrogen for 7 years or longer (Ziel & Finkle, 1975).

A subsequent study, of patients with newly-diagnosed endometrial cancer in a large retirement community, utilized both health-plan records and personal interviews and achieved essentially the same results. In addition, this study indicated that excess risk was apparent both for users of conjugated oestrogens and for women who had used other types of oestrogens, and that a greater risk occurred among women using tablets containing higher doses of oestrogen than among those using lower dose tablets (Mack *et al.*, 1976).

Six other studies have corroborated these findings, indicating excess risk for users of a variety of types of oestrogen preparations and evidence of a dose-response relationship with strength of the tablet and duration of use; these studies consist of two case-control interview studies (Antunes *et al.*, 1979; Wigle *et al.*, 1978), two case-control studies involving a review of medical records (Gray *et al.*, 1977; Horwitz & Feinstein, 1978), a case-control record-linkage study of a large group practice (McDonald *et al.*, 1977), and a cohort study of the frequency of a subsequent primary malignancy of the endometrium among breast cancer patients treated with nonsteroidal oestrogens (Hoover *et al.*, 1976a).

To date, no adequate evaluation has been made of the influence on cancer risks of the addition of progestational agents to compounds used for hormone replacement therapy. As noted in the discussion of endogenous hormones (pp. 92-93), such evaluation is important, since it has been suggested that this addition might at least partially diminish the risk of endometrial cancer in women undergoing oestrogen therapy. It should be noted, however, that the sequential, cyclic use of oestrogens and progestins in oral contraceptives may also be associated with an increased risk of endometrial cancer (see pp. 111-112).

The methods employed in the studies outlined above have been criticized and questioned in various ways. These criticisms can be presented and answered as follows:

1. Women chosen as controls had diseases with risk factors different from those for endometrial cancer. However, a wide variety of control groups were used in the studies done to date, and these have yielded essentially the same results.

2. The risk factors for endometrial cancer were not adequately controlled in the analyses. However, adequate control for endometrial cancer risk factors, particularly obesity and hypertension, tends to increase rather than decrease the strength of the association (Gray *et al.*, 1977).

3. The interval between first exposure and diagnosis (latent period) was too short to be consistent with current concepts of carcinogenesis. However, the latent period for an exposure-disease association is variable, and there is no reason to believe that the mechanism by which endometrial cancer is produced by oestrogenic agents should be particularly long.

4. The increase in endometrial cancer rates was not observed until 1970. However, widespread use of oestrogen replacement therapy began only in the mid-1960s, and the rising rates of hysterectomy over the past 25 years have reduced the population at risk for developing endometrial cancer. Furthermore, the increase in incidence of endometrial cancer during the 1970s parallels the rise in use of oestrogens during the preceding decade (Weiss *et al.*, 1976).

5. If oestrogens are the cause of the excess risk, why were only conjugated oestrogens implicated? As noted previously, every oestrogenic drug that has been adequately investigated has been associated positively with endometrial cancer.

6. Women who had had a hysterectomy (a group more likely to have used oestrogens) were excluded from the control groups. However, this is a misconception: all that was required in these studies was that the

controls had had an intact uterus at the age at which their matched cases were diagnosed. This follows the standard epidemiological practice in which comparability of cases and controls is assured by including as controls only those individuals who would have been included in the case group had they developed the disease in question. A recent study in which controls were only women who had undergone a hysterectomy achieved results similar to those of the other studies (Gray *et al.*, 1977).

7. The 'cancers' were not really cancer but were misdiagnosed hyperplasia, a condition known to be associated with oestrogen use. However, when the pathological material from oestrogen-exposed and non-oestrogen-exposed cases was reviewed by pathologists expert in the area of uterine pathology, the findings were essentially the same as those of the original reports (Gordon *et al.*, 1977).

8. The fact that the oestrogen-associated cancers were found at an early stage may indicate that the lesions were only diagnosed because the oestrogen therapy caused them to bleed, and that these cancers would have been diagnosed later or not at all among non-users. However, while in most studies the strength of the association was found to be greater among patients with earlier stage and/or lower grade malignancies, substantial excess risk has also been found for the more advanced stages and grades. Interpretation of these associations will be greatly facilitated when studies large enough to investigate differences in risk between current and former users are reported.

9. A criticism related to #8 contends that the association between oestrogen use and endometrial cancer results from increased medical attention and, therefore, a higher rate of detection of the cancer among oestrogen users, since such women commonly have oestrogen-induced vaginal bleeding and consequently come under close medical surveillance. Indeed, in two studies, control groups were comprised of women who underwent dilatation and curettage for benign conditions (Dunn & Bradbury, 1967; Horwitz & Feinstein, 1978). However, the control series in these studies (including women with benign conditions such as uterine polyps, leiomyomas and various conditions of uterine overdevelopment) are subject to selection bias, while the case series (consisting of women with a progressive neoplastic condition) is comparatively unbiased (Hutchinson & Rothman, 1978). In addition, oestrogen use is known to be a major cause of abnormal uterine bleeding. It is considered poor design to include in a control group individuals with conditions caused by the exposure under study.

10. Women who develop symptoms of the climacteric are predisposed to develop endometrial cancer, and oestrogen therapy merely identifies this subgroup of women. However, there appears to be no relationship between either the presence or the severity of symptoms of the climacteric and risk of endometrial cancer, when confounding factors are controlled for (Mack *et al.*, 1976). In addition, the strength of the association

between oestrogen use and endometrial cancer in the USA is similar in populations with a low frequency of exposure (McDonald *et al*., 1977) and in those with a high frequency of exposure (Mack *et al*., 1976). If the predisposition hypothesis were true, the risk should be higher among the high-exposure group. Finally, the rise in the incidence rates for this disease is too rapid to be consistent with genetic changes in the population.

In summary, a number of recent studies, utilizing a variety of designs, have found a consistent, strongly positive association between exposure to a number of oestrogenic substances and risk of endometrial cancer, with evidence of positive dose-response relationships both for strength of medication and duration of use. The conclusions of these studies are supported by evidence of rising incidence rates of endometrial cancer following the dramatic increase in use of oestrogens for symptoms of the climacteric in the USA (Greenwald *et al*., 1977; Weiss *et al*., 1976).

Recently, in the USA, these incidence rates have reached a plateau and are possibly declining; this follows closely a reduction in both the frequency of use and the average dose of oestrogens for symptoms of the climacteric. A recent cohort study (Jick *et al*., 1979) indicates that this decline in incidence is due to the reduction in use of oestrogens for symptoms of the climacteric, rather than to changing diagnostic practices. In this study, the incidence rate of endometrial cancer among the entire population studied declined following the reduction in oestrogen use; however, the incidence rate among those using oestrogens remained at a high level. This rapid effect of reduction in oestrogen use, if confirmed, has great significance for its immediate relevance to cancer prevention.

(b) Breast cancer

Since 1970, new observations have been made with respect to the relationship between use of oestrogens for symptoms of the climacteric and breast cancer. A cohort study carried out in Nashville, Tennessee was first reported in 1971 (Burch & Byrd, 1971) and subsequently (Burch *et al*., 1974, 1975; Byrd *et al*., 1973). Although this study had some of the same faults as those described under *'Early studies'* it was better designed and analysed. Among the 735 women who were followed for 9 years or more and who had had a hysterectomy, 21 cases of breast cancer were observed *versus* 18 expected. However, half of the total group had undergone bilateral oophorectomy, and the anticipated protection against breast cancer did not occur in this group. In addition, although the study was limited to those who had received oestrogens for 5 or more years, the first 5 years of experience were incorrectly included in the calculation of the expected value, and therefore the number of expected cases was overestimated.

In 1976, another cohort study was reported, in which 1891 women in Louisville, Kentucky who had been given conjugated oestrogens for symptoms of the climacteric were followed for an average of 12 years (Hoover *et al.*, 1976b). Breast cancer was observed in 49, whereas 39.1 were expected on the basis of rates in the general population (relative risk, 1.3; P=0.06). The relative risk increased with duration of follow-up, progressing to 2.0 after 15 years (13/6.6; P=0.01). However, risk was not related to duration of use. In addition, after 10 years of follow-up observation, two factors related to a low risk of breast cancer, multiparity and oophorectomy, were no longer so related. In this study, oestrogen use was also related to an increased risk of breast cancer among women in whom benign disease developed after they started using the drug.

A number of recent case-control studies of breast cancer show no significant association with oestrogen use; however, none of these has satisfactorily been able to address the question of long-term use (Boston Collaborative Drug Surveillance Program, 1974; Casagrande *et al.*, 1976; Craig *et al.*, 1974; Mack *et al.*, 1975; Ravnihar *et al.*, 1979; Sartwell *et al.*, 1977). While these studies do not contribute much to the elucidation of the association between long-term use of oestrogens for symptoms of the climacteric and breast cancer, the discussion of the problems involved in conducting studies of this type is useful: for example, investigators have pointed out the confounding that may exist among type of menopause, age at menopause, age, oestrogen use and breast cancer.

In summary, results of prospective studies of women who have used oestrogens for symptoms of the climacteric raise the possibility of an increased risk of breast cancer and indicate that a thorough evaluation is necessary. A full investigation of these agents will be difficult and will necessitate detailed information on such factors as latent period, risk indicators for breast cancer and type of therapeutic regimen, and will, in addition, require sophisticated design and analytical techniques.

Breast cancer has also been reported in two male transvestites who took oestrogens in large doses to produce gynaecomastia (Symmers, 1968). The disease in young men and the treatment are both so rare that it is difficult to believe that the events were not causally related. The possible relationship between diethylstilboestrol therapy for carcinoma of the prostate and cancer of the male breast is discussed in the monograph on diethylstilboestrol, p. 173.

Although an excess of breast cancer has been observed in one follow-up study of pregnant women exposed to diethylstilboestrol, the difference in rates was not statistically significant from that in controls (Bibbo *et al.*, 1978).

(c) Other cancers

In a recent prospective study, a statistically significant excess risk of ovarian cancer was reported among a small group of women who had been treated with diethylstilboestrol and conjugated oestrogens for symptoms of the climacteric (Hoover et al., 1977). There was no significant elevation of risk for those women who had received only conjugated oestrogens. In another follow-up study (Bibbo et al., 1978), 4 women treated with diethylstilboestrol during pregnancy subsequently developed ovarian cancers, compared with 1 in a control group of comparable size; the numbers are small and are not statistically significant. However, these observations, taken together with the suggestion from some animal studies of an association of diethylstilboestrol with the development of ovarian cancers, indicate the need for further investigation.

A cohort study (Burch & Byrd, 1971; Burch et al., 1974, 1975; Byrd et al., 1973) has shown lower than expected numbers of cancers other than those of the breast and reproductive system, and especially of colon cancer. The deficiency of malignancies at this site cannot obviously be explained by any apparent bias in this study. While the lack of any evidence of a dose-response relationship weakens arguments in favour of a protective effect, additional studies need to be done to explain these observations.

(d) Benign breast disease

The only benign neoplasm that has been evaluated for its relation to the use of oestrogens for symptoms of the climacteric is benign breast disease. Three case-control studies (Boston Collaborative Drug Surveillance Program, 1974; Ravnihar et al., 1979; Sartwell et al., 1973) found no association between oestrogen use and the risk of surgically confirmed benign breast disease, but one (Nomura & Comstock, 1976) found a $2\frac{1}{2}$-fold excess risk. However, the method of case and control selection in the latter study may not have been comparable.

Androgens used in treatment

Johnson et al. (1972) described 4 patients with aplastic anaemia who developed hepatocellular carcinoma after long-term chemotherapy with androgenic-anabolic steroids. Similar case reports in patients with various conditions were published subsequently (Boyd & Mark, 1977; Cattan et al., 1974; Farrell et al., 1975; Henderson et al., 1973; Kew et al., 1976; Meadows et al., 1974; Sale & Lerner, 1977; Shapiro et al., 1977; Ziegenfuss & Carabasi, 1973), but doubt has been raised about the diagnosis in some patients, since the clinical and pathological details described have not always provided convincing evidence of malignancy; for example, some authors (e.g., Farrell et al., 1975) have reported regression of the lesions after discontinuation of therapy.

These findings are difficult to interpret, because liver conditions such as haemosiderosis and hepatitis, which may be associated with hepatocellular carcinoma, have frequently been described in patients with aplastic anaemia.

One case report describes a Wilms tumour that developed in an adult man who used large quantities of anabolic-androgenic steroids as part of a body-building programme (Prat *et al.*, 1977).

Hormonal contraception

In many of the reports cited below concerning use of oral contraceptives and carcinogenesis in humans, neither the specific steroid hormones contained in the contraceptives nor the dose levels were specified. This information (see Table 7, p. 57) is important for determining whether some combinations of hormones are more specifically related to carcinogenesis at a particular anatomical site than others and for the purpose of estimating dose responses. For future studies, it will be helpful to know the specific doses and combinations used, as well as the duration of their use and dates of their availability on the market.

Breast

(a) Gross and microscopic changes: Fechner (1977) has summarized the literature on gross and microscopic changes in normal breast and on benign and malignant breast tumours in response to oral contraceptives. Alterations in breast volume were similar during cycles with oral contraceptives and during spontaneous menstrual cycles in the same women; however this increased volume may not return completely to pretreatment size in adolescents. No changes unique to users of oral contraceptives were found, either by mammograms or by histological examination of the normal breast and of benign and malignant lesions of the breast. Lobular hyperplasia and secretory changes that have been described in oral contraceptive users who have never been pregnant also occur in non-users. Epithelial hyperplasia in fibroadenomas removed from oral contraceptive users is no different from that seen in non-users. Evaluation of changes unique to oral contraceptive users with fibrocystic disease is more difficult because of the wide spectrum of epithelial and stromal changes, but in general no significant difference from age-matched controls in the percentages showing hyperplasia or other changes has been observed. However, one report has suggested that lesions in which epithelial atypia are minimal or absent are relatively less common in users of oral contraceptives (LiVolsi *et al.*, 1978). No differences in cell proliferation in normal breast ducts, fibroadenomas and other ductal hyperplasias from oral contraceptive users compared with those from non-users was found by nuclear labelling. Fechner also pointed out that a shift in cell type or histological pattern may be evidence of an association of oral contraceptives with breast cancer, even if no histological changes unique to oral contraceptives are seen. There is no

evidence as yet of any qualitative difference between cancers from oral contraceptive users and those from non-users, nor is there a disproportion in cell types.

(b) Benign breast disease: With one exception (Nomura & Comstock, 1976), retrospective case-control and cohort epidemiological studies have been consistent in finding a deficit of benign breast disease (fibrocystic disease and/or fibroadenoma) in current oral contraceptive users (Boston Collaborative Drug Surveillance Programme, 1973; Kelsey *et al.*, 1978; Ory *et al.*, 1976; Royal College of General Practitioners, 1974; Sartwell *et al.*, 1973; Vessey *et al.*, 1972). In 2 of 4 studies in which the type of benign breast disease was specified, the protective effect was noted consistently for fibrocystic disease and then for fibroadenoma (Ory *et al.*, 1976; Vessey *et al.*, 1972). The apparent protective effect is related to duration of use and may persist after cessation of use. For current users of oral contraceptives, with total exposure for longer than 2 years, the risk of being hospitalized for breast biopsy is only 25% that of those who have never used oral contraceptives (Vessey *et al.*, 1972).

Janerich *et al.* (1977) have raised the interesting question of possible negative bias in women with a history of benign breast disease: a smaller number of users of oral contraceptives would be found among cases of benign breast disease if women with a history of such disease had been advised not to use oral contraceptives. One third of physicians considered benign breast disease to be a contraindication for beginning use of oral contraceptives, and nearly one-half of them thought that continued use of these contraceptives is contraindicated in patients who develop benign breast disease. However, in one cohort study, the protective effect of oral contraceptive use against benign breast tumour was statistically significant in women with and without prior benign breast disease (Vessey *et al.*, 1976).

The cohort study of the Royal College of General Practitioners (1974) provides additional evidence of the protective effect of oral contraceptive use against benign breast disease. This effect became apparent after 2 years of exposure to oral contraceptives and was related to the strength of the progestin component. Little is known about the natural history of benign breast tumours and fibrocystic disease; but women with a history of fibrocystic disease may be at increased risk for breast cancer. The important question is whether the apparent protective effect of oral contraceptives against benign breast disease is relevant to malignant neoplasms of the breast. Women with fibrocystic lesions characterized by epithelial atypia are at increased risk of breast cancer (Black *et al.*, 1972; Kodlin *et al.*, 1977); and one study has shown that oral contraceptives do not protect against such lesions (LiVolsi *et al.*, 1978).

(c) Breast cancer: Studies to date on the relationship of oral contraceptive use to breast cancer have yielded no conclusive results. Most of the available information comes from retrospective case-control studies, but in none of the studies have sufficient numbers of people been exposed long enough to provide unequivocal evidence of any association.

Cohort studies provide only limited information, due to the small numbers of incident cases so far. In one study (Vessey *et al.*, 1976), 16 cases of breast tumours were reported, and the lowest rate was in those using oral contraceptives; however, the differences are not statistically significant. In the Royal College of General Practitioners' (1974) cohort study, 31 cancers were reported (11 cases in users, 4 in ex-users and 16 in non-users of oral contraceptives), and the standardized rates were no different; however, only 5% of women had used hormones for more than 5 years. The authors concluded that 'the number of cases of breast cancer, though small, is not negligible and shows no association with pill usage'. A cohort study in Boston (Ory *et al.*, 1976) compared rates of hospitalization for breast cancer in users and non-users of oral contraceptives. There were 137 cases of breast cancer collected over a 30-month period; the hospitalization rate was lower for users than for non-users, but the difference was not statistically significant and was not related to the duration of use.

A number of case-control studies have been reported. Vessey *et al.*. (1972) studied married women, 16-39-years old; between 1968 and 1971 there were 90 cases and 180 controls matched for age and parity. The controls were selected from women with acute medical and acute or elective surgical conditions. No association was found between breast cancer and oral contraceptive use. Additional cases were collected from 1972-1974, with the age range extended to 45 years and one control matched to each case (Vessey *et al.*, 1975). The results of the analyses on interval since last use, interval since first use and total duration of use for the additional group of 232 cancers and 232 matched controls were comparable with the earlier results. The lack of association was not affected by separate analyses for nulliparous women and parous women, for those younger and older than 36 years of age, or for brand of oral contraceptive used. Adjustment for the effects of factors such as social class, age at first childbirth, menopausal status and history of previous breast biopsy, which differed between the groups, produced little change in the findings. However, of the 322 women included in the study (90 + 232), only 7.5% of cases had first used oral contraceptives more than 8 years before a lump was first noticed, and only 14.3% had used them for more than 2 years. Additional studies have produced similar negative results (Kelsey *et al.*, 1978; Sartwell *et al.*, 1977).

The case-control study reported by Paffenbarger *et al.* (1977) extended the analysis of data reported by the same group (Fasal & Paffenbarger, 1975). Patients under 50 years of age with breast cancer were identified from 1970-1972 in 19 hospitals in the San Francisco area; 2 controls were selected for each case from the same hospital, one from a medical and the other from a surgical service. The 452 cancer patients and 872 controls matched for age, race, religion and time of hospitalization were interviewed in their homes. Results were expressed as relative risk and were adjusted for differences in age, race, religion, education, menopause status, history of benign breast disease and age at first childbirth. No significant difference was found in risk of breast cancer between cases and controls who had ever used oral contraceptives; the risk did not differ during time periods when the oral contraceptives changed in potency and composition. However, there was an increased risk of breast cancer among current users, in women who had used oral contraceptives for 2-4 years, and in women with previously diagnosed breast disease who had used them for more than 6 years. An additional finding in this updated report was that use of oral contraceptives before first childbirth increased the risk of breast cancer, the greatest effect being in women who were 25 years or older at birth of first child. There was no increased risk associated with use of oral contraceptives in nulliparous women. This report thus suggests that the risk of breast cancer is increased in users of oral contraceptives who are already at high risk because of a history of benign breast disease, and in women who may have been put at a high risk because they used oral contraceptives prior to first childbirth after the age of 25 years. Similar results were reported by Lees *et al*. (1978).

Uterus

(a) *Non-neoplastic changes in the cervix*: Among the earliest reported effects of steroid contraceptives were the changes described as 'polyploid endocervical hyperplasia' and 'microglandular hyperplasia of the cervix'. In one biopsy series (Friedrich, 1973; Moghissi, 1977), basal-cell hyperactivity, squamous metaplasia and microglandular hyperplasia were observed more frequently in specimens from women using sequential rather than combination oral contraceptives, and least frequently in non-users. These and other changes, which include increased vascularity and oedema, are qualitatively similar to changes that occur during pregnancy and are usually reversible upon discontinuation of hormonal contraceptives. Although they are occasionally sufficiently atypical in gross or microscopic appearance to raise the question of neoplastic changes, these lesions are considered to be non-neoplastic responses.

(b) *Cervical neoplasia*: A large number of studies have been reported on the possible carcinogenic effects of oral contraceptive use on the cervix. In many studies, the data utilized in the analyses were extracted from programmes for the cytological detection of cervical neoplasia (Attwood, 1966; Berget & Weber, 1974; de Brux, 1974; Chai *et al*., 1970; Collette *et al*., 1978; Kline *et al*., 1970; Liu *et al*., 1967; Melamed *et al*., 1969; Pincus & Garcia, 1965; Sandmire *et al*., 1976), and a comparison was made of the prevalence of cervical neoplasia in users and non-users of oral contraceptives. The studies are therefore all based on routinely collected data, are difficult to interpret and have yielded conflicting results. Three recent studies of this type have been selected and are described below.

A study in Denmark reported on 13,224 women, aged 30-49 years, who participated in a screening programme: no significant differences were found in cytological abnormalities or in biopsy-verified dysplasia, cancer *in situ* or invasive cancer between oral contraceptive users and non-users (Berget & Weber, 1974). Average duration of exposure was 24 months. The frequency of abnormal smears and of cancer *in situ* in oral contraceptive users and non-users did not vary with age, age at first pregnancy, number of pregnancies or socio-economic status, except that oral contraceptive users of the middle social class had significantly higher rates than non-users of that class. The meaning of this latter finding is uncertain because multiple comparisons were made and some differences between subgroups could have been statistically significant by chance alone.

In a study in France (de Brux, 1974), no difference was seen in frequency of cellular atypia and cancer *in situ* in women using high-dose oral contraceptives compared with pregnant women; cellular atypia and cancer *in situ* were least frequent in women using low-dose oral contraceptives. The duration of use was from 6 months to 4 years.

In a report from The Netherlands (Collette *et al.*, 1978), it was concluded that women in that country who choose oral contraceptives as their method of contraception are not likely to be at higher risk for cervical cancer than other women. There was no significant difference in prevalence of cancer between current oral contraceptive users and non-users among women attending a mass screening programme for cervical cancer.

Retrospective case-control studies have also utilized rosters of cytological screening programmes to ascertain cases mainly of dysplasia and cancer *in situ*. In one study in the USA (Thomas, 1972), the controls used were a probability sample from the screened population from which the cases originated. Although exposure to oral contraceptives was the same in cases and controls, the mean duration of exposure was less than 2 years, and the mean interval from first starting the contraceptives to detection of neoplasia was less than 3 years.

A Canadian report, utilizing data from the British Columbia cytological screening programme, was restricted to cases of preclinical cervical cancer detected in 1970 in women who were in their third decade, and to age-matched controls (Worth & Boyes, 1972). Cases did not differ from controls in mean duration of exposure to oral contraceptives (2 years for ages 20-24, and 3 years for ages 25-29). Cases had histories of increased frequency of divorce and common-law relationships compared with controls, but these high-risk factors were not considered in the analysis. Adjustment for these factors would tend to reinforce the lack of association in this report between oral contraceptive use and cervical cancer.

In another retrospective case-control study (Boyce *et al*., 1977), an updating of a previous report compared oral contraceptive use in 689 consecutive cases of cervical cancer of all stages with that of an equal number of controls, interviewed in the same hospital, matched for age, race, age at first intercourse, age at first pregnancy and socio-economic status, and with negative cytological tests. No differences between cases and controls with regard to exposure to oral contraceptives were found, nor were there differences in the type or dose of oestrogen in the oral contraceptives between cases and controls. The mean duration of oral contraceptive use for cases and controls was approximately 16 months. Some underestimation of differences could have resulted from failure to maintain the paired matching in the analyses.

The only case-control study that has shown a positive association between use of oral contraceptives and cervical cancer is that of Ory *et al*. (1977). The cases were ascertained from a file of cytological tests performed on black women in a family planning programme. The cases chosen were women aged 15-44, who had entered the programme between 1967 and 1972, who had had 2 consecutive negative tests and then an abnormal test result between 1970 and 1972. The diagnosis of dysplasia or cancer *in situ* was confirmed by biopsy within a year after the finding of abnormal cytology. The controls were other screened women, aged 15-44, with the same entry dates, who had had 3 consecutive negative tests. All subjects used either oral contraceptives or an intrauterine device. Estimates of relative risk were standardized for a number of factors, including age, age at first childbirth and number of pregnancies, but no information was available on other confounding factors more directly related to sexual activity. Another problem, which may have biassed the results, was the substantial disagreement with the original histological diagnosis of cancer *in situ* on the part of one of the two pathologists who reviewed the slides. The risk of developing cancer *in situ* in women using oral contraceptives increased significantly with duration of exposure: for a duration of 3 years or more, the risk was almost 5 times that of women using an intrauterine device. In women using oral contraceptives, the increase in the risk for dysplasia was not as large as for cancer *in situ*, but it was significantly higher than in women using an intrauterine device.

Three cohort studies have examined the incidence of dysplasia, cancer *in situ* and invasive cancer. In two, the cohorts were women who used some form of birth control (oral contraceptives, intrauterine devices and/or diaphragms), thus increasing the likelihood that the groups were comparable with regard to sexual activity (Melamed & Flehinger, 1973; Vessey *et al*., 1976). In the other study, the cohort also included women who used no method and women who used other methods of contraception (Peritz *et al*., 1977).

Melamed *et al*. (1969) had originally reported an excess of cervical cancer *in situ* in women who chose and used oral contraceptives, compared with matched groups of diaphragm users. The rate estimates were based on the combined prevalent and incident cases. In a more recent study (Melamed & Flehinger, 1973), only women with initially negative cytological tests were entered into the cohort. To be included in the analysis of rates, subjects had to have had negative results for 2 successive routine cytological examinations and to have returned to a third examination at which cancer or precancerous lesions were detected and to have continued to use contraceptives during this time. Then, 2 pairs of contraceptive groups were established by matching 3 oral contraceptive users to 1 person with an intrauterine device, and 3 oral contraceptive users to 1 diaphragm user. All contraceptive groups were examined and tested equally, thus ensuring equal probability of detecting abnormalities and overcoming the bias of preferential testing of users of oral contraceptives. Women with dysplasia, as well as those with cancer *in situ*, were removed from further follow-up at the time of detection. The average exposure time was 3 years. No significant differences in rates of cancer *in situ* or precancerous cervical lesions were found.

A cohort study in the UK is following 17,032 married women, aged 25-39 years, originally recruited at 17 family planning clinics (Vessey *et al*., 1976; Wright *et al*., 1978). Incidence rates of cervical neoplasia are estimated according to the method of contraception in use at entry into the study in terms of woman-years of observation; 56% were using oral contraceptives, 25% a diaphragm and 19% an intrauterine device. About 25% had discontinued use of oral contraceptives by the end of the first year, and during the fourth year only about 50% of the original oral contraceptive group were still using this method. The incidence rates of dysplasia and of cancer *in situ* were similar in users of oral contraceptives and in users of intrauterine devices; only a few cases of either condition were observed in diaphragm users. All 6 cases of invasive cancer were seen in oral contraceptive users. By September 1977, a total of 65 women had developed biopsy-proven cervical dysplasia (26 cases), cancer *in situ* (33 cases) and invasive cancer (6 cases). In the data analysis, the 3 conditions are considered together as cervical neoplasia. The incidence rate of cervical neoplasia in diaphragm users (0.17 per thousand woman-years of observation) was much lower than those in users of oral contraceptives and intrauterine devices (0.95 and 0.87, respectively). The difference could not be explained in terms of potentially confounding variables (age, social class, cigarette smoking, age at marriage, age at first pregnancy). Detailed sexual histories were collected from 52 of the patients with cervical neoplasia and from 139 controls. Diaphragm users were found to be less likely to have had coitus at an early age and had had fewer sexual partners than users of

the other two methods, but the risk of cervical neoplasia in diaphragm
users was still only one quarter of that in users of the other two
methods after adjusting for the effects of these variables.

The incidence of cervical neoplasia in 17,942 women, 18-58 years of
age, enrolled in a health plan and followed for 37,373 woman-years
has been reported (Peritz *et al*., 1977). A number of factors were taken
into account in the analyses, but information on risk factors relating
to sexual activity was not available. The relative risk of cancer *in
situ* in oral contraceptive users increased significantly with duration
of exposure, the increased risk being less evident in women with dysplasia.

One cohort study in the USA (Stern *et al*., 1977) was concerned with
direct observation of development of cancer *in situ* in women with dysplasia.
The cohort was chosen from approximately 11,000 women attending family
planning clinics, from those who had had no prior use of oral contraceptives
and no illness or history of illness that would bias the choice of
method. Of the 6000 eligible women, 14-49 years of age, 300 (approximately
5%) were found to have dysplasia and were entered into the follow-up
study, with a sample of 5% of women without dysplasia. The average age
of women with dysplasia was 23 years. All of the women were given
either oral contraceptives (203 cases) or other methods of contraception
(97). One oral contraceptive combination at one dose level was used
throughout; of the non-oral contraceptive users, 90% used an intrauterine
device. All groups were examined and tested uniformly at 2 months, at 6
months, and then every 6 months. Readings of cytological smears were
done on a 'blind' basis and found to be reliable by analysis of replicate
readings. A cytological scale of increasing degree of abnormality was
constructed, and average scores for oral contraceptive users and non-
users were compared at each time interval, so that small changes could
be measured. The scores were adjusted for a number of variables, including
age, race, parity and age at first intercourse. Significant differences
in severity of dysplasia between oral contraceptive users and the users
of other methods were first observed after 3 years of exposure. By this
time, more than half of the women were lost to follow-up, having moved
or refused to return to the clinic, or because they were excluded from
the analysis after they became pregnant, or changed or discontinued use
of their contraceptive method. Analysis of the reasons for dropping out
and a comparison of the characteristics and cytological scores of those
who remained and those who dropped out at each time interval yielded
no evidence that a bias of differential drop-out was introduced into the
analysis. By about 7 years after the study was started, 13 women had
developed cancer *in situ* (10 in oral contraceptive users, 3 in users of
other methods); life-table analysis showed a 6-fold increase in risk for
cancer *in situ* in those who had had dysplasia among oral contraceptive
users compared with the users of other methods. Six of the 10 conversions
from dysplasia to cancer *in situ* in oral contraceptive users occurred
after 5 years of exposure. In the cohorts of women without dysplasia,
there was no evidence of differential change when average scores of oral
contraceptive users were compared with those of users of other methods
over time.

The results suggest a promoting rather than an initiating effect of steroid contraception on the development of cancer of the cervix. The observation of prolonged latency in the development of cancer *in situ*, even in women who already had dysplasia, is a strong reminder that sufficient time must be allowed from onset of exposure in studies of carcinogenesis in humans.

Evaluation of studies on the relationship of oral contraceptive use to cervical cancer is complicated by the widespread practice of cytological screening. In screened populations, the presumed natural progression from normal to dysplasia to cancer *in situ* to invasive cancer is obscured by the detection and treatment of precancerous and preinvasive lesions. Oral contraceptive users may be tested preferentially, which could lead to a spurious excess of detected neoplastic lesions when compared with non-users. This bias can be avoided by equal testing of oral contraceptive users and non-users. Paradoxically, the removal of dysplasia cases at the time of detection may lead to an underestimate of cancer *in situ* in oral contraceptive users, if the increased incidence of carcinoma *in situ* in women with dysplasia is differentially affected by exposure to oral contraceptives (Stern *et al.*, 1977).

(c) Endometrial cancer: The normal, cyclic changes in the endometrium are modified during use of oral contraceptives, and the alterations vary, depending on whether a combination or sequential regimen is used. With combination oral contraceptives, the endometrium becomes progressively thinner and inactive, and the monthly withdrawal bleeding tends to be scanty; whereas with the sequential regimen, the endometrium more closely approximates the proliferative and secretory phases of the cycle.

In one biopsy series of 111 asymptomatic young women, aged 21-32, who were long-term users of a sequential oral contraceptive containing ethinyloestradiol and dimethisterone (Oracon), focal adenomatous endometrial hyperplasia was noted in 13.5%, and there was an association with duration of use. The lesions showed no atypia, but these patients are being followed up (Kreutner *et al.*, 1976). This finding is of special interest, since case reports linking endometrial cancer in young women with oral contraceptive use have been appearing in the literature since 1975 (Lyon, 1975; Lyon & Frisch, 1976), and the majority of the cases had used the same preparation for long periods of time. Of a series of 30 cases of endometrial cancer in oral contraceptive users under the age of 40, two-thirds had been using sequentials and the remainder combination types. This represents a higher than expected level of use of sequentials in women with endometrial cancer, since less than 10% of total oral contraceptive use in the USA was of the sequential type. The usual risk factors and conditions that predispose to endometrial cancer (nulliparity, obesity or polycystic ovaries) were absent in most of these cases; on the other hand, many of the women with endometrial cancer who used combination oral contraceptives exhibited one or more of these characteristics and are thus comparable with young women with endometrial cancer who never used oral contraceptives (Silverberg *et al.*, 1977). This absence of the usual risk factors in women with endometrial cancer who used sequential oral contraceptives has been reported by others (Cohen & Deppe, 1977; Kaufman *et al.*, 1976; Kelley *et al.*, 1976). The absence of predisposing factors for endometrial cancer in users of sequential oral contraceptives suggests that these women would not have been at high risk for developing endometrial cancer under age 40 had they not used oral contraceptives. The excess of endometrial cancer in women using sequentials applies mainly to use of one of the first of the sequentials to be marketed in the USA (1965), which was also one of the last to be withdrawn (1976).

There has been no estimate of risk of endometrial cancer in oral contraceptive users.

(d) Trophoblastic tumours: Following the removal of a benign hydatidiform mole, trophoblastic activity should be monitored for 2 years to ensure that no invasive lesions have developed. Since this involves assay of human chorionic gonadotropin levels, and since interpretation of these levels would be obscured by an intervening pregnancy, women are cautioned to avoid pregnancy for 2 years. Of 611 women with a history of benign hydatidiform mole, approximately 10% subsequently developed invasive mole; of these, a higher proportion (double) of women who used oral contraceptives before their assay results returned to normal developed invasive mole than of the women who never started using them. This suggests that increased development of invasive trophoblastic disease may be due to the use of oral contraceptives (Stone *et al.*, 1976).

(e) Uterine fibroids: A lower rate of uterine fibroids was found in oral contraceptive users (Royal College of General Practitioners, 1974); however, it is not clear whether this was a true protective effect or was due to self-selection, since women with fibroids are usually not given combination oral contraceptives because their oestrogenic component can stimulate fibroid growth. In another study (Vessey *et al.*, 1976), there was no evidence of a protective effect against uterine fibroids.

Ovary

(a) Non-neoplastic and benign lesions: A negative association has been observed between use of oral contraceptives and functional ovarian cysts (Ory, 1974; Royal College of General Practitioners, 1974). This beneficial action is probably directly related to suppression by oral contraceptives of the development of ovarian follicles and of ovulation. No association or protective effect was noted for benign tumours of the ovary (Vessey *et al.*, 1976).

In a study in Finland, the incidence of functional ovarian cysts was increased in women using low-dose, progestin-only oral contraceptives, compared with non-users; follicular (functional ovarian) cysts did not occur in women using combination oral contraceptives. The results confirm the protective effect of combination oral contraceptives against functional cysts but indicate that the use of continuous low-dose progestin-only oral contraceptives may increase the risk. Low-dose progestins account for one-third of all hormonal contraceptives used in Finland, and they are often recommended for young women. The women with follicular cysts who had used low-dose progestin-only preparations were 16-26 years of age and had been free of ovarian cysts on pelvic examination at the time the medication was started (Ylikorkala, 1977).

(b) Ovarian cancer: One study in the UK (Newhouse *et al.*, 1977) suggests that use of oral contraceptives has a protective effect against ovarian cancer. This was a retrospective case-control study of 300 cases of ovarian cancer collected from a number of medical centres; about half of the cases were under 55 years of age. There were two groups of age-matched controls, from hospitals and neighbourhoods. Cases and controls were similar with regard to mean age at menarche, mean age at birth of first child, and mean age at both surgical and natural menopause. However, family size was smaller in the cases, and more cases had never been married or pregnant. The risk for ovarian cancer was significantly lower in women with a history of oral contraceptive use; but there was no information on duration of use.

Pituitary

A number of series of cases of adenoma of the pituitary have been reported in young women, a high proportion of whom had recently stopped using oral contraceptives (e.g., Chang *et al.*, 1977; Sherman *et al.*, 1978). However, these findings are inconclusive. A case-control study revealed no association of prior use of oral contraceptives with development of pituitary tumours (Coulam *et al.*, 1979).

Malignant melanoma

Evidence for a possible association between oral contraceptive use and melanoma of the skin is based on an analysis of incidence of melanoma in a cohort of women, 17-59 years of age, who were enrolled in a health plan between December 1968 and February 1972 and followed through 1975. Information on previous and current oral contraceptive use was obtained at entry and was monitored subsequently. A total of 22 cases were found among 17,942 women with 90,000 person-years of observation. The age-adjusted rates per 100,000 person-years were 17.6 for those who had never used oral contraceptives, 24.1 for less than 4 years' use and 29.5 for more than 4 years' use. These differences were not statistically significant (Beral *et al.*, 1977).

A case-control study identified 37 additional melanoma cases in the tumour registry of the same health plan between 1968 and 1976, in women aged 20-59 years. None of these women had been included in the above analysis of incidence rates. Two controls were selected at random for each case from the health plan file. The estimated relative risk in women who had ever used oral contraceptives was 1.8, compared with women who had never used them, but the difference was not statistically significant. Users of oral contraceptives showed an excess of melanomas localized on the lower limbs (Beral *et al.*, 1977).

In neither study was any information given about solar exposure, which is the most important known risk factor for melanoma. If users of oral contraceptives are more likely to spend time outdoors than non-users, this would have a strong influence on the interpretation of these results.

Liver

(a) *Benign neoplasms*: Increasing numbers of reports of hepatocellular adenomas in young women have appeared since the initial publication by Baum *et al.* (1973) called attention to a possible relationship between liver-cell adenomas and oral contraceptive use in 7 women. From a review of the world medical literature, it was estimated that 137 cases of benign hepatic-cell tumours had been reported by 1976 (Mahboubi & Shubik, 1977) and 172 cases by 1977 (Letoublon *et al.*, 1978); however, these tumours were rare prior to the 1960s (Nissen *et al.*, 1978). If the increased number of reports in young women represents a true increase in incidence, then exposure to new factors such as steroid contraceptives must be considered.

Considering the millions of women using oral contraceptives, the proportion of those reported with liver tumours is small; however, the numbers are probably underestimated due to the difficulty of detecting occult nodules in the liver. Even though liver adenomas are infrequent and are considered to be benign, they may be fatal due to haemorrhage and rupture. All of the reports stress a prolonged duration of exposure to oral contraceptives: an average of 5 years, with a range of 6 months to 11 years (Mahboubi & Shubik, 1977).

Results of two retrospective case-control studies have been reported. In the first study (Edmondson *et al.*, 1976a), 42 cases of liver-cell adenoma diagnosed since 1955 were collected from all over the USA and compared with age-matched neighbourhood controls; complete information for analysis was available for 34 case-control pairs. The results indicated a significant association of the tumours with prolonged exposure to oral contraceptives and with the use of a combination containing mestranol as the oestrogen component. The authors commented that cases of liver tumours have also been associated with combinations containing ethinyloestradiol. Mestranol has been sold for a longer period of time than ethinyloestradiol, and this could account in part for the association. Subsequent analysis of the data, taking these trends into account, did not alter the results (Edmondson *et al.*, 1976b).

The other case-control study utilized cases registered with the Armed Forces Institute of Pathology between 1960 and 1976; 79 surviving cases were compared with 220 age-matched, neighbourhood controls. A significant increase in risk of developing hepatocellular adenoma was found with prolonged duration of use. Use of high-potency oral contraceptives was also associated with higher risk (Rooks *et al.*, 1977). No detailed analysis of the data was provided.

Although there is not complete agreement on the criteria for classifying liver tumours, hepatocellular adenoma seems to be a distinct entity. Some of its features are increased vascularity and tendency to rupture (Ameriks *et al.*, 1975; Christopherson, 1975), often the first clinical indication, and there have been reports of spontaneous regression after cessation of oral contraceptive use. The incidence of these tumours is not known and is difficult to estimate since the majority may be clinically silent.

In assessing the association between oral contraceptives and liver tumours, a detection bias must be considered if the cases were mostly collected after 1973, when the medical profession was alerted to a possible relation (Baum *et al.*, 1973). Nodules in oral contraceptive users would not only be diagnosed more readily, but doctors would be more apt to report them in the literature and to refer them to a registry. This possible bias is not as likely to apply to the two case-control studies, since many cases were collected prior to the report of Baum *et al.*

The important role of the liver in metabolizing steroid hormones, as well as in detoxifying drugs and other chemicals, must be taken into account. Some hepatotoxic drugs and chemicals have recently been introduced into the environment, and possible interactions between these and the exogenous sex hormones should be considered.

(b) Malignant tumours: Hepatocellular carcinomas have been reported in users of oral contraceptives (Gattanell *et al.*, 1978; Glassberg & Rosenbaum, 1976; Ham *et al.*, 1978; Menzies-Gow, 1978; Meyer *et al.*, 1974; Schmidt, 1977; Thalassinos *et al.*, 1974), but less frequently than benign tumours. The duration of exposure to oral contraceptives was short, in some cases less than one year; and no controlled studies have been reported.

Benign tumour of the liver has not been considered to be a precursor of malignancy; however, malignant tissue was found in 2 hepatic adenomas in oral contraceptive users (Chevrel, 1976; Davis *et al.*, 1975).

References

Aiman, J., Nalick, R.H., Jacobs, A., Porter, J.C., Edman, C.D., Vellios, F. & MacDonald, P.C. (1977) The origin of androgen and estrogen in a virilized postmenopausal woman with bilateral benign cystic teratomas. Obstet. Gynecol., 49, 695-704

Aiman, J., Edman, C.D., Worley, R.J., Vellios, F. & MacDonald, P.C. (1978) Androgen and estrogen formation in women with ovarian hyperthecosis. Obstet. Gynecol., 51, 1-9

Ameriks, J.A., Thompson, N.W., Frey, C.F., Appelman, H.D. & Walter, J.F. (1975) Hepatic cell adenomas, spontaneous liver rupture, and oral contraceptives. Arch. Surg., 110, 548-557

Anderson, J.N., Peck, E. J., Jr & Clark, J.H. (1975) Estrogen-induced uterine responses and growth: relationship to receptor estrogen binding by uterine nuclei. Endocrinology, 96, 160-167

Anon. (1977) Oral contraceptives. Debate on oral contraceptives and neoplasia continues; answers remain elusive. Population Reports, Series A, No. 4, Washington DC, George Washington University Medical Center, Department of Medical & Public Affairs, pp. A-69-A-100

Antunes, C.M.F., Stolley, P.D., Rosenshein, N.B., Davies, J.L., Tonascia, J.A., Brown, C., Burnett, L., Rutledge, A., Pokempher, M. & Garcia, R. (1979) Endometrial cancer and estrogen use. New Engl. J. Med., 300, 9-13

Arthes, F.G., Sartwell, P.E. & Lewison, E.F. (1971) The pill, estrogens, and the breast. Epidemiologic aspects. Cancer, 28, 1391-1394

Attwood, M.E. (1966) Cytology and the contraceptive pill. J. Obstet. Gynaec. Br. Commonw., 73, 662-665

Baird, D., Horton, R., Longcope, C. & Tait, J.F. (1968) Steroid pre-hormones. Perspect. Biol. Med., 11, 384-421

Baird, D.T., Horton, R., Longcope, C. & Tait, J.F. (1969) Steroid dynamics under steady-state conditions. Recent Prog. Horm. Res., 25, 611-664

Bakke, J.L. (1963) A teaching device to assist active therapeutic intervention in the menopause. West. J. Surg. Obst. Gynecol., 71, 241-245

Baum, J.K., Holtz, F., Bookstein, J.J. & Klein, E.W. (1973) Possible association between benign hepatomas and oral contraceptives. Lancet, ii, 926-929

Benjamin, F. & Deutsch, S. (1976) Plasma levels of fractionated estrogens and pituitary hormones in endometrial carcinoma. Am. J. Obstet. Gynecol., 126, 638-647

Beral, V., Ramcharan, S. & Faris, R. (1977) Malignant melanoma and oral contraceptive use among women in California. Br. J. Cancer, 36, 804-809

Berget, A. & Weber, T. (1974) Influence of oral contraception on cytology and histology of the cervix uteri. Dan. med. Bull., 21, 172-176

Bibbo, M., Haenszel, W.M., Wied, G.L., Hubby, M. & Herbst, A.L. (1978) A twenty-five-year follow-up study of women exposed to diethylstilbestrol during pregnancy. New Engl. J. Med., 298, 763-767

Black, M.M., Barclay, T.H.C., Cutler, S.J., Hankey, B.F. & Asire, A.J. (1972) Association of atypical characteristics of benign breast lesions with subsequent risk of breast cancer. Cancer, 29, 338-343

Boston Collaborative Drug Surveillance Program (1974) Surgically confirmed gallbladder disease, venous thromboembolic disease, and breast tumours, in relation to postmenopausal estrogen therapy. New Engl. J. Med., 290, 15-18

Boston Collaborative Drug Surveillance Programme (1973) Oral contraceptives and venous thromboembolic disease, surgically confirmed gallbladder disease, and breast tumours. Lancet, i, 1399-1404

Boyce, J.G., Lu, T., Nelson, J.H., Jr & Fruchter, R.G. (1977) Oral contraceptives and cervical carcinoma. Am. J. Obstet. Gynecol., 128, 761-766

Boyd, P.R. & Mark, G.J. (1977) Multiple hepatic adenomas and a hepatocellular carcinoma in a man on oral methyl testosterone for eleven years. Cancer, 40, 1765-1770

Brecher, P.I. & Witiz, H.H. (1967) Competition between estradiol and estriol for end organ receptor proteins. Steroids, 9, 431-442

Brown, J.B. & Matthew, G.D. (1962) IV. Steroid hormones. The application of urinary estrogen measurements to problems in gynecology. Recent Prog. Horm. Res., 18, 337-385

Brown, J.B. & Strong, J.A. (1965) The effect of nutritional status and thyroid function on the metabolism of oestradiol. J. Endocrinol., 32, 107-115

de Brux, J. (1974) Lesions of the uterine cervix during oral contra-
    ception (Fr.). Sem. Hôp. Paris, 50, 1491-1495

Bulbrook, R.D, Hayward, J.L. & Thomas, B.S. (1964) The relation
    between the urinary 17-hydroxycorticosteroids and 11-deoxy-17-
    oxosteroids and the fate of patients after mastectomy. Lancet,
    i, 945-947

Burch, J.C. & Byrd, B.F., Jr (1971) Effects of long-term administration
    of estrogen on the occurrence of mammary cancer in women   Ann. Surg.,
    174, 414-418

Burch, J.C., Byrd, B.F., Jr & Vaughn, W.K. (1974) The effects of long-
    term estrogen on hysterectomized women. Am. J. Obstet. Gynecol.,
    118, 778-782

Burch, J.C., Byrd, B.F. & Vaughn, W.K. (1975) The effects of long-term
    estrogen administration to women following hysterectomy. In:
    Van Keep, P.A. & Lauritzen, C., eds, Estrogens in the Post-Menopause
    (Frontiers of Hormone Research Ser., Vol. 3), Basel, Karger, pp. 208-214

Byrd, B.F., Jr, Burch, J.C. & Vaughn, W.K. (1973) Significance of post-
    operative estrogen therapy on the occurrence and clinical course of
    cancer. Ann. Surg., 177, 626-631

Casagrande, J., Gerkins, V., Henderson, B.E., Mack, T. & Pike, M.C.
    (1976) Exogenous estrogens and breast cancer in women with natural
    menopause. J. natl Cancer Inst., 56, 839-841

Cattan, D., Vesin, P., Wautier, J., Kalifat, R. & Meignan, S. (1974)
    Liver tumours and steroid hormones. Lancet, i, 878

Chai, M.S., Johnson, W.D. & Tricomi, V. (1970) Five years' experience
    with contraceptive pills. Cervical epithelial changes. N.Y. State
    J. Med., 70, 2663-2666

Chang, R.J., Keye, W.R., Jr, Young, J.R., Wilson, C.B. & Jaffe, R.B. (1977)
    Detection, evaluation, and treatment of pituitary microadenomas in
    patients with galoctorrhoea and amenorrhea. Am. J. Obstet. Gynecol.,
    128, 356-363

Chevrel, B. (1976) Responsibility of steroid hormones in the development
    of malignant tumours (Fr.). Nouv. Presse méd., 5, 1145

Christopherson, W.M. (1975) Liver tumours and the pill. Br. med. J.,
    iv, 756

Cohen, C.J. & Deppe, G. (1977) Endometrial carcinoma and oral contra-
    ceptive agents. Obstet. Gynecol., 49, 390-392

Cole, P., Brown, J.B. & MacMahon, B. (1976) Oestrogen profiles of parous and nulliparous women. Lancet, ii, 596-598

Collette, H.J.A., Linthorst, G. & de Waard, F. (1978) Cervical carcinoma and the pill. Lancet, i, 441-442

Coulam, C.B., Annegers, J.F., Abboud, C.F., Laws, E.R., Jr & Kurland, L.T. (1979) Pituitary adenoma and oral contraceptives: a case-control study. Fertil. Steril., 31, 25-28

Craig, T.J., Comstock, G.W., & Geiser, P.B. (1974) Epidemiologic comparison breast cancer patients with early and late onset of malignancy and general population controls. J. natl Cancer Inst., 53, 1577-1581

Davis, M., Portmann, B., Searle, M., Wright, R. & Williams, R. (1975) Histological evidence of carcinoma in a hepatic tumour associated with oral contraceptives. Br. med. J., iv, 496-498

Defares, J.G. (1971) Is cancer preventible? Lancet, i, 135-136

Dickinson, L.E., MacMahon, B., Cole, P. & Brown, J.B. (1974) Estrogen profiles of Oriental and Caucasian women in Hawaii. New Engl. J. Med., 291, 1211-1213

Dunn, L.J. & Bradbury, J.T. (1967) Endocrine factors in endometrial carcinoma. A preliminary report. Am. J. Obstet. Gynecol., 97, 465-471

Edman, C.D. & MacDonald, P.C. (1978) Effect of obesity on conversion of plasma androstenedione to estrone in ovulatory and anovulatory young women. Am. J. Obstet. Gynecol., 130, 456-461

Edman, C.D., Aiman, E.J., Poeter, J.C. & MacDonald, P.C. (1978) Identification of the estrogen product of extraglandular aromatization of plasma androstenedione. Am. J. Obstet. Gynecol., 130, 439-447

Edmondson, H.A., Henderson, B. & Benton, B. (1976a) Liver-cell adenomas associated with the use of oral contraceptives. New Engl. J. Med., 294, 470-472

Edmondson, H.A., Henderson, B.E. & Benton, B. (1976b) Liver-cell adenomas and oral contraceptives. New Engl. J. Med., 294, 1064

Farrell, G.C., Joshua, D.E., Uren, R.F., Baird, P.J., Perkins, K.W. & Kronenberg, H. (1975) Androgen-induced hepatoma. Lancet, i, 430-432

Fasal, E. & Paffenbarger, R.S., Jr (1975) Oral contraceptives as related
    to cancer and benign lesions of the breast. J. natl Cancer Inst.,
    55, 767-773

Fechner, R.E. (1977) Influence of oral contraceptives on breast diseases.
    Cancer, 39, 2764-2771

Friedrich, E.R. (1973) The effects of oral contraceptives on the cytology
    of the secretory cells of the cervix. In: Blandau, R.J. & Moghissi,
    K., eds, The Biology of the Cervix, Chicago, IL, University of
    Chicago Press, pp. 367-384

Gattanell, P.N., Perloff, M. & Holland, J.F. (1978) Hepatocellular
    carcinoma in a young woman with prolonged exposure to oral contra-
    ceptives. Med. ped. Oncol., 4, 99-103

Geist, S.H., Walter, R.I. & Salmon, U.J. (1941) Are estrogens carcino-
    genic in the human female? II. Atypical endometrial proliferation
    in a patient treated with estrogens. Am. J. Obstet. Gynecol., 42,
    242-248

Glassberg, A.B. & Rosenbaum, E.H. (1976) Oral contraceptives and
    malignant hepatoma. Lancet, i, 479

Gordan, G.S. (1961) Osteoporosis. Diagnosis and treatment. Texas State
    J. Med., 57, 740-747

Gordon, G.G., Olivo, J., Rafii, F. & Southren, A.L. (1975) Conversion
    of androgens to estrogens in cirrhosis of the liver. J. clin.
    Endocrinol. Metab., 40, 1018-1026

Gordon, J., Reagen, J.W., Finkle, W.D. & Ziel, H.K. (1977) Estrogen
    and endometrial carcinoma. An independent pathology review
    supporting original risk estimate. New Engl. J. Med., 297, 570-571

Gray, L.A., Christopherson, W.M. & Hoover, R.N. (1977) Estrogens and
    endometrial carcinoma. Obstet. Gynecol., 49, 385-389

Greenwald, P., Caputo, T.A. & Wolfgang, P.E. (1977) Endometrial cancer
    after menopausal use of estrogens. Obstet. Gynecol., 50, 239-243

Ham, J.M., Stevenson, D. & Liddelow, A.G. (1978) Hepatocellular carcinoma
    possibly induced by oral contraceptives. Am. J. dig. Dis., 23,
    38s-40s

Hayward, J. (1970) Hormones and Human Breast Cancer. An Account of 15
    Years Study, Berlin, Springer, pp. 124-131

Hemsell, D.L., Grodin, J.M., Brenner, P.F., Siiteri, P.K. & MacDonald, P.C. (1974) Plasma precursors of estrogen. II. Correlation of the extent of conversion of plasma androstenedione to estrone with age. J. clin. Endocrinol. Metab., 38, 476-479

Henderson, J.T., Richmond, J. & Sumerling, M.D. (1973) Androgenic-anobolic steroid therapy and hepatocellular carcinoma. Lancet, i, 934

Hisaw, F.L., Velardo, J.T. & Goolsby, C.M. (1954) Interaction of estrogens on uterine growth. J. clin. Endocrinol. Metab., 14, 1134-1143

Hoover, R., Fraumeni, J.F., Jr, Everson, R. & Myers, M.H. (1976a) Cancer of the uterine corpus after hormonal treatment for breast cancer. Lancet, i, 885-887

Hoover, R., Gray, L.A., Sr, Cole, P. & MacMahon, B. (1976b) Menopausal estrogens and breast cancer. New Engl. J. Med., 295, 401-405

Hoover, R., Gray, L.A., Sr & Fraumeni, J.F., Jr (1977) Stilboestrol (diethylstilbestrol) and the risk of ovarian cancer. Lancet, ii, 533-534

Horwitz, R.I. & Feinstein, A.R. (1978) Alternative analytic methods for case-control studies of estrogens and endometrial cancer. New Engl. J. Med., 299, 1089-1094

Huggins, C. & Jensen, E.V. (1955) The depression of estrone-induced uterine growth by phenolic estrogens with oxygenated functions at positions 6 or 16: the impeded estrogens. J. exp. Med., 102, 335-346

Hutchinson, G.B. & Rothman, K.J. (1978) Correcting a bias? New Engl. J. Med., 299, 1129-1130

Janerich, D.T., Glebatis, D.M. & Dugan, J.M. (1977) Benign breast disease and oral contraceptive use. J. Am. med. Assoc., 237, 2199-2201

Jensen, E.I. & Østergaard, E. (1954) Clinical studies concerning the relationship of estrogens to the development of cancer of the corpus uteri. Am. J. Obstet. Gynecol., 67, 1094-1102

Jick, H., Watkins, R.N., Hunter, J.R., Dinan, B.J., Madsen, S., Rothman, K.J. & Walker, A.M. (1979) Replacement estrogens and endometrial cancer. New Engl. J. Med., 300, 218-222

Johnson, F.L., Feagler, J.R., Lerner, K.G., Majerus, P.W., Siegel, M., Hartmann, J.R. & Thomas, C.D. (1972) Association of androgenic-anabolic steroid therapy with development of hepatocellular carcinoma. Lancet, ii, 1273-1276

Judd, H.L., Lucas, W.E. & Yen, S.S.C. (1976) Serum 17β-estradiol and estrone levels in postmenopausal women with and without endometrial cancer. J. clin. Endocrinol. Metab., 43, 272-278

Kaufman, R.H., Reeves, K.O. & Dougherty, C.M. (1976) Severe atypical endometrial changes and sequential contraceptive use. J. Am. med. Assoc., 236, 923-926

Kelley, H.W., Miles, P.A., Buster, J.E. & Scragg, W.H. (1976) Adenocarcinoma of the endometrium in women taking sequential oral contraceptives. Obstet. Gynecol., 47, 200-202

Kelsey, J.L., Holford, T.R., White, C., Mayer, E.S., Kilty, S.E. & Acheson, R.M. (1978) Oral contraceptives and breast disease. An epidemiological study. Am. J. Epidemiol., 107, 236-244

Kew, M.C., Van Coller, B., Prowse, C.M., Skikne, B., Wolfsdorf, J.I., Ysdale, T., Krawitz, S., Altman, H., Levin, S.E. & Bothwell, T.H. (1976) Occurrence of primary hepatocellular cancer and peliosis hepatis after treatment with androgenic steroids. S. Afr. med. J., 50, 1233-1237

Kim, M.H., Hosseiniam, A.H. & Dupon, C. (1974) Plasma levels of estrogens, androgens and progesterone during normal and dexamethasone-treated cycles. J. clin. Endocrinol. Metab., 39, 706-712

Kline, T.S., Holland, M. & Wemple, D. (1970) Atypical cytology with contraceptive hormone medication. Am. J. clin. Pathol., 53, 215-222

Kodlin, D., Winger, E.E., Morgenstern, N.L. & Chen, U. (1977) Chronic mastopathy and breast cancer. A follow-up study. Cancer, 39, 2603-2607

Kreutner, A., Jr, Johnson, D. & Williamson, H.O. (1976) Histology of the endometrium in long-term use of a sequential oral contraceptive. Fertil. Steril., 27, 905-910

Laverty, C.R.A., Brown, J.B. & Fortune, D.W. (1975) Hormonal function of ovarian tumors. Contemp. Obstet. Gynecol., 5, 77-81

Lees, A.W., Burns, P.E. & Grace, M. (1978) Oral contraceptives and breast disease in premenopausal Northern Albertan women. Int. J. Cancer, 22, 700-707

Leis, H.P., Jr (1966) Endocrine prophylaxis of breast cancer with cyclic estrogen and progesterone. Int. Surg., 45, 496-503

Lemon, H.M. (1970) Abnormal estrogen metabolism and tissue estrogen receptor proteins in breast cancer. Cancer, 25, 423-435

Letoublon, C., Champetier, J., Benbassa, A., Durand, A., Laborde, Y. & Pasquier, D. (1978) Benign liver tumours and oral contraceptives (Fr.). Lyon chir., 74, 121-124

Liu, W., Koebel, L., Shipp, J. & Prisby, H. (1967) Cytologic changes following the use of oral contraceptives. Obstet. Gynecol., 30, 228-232

LiVolsi, V.A., Stadel, B.V., Kelsey, J.L., Holford, T.R. & White, C. (1978) Fibrocystic breast disease in oral contraceptive users. A histopathological evaluation of epithelial atypia. New Engl. J. Med., 299, 381-385

Longcope, C., Pratt, J.H., Schneider, S.H. & Fineberg, S.E. (1978) Aromatization of androgens by muscle and adipose tissue *in vivo*. J. clin. Endocrinol. Metab., 46, 146-152

Lyon, F.A. (1975) The development of adenocarcinoma of the endometrium in young women receiving long-term sequential oral contraception. Am. J. Obstet. gynecol., 123, 299-301

Lyon, F.A. & Frisch, M.J. (1976) Endometrial abnormalities occurring in young women on long-term sequential oral contraception. Obstet. Gynecol., 47, 639-643

MacDonald, P.C., Grodin, J.M., Edman, C.D., Vellios, F. & Siiteri, P.K. (1976) Origin of estrogen in a postmenopausal woman with a non-endocrine tumor of the ovary and endometrial hyperplasia. Obstet. Gynecol., 47, 644-650

MacDonald, P.C., Edman, C.D., Hemsell, D.L., Porter, J.C. & Siiteri, P.K. (1978) Effect of obesity on conversion of plasma androstenedione to estrone in postmenopausal women with and without endometrial cancer. Am. J. Obstet. Gynecol., 130, 448-455

Mack, T.M., Henderson, B.E., Gerkins, V.R., Arthur, M., Baptista, J. & Pike, M.C. (1975) Reserpine and breast cancer in a retirement community. New Engl. J. Med., 292, 1366-1371

Mack, T.M., Pike, M.C., Henderson, B.E., Pfeffer, R.I., Gerkins, V.R., Arthur, M. & Brown, S.E. (1976) Estrogens and endometrial cancer in a retirement community. New Engl. J. Med., 294, 1262-1267

MacMahon, B., Cole, P. & Brown, J. (1973) Etiology of human breast cancer: a review. J. natl Cancer Inst., 50, 21-42

MacMahon, B., Cole, P., Brown, J.B., Aoki, K., Lin, T.M., Morgan, R.W. & Woo, N.-C. (1974) Urine oestrogen profiles of Asian and North American women. Int. J. Cancer, 14, 161-167

Mahboubi, E. & Shubik, P. (1977) Epidemiological relationship between
    steroid hormones and liver lesions. J. Toxicol. environ. Health,
    3, 207-218

Marmorston, J., Crowley, L.G., Myers, S.M., Stern, E. & Hopkins, C.E.
    (1965) I. Urinary excretion of neutral 17-ketosteroids and
    pregnanediol by patients with breast cancer and benign breast disease.
    Am. J. Obstet. Gynecol., 92, 447-459

McDonald, T.W., Annegers, J.F., O'Fallon, W.M., Dockerty, M.B., Malkasian,
    G.D., Jr, & Kurland, L.T. (1977) Exogenous estrogen and endometrial
    carcinoma: case-control and incidence study. Am. J. Obstet. Gynecol,,
    127, 572-580

Meadows, A.T., Nalman, J.L. & Valdes-Dapena, M. (1974) Hepatoma
    associated with androgen therapy for aplastic anemia. J. Pediatr.,
    84, 109-110

Melamed, M.R. & Flehinger, B.J. (1973) Early incidence rates of precancerous
    cervical lesions in women using contraceptives. Gynecol. Oncol., 1,
    290-298

Melamed, M.R., Koss, L.G., Flehinger, B.J., Kelisky, R.P. & Dubrow, H.
    (1969) Prevalence rates of uterine cervical carcinoma in situ
    for women using the diaphragm or contraceptive oral steroids.
    Br. med. J., iii, 195-200

Menzies-Gow, N. (1978) Hepatocellular carcinoma associated with oral
    contraceptives. Br. J. Surg., 65, 316-317

Meyer, P., LiVolsi, V.A. & Cornog, J.L. (1974) Hepatoblastoma
    associated with an oral contraceptive. Lancet, ii, 1387

Mishell, D.R., Jr, Nakamura, R.M., Crosignani, P.G., Stone, S.,
    Kharma, K., Nagata, Y. & Thorneycroft, I.H. (1971) Serum
    gonadotropin and steroid patterns during the normal menstrual
    cycle. Am. J. Obstet. Gynecol., 111, 60-65

Moghissi, K.S. (1977) Oral contraceptives and endometrial and cervical
    cancer. J. Toxicol. environ. Health, 3, 243-265

Newhouse, M.L., Pearson, R.M., Fullerton, J.M., Boesen, E.A.M. &
    Shannon, H.S. (1977) A case control study of carcinoma of the ovary.
    Br. J. prev. soc. Med., 31, 148-153

Nimrod, A. & Ryan, K.J. (1975) Aromatization of androgens by human
    abdominal and breast fat tissue. J. clin. Endocrinol. Metab., 40,
    367-372

Nissen, E.D., Nissen, S.A. & Kent, D.R. (1978) Liver neoplasia and oral contraceptives. In: Sciarra, J.J., Zatuchni, G. & Speidal, J.J., eds, Risks, Benefits, and Controversies in Fertility Control, Hagerstown, MD, Harper & Row, pp. 176-184

Nomura, A. & Comstock, G.W. (1976) Benign breast tumor and estrogenic hormones: a population-based retrospective study. Am. J. Epidemiol., 103, 439-444

Ory, H. (1974) Functional ovarian cysts and oral contraceptives. Negative association confirmed surgically. A cooperative study. J. Am. med. Assoc., 228 68-69

Ory, H., Cole, P., MacMahon, B. & Hoover, R. (1976) Oral contraceptives and reduced risk of benign breast diseases. New Engl. J. Med., 294, 419-422

Ory, H.W., Conger, S.B., Naib, Z., Tyler, C.W., Jr & Hatcher, R.A. (1977) Preliminary analysis of oral contraceptive use and risk for developing premalignant lesions of the uterine cervix. In: Garattini, S. & Berendes, H.W., eds, Pharmacology of Steroid Contraceptive Drugs, New York, Raven Press, pp. 211-218

Östör, A.G., Fortune, D.W., Evans, J.H. & Kneale, B.L. (1978) Endometrial carcinoma in gonadol dysgenesis with and without estrogen therapy. Gynecol. Oncol., 6, 316-327

Paffenbarger, R.S., Jr, Fasal, E., Simmons, M.E. & Kampert, J.B. (1977) Cancer risk as related to use of oral contraceptives during fertile years. Cancer, 39, 1887-1891

Peritz, E., Ramcharan, S., Frank, J., Brown, W.L., Huang, S. & Ray, R. (1977) The incidence of cervical cancer and duration of oral contraceptive use. Am. J. Epidemiol., 106, 462-469

Pincus, G. & Garcia, C.-R. (1965) Studies on vaginal, cervical and uterine histology. Metabolism, 14, 344-347

Poortman, J., Thijssen, J.H.H. & Schwarz, F. (1973) Androgen production and conversion to estrogens in normal postmenopausal women and in selected breast cancer patients. J. clin. Endocrinol. Metab., 37, 101-109

Prat, J., Gray, G.F., Stolley, P.D. & Coleman, J.W. (1977) Wilms tumor in an adult associated with androgen abuse. J. Am. med. Assoc., 237, 2322-2323

Raju, U., Ganguly, M., Weiss, G., Zarkin, A. & Levitz, M. (1975) Serum unconjugated estriol in the menstrual cycle and early pregnancy. Gynecol. Invest., 6, 356-364

Raju, U., Ganguly, M. & Levitz, M. (1977) Estriol conjugates in human breast cyst fluid and in serum of premenopausal women. J. clin. Endocrinol. Metab., 45, 429-434

Ravnihar, B., Seigel, D.G. & Lindtner, J. (1979) An epidemiologic study of breast cancer and benign breast neoplasias in relation to the oral contraceptive and estrogen use. Eur. J. Cancer, 15, 395-405

Reti, L.L., Rome, R.M., Jr, Brown, J.B. & Fortune, D.W. (1978) Urinary oestrogen and pregnanediol excretion, endometrial and ovarian pathology and body weight in women with postmenopausal bleeding. Br. J. Obstet. Gynaecol., 85, 857-861

Rizkallah, T.H., Tovell, H.M.M. & Kelly, W.G. (1975) Production of estrone and fractional conversion of circulating androstenedione to estrone in women with endometrial cancer. J. clin. Endocrinol. Metab., 40, 1045-1056

Rome, R.M., Laverty, C.R. & Brown, J.B. (1973) Ovarian tumours in post-menopausal women. Clinicopathological features and hormonal studies. J. Obstet. Gynaecol. Br. Commonw., 80, 984-991

Rome, R.M., Brown, J.B., Mason, T., Smith, M.A., Laverty, C. & Fortune, D. (1977) Oestrogen excretion and ovarian pathology in post-menopausal women with atypical hyperplasia, adenocarcinoma and mixed adenosquamous carcinoma of the endometrium. Br. J. Obstet. Gynaecol., 84, 88-97

Rooks, J.B., Ory, H.W., Ishak, K.G., Strauss, L.T., Greenspan, J.R. & Tyler, G.W., Jr (1977) The association between oral contraception and hepatocellular adenoma - a preliminary report. Int. J. Gynaecol. Obstet., 15, 143-144

Rotti, K., Stevens, J., Watson, D. & Longcope, C. (1975) Estriol concentrations in plasma of normal, non-pregnant women. Steroids, 25, 807-816

Royal College of General Practitioners (1974) Oral Contraceptives and Health, London, Pitman Medical

Sale, G.E. & Lerner, K.G. (1977) Multiple tumors after androgen therapy. Arch. Pathol. lab. Med., 101, 600-603

Sandmire, H.F., Austin, S.D. & Bechtel, R.C. (1976) Carcinoma of the cervix in oral contraceptive steroid and IUD users and nonusers. Am. J. Obstet. Gynecol., 125, 339-345

Sartwell, P.E., Arthes, F.G. & Tonascia, J.A. (1973) Epidemiology of benign breast lesions: lack of assocation with oral contraceptive use. New Engl. J. Med., 288, 551-554

Sartwell, P.E., Arthes, F.G. & Tonascia, J.A. (1977) Exogenous hormones, reproductive history, and breast cancer. J. natl Cancer Inst., 59, 1589-1592

Schleyer-Saunders, E. (1960) The management of the menopause: a new approach. Med. Press, 244, 337-346

Schmidt, G. (1977) Hepatocellular carcinoma. A possible complication of oral contraceptive steroids. Med. J. Aust., 1, 215-217

Shapiro, P., Ikeda, R.M., Ruebner, B.H., Connors, M.H., Halsted, C.C & Abildgaard, C.F. (1977) Multiple hepatic tumors and peliosis hepatis in Fanconi's anemia treated with androgens. Am. J. Dis. Child., 131, 1104-1106

Sherman, B.M., Harris, C.E., Schlechte, J., Duello, T.M., Halmi, N.S., VanGilder, J., Chapler, F.K. & Granner, D.K. (1978) Pathogenesis of prolactin-secreting pituitary adenomas. Lancet, ii, 1019-1021

Siiteri, P.K. (1978) Steroid hormones and endometrial cancer. Cancer Res., 38, 4360-4366

Siiteri, P.K. & MacDonald, P.C. (1973) Role of extraglandular estrogen in human endocrinology. In: Greep, R.O. & Astwood, E.B., eds, Handbook of Physiology, Vol. 2, Bethesda, MD, American Physiological Society, pp. 615-629

Siiteri, P.K., Schwarz, B.E. & MacDonald, P.C. (1974) Estrogen receptors and the estrone hypothesis in relation to endometrial and breast cancer. Gynecol. Oncol., 2, 228-238

Silverberg, S.G., Makowski, E.L. & Roche, W.D. (1977) Endometrial carcinoma in women under 40 years of age. Comparison of cases in oral contraceptive users and non-users. Cancer, 39, 592-598

Smith, D.C., Prentice, R., Thompson, D.J. & Herrmann, W.L. (1975) Association of exogenous estrogen and endometrial carcinoma. New Engl. J. Med., 293, 1164-1167

Stern, E., Hopkins, C.E., Weiner, J.M. & Marmorston, J. (1964) Hormone excretion patterns in breast and prostate cancer are abnormal. Science, 145, 716-719

Stern, E., Forsythe, A.B., Youkeles, L. & Coffelt, C.F. (1977) Steroid contraceptive use and cervical dysplasia: increased risk of progression. Science, 196, 1460-1462

Stone, M., Dent, J., Kardana, A. & Bagshawe, K.D. (1976) Relationship of oral contraception to development of trophoblastic tumour after evacuation of a hydatidiform mole. Br. J. Obstet. Gynaecol., 83, 913-916

Symmers, W.St C. (1968) Carcinoma of breast in trans-sexual individuals after surgical and hormonal interference with the primary and secondary sex characteristics. Br. med. J., ii, 83-85

Terenius, L. (1971) Effect of anti-oestrogens on initiation of mammary cancer in the female rat. Eur. J. Cancer, 7, 65-70

Thalassinos, N.C., Lymberatos, C., Hadjioannou, J. & Gardikas, C. (1974) Liver-cell carcinoma after long-term oestrogen-like drugs. Lancet, i, 270

Thomas, D.B. (1972) Relationship of oral contraceptives to cervical carcinogenesis. Obstet. Gynecol., 40, 508-518

Thomas, D.B. (1978) Role of exogenous female hormones in altering the risk of benign and malignant neoplasms in humans. Cancer Res., 38, 3991-4000

Trichopoulos, D., MacMahon, B. & Cole, P. (1972) Menopause and breast cancer risk. J. natl Cancer Inst., 48, 605-613

Tseng, L. & Gurpide, E. (1974) Estradiol and 20α-dihydroprogesterone dehydrogenase activities in human endometrium during the menstrual cycle. Endocrinology, 94, 419-423

Vessey, M.P., Doll, R. & Sutton, P.M. (1972) Oral contraceptives and breast neoplasia: a retrospective study. Br. med. J., iii, 719-724

Vessey, M.P., Doll, R. & Jones, K. (1975) Oral contraceptives and breast cancer. Lancet, i, 941-944

Vessey, M., Doll, R., Peto, R., Johnson, B. & Wiggins, P. (1976) A long-term folow-up study of women using different methods of contraception - an interim report. J. biosoc. Sci., 8, 373-427

Wallach, S. & Henneman, P.G. (1959) Prolonged estrogen therapy in post-menopausal women. J. Am. med. Assoc., 171, 1637-1642

Weiss, N.S., Szekely, D.R. & Austin, D.F. (1976) Increasing incidence of endometrial cancer in the United States. New Engl. J. Med., 294, 1259-1262

WHO (1978) Steroid contraception and the risk of neoplasia. Report of a WHO Scientific Group. World Health Org. tech. Rep. Ser., No. 619, Geneva

Wigle, D.T., Grace, M. & Smith, E.S.O. (1978)   Estrogen use and cancer of the uterine corpus in Alberta. Can. med. Assoc. J., 118, 1276-1278

Wilson, R.A. (1962)   The roles of estrogen and progesterone in breast and genital cancer. J. Am. med. Assoc., 182, 327-331

Worth, A.J. & Boyes, D.A. (1972)   A case control study into the possible effects of birth control pills on pre-clinical carcinoma of the cervix. J. Obstet. Gynaecol. Br. Commonw., 79, 673-679

Wright, N.H., Vessey, M.P., Kenward, B., McPherson, K. & Doll, R. (1978) Neoplasia and dysplasia of the cervix uteri and contraception: a possible protective effect of the diaphragm. Br. J. Cancer, 38, 273-279

Wynder, E.L., Bross, I.Y. & Hirayama, T. (1960)   A study of the epidemiology of cancer of the breast. Cancer, 13, 559-601

Wynder, E.L., Escher, G.C. & Mantel, N. (1966)   An epidemiological investigation of cancer of the endometrium. Cancer, 19, 489-520

Ylikorkala, O. (1977)   Ovarian cysts and hormonal contraception. Lancet, i, 1101-1102

Ziegenfuss, J. & Carabasi, R. (1973)   Androgens and hepatocellular carcinoma. Lancet, i, 262

Ziel, H.K. & Finkle, W.D. (1975)   Increased risk of endometrial carcinoma among users of conjugated estrogens. New Engl. J. Med., 293, 1167-1170

GENERAL CONCLUSIONS ON SEX HORMONES

Steroid hormones are essential for the growth, differentiation and function of many tissues in both animals and humans. It has been established by animal experimentation that modification of the hormonal environment by surgical removal of endocrine glands, by pregnancy or by exogenous administration of steroids can increase or decrease the spontaneous occurrence of tumours or the induction of tumours by applied carcinogenic agents. In humans, endogenous hormones are important in the initiation and progression of tumours. The incidence of tumours in humans could be altered by exposure to various exogenous hormones, singly or in combination.

For an administered oestrogen seriously to influence the human hormonal environment, its intake must be equal to, or greater than, the amounts of oestrogens produced endogenously (p. 47). For contraceptive medication to be effective, the intake of steroids must be sufficient to alter the hormonal environment. The doses at which steroids are administered for other therapeutic purposes are considerably higher; the possibility that a carcinogenic risk may be involved in such medication must therefore be considered. For example, the minimum effective dose of diethylstilboestrol that produces mammary carcinogenesis in mice is of the same order as the doses used in women for therapy of the climacteric or following ovariectomy.

Animal data

Administration of the naturally occurring oestrogens, oestradiol-17β and oestrone, increases the incidence of tumours in a number of organs in a variety of animal species. There is limited evidence for the carcinogenicity of oestriol, whereas insufficient evidence was available concerning the conjugated oestrogens. Diethylstilboestrol has a carcinogenic potential comparable with those of oestradiol-17β and of oestrone, and there is no evidence to support the suggestion that its carcinogenic properties are due to some special biological function other than its oestrogenic activity. Ethinyloestradiol and mestranol have been shown to be carcinogenic in animals, but there is no evidence that they are more or less carcinogenic than are other oestrogens with comparable levels of oestrogenic activity. Insufficient data were available to evaluate the carcinogenicity of dienoestrol and chlorotrianisene, which are structurally similar to diethylstilboestrol. Because of lack of experimental data, no attempt has been made to show a relationship between carcinogenic potential and oestrogenic activity for any of the compounds considered.

In the majority of experiments in which animals were treated with oestrogens and which resulted in carcinogenesis, high dose levels were used. The information currently available is, however, inadequate to indicate the minimum doses required to produce carcinogenesis, and these could be much lower than those commonly employed in animal studies.

There is limited evidence that natural progestins have a carcinogenic potential. There is, however, evidence that low doses of progesterone administered over long periods act in combination with carcinogenic agents, such as some viruses or chemicals, to enhance tumour development. In part, therefore, long-term administration of synthetic progestins may produce a comparable hazard by increasing the incidence of tumours due to other agents. This is dependent on the degree of progestational activity possessed by the compound in question relative to its other hormonal characteristics.

Animal data concerning the synthetic progestins provide either insufficient or limited evidence of their carcinogenic potential. Combination with oestrogens seems to enhance their carcinogenic potential. There is limited evidence for the carcinogenicity of some progestins (chlormadinone acetate, medroxyprogesterone acetate, megestrol acetate) in dogs, which is associated with the production of mammary tumours.

There is sufficient evidence for the carcinogenicity of testosterone in mice and rats.

The mechanism(s) by which hormones act in the induction of cancer is not understood. Although many carcinogens show a mutagenic action, no sex hormones, including diethylstilboestrol, nor any of their metabolic products, have so far convincingly been shown to be mutagenic; however, covalent binding of their metabolites to DNA and other results from short-term tests that indicate interaction with DNA have been reported.

The evidence suggests that steroid hormones may stimulate carcinogenesis in several ways and, in addition, provide a background for subsequent tumorigenesis by chemical, physical or viral agents and promote the growth and metastasis of tumours once they have been initiated.

The administration of sex steroids and diethylstilboestrol prenatally or neonatally, especially to mice, results in teratogenic changes and altered endocrine function. Carcinogenesis may occur consequent to these alterations. Both in neonates and adults, sex steroid-stimulated prolactin secretion may lead to increased mammary carcinogenesis.

Human data

Sex hormones, such as those considered in this monograph, have been and are used extensively in human therapy. When they are used for the treatment of disseminated cancer, such as that of the breast, prostate and endometrium, their effect on tumour growth and the severity of their side-effects are the major considerations. The use of sex hormones in therapy for other conditions (for example, menstrual disorders, climacteric syndrome, pregnancy maintenance, osteoporosis, abnormal protein metabolism, gonadal deficiency) makes the question of carcinogenic hazard more pertinent. With the continuing development of steroid use for the control of conception, the question of possible carcinogenic hazards has become of major importance.

Epidemiological studies to evaluate possible carcinogenic effects of administered oestrogens and progestins in humans suffer from two major difficulties. Firstly, the interval between the commencement of administration and the possible appearance of cancer may be long. Secondly, to detect a small or moderate change in risk, observations on large numbers of subjects are required.

With these reservations in mind, the following conclusions can be made:

1. <u>Intrauterine exposure to diethylstilboestrol</u> - The administration of diethylstilboestrol to women during pregnancy is causally associated with an increased risk of vaginal and cervical clear-cell adenocarcinoma in exposed daughters. Non-neoplastic changes of the female genital tract, including transverse fibrous septae, vaginal adenosis and cervical ectropion, have been observed frequently; non-malignant structural changes in the male reproductive tract have also been reported.

2. <u>Oestrogens administered to adults</u> - The administration of oestrogens (including diethylstilboestrol) to adult women is causally associated with an increased incidence of endometrial cancer. There is also a possibility that the risk of breast cancer is increased by such therapy, but the evidence is not conclusive. There is good evidence that factors which increase or prolong exposure of the uterus to endogenous oestrogens result in an increased risk of developing endometrial cancer. At present, the specific role of endogenous hormones in the development of breast cancer is unclear.

3. <u>Progestins</u> - There are no adequate data in humans to assess whether progestins used as contraceptives (either as pills or as injections) alter the risk of developing cancer.

4. <u>Androgens</u> - Prolonged androgen therapy may be associated with an increased risk of hepatocellular tumours, but the evidence is not conclusive.

5. <u>Oral contraceptives</u> - Oral contraceptive use decreases the risk of benign breast disease. There is no clear evidence that their use alters the risk of breast cancer, although limited data suggest that the preparations may interact with other risk factors (e.g., late age at first pregnancy, presence of benign breast lesions) in the development of the disease. Oral contraceptives may increase the risk of cervical dysplasia and carcinoma *in situ* after long-term use. Few data are available concerning invasive cancer of the cervix. Sequential oral contraceptives may increase the risk of endometrial cancer, but the evidence is not conclusive.

Long-term use of oral contraceptives markedly increases the relative risk of hepatocellular adenoma. The effect is greater in older women and in those using preparations containing high doses of steroids.

Oral contraceptives may increase the risk of malignant melanoma and of pituitary adenoma and decrease the risk of ovarian cancer, but the available data are inadequate for a proper assessment.

THE MONOGRAPHS

OESTROGENS

CHLOROTRIANISENE

1. Chemical and Physical Data

1.1 Synonyms and trade names

Chem. Abstr. Services Reg. No.: 569-57-3

Chem. Abstr. Name: 1,1',1"-(1-Chloro-1-ethenyl-2-ylidene)-
tris(4-methoxybenzene)

Synonyms: Chlorotrianisine; chlorotrianizen; chlorotris-
(*para*-methoxyphenyl)ethylene; chlortrianisen; khlortrianizen;
tri-*para*-anisylchloroethylene; tris(*para*-methoxyphenyl)chloro-
ethylene

Trade names: Anisene; Chlorestrolo; Chlorotrisin; Clorestrolo;
Clorotrisin; Hormonisene; Merbentul; Metace; NSC-10108; Rianil;
Tace; TACE; Tace-FN

1.2 Structural and molecular formulae and molecular weight

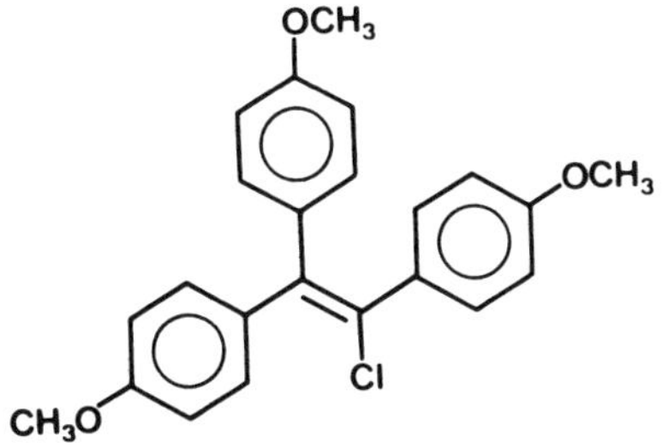

$C_{23}H_{21}ClO_3$ Mol. wt: 380.9

1.3 Chemical and physical properties

From Wade (1977) and Windholz (1976)

(<u>a</u>) Description: Small, white crystals

(<u>b</u>) Melting-point: 114-116°C; softens at 108°C

(c) Spectroscopy data: λ_{max} 310 nm (E_1^1 423), λ_{min} 278 nm in chloroform

(d) Solubility: Soluble in water (1 in 4200), ethanol (1 in 360), methanol (1 in 360), acetone (1 in 7), chloroform (1 in 1.5), diethyl ether (1 in 28) and fixed oils (1 in 100); practically insoluble in 2,2,4-trimethylpentane. Also soluble in glacial acetic acid, carbon tetrachloride and benzene

(e) Stability: Unstable to light and air

1.4 Technical products and impurities

Various national and international pharmacopoeias give specifications for the purity of chlorotrianisene in pharmaceutical products. For example, chlorotrianisene is available in the US as a NF grade containing 97-103% active ingredient on a dried basis and not more than 0.002% heavy metals. Capsules in 12, 24 and 72 mg doses contain 93-107% of the stated amount of chlorotrianisene (National Formulary Board, 1975).

Chlorotrianisene is available in the UK in 12 mg capsules and 24 mg tablets (Wade, 1977).

2. Production, Use, Occurrence and Analysis

2.1 Production and use

(a) Production

A method for synthesizing chlorotrianisene was first patented in 1944 by Basford, by reacting tri-*para*-anisylethylene or tri-*para*-anisylethanol with chlorine in an inert solvent. Another method was patented in 1947 by Shelton and Van Campen, involving synthesis from *para*(*para*-anisoyl)anisole (Windholz, 1976). Chlorotrianisene can be prepared by the following method: (1) anisaldehyde is reacted with potassium cyanide to produce anisoin, which is reduced with zinc and hydrochloric acid to deoxyanisoin; (2) a Grignard reaction of deoxyanisoin with *para*-methoxyphenyl-magnesium bromide gives 1,1,2-tri-*para*-anisyl-ethanol, which is dehydrated with phosphoric acid to 1,1,2-tri-*para*-anisylethylene; (3) chlorination of 1,1,2-tri-*para*-anisylethylene yields chlorotrianisene (Harvey, 1975). It is not known whether this is the process used for commercial production.

Commercial production of chlorotrianisene in the US was first
reported in 1952 (US Tariff Commission, 1953). In 1975 and 1976, two US
companies reported production of an undisclosed amount (see preamble,
p. 20) (US International Trade Commission, 1977a,b); however, in 1975,
US production of 13 oestrogen and progestin substances, including
chlorotrianisene, amounted to 10.5 thousand kg (US International Trade
Commission, 1977b).

No data on its production in Europe were available to the Working
Group.

Chlorotrianisene is not produced in Japan, and there is no evidence
that it has been imported in recent years.

(b) Use

Chlorotrianisene is not used extensively in human medicine (Murad &
Gilman, 1975). It has been used for the treatment of symptoms of the
climacteric and of prostatic carcinoma, in a dose of 12-25 mg daily;
for vulvar dystrophies, in a dose of 12-25 mg daily for 30-60 days; to
prevent post-partum breast engorgement, in a dose of 12 mg 4 times daily
for 7 days or 25 mg every 6 hrs for 6 doses, the first dose given within
8 hrs of delivery; and for the treatment of female hypogonadism, in a
dose of 12-25 mg daily for 21 days, with a progestin given on days 17 to
21, and repeated after the 5th day of induced menstruation (Harvey,
1975).

Chlorotrianisene is used in the US and the UK but does not appear
to have been used in Japan in recent years.

The US Food & Drug Administration (1977) has ruled that, with
effect from 20 September 1977, oestrogens for general use must carry
patient and physician warning labels concerning use, risks and contraindications.

2.2 Occurrence

Chlorotrianisene is not known to occur naturally.

2.3 Analysis

Typical analytical procedures for the determination of chlorotrianisene are summarized in Table 1. Abbreviations used are: HPLC, high-
pressure liquid chromatography; CC, column chromatography; TLC, thin-
layer chromatography; and UV, ultra-violet spectrometry. See also
'General Remarks on Sex Hormones', p. 60.

TABLE 1

Analytical methods for chlorotrianisene

Sample matrix	Sample preparation	Assay procedure	Reference
Bulk chemical	Dissolve (anhydrous ethanol); add sodium; reflux; add nitric acid & aqueous silver nitrate	Titration (ammonium thiocyanate)	British Pharmacopoeia Commission (1973) National Formulary Board (1975)
Bulk chemical	Dissolve (methanol-water); CC (diatomaceous earth-acetonitrile column); elute (heptane); evaporate & dissolve in ethanol	UV	Graham & Kenner (1973)
Hard capsules	Dissolve (heptane); CC (silica gel-nitromethane column); elute (heptane); evaporate & dissolve in chloroform	UV (310 nm)	National Formulary Board (1975)
Soft capsules	Dissolve (dimethylformamide); dilute with methanol	HPLC (reversed-phase); UV (254 nm)	Roos (1974)
Tablets	Powder; dissolve (chloroform)	TLC (silica gel); UV (310 nm)	British Pharmacopoeia Commission (1973)

3. Biological Data Relevant to the Evaluation
    of Carcinogenic Risk to Humans

3.1 Carcinogenicity studies in animals

Oral administration

Rat: Groups of 20 male and 20 female weanling Sprague-Dawley rats
were fed diets containing chlorotrianisene at concentrations resulting
in intakes of 0, 0.05, 0.2 and 2 mg/kg bw per day for 2 years. The
numbers of survivors at 24 months were 9 male and 12 female controls,
15 males and 19 females given 0.05 mg/kg bw, 18 males and 17 females
given 0.2 mg/kg bw and 12 males and 11 females given 2 mg/kg bw. Mammary
tumours, mainly fibroadenomas, occurred in 1 male rat treated with the
highest dose compared with 0 in male controls, and in 2, 0 and 2 females
in the treated groups, compared with 8 in female controls. The incidences
of pituitary tumours were 1, 1 and 0 in treated males, compared with 4
in male controls, and 2, 0 and 0 in treated females, compared with 4 in
female controls (Gibson et al., 1967).

3.2 Other relevant biological data

In the Allen-Doisy test in mice, chlorotrianisene has about 1/10-
1/20 of the activity of oestradiol-17β when given by s.c. administration
and about 1/3-2/3 of the activity of oestradiol-17β when given orally
(Emmens & Martin, 1964). In the uterine growth test (Rubin's test) in
mice, it is 0.14 times more active than oestradiol-17β (Brotherton,
1976). In humans, when given orally the compound has about 1/5-1/3 the
activity of oestradiol-17β (Emmens & Martin, 1964; Kupperman et al.,
1953) and 1/8 the activity of diethylstilboestrol (Murad & Gilman,
1975).

No data on the toxicity of chlorotrianisene were available.

Chlorotrianisene is stored preferentially in adipose tissue (Murad
& Gilman, 1975); no other data on its metabolism were available.

No data on its embryotoxicity or mutagenicity were available.

3.3 Case reports and epidemiological studies

See the section, 'Oestrogens and Progestins in Relation to Human
Cancer', p. 83.

4. Summary of Data Reported and Evaluation[1]

4.1 Experimental data

Chlorotrianisene was tested in only one experiment in rats by oral administration. The data were insufficient to evaluate the carcinogenicity of this compound.

4.2 Human data

No case reports or epidemiological studies on chlorotrianisene alone were available to the Working Group.

Case reports and epidemiological studies on steroid hormones used in oestrogen treatment have been summarized in the section, 'Oestrogens and Progestins in Relation to Human Cancer', p. 83.

4.3 Evaluation

The available experimental data are insufficient to evaluate the carcinogenicity of chlorotrianisene in animals. Studies in humans strongly suggest that the administration of oestrogens is causally related to an increased incidence of endometrial carcinoma; there is no evidence that chlorotrianisene is different from other oestrogens in this respect.

---

[1]This section should be read in conjunction with pp. 62–64 in the 'General Remarks on Sex Hormones' and with the 'General Conclusions on Sex Hormones', p. 131.

5. References

British Pharmacopoeia Commission (1973) British Pharmacopoeia, London,
    HMSO, pp. 103-104

Brotherton, J. (1976) Sex Hormone Pharmacology, London, Academic Press,
    p. 49

Emmens, C.W. & Martin, L. (1964) Estrogens. In: Dorfman, R.I., ed.,
    Methods in Hormone Research, Vol. 3/A, London, Academic Press,
    pp. 1-75

Gibson, J.P., Newberne, J.W., Kuhn, W.L. & Elsea, J.R. (1967) Comparative
    chronic toxicity of three oral estrogens in rats. Toxicol. appl.
    Pharmacol., 11, 489-510

Graham, R.E. & Kenner, C.T. (1973) Acetonitrile-diatomaceous earth column
    for separation of steroids and other compounds. J. pharm. Sci., 62,
    1845-1849

Harvey, S.C. (1975) Hormones. In: Osol, A. et al., eds, Remington's
    Pharmaceutical Sciences, 15th ed., Easton, PA, Mack, p. 918

Kupperman, H.S., Blatt, H.G.H., Wiesbader, H. & Filler, W. (1953)
    Comparative clinical evaluation of estrogenic preparations by
    the menopausal and amenorrheal indices. J. clin. Endocrinol.
    Metab., 13, 688-703

Murad, F. & Gilman, A.G. (1975) Estrogens and progestins. In: Goodman,
    L.S. & Gilman, A., eds, The Pharmacological Basis of Therapeutics,
    5th ed., New York, Macmillan, p. 1431

National Formulary Board (1975) National Formulary, 14th ed.,
    Washington DC, American Pharmaceutical Association, pp. 138-140

Roos, R.W. (1974) Identification and determination of synthetic estrogens
    in pharmaceuticals by high-speed, reversed-phase partition chromato-
    graphy. J. pharm. Sci., 63, 594-599

US Food & Drug Administration (1977) Patient labeling for estrogens for
    general use. Drugs for human use; drug efficacy study implementation.
    Fed. Regist., 42, 37645-37646

US International Trade Commission (1977a) Synthetic Organic Chemicals, US
    Production and Sales, 1976, USITC Publication 833, Washington DC,
    US Government Printing Office, p. 148

US International Trade Commission (1977b) Synthetic Organic Chemicals, US Production and Sales, 1975, USITC Publication 804, Washington DC, US Government Printing Office, pp. 90, 102

US Tariff Commission (1953) Synthetic Organic Chemicals, US Production and Sales, 1952, Report No. 190, Second Series, Washington DC, US Government Printing Office, p. 100

Wade, A., ed. (1977) Martindale, The Extra Pharmacopoeia, 27th ed., London, The Pharmaceutical Press, p. 1392

Windholz, M., ed. (1976) The Merck Index, 9th ed., Rahway, NJ, Merck & Co., p. 278

CONJUGATED OESTROGENS

1. Chemical and Physical Data

1.1 Synonyms and trade names

Conjugated oestrogens

Chem. Abstr. Services Reg. No.: Not available

Chem. Abstr. Name: Not available

Conjugated oestrogens are an amorphous mixture obtained from the urine of pregnant mares containing naturally occurring, water-soluble, conjugated forms of mixed oestrogens (principally sodium oestrone sulphate and sodium equilin sulphate). Piperazine oestrone sulphate, a synthetic conjugated oestrogen, is also available (Wade, 1977).

Trade names: Amnestrogen; Ces; Climestrone; Co-Estro; Conest; Conestron; Conjes; Equigyne; Estratab; Estrifol; Estroate; Estrocon; Estromed; Estropan; Evex; Femacoid; Femest; Fem H; Femogen; Formatrix; Ganeake; Genisis; Glyestrin; Kestrin; Menest; Menogen; Menotab; Menotrol; Milprem; MsMed; Neo-Estrone; Novoconestron; Oestrilin; Oestro-Feminal; Oestropak Morning; Ovest; Palopause; Par Estro; PMB; Premarin; Presomen; Promarit; SK-Estrogens; Sodestrin-H; Tag-39; Transannon; Trocosone; Zeste

Sodium oestrone sulphate

Chem. Abstr. Services Reg. No.: 438-67-5

Chem. Abstr. Name: 3-(Sulfooxy)estra-1,3,5(10)-trien-17-one sodium salt

Synonyms: Estrone hydrogen sulfate sodium salt; estrone sodium sulfate; estrone sulfate sodium; oestrone hydrogen sulphate sodium salt; oestrone sodium sulphate; oestrone sulphate sodium; sodium estrone 3-monosulfate; sodium estrone sulfate; sodium estrone-3-sulfate; sodium oestrone 3-monosulphate; sodium oestrone sulphate; sodium oestrone-3-sulphate

Trade names: Conestoral; Evex; Morestin

Sodium equilin sulphate

Chem. Abstr. Services Reg. No.: 16680-47-0

Chem. Abstr. Name: 3-(Sulfooxy)estra-1,3,5(10),7-tetraen-17-one
sodium salt

Synonyms: Equilin sodium sulfate; equilin sodium sulphate; estra-
1,3,5(10),7-tetraen-17-one hydrogen sulfate sodium salt; oestra-1,3,
5(10),7-tetraen-17-one hydrogen sulphate sodium salt; sodium
equilin 3-monosulfate; sodium equilin 3-monosulphate; sodium equilin
sulfate

Piperazine oestrone sulphate

Chem. Abstr. Services Reg. No: 7280-37-7

Chem. Abstr. Name: 3-(Sulfooxy)estra-1,3,5(10)-trien-17-one compd.
with piperazine (1:1)

Synonyms: Estrone, hydrogen sulfate, compd. with piperazine (1:1);
oestrone, hydrogen sulphate, compd. with piperazine (1:1); piperazine
estrone sulfate; piperazine 17-oxo-oestra-1,3,5(10)-trien-3-yl
sulphate

Trade names: Harmogen; Ogen; Sulestrex; Sulestrex Piperazine

1.2 Structural and molecular formulae and molecular weights

Sodium oestrone sulphate

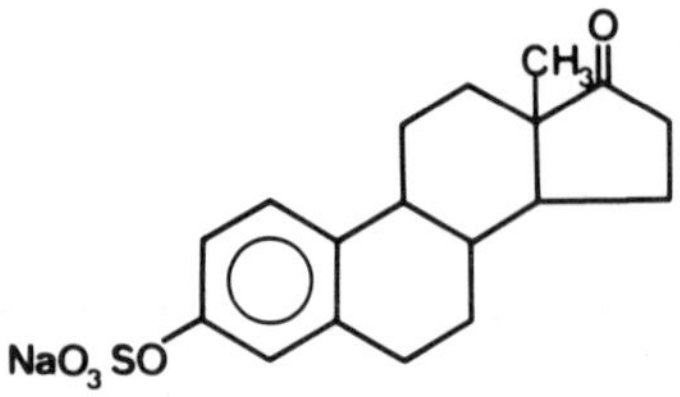

$C_{18}H_{21}NaO_5S$ Mol. wt: 372.4

Sodium equilin sulphate

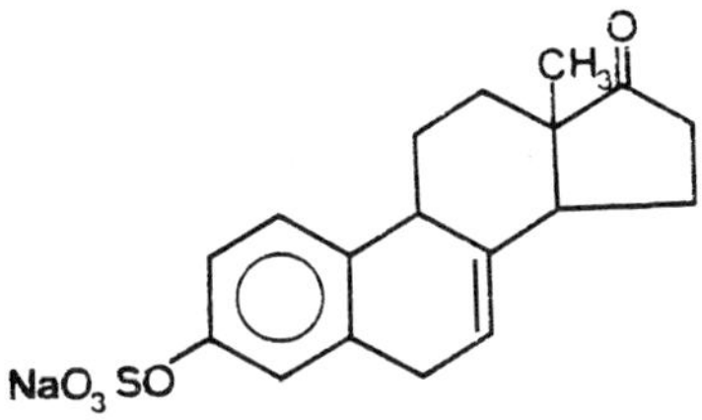

$C_{18}H_{19}NaO_5S$ Mol. wt: 370.4

Piperazine oestrone sulphate

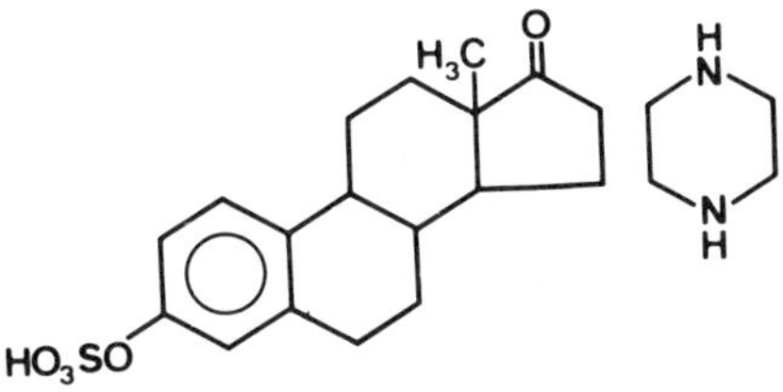

$C_{18}H_{22}O_5S.C_4H_{10}N_2$ Mol. wt: 436.6

1.3 Chemical and physical properties

Conjugated oestrogens

From Harvey (1975)

(a) Description: Buff-coloured powder

(b) Solubility: Soluble in water

(c) Stability: The sodium equilin sulphate component is unstable to
     light and air.

Piperazine oestrone sulphate

From Chang (1976) and Wade (1977)

(a) Description: White to yellowish-white crystalline powder

(b) Melting point: 190°C; solidifies on further heating and melts
     at 245°C with decomposition

(c) Spectroscopy data: λ_{max} 268 nm ($E^1_1 = 19.5$) and 275 nm
($E^1_1 = 19.1$) in 0.04% NaOH; infrared, nuclear magnetic
resonance, Raman and mass spectral data have been tabulated.

(d) Optical rotation: $[\alpha]^{25}_D + 87.8°$ (1.0% in 0.4% aqueous NaOH)

(e) Solubility: Very slightly soluble in water (8 mg/ml); practically
insoluble in diethyl ether, benzene and isopropanol; very
slightly soluble in 95% ethanol, chloroform, acetone, methylene
dichloride, mineral oil and sesame oil; soluble in 0.1 N
sodium hydroxide (57 mg/ml) and propylene glycol (35 mg/ml)

(f) Stability: Not hygroscopic when exposed to 40-50% relative
humidity for 3 weeks. When refluxed for 3 hrs, it was stable in
water, produced less than 10% free oestrone in 1 N NaOH and was
hydrolysed completely in 1 N HCl. When heated at 105°C for one
month, about 10% free oestrone was produced.

1.4 Technical products and impurities

Conjugated oestrogens are available in the US as a USP grade containing
90-110% active ingredient, consisting of 50-65% sodium oestrone sulphate
and 20-35% sodium equilin sulphate, calculated on the basis of the total
conjugated oestrogen content, and not more than 2.5% free steroids.
Tablets in 0.3, 0.625, 1.25 and 2.5 mg doses contain 90-115% of the
stated amount of conjugated oestrogens (US Pharmacopeial Convention
Inc., 1975). Conjugated oestrogens are also available as a 5 mg/ml
injectable preparation (Murad & Gilman, 1975). Vaginal creams are also
available in the US, containing 625 mg/kg conjugated oestrogens (Murad &
Gilman, 1975). Combinations of conjugated oestrogens with methyltestosterone, or with phenobarbital or meprobamate, are available in tablet
form (Kastrup, 1976, 1977, 1978).

In the UK, conjugated oestrogens are available in tablets in 0.625,
1.25 and 2.5 mg doses; in creams containing 625 mg/kg; and as a water-
soluble preparation in vials of 25 mg with 5 ml of sterile diluent
(Wade, 1977).

Piperazine oestrone sulphate is available in the US as a NF grade
containing 97-103% active ingredient on a dried basis and no more than
2% free oestrone. Tablets in 0.75, 1.5, 3 and 6 mg doses contain 90-
110% of the stated amount of piperazine oestrone sulphate (National
Formulary Board, 1975). It is available in the UK as tablets of 1.5 mg
(Wade, 1977).

2. Production, Use, Occurrence and Analysis

2.1 Production and use

(a) Production

Conjugated oestrogens are obtained by subjecting pregnant mares' urine to a solvent extraction process (Harvey, 1975). In an extraction method first patented in the US in 1951, the solids were extracted with aqueous acetone from the urine of mares that were at least 5 months pregnant (Bates & Cohen, 1951).

Piperazine oestrone sulphate can be prepared by reacting oestrone with SO_3 in N,N-dimethylformamide, followed by the addition of piperazine (Harvey, 1975).

Commercial production of conjugated oestrogens in the US was first reported in 1968 (US Tariff Commission, 1970), although production of natural equine oestrone was reported in 1959 (US Tariff Commission, 1960). In 1975 and 1976, only one US company reported production of an undisclosed amount (see preamble, p. 20) (US International Trade Commission, 1977a,b); however, in 1975, US production of 13 oestrogen and progestin substances, including conjugated oestrogens, amounted to 10.5 thousand kg (US International Trade Commission, 1977a). Data on US imports and exports of conjugated oestrogens are not available.

Commercial production of piperazine oestrone sulphate in the US was first reported in 1950 (US Tariff Commission, 1951) and was last reported in 1975, when production of 13 oestrogen and progestin substances, including piperazine oestrone sulphate, amounted to 10.5 thousand kg (US International Trade Commission, 1977a).

No information on the production of conjugated oestrogens or piperazine oestrone sulphate in Europe was available to the Working Group.

Conjugated oestrogens are not produced in Japan, and only negligible quantities have been imported in recent years.

(b) Use

Conjugated oestrogens have been used in human medicine and were generally administered orally in a cyclic regimen every day for 3 weeks followed by one week without. They have been used: (1) for the treatment of symptoms of the climacteric and following ovariectomy; (2) for vulvar dystrophies, in a dose of 1.25 mg per day; (3) for female hypogonadism, in a dose of 2.5-7.5 mg per day for 20 days (combined with a progestin on days 16-20) followed by 10 days without; (4) for chemotherapy of mammary carcinoma, in a dose of 10 mg 3 times per day for at least 3 months, and of prostatic carcinoma, in a dose of 1.25-2.5 mg 3 times per day;   (5) for the prevention of post-partum breast engorgement, in a dose of 3.75 mg every 4 hrs for 5 doses or 1.25 mg every 4 hrs for 5 days, and may also be given in combination with methyltestosterone; and (6) for dysfunctional uterine bleeding, in an i.m. or i.v. dose of 25 mg, repeated within 6-12 hrs if necessary (Harvey, 1975;   Wade, 1977).

Unspecified oestrogens, believed to include substances such as conjugated oestrogens (Miller, 1976), have been used in the following cosmetic preparations: hormonal skin care preparations (at levels of less than 0.1-5%);   moisturizing lotions (1-5%);   and wrinkle-smoothing compounds, hair conditioners, hair straighteners, shampoos and grooming aid tonics (<0.1%).

Piperazine oestrone sulphate is used orally (1) for the treatment of symptoms of the climacteric and following ovariectomy, in a dose of 1.5-3 mg per day;   (2) for dysfunctional uterine bleeding, in a dose of 4.5-9 mg per day until bleeding stops, followed by a cyclic regimen of 1.5-3 mg per day for 20 days, with a progestin added during the 11th-20th or 16th-20th day, and a rest of 10 days;   (3) for the prevention of post-partum breast engorgement, in a dose of 4.5 mg every 4 hrs for a total of 5 doses (Harvey, 1975);   (4) for atrophic vaginitis and vulvar dystrophies;   (5) for female hypogonadism;   and (6) for chemotherapy of prostatic carcinoma (Kastrup, 1976).

The US Food & Drug Administration (1977) has ruled that with effect from 20 September 1977 oestrogens for general use must carry patient and physician warning labels concerning use, risks and contraindications.

2.2   Occurrence

Conjugated oestrogens are naturally occurring substances excreted in the urine of pregnant mares (Windholz, 1976).

Piperazine oestrone sulphate is not known to occur naturally.

2.3   Analysis

(a)   Conjugated oestrogens

Typical analytical methods for the determination of conjugated oestrogens are summarized in Table 1.   Abbreviations used are: GC/FID, gas chromatography/flame-ionization detection;   HPLC, high-pressure liquid chromatography;   CC, column chromatography;   TLC, thin-layer chromatography;   and UV, ultra-violet spectrometry.   See also the section, 'General Remarks on Sex Hormones', p. 60.

Table 1

Analytical methods for conjugated oestrogens

Sample matrix	Sample preparation	Assay procedure	Reference
Bulk chemical	Dissolve (water)	TLC (Silica gel G coated with silver nitrate; acid spray)	Crocker & Lodge (1972)
Bulk chemical	Dissolve (aqueous methanol)	HPLC (UV, 254 nm)	Musey et al. (1978)
Tablets; lyophilized cake & bulk chemical	Powder; dissolve (pH 5.2; acetate buffer); hydrolyse (sulphatase enzyme); extract (1,2-dichloroethane); derivatize (trimethylsilyl)	GC/FID	Johnson et al. (1975)
Tablets	Powder; CC (diatomaceous earth); hydrolyse; perform a complex series of extractions and washings	HPLC (UV, 280 nm)	Roos (1976)
Tablets	Powder; CC (diatomaceous earth); hydrolyse; perform a series of extractions and washings; treat with iron-phenol reagent	Colorimetry (350 nm–800 nm)	Horwitz (1975) US Pharmacopeial Convention Inc. (1975)
Pharmaceutical products	Dissolve	TLC (Silica gel G coated with silver nitrate); expose to sulphuryl chloride vapours & steam; UV (412 nm)	Schlemmer (1971)
Conjugated oestrogens added to urine	Add conjugated oestrogens to urine pretreated with an ion-exchange resin; evaporate & dissolve (aqueous methanol)	HPLC (UV, 254 nm)	Musey et al. (1978)

(b) Piperazine oestrone sulphate

Analytical methods for the determination of piperazine oestrone sulphate as a bulk chemical and in pharmaceutical preparations have been reviewed (Chang, 1976). Typical methods are summarized in Table 2. The abbreviation used is: UV, ultra-violet spectrometry.

TABLE 2

Analytical methods for piperazine oestrone sulphate

Sample matrix	Sample preparation	Assay procedure	Reference
Bulk chemical	Dissolve (sodium hydroxide); wash (chloroform); acidify (hydrochloric acid); neutralize (sodium hydroxide)	UV (238 nm)	National Formulary Board (1975)
Tablets	Powder; dissolve (water); wash (chloroform); acidify (hydrochloric acid); extract (chloroform); wash (sodium carbonate-water); filter; evaporate; dissolve (potassium hydroxide in 80% aqueous methanol)	UV (241 nm)	National Formulary Board (1975)

3.   Biological Data Relevant to the Evaluation
of Carcinogenic Risk to Humans

3.1   Carcinogenicity studies in animals

Oral administration

Rat: Groups of 20 male and 20 female weanling Sprague-Dawley rats were fed diets containing conjugated oestrogens (Premarin®) at concentrations resulting in intakes of 0, 0.07 and 0.7 mg/kg bw per day for 2 years. Survivors at 24 months were 9 male and 12 female controls, 13 males and 14 females given 0.07 mg/kg bw and 5 males and 6 females given 0.7 mg/kg bw. Mammary tumours, mainly fibroadenomas, occurred in 1 male rat treated with the low dose and in 3 treated with the high dose, compared with 0 in male controls, and in 4 females treated with the low dose and in 7 treated with the high dose, compared with 8 in female controls. The incidences of pituitary tumours in males were 2 in those given the low dose and 7 in those given the high dose, compared with 4 in controls; in females, the respective incidences were 9, 7 and 4. Thyroid carcinomas occurred in 2 females that received the low dose and in 1 female that received the high dose; no such tumours occurred in controls (Gibson *et al.*, 1967).

3.2   Other relevant biological data

No data were available on sodium equilin sulphate, a principal component of conjugated oestrogens, or on piperazine oestrone sulphate. Oestrone sulphate is rapidly taken up by isolated rat liver cells and hydrolysed to the free oestrogen. The oestrone formed is further converted *via* the pathways used by natural oestrogens (see monograph on oestradiol-17β, p. 279) (Höller *et al.*, 1977; Schwenk *et al.*, 1978).

Oestrone sulphate is a major oestrogen found in human plasma (Longcope, 1972; Ruder *et al.*, 1972). The metabolism of natural oestrogens in humans is discussed in the monograph on oestradiol-17β (p. 279).

No data on the toxicity, embryotoxicity or mutagenicity of conjugated oestrogens were available.

3.3   Case reports and epidemiological studies

See the section, 'Oestrogens and Progestins in Relation to Human Cancer', p. 83 and the monograph on diethylstilboestrol, p. 173.

4.   Summary of Data Reported and Evaluation[1]

4.1   Experimental data

Conjugated oestrogens (Premarin®) were tested in only one experiment in rats by oral administration. The data were insufficient to evaluate the carcinogenicity of this compound.

4.2   Human data

Case reports and epidemiological studies on steroid hormones used in oestrogen treatment have been summarized in the section, 'Oestrogens and Progestins in Relation to Human Cancer', p. 83. Because most of the studies which concerned endometrial carcinoma involved the use of conjugated oestrogens, the evidence in humans that administration of these agents is causally related to an increased risk of developing this cancer is particularly convincing.

4.3   Evaluation

The available experimental data are insufficient to evaluate the carcinogenicity of conjugated oestrogens in animals. Studies in humans strongly suggest that the administration specifically of conjugated oestrogens is causally related to an increased incidence of endometrial carcinoma.

---

[1]This section should be read in conjunction with pp. 62-64 in the 'General Remarks on Sex Hormones' and with the 'General Conclusions on Sex Hormones', p. 131.

5. References

Bates, R.W. & Cohen, H. (1951) Conjugated estrogen preparation. US
    Patent 2,565,115 (to E.R. Squibb & Sons) [Chem. Abstr., 46, 222h]

Chang, Z.L. (1976) Piperazine estrone sulfate. In: Florey, K., ed.,
    Analytical Profiles of Drug Substances, Vol. 5, New York, Academic
    Press, pp. 375-402

Crocker, L.E. & Lodge, B.A. (1972) Thin-layer chromatographic separation
    of conjugated estrogens on Silica Gel G-silver nitrate plates.
    J. Chromatogr., 69, 419-420

Gibson, J.P., Newberne, J.W., Kuhn, W.L. & Elsea, J.R. (1967) Comparative
    chronic toxicity of three oral estrogens in rats. Toxicol. appl.
    Pharmacol., 11, 489-510

Harvey, S.C. (1975) Hormones. In: Osol, A. et al., eds, Remington's
    Pharmaceutical Sciences, 15th ed., Easton, PA, Mack, pp. 915-917

Hüller, M., Grochtmann, W., Napp, M. & Breuer, H. (1977) Studies on the
    metabolism of estrone sulphate. Comparative perfusions of oestrone
    and oestrone sulphate through isolated rat livers. Biochem. J., 166,
    363-371

Horwitz, W., ed (1975) Official Methods of Analysis of the Association
    of Official Analytical Chemists, 12th ed., Washington DC, Association
    of Official Analytical Chemists, pp. 742-743

Johnson, R., Masserano, R., Haring, R., Kho, B. & Schilling, G. (1975)
    Quantitative GLC determination of conjugated estrogens in raw materials
    and finished dosage forms. J. pharm. Sci., 64, 1007-1011

Kastrup, E.K., ed. (1976) Facts and Comparisons, St Louis, MO, Facts &
    Comparisons Inc., pp. 100c, 102

Kastrup, E.K., ed. (1977) Facts and Comparisons, St Louis, MO, Facts &
    Comparisons Inc., pp. 99a, 100, 114

Kastrup, E.K., ed. (1978) Facts and Comparisons, St Louis, MO, Facts &
    Comparisons Inc., p. 103

Longcope, C. (1972) The metabolism of estrone sulfate in normal males.
    J. clin. Endocrinol. Metab., 34, 113-122

Miller, A. (1976) Cosmetic ingredients. Household and Personal Products
    Industry, October, p. 62

Murad, F. & Gilman, A.G. (1975) Estrogens and progestins. In: Goodman, L.S. & Gilman, A., eds, The Pharmacological Basis of Therapeutics, 5th ed., New York, Macmillan, p. 1423

Musey, P.I., Collins, D.C. & Preedy, J.R.K. (1978) Separation of estrogen conjugates by high pressure liquid chromatography. Steroids, 31, 583-592

National Formulary Board (1975) National Formulary, 14th ed., Washington DC, American Pharmaceutical Association, pp. 579-581

Roos, R.W. (1976) Determination of conjugated and esterified estrogens in pharmaceutical tablet dosage forms by high-pressure, normal-phase partition chromatography. J. chromatogr. Sci., 14, 505-512

Ruder, H.J., Loriaux, L. & Lipsett, M.B. (1972) Estrone sulfate: production rate and metabolism in man. J. clin. Invest., 51, 1020-1033

Schlemmer, W. (1971) Quantitative thin-layer chromatography. Assay of drug mixtures by scanning of remission peaks. J. Chromatogr., 63, 121-129

Schwenk, M., López del Pino, V. & Bolt, H.M. (1978) Metabolism and disposition of 17α-ethinyloestradiol and oestrone sulfate in isolated rat liver cells (Abstract no. 39). Acta endocrinol., Suppl. 215, 42-43

US Food & Drug Administration (1977) Patient labeling for estrogens for general use. Drugs for human use; drug efficacy study implementation. Fed. Regist., 42, 37645-37646

US International Trade Commission (1977a) Synthetic Organic Chemicals, US Production and Sales, 1975, USITC Publication 804, Washington DC, US Government Printing Office, pp. 90, 102

US International Trade Commission (1977b) Synthetic Organic Chemicals, US Production and Sales, 1976, USITC Publication 833, Washington DC, US Government Printing Office, p. 148

US Pharmacopeial Convention Inc. (1975) The US Pharmacopeia, 19th rev., Rockville, MD, pp. 181-183

US Tariff Commission (1951) Synthetic Organic Chemicals, US Production and Sales, 1950, Report No. 173, Second Series, Washington DC, US Government Printing Office, p. 102

US Tariff Commission (1960) Synthetic Organic Chemicals, US Production and Sales, 1959, Report No. 206, Second Series, Washington DC, US Government Printing Office, p. 116

US Tariff Commission (1970) Synthetic Organic Chemicals, US Production
    and Sales, 1968, TC Publication 327, Washington DC, US Government
    Printing Office, p. 125

Wade, A., ed. (1977) Martindale, The Extra Pharmacopoeia, 27th ed., London,
    The Pharmaceutical Press, pp. 1419-1420, 1422

Windholz, M., ed. (1976) The Merck Index, 9th ed., Rahway, NJ, Merck &
    Co., p. 323

DIENOESTROL

1. Chemical and Physical Data

1.1 Synonyms and trade names

Chem. Abstr. Services Reg. No.: 84-17-3

Chem. Abstr. Name: 4,4'-(1,2-Diethylidene-1,2-ethanediyl)bisphenol

Synonyms: 3,4-Bis(4-hydroxyphenyl)-2,4-hexadiene; 3,4-bis(*para*-hydroxyphenyl)-2,4-hexadiene; dehydrostilbestrol; dehydrostilboestrol; dienestrol; 4,4'-(diethylideneethylene)diphenol; *para,para*'-(diethylideneethylene)diphenol; 4,4'-dihydroxy-γ,δ-diphenyl-β,δ-hexadiene; di(*para*-oxyphenyl)-2,4-hexadiene; estrodienol; oestrodienol

Trade names: Agaldog; Cycladiène; Dienol; Dinovex; DV; Estraguard; Estroral; Follidiene; Follormon; Gynefollin; Hormofemin; Isodienestrol; Oestrasid; Oestrodiene; Oestroral; Oestrovis; Para-dien; Restrol; Retalon; Sexadien; Synestrol; Teserene; Willnestrol

1.2 Structural and molecular formulae and molecular weight

$C_{18}H_{18}O_2$ Mol. wt: 266.3

1.3 Chemical and physical properties

From Wade (1977) and Windholz (1976)

(a) Description: White needles (from ethanol)

(b) Melting-point: 227-228°C; sublimes at 130°C and 1 mm; sublimate melting-point, 231-234°C

(c) Solubility: Practically insoluble in water; soluble in ethanol (1 in 8), acetone (1 in 5) and diethyl ether (1 in 15); also soluble in methanol, propylene glycol, fixed oils and solutions of alkaline hydroxides; slightly soluble in chloroform

1.4 Technical products and impurities

Various national and international pharmacopoeias give specifications for the purity of dienoestrol in pharmaceutical products. For example, dienoestrol is available in the US as a NF grade containing 98.0-100.5% active ingredient on a dried basis. Creams in 0.01% doses and tablets in 0.1 and 0.5 mg doses contain 90-110% of the stated amount of dienoestrol (National Formulary Board, 1975). It is also available in the US in 0.25 mg tablets and in foam (0.01%) in an oil-in-water emulsion (Kastrup, 1976, 1978).

Dienoestrol available in Europe contains 98.5-101.5% active ingredient on a dried basis (Council of Europe, 1975).

In the UK, dienoestrol is available in creams (0.1 mg/g and 0.16% doses) and compounded (0.16 mg) with phenobarbitone (10 mg), theobromine (50 mg), calcium lactate (150 mg) or bromvaletone (30 mg) (Wade, 1977).

2. Production, Use, Occurrence and Analysis

2.1 Production and use

(a) Production

A method for synthesizing dienoestrol was first reported in 1939 (Dodds *et al.*, 1939). It can be prepared from diethylstilboestrol diacetate by bromination to the dibromo derivative, which is dehydro-brominated (by refluxing with pyridine) to dienoestrol diacetate and saponified to yield dienoestrol (Harvey, 1975). It is not known whether this method is used for commercial production.

Commercial production of dienoestrol diacetate in the US was first reported in 1964 (US Tariff Commission, 1965) and was last reported in 1972 (US Tariff Commission, 1974). US imports of dienoestrol through principal US customs districts amounted to 20 kg in 1974 and 1975 (US International Trade Commission, 1976, 1977a) and to 19 kg in 1976 (US International Trade Commission, 1977b).

Dienoestrol is believed to be produced commercially in Italy and the UK, and its acetate is manufactured in Italy, but no information was available on the quantities produced.

Dienoestrol is not produced in Japan, and there is no evidence that it has been imported in recent years.

(b) Use

Dienoestrol is used in human medicine for treatment of postmenopausal symptoms and for replacement therapy following ovariectomy, in oral doses of 0.1-0.5 mg per day for mild to moderate symptoms and 1-1.5 mg per day for severe symptoms, with gradual downward adjustment to the lowest effective maintenance dose. Creams and suppositories are used locally to treat vulvar dystrophies associated with the climacteric, in doses of 0.01% cream or 0.7 mg suppositories 1 or 2 times a day for 7-14 days, gradually diminished to 1-3 times a week. Dienoestrol is also administered orally: (1) for the treatment of dysfunctional uterine bleeding, in doses of 5-20 mg 4 times per day until bleeding stops, followed by 10 mg per day for 25 days (which may be repeated for another 25 days if withdrawal bleeding is excessive); (2) to prevent post-partum breast engorgement, in a dose of 1.5 mg per day for 3 days, then 0.5 mg per day for 7 days; (3) for the treatment of breast cancer in postmenopausal women, in a dose of 15 mg daily; and (4) for treatment of prostatic cancer, in a dose of 5-15 mg daily (Harvey, 1975).

Dienestrol does not appear to have been used in Japan in recent years. No data on its use in Europe were available.

The US Food & Drug Administration (1977) has ruled that with effect from 20 September 1977 oestrogens for general use must carry patient and physician warning labels concerning use, risks and contraindications.

2.2 Occurrence

Dienoestrol is not known to occur naturally.

2.3 Analysis

Typical analytical methods for the determination of dienoestrol are summarized in Table 1. Abbreviations used are: HPLC, high-pressure liquid chromatography; CC, column chromatography; TLC, thin-layer chromatography; and UV, ultra-violet spectrometry. See also section, 'General Remarks on Sex Hormones', p. 60.

Table 1

Analytical methods for dienoestrol

Sample matrix	Sample preparation	Assay procedure	Sensitivity or limit of detection	Reference
Bulk chemical	Acetylate (acetic anhydride-pyridine); add water	Titration (sodium hydroxide)	–	British Pharmacopoeia Commission (1973) Council of Europe (1975)
Bulk chemical	Dissolve (acetonitrile-heptane); CC (diatomaceous earth-acetonitrile column); elute (heptane-chloroform); evaporate; dissolve in ethanol	UV	–	Graham & Kenner (1973)
Bulk chemical	Add 0.3M tripotassium phosphate; CC (2 diatomaceous earth columns in series); evaporate; dissolve (methanol); add methanolic sulphuric acid	UV (240-400 nm)	–	Horwitz (1975, 1977)
Bulk chemical	Acetylate (acetic anhydride-pyridine); add water; refrigerate; collect precipitate	Gravimetry	–	National Formulary Board (1975)
Tablets	Powder; dissolve (diethyl ether); evaporate; dissolve (aqueous ethanol); add hydrochloric acid & sodium molybdotungstophosphate solution; add sodium carbonate solution	Colorimetry (750 nm)	–	British Pharmacopoeia Commission (1973)

Table 1 (continued)

Sample matrix	Sample preparation	Assay procedure	Sensitivity or limit of detection	Reference
Tablets	Powder; CC (silica gel); evaporate; dissolve (acetate buffer, sulphuric acid & sodium nitrite); add electrolyte solution	Polarography	–	National Formulary Board (1975)
Tablets	Powder; dissolve (methanol)	HPLC (UV, 254 nm)	ng level	Roos (1974)
Cream	Separate (a complex series of extractions & washings); CC (silica gel); dissolve (acetic acid, sulphuric acid & sodium nitrate); add electrolyte solution	Polarography	–	National Formulary Board (1975)
Creams	Dissolve (methanol:diethyl ether, 1:1)	HPLC (UV, 254 nm)	ng level	Roos (1974)
Cottonseed-oil formulation	Dissolve (dimethylformamide: methanol, 1:1)	HPLC (UV, 254 nm)	ng level	Roos (1974)
Suppositories	Dissolve (methanol:diethyl ether, 1:1)	HPLC (UV, 254 nm)	ng level	Roos (1974)
Serum	Extract	HPLC	2 ng/20 mm^3	Hesse et al. (1977)
Serum	Extract	TLC; UV-densitometry (287 nm) High-performance TLC; UV-densitometry (287 nm)	50 ng 10 ng	Jarc et al. (1977)
Animal tissue	Extract	TLC; UV-densitometry (287 nm) High-performance TLC; UV-densitometry (287 nm)	50 ng 10 ng	Jarc et al. (1977)

3. Biological Data Relevant to the Evaluation of Carcinogenic Risk to Humans

3.1 Carcinogenicity studies in animals

(a) Subcutaneous and/or intramuscular administration

Guinea-pig: One hundred and twenty-five female guinea-pigs (65 ovariectomized and 60 intact) were given dienoestrol subcutaneously in daily doses of 1 mg/kg bw and sacrificed at different times. Uterine leiomyomas were found microscopically in 8/23 animals killed between 31-60 days, in 12/18 animals killed between 61-90 days and in 12/25 animals killed after 90 days of treatment. Such tumours were observed only in 2/18 ovariectomized animals killed between 61-90 days and in 6/25 killed after 90 days. In addition, 6 extragenital tumours were found, but their localization was not specified. No tumours were found in a total of 20 intact and 20 ovariectomized controls sacrificed at similar times (Zhuravleva & Melnikov, 1973) [The Working Group questioned the basis for tumour diagnosis].

(b) Other experimental systems

Vaginal instillation: Thirty-seven female virgin CC57W mice received dienoestrol in polyurethane tampons once or twice weekly in the vagina as either 30 insertions within 120 days (total mean dose, 0.46 mg/mouse) or 60 insertions within 273 days (total mean dose, 0.735 mg/mouse). Of 28 cases of hyperplasia of ovarian granulosa cells, 15 were classified as ovarian tumours (folliculomas); no such lesions were seen among 41 controls given polyurethane tampons alone. The incidence of tumours in relation to duration of experiment and dose received was not specified. Papillomas of the vagina were found in 29/29 treated mice and in 28/41 controls (Volfson, 1974, 1976) [The Working Group noted the insufficient reporting of the experiment].

3.2 Other relevant biological data

No data on the toxicity of dienoestrol were available to the Working Group.

Dienoestrol is a known metabolite of diethylstilboestrol in primates and mice; it is converted to ω-hydroxy-dienoestrol, which is excreted in conjugated form (predominantly as glucuronides) (Metzler & McLachlan, 1978; Metzler et al., 1977; and see monograph on diethylstilboestrol, p. 173). Rabbits given oral doses of dienoestrol excreted dienoestrol glucuronide in their urine (Dodgson et al., 1948).

Dienoestrol induced sister chromatid exchanges in cultured human fibroblasts; however, it was not mutagenic in 4 *Salmonella typhimurium* strains either in the presence or absence of a rat liver homogenate (Glatt *et al.*, 1979; Rüdiger *et al.*, 1979).

Dienoestrol is chemically similar to diethylstilboestrol and has also been used, although to a smaller extent, in pregnancy therapy. It is believed to be associated with the same abnormalities as occur in offspring exposed *in utero* to diethylstilboestrol (see monograph p. 173). However, no data on the embryotoxicity or teratogenicity of dienoestrol were available.

3.3 Case reports and epidemiological studies

One case of adenocarcinoma of the vagina has been reported in a young girl, 17-years old, whose mother had taken 5 mg per day dienoestrol orally and 2 i.m. doses of oestrone during the 3rd month of pregnancy (Greenwald *et al.*, 1971).

See also the section, 'Oestrogens and Progestins in Relation to Human Cancer', p. 83.

4. Summary of Data Reported and Evaluation[1]

4.1 Experimental data

Dienoestrol was tested in female guinea-pigs by subcutaneous injection and in female mice by intravaginal administration. Although pointing to the induction of 'uterine tumours' in guinea-pigs and ovarian tumours in mice, these experiments were insufficient to evaluate the carcinogenicity of this compound.

4.2 Human data

No case reports or epidemiological studies on dienoestrol alone were available to the Working Group. Case reports and epidemiological studies on steroid hormones used in oestrogen treatment have been summarized in the section, 'Oestrogens and Progestins in Relation to Human Cancer', p. 83.

---

[1]This section should be read in conjunction with pp. 62-64 of the 'General Remarks on Sex Hormones' and with the 'General Conclusions on Sex Hormones', p. 131.

4.3 <u>Evaluation</u>

The available experimental data are insufficient to evaluate the
carcinogenicity of dienoestrol in animals. Studies in humans strongly
suggest that the administration of oestrogens is causally related to an
increased incidence of endometrial carcinoma; there is no evidence that
dienoestrol is different from other oestrogens in this respect.

5. References

British Pharmacopoeia Commission (1973) British Pharmacopoeia, London, HMSO, pp. 159160

Council of Europe (1975) European Pharmacopoeia, Vol. III, Sainte-Ruffine, France, pp. 207-208

Dodds, E.C., Golberg, L., Lawson, W. & Robinson, R. (1939) Synthetic estrogenic compounds related to stilbene and diphenylethane. I. Proc. R. Soc. (Lond.), B127, 140-167 [Chem. Abstr., 33, 6412(5)]

Dodgson, K.S., Garton, G.A., Stubbs, A.L. & Williams, R.T. (1948) Studies in detoxication. XV. On the glucuronides of stilboestrol, hexoestrol and dienoestrol. Biochem. J., 42, 357-365

Glatt, H.R., Metzler, M. & Oesch, F. (1979) Diethylstilbestrol and 11 derivatives. A mutagenicity study with Salmonella typhimurium. Mutat. Res., 67, 113-121

Graham, R.E. & Kenner, C.T. (1973) Acetonitrile-diatomaceous earth column for separation of steroids and other compounds. J. pharm. Sci., 62, 1845-1849

Greenwald, P., Barlow, J.J., Nasca, P.C. & Burnett, W.S. (1971) Vaginal cancer after maternal treatment with synthetic estrogens. N. Engl. J. Med., 285, 390-392

Harvey, S.C. (1975) Hormones. In: Osol, A. et al., eds, Remington's Pharmaceutical Sciences, 15th ed., Easton, PA, Mack, p. 918

Hesse, C., Pietrzik, K. & Hützel, D. (1977) Identification and estimation of diethylstilboestrol and dienoestrol by high-speed liquid chromatograpy (Ger.). Chromatographia, 10, 256-261

Horwitz, W., ed. (1975) Official Methods of Analysis of the Association of Official Analytical Chemists, 12th ed., Washington DC, Association of Official Analytical Chemists, p. 746

Horwitz, W. (1977) Dienestrol. J. Assoc. off. anal. Chem., 60, 482

Jarc, H., Ruttner, O. & Krocza, W. (1977) The quantitative detection of oestrogens and antithyroid drugs by thin-layer and high-performance thin-layer chromatography in animal tissue (Ger.). J. Chromatogr., 134, 351-358

Kastrup, E.K., ed. (1976) Facts and Comparisons, St Louis, MO, Facts & Comparisons Inc., p. 101a

Kastrup, E.K., ed. (1978) Facts and Comparisons, St Louis, MO, Facts &
    Comparisons Inc., p. 103

Metzler, M. & McLachlan, J.A. (1978) Oxidative metabolites of
    diethylstilbestrol in the fetal, neonatal and adult mice. Biochem.
    Pharmacol., 27, 1087-1094

Metzler, M., Müller, W. & Hobson, W.C. (1977) Biotransformation of
    diethylstilbestrol in the rhesus monkey and the chimpanzee. J.
    Toxicol. environ. Health, 3, 439-450

National Formulary Board (1975) National Formulary, 14th ed.,
    Washington DC, American Pharmaceutical Association, pp. 200-203

Roos, R.W. (1974) Identification and determination of synthetic estrogens
    in pharmaceuticals by high-speed, reversed-phase partition chroma-
    tography. J. pharm. Sci., 63, 594-599

Rüdiger, H.W., Haenisch, F., Metzler, M., Glatt, H.R. & Oesch, F. (1979)
    Activation of diethylstilbestrol to metabolites which induce sister
    chromatid exchanges in human cultured fibroblasts. Science (in
    press)

US Food & Drug Administration (1977) Patient labeling for estrogens
    for general use. Drugs for human use; drug efficacy study
    implementation. Fed. Regist., 42, 37645-37646

US International Trade Commission (1976) Imports of Benzenoid Chemicals
    and Products, 1974, USITC Publication 762, Washington DC, US
    Government Printing Office, p. 82

US International Trade Commission (1977a) Imports of Benzenoid Chemicals
    and Products, 1975, USITC Publication 806, Washington DC, US
    Government Printing Office, p. 83

US International Trade Commission (1977b) Imports of Benzenoid Chemicals
    and Products, 1976, USITC Publication 828, Washington DC, US
    Government Printing Office, p. 88

US Tariff Commission (1965) Synthetic Organic Chemicals, US Production
    and Sales, 1964, TC Publication 167, Washington DC, US Government
    Printing Office, p. 130

US Tariff Commission (1974) Synthetic Organic Chemicals, US Production
    and Sales, 1972, TC Publication 681, Washington DC, US Government
    Printing Office, p. 116

Volfson, N.I. (1974) The blastomogenic action of sinestrol during intra-
    vaginal insertions. Neoplasma, 21, 569-576

Volfson, N.I. (1976) On the genesis of experimental granulosa cell tumors of the ovary. Vop. Onkol., 22, 68-75

Wade, A., ed. (1977) Martindale, The Extra Pharmacopoeia, 27th ed., London, The Pharmaceutical Press, p. 1395

Windholz, M., ed. (1976) The Merck Index, 9th ed., Rahway, NJ, Merck & Co., p. 410

Zhuravleva, T.B. & Melnikov, Y.G. (1973) Morphogenesis of experimental myomas of the uterus. Arkhiv. Patol., 35, 38-44

DIETHYLSTILBOESTROL and DIETHYLSTILBOESTROL DIPROPIONATE

A monograph on diethylstilboestrol was published previously (IARC, 1974). Relevant data that have appeared since that time have been evaluated in the present monograph.

A review is available (Young, 1978).

1. Chemical and Physical Data

Diethylstilboestrol

1.1 Synonyms and trade names

Chem. Abstr. Services Reg. No.: 56-53-1

Chem. Abstr. Name: (E)-4,4'-(1,2-Diethyl-1,2-ethenediyl)bisphenol

Synonyms: 3,4-Bis(*para*-hydroxyphenyl)-3-hexene; DEB; DES; α,α'-diethylstilbenediol; (E)-α,α'-diethyl-4,4'-stilbenediol; *trans*-α,α'-diethyl-4,4'-stilbenediol; *trans*-diethylstilbesterol; diethylstilbestrol; *trans*-diethylstilbestrol; *trans*-diethyl-stilboestrol; 4,4'-dihydroxydiethylstilbene; 4,4'-dihydroxy-α,β-diethylstilbene; stilbestrol; stilboestrol

Trade names[1]: Acnestrol; Antigestil; Bio-des; Bufon; [Climaterine]; Comestrol; Cyren; Cyren A; Dawe's destrol; Desma; Destrol; DiBestrol '2' Premix; Dicorvin; DiEstryl; Distilbene; Domestrol; [Estilben]; Estilbin 'MCO'; [Estril]; Estrobene; Estromenin; Estrosyn; [Follidiene]; Fonatol; Grafestrol; Gynopharm; Hi-Bestrol; Idroestril; Iscovesco; Menostilbeen; Microest; Milestrol; Neo-Oestranol I; Oekolp; Oestrogen; Oestrogenine; Oestrol Vetag; Oestromenin;

---

[1]Those in square brackets are preparations that are no longer produced commercially.

[Oestromensil]; Oestromensyl; [Oestromienin]; Oestromon;
Pabestrol; Palestrol; Percutatrine Oestrogénique Iscovesco;
[Protectona]; Rumestrol 1; Rumestrol 2; Sedestran; Serral;
Sexocretin; Sibol; Sintestrol; Stibilium; Stil;
Stilbetin; Stilboefral; Stilboestroform; Stilbofollin; Stilbol;
Stilkap; Stil-Rol; Synestrin; Synthoestrin; Synthofolin;
Syntofolin; Tampovagan Stilboestrol; Tylosterone; Vagestrol

1.2 Structural and molecular formulae and molecular weight

$C_{18}H_{20}O_2$ Mol. wt: 268.3

1.3 Chemical and physical properties

From Windholz (1976), unless otherwise specified

(a) Description: White platelets (from benzene)

(b) Melting-point: 169-172°C

(c) Spectroscopy data: Infra-red spectral data have been tabulated
(Grasselli & Ritchey, 1975).

(d) Solubility: Practically insoluble in water (1 in 40,000)
(Madan & Cadwallader, 1973); soluble in ethanol (1 in 5),
chloroform (1 in 200), diethyl ether (1 in 3), arachis oil
(1 in 40) and olive oil (1 in 90); also soluble in acetone,
dioxane, ethyl acetate, fixed oils, methanol and aqueous
solutions of alkaline hydroxides (Wade, 1977)

(e) Stability: The diethylstilboestrol (DES) used commercially is the *trans*-isomer; the *cis*-isomer is obtained with difficulty and tends to revert to the *trans*-form (Stecher, 1968).

1.4 Technical products and impurities

Various national and international pharmacopoeias give specifications for the purity of DES in pharmaceutical products. For example, it is available in the US as a USP grade containing 97.0–100.5% active ingredient on a dried basis. Injections in 5 and 25 mg/ml doses in vegetable oil, suppositories in 0.1, 0.5 and 1 mg doses and tablets in 0.1, 0.25, 0.5, 1, 5, 10, 25, 50 and 100 mg doses contain 90–110% of the stated amount of DES (US Pharmacopeial Convention Inc., 1975). It is also available in the US in tablets combined with methyltestosterone (Kastrup, 1976, 1977, 1978). It is formulated as pellet implants and as a feed additive to stimulate growth in food animals for human consumption (Young, 1978).

In the UK, DES is available in 0.5, 1.5 and 25 mg tablets and combined (0.1 mg) with 16 mg phenobarbitone; it is also available in pessaries containing 0.5 mg DES (Wade, 1977).

Diethylstilboestrol dipropionate

1.1 Synonyms and trade names

Chem. Abstr. Services Reg. No.: 130-80-3

Chem. Abstr. Name: (E)-4,4'-(1,2-Diethyl-1,2-ethenediyl)bisphenol dipropionate

Synonyms: α,α'-Diethyl-4,4'-stilbenediol dipropionate; (E)-α,α'-diethyl-4,4'-stilbenediol dipropionate; α,α'-diethyl-4,4'-stilbenediol *trans*-dipropionate; α,α'-diethyl-4,4'-stilbenediol dipropionyl ester; diethylstilbene dipropionate; diethylstilbesterol dipropionate; diethylstilbestrol dipropionate; diethylstilbestrol propionate; diethylstilboestrol dipropionate; diethylstilboestrol propionate; dihydroxydiethylstilbene dipropionate; *para*, *para*'-dipropionoxy-*trans*-α,β-diethylstilbene; stilbestrol dipropionate; stilbestrol propionate; stilboestrol dipropionate

Trade names: Clinestrol; Cyren B; Dibestil; Estilben; Estilbin; Estroben DF; Estrobene DP; Estrogenin; Estrostilben; Euvestin; Gynolett; Horfemine; Neo-Oestranol II; Neo-Oestronol II; New-Oestranol 11; Oestrogynaedron; Orestol; Pabestrol D; Sinciclan; Stilbestronate; Stilboestrol DP; Stilbofax; Stilronate; Synoestron; Syntestrin; Syntestrine; Willestrol

1.2 Structural and molecular formulae and molecular weight

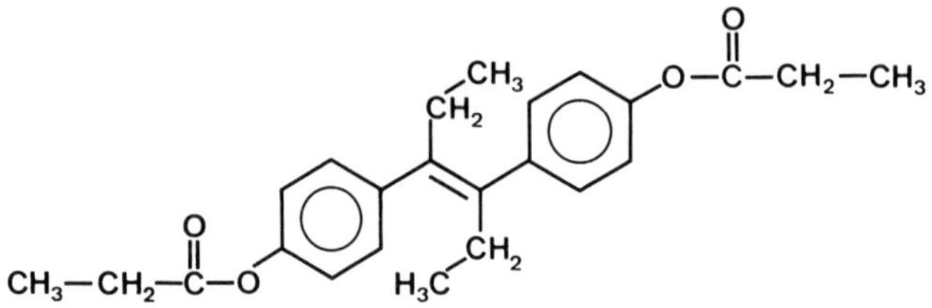

$C_{24}H_{28}O_4$ Mol. wt: 380.41

1.3 Chemical and physical properties

From Wade (1977)

(a) Description: Odourless, tasteless, colourless crystals or white crystalline powder

(b) Melting-point: 105-107°C

(c) Solubility: Soluble in 90% ethanol (1 in 100), diethyl ether (1 in 6), olive oil (1 in 45); also soluble in fixed oils, acetone and chloroform; very slightly soluble in water; insoluble in solutions of alkaline hydroxides

1.4 Technical products and impurities

Various national and international pharmacopoeias give specifications for the purity of diethylstilboestrol dipropionate in pharmaceutical products. For example, it is available in the US as a NF grade containing 98.0-100.5% active ingredient on a dried basis. Tablets in 0.5, 1 and 5 mg doses contain 90-110% of the stated amount (National Formulary Board, 1975).

2. Production, Use, Occurrence and Analysis

2.1 Production and use

(a) Production

Synthesis of DES was first reported by Dodds *et al.* (1938). The following starting materials can be used in its preparation: deoxy-anisoin, *para*-anisaldehyde, anisole or anethole hydrobromide (Dorfman, 1966; Windholz, 1976). It has been produced commercially in the US by converting *para*-anisoin to ethyldeoxyanisoin and further rearrangement to DES (Young, 1978).

The synthesis of diethylstilboestrol dipropionate was first reported in 1939 (Dodds *et al.*, 1939). It can be prepared by treatment of DES with propionic anhydride in the presence of pyridine.

Commercial production of DES in the US was first reported in 1941 (US Tariff Commission, 1945). In 1975, only two US companies reported production of an undisclosed amount (see preamble, p. 20); however, production of 13 oestrogen and progestin substances, including DES, in that year amounted to 10.5 thousand kg (US International Trade Commission, 1977a). In 1976, only one US company reported production of an undisclosed amount (US International Trade Commission, 1977b).

In 1966 and 1967, only one US company reported commercial production of diethylstilboestrol dipropionate (US Tariff Commission, 1968, 1969).

US imports of DES through principal US customs districts amounted to 6.2 thousand kg in 1974 (US International Trade Commission, 1976), 5.6 thousand kg in 1975 (US International Trade Commission, 1977c) and 5.9 thousand kg in 1976 (US International Trade Commission, 1977d). Data on US exports are not available.

Between 10-100 thousand kg DES are believed to be produced annually in western Europe. Italy is believed to be the major producer, with 1-10 thousand kg produced in France, less than 1 thousand kg in the Federal Republic of Germany and an unknown quantity in the UK.

Diethylstilboestrol dipropionate is believed to be produced commercially in Italy and the UK, but no information was available on the quantities produced.

DES is not produced in Japan, and there is no evidence that it has been imported recently.

(b) Use

In human medicine, DES is used for the treatment of symptoms arising
during the climacteric and following ovariectomy, in an oral dose of
0.1-0.5 mg per day in a cyclic regimen. For senile vaginitis and vulvar
dystrophy, it is given in an oral dose of 1 mg per day, or, for vulvar
dystrophies and atrophic vaginitis, in suppository form in a dose of up
to 1 mg per day. DES is employed as a post-coital emergency contraceptive
('morning-after pill') in an oral dose of 25 mg twice a day for 5 days
starting within 72 hours of insemination. It has been used for the
prevention of post-partum breast engorgement, in an oral dose of 5 mg 1-
3 times per day for a total of 30 mg and may be given in combination
with methyltestosterone. It is used for chemotherapy of advanced carcinoma
of the breast in an oral dose of 15 mg per day, and for carcinoma of the
prostate in an initial oral dose of 1-3 mg per day, which may be reduced
to 1 mg per day. For dysfunctional uterine bleeding, DES is given in an
oral dose of 5 mg 3-5 times per day until bleeding stops. It is also
used for the treatment of female hypogonadism, in an oral dose of 1 mg
per day (Harvey, 1975; Wade, 1977).

Diethylstilboestrol dipropionate is transformed to DES in the body
and has similar uses in human medicine; the only differences between
the two are in the solubility and rate of absorption. It is given most
often in cases where DES is not tolerated. The usual dose is 0.1-1 mg
daily, given orally, by i.m. injection or applied locally in ointments
(Wade, 1977).

Fosfestrol (diethylstilboestrol diphosphate; Honvan$^{®}$), a
derivative of DES, is also used in chemotherapy of prostatic cancer
(Harvey, 1975). It was first used for the maintenance of pregnancy in
1948 (see also section 3.3).

DES is used in veterinary medicine in replacement therapy for
underdeveloped females, in incontinence and vaginitis of spayed bitches,
to induce heat in anoestrus, for uterine inertia and pyometra, to prevent
conception in mismated bitches and to check milk secretion in pseudopregnancy. It is used for prostatic hypertrophy in dogs. I.m. doses
for these purposes are as follows: horses (10-25 mg), cows, heifers and
small breeds (10-20 mg), large breeds (20-25 mg), sheep (2-3 mg), swine
(3-10 mg) and dogs (0.2-1 mg; may also be given orally) (Harvey, 1975).

It was first used as a growth promoter in poultry (McMartin et al.,
1978) and in beef cattle (Jukes, 1976). New drug applications were
approved in 1954 and 1955 for feeding of DES at the rate of 10 mg per
head per day and for the s.c. implantation of 72 mg DES to beef cattle
(Umberger, 1975). DES is now used in only 60% of steers, rather than in
90% as reported earlier (Anon., 1978).

As of June 1978, DES was permitted for use in human medicine as follows: (1) replacement therapy of oestrogen deficiencies associated with the climacteric and other hormone-related conditions; (2) control of functional menstrual disorders; (3) prevention of post-partum breast engorgement; (4) chemotherapy of prostate cancer and breast cancer in postmenopausal women; and (5) as a 'morning-after pill' in emergency situations such as rape and incest. It is also permitted as a growth promoter for cattle and sheep under the following conditions: (1) when used as a feed additive, levels used may not exceed 20 mg per day for cattle and 2 mg per day for sheep, and DES must be withdrawn from the diet at least 14 days prior to slaughter; and (2) ear implants in sheep and cattle should be inserted no less than 120 days before slaughter (Young, 1978). No residues should occur in the uncooked edible tissue of cattle and sheep after slaughter or in any food derived from the living animal (US Food & Drug Administration, 1978). However, its use in other applications is believed to be continuing, pending the outcome of a court action.

In the UK, DES is not permitted to be added to animal feed but is available as an implant for growth promotion. The use of DES as a growth promoter for cattle is reported to have been banned in Australia, Canada, the Federal Republic of Germany, Japan (Maugh, 1976) and Austria (Stöckl *et al.*, 1978).

The US Food & Drug Administration (1977) has ruled that with effect from 20 September 1977 oestrogens for general use must carry patient and physician warning labels concerning use, risks and contraindications.

2.2 Occurrence

DES and diethylstilboestrol dipropionate are not known to occur naturally.

(a) Occupational exposure

Air samples collected inside the plastic suits of full-time workers in a plant manufacturing DES contained concentrations of 0.4-1.8 $\mu g/m^3$ DES; two sets of air samples collected in areas outside the main workroom contained 0.2 $\mu g/m^3$ and 12.8 $\mu g/m^3$ (Young, 1978). An air sample taken in a finishing room contained 24 $\mu g/m^3$ DES. Air samples taken in the ambient air of three plants where DES was mixed with animal feed contained 0.02-1.03 $\mu g/m^3$ (Young, 1978).

(b) Food residues

DES residues were detected at levels of less than 2 $\mu g/kg$ in 2 and 0.5% of beef livers assayed in 1972 and 1973 by the US Department of Agriculture (Jukes, 1976; Mussman, 1975); it was estimated that the

possible level in beef muscle is about 1/10 that found in the liver
(Jukes, 1974). In the same years, residues were detected in less than
2% of 1900 sheep livers examined (Mussman, 1975). From 1973 to June
1976, no residues of DES were detected at the 0.5 µg/kg level of sensitivity
in 99.4% of 9426 beef livers analysed (Anon., 1977).

(c) Water

DES has been found in certain drinking-water samples at levels of
0.11-0.26 ng/l (Rurainski *et al*., 1977). However, it did not appear on
a list of carcinogens and mutagens identified in water supplies in the
US and Europe, in which 1728 contaminants were identified (Kraybill *et
al*., 1977).

2.3 Analysis

Typical analytical methods for determination of DES are summarized
in Table 1. Abbreviations used are: GC/FID, gas chromatography/flame-
ionization detection; GC/ECD, gas chromatography/electron-capture
detection; GC/MS, gas chromatography/mass spectrometry; HPLC, high-
pressure liquid chromatography; CC, column chromatography; TLC, thin-
layer chromatography; UV, ultra-violet spectrometry; FL, fluorimetry;
and RIA, radioimmunoassay. See also 'General Remarks on Sex Hormones',
p. 60.

TABLE 1

Analytical methods for Diethylstilboestrol

Sample matrix	Sample preparation	Assay procedure	Sensitivity or limit of detection	Reference
Bulk chemical	Dissolve (ethanol); add aqueous dipotassium phosphate solution & irradiate	UV (418 nm)	—	British Pharmacopoeia Commission (1973); Council of Europe (1975); US Pharmacopeial Convention Inc. (1975)
Tablets	Powder; extract (ethanol); centrifuge; add dipotassium phosphate solution & irradiate	UV (418 nm)	—	British Pharmacopoeia Commission (1973)
Tablets	Powder; extract (chloroform-aqueous acid); wash (water); evaporate; dissolve (ethanol); add dipotassium phosphate solution & irradiate	UV (418 nm)	—	Horwitz (1975)
Tablets	Powder; dissolve (methanol)	HPLC (UV, 254 nm)	—	Roos (1974)
Tablets	Powder; dissolve (ethanol); extract (chloroform-aqueous acid); wash (water); evaporate; dissolve (ethanol); add dipotassium phosphate solution & irradiate	UV (418 nm)	—	US Pharmacopeial Convention Inc. (1975)
Suppositories	Dissolve (water-ethanol); extract (chloroform-sodium hydroxide); evaporate; dissolve (ethanol); add dipotassium phosphate solution & irradiate	UV (418 nm)	—	US Pharmacopeial Convention Inc. (1975)

Table 1 (continued)

Sample matrix	Sample preparation	Assay procedure	Sensitivity or limit of detection	Reference
Creams and suppositories	Dissolve (methanol:diethyl ether, 1:1)	HPLC (UV, 254 nm)	-	Roos (1974)
Cottonseed oil formulation	Dissolve (dimethylformamide: methanol, 1:1)	HPLC (UV, 254 nm)	-	Roos (1974)
Vegetable oil formulation	Extract (isooctane-aqueous sodium hydroxide); wash (chloroform); adjust to pH 9.5; extract (chloroform); evaporate; dissolve (ethanol); add aqueous dipotassium phosphate solution & irradiate	UV (418 nm)	-	Horwitz (1975); US Pharmacopeial Convention Inc. (1975)
Drinking-water	Extract; separate (TLC)	TLC; radiometry	-	Rurainski et al. (1977)
Feeds	Isolate by a series of extractions; CC (diatomaceous earth-tripotassium phosphate) & irradiate	TLC (2,4-dinitro-phenylhydrazine spray) or UV (415 nm)	0.07 mg/kg 0.55 mg/kg	Jeffus & Kenner (1972)
Feeds	Separate (a complex series of extractions & washings); CC (diatomaceous earth-tripotassium phosphate); irradiate; extract; oxidize (acidic bisulphite solution) & extract	FL (385 nm)	5 µg/kg (20 g sample)	Jeffus & Kenner (1973)
Animal chow	Extract (methanol); CC (Sephadex LH-20); extract (sodium hydroxide-benzene; carbonate buffer-benzene); CC (silica gel); derivatize (pentafluoropropionyl)	GC/ECD HPLC (UV, 254 nm)	1 µg/kg (20 g sample)	King et al. (1977)
Serum	Extract	High-performance TLC; UV densitometry (287 nm)	10 ng	Jarc et al. (1977)

Table 1 (continued)

Sample matrix	Sample preparation	Assay procedure	Sensitivity or limit of detection	Reference
Urine	Filter; dissolve (buffer solution); add antiserum & tracer solution; incubate; add second antibody solution; incubate & centrifuge	RIA	–	Gutierrez-Cernosek & Cernosek (1977)
Biological fluids & animal tissues	Hydrolyse (β-glucuronidase-catalysed); extract (aqueous sodium carbonate-toluene); separate; add trimethyl-phenylammonium hydroxide & separate	GC/FID	8 μg/l (1 ml sample)	Kohrman & MacGee (1977)
Beef muscle, liver & kidney	Extract (methanol); hydrolyse (β-glucuronidase); extract (sodium hydroxide-chloroform, carbonate buffer-chloroform) & derivatize (dichloroacetyl)	GC/ECD	1 μg/kg (80 g sample)	Donoho et al. (1973)
Animal tissue	Homogenize (aqueous aceto-nitrile); hydrolyse (hydro-chloric acid); perform a series of extractions & washings	TLC; UV densitometry (287 nm)	150 ng	Jarc et al. (1977)
Beef liver	Extract (methanol); hydrolyse (β-glucuronidase); extract (sodium hydroxide-chloroform, carbonate buffer-chloroform) & derivatize (dichloroacetyl)	GC/ECD GC/MS	–	Day et al. (1975)

Table 1 (continued)

Sample matrix	Sample preparation	Assay procedure	Sensitivity or limit of detection	Reference
Beef liver	Isolate by a series of extrac- tions; hydrolyse (hydro- chloric acid); CC; derivatize (heptafluorobutyryl)	GC/ECD GC/electrolytic conductivity	—	Lawrence & Ryan (1977)
Beef liver	Separate (a complex series of extractions, washings & hydrolysis); irradiate; extract; oxidize (acidified bisulphite solu- tion); extract; evaporate & dissolve (methanol)	FL (380 nm)	—	Ponder (1974)

3. Biological Data Relevant to the Evaluation
of Carcinogenic Risk to Humans

3.1 Carcinogenicity studies in animals

(a) Oral administration

Mouse: Of 22 effective male C3H mice (MTV[+])[1] administered 0.125-
0.75 mg DES in sesame oil by stomach tube twice weekly for total doses
of 4.25-14.25 mg, 18 developed mammary carcinomas. The average induction
time was 24-28 weeks. No information was available on the controls
(Shimkin & Grady, 1941).

In male mice of two hybrid stocks (ZD$_8$F and AZF$_1$), feeding of a
semisynthetic diet containing DES (average intake, 0.5 µg/animal per day)
resulted in the appearance of mammary tumours. The incidences of tumours
were lower (11/30 and 12/37) and the average induction times longer
(14.6 months and 18.8 months) in intact males than in castrates (incidences,
33/34 and 19/20; induction times, 10.7 months and 14.3 months) (Huseby,
1953).

Dietary restriction to 1/3 of the caloric intake reduced the mammary
tumour incidence from 25 to 0% in virgin female A strain mice on a DES-
containing diet fed *ad libitum*. The mammary glands of the mice on the
restricted diet were considerably less well developed than those of the
controls (Ball *et al.*, 1946).

C3H and A strain mice (MTV[+]) received DES in the diet at levels of
6.25-1000 µg/kg diet. A dose level of 25 µg/kg resulted in a calculated
daily intake of 0.06-0.09 µg DES/mouse, which is comparable to the
intake of 0.066 µg found necessary to maintain oestrus. The incidence
of mammary carcinomas in virgin female C3H mice maintained on a control
diet was 40/121; this incidence was slightly greater in mice given
levels of 6.25-25 µg/kg DES in the diet; and with 50 µg/kg the incidence
was 36/68 (P<0.01). In those given 500 and 1000 µg/kg, the incidences
of mammary carcinomas were 50/59 and 49/58. The tumour induction times
decreased progressively with increased DES concentrations, from 49 weeks
in those on the control diet to 31 weeks in those given the 1000 µg/kg
level [It is noteworthy that ovarian weights showed a marked decline
with DES concentrations of 25 µg/kg or more]. Intact male C3H mice
developed a significant number of mammary carcinomas (23/60) only when

---

[1]MTV[+]: mammary tumour virus expressed (see p. 62)

given 500 µg/kg DES in the diet or more (30/71 developed in those given
1000 µg/kg), although some mammary tumours occurred in those given lower
concentrations. Castrated A strain males were less susceptible to all
dietary concentrations of DES. No mammary tumours occurred in control
groups of 115 intact male C3H mice or 136 castrated male A strain mice
(Gass et al., 1964).

Groups of 85-97 castrated male C3H mice (MTV[+]) were given diets
containing 500 or 1000 µg/kg DES during 2-, 7-, 14- or 28-day cycles,
alternating with similar durations on a control diet; the mammary
carcinoma incidences were similar in all groups, at both dose levels,
irrespective of the cycle length. However, the incidence of tumours was
significantly higher in animals receiving continuous administration of
250 or 500 µg/kg DES. Lower incidences of mammary carcinomas were found
in groups of similarly treated intact male mice (Okey & Gass, 1968).

Groups of 50 castrated male C3H/An mice (MTV[+]) and C3H/Anf mice
(MTV[-])[1] were fed diets containing 0 (control) and 250 µg/kg diet DES for
18 months. The incidence of mammary adenocarcinomas in C3H/An controls
was 0/50, compared with 36/50 [P<0.01] in treated mice; the incidence
in C3H/Anf controls was 1/50, compared with 5/50 (not significant) in
treated animals. In a further experiment, similar groups of 30 castrated
male mice of both strains were fed DES for 12 months. No mammary tumours
occurred in C3H/Anf mice or in C3H/An controls. In C3H/An treated mice,
the incidence of mammary adenocarcinomas was 9/30 [P<0.01] within the
12-month observation period (Gass et al., 1974).

Groups of virgin female C3H/HeJ mice (MTV[+]) and female C3HeB/FeJ
mice (MTV[-]) were fed 0, 10, 100 or 500 µg/kg diet DES for 52 or more
weeks. At 52 weeks, no mammary tumours were seen in the C3HeB/FeJ mice;
adenocarcinomas of the mammary gland occurred in 2/47, 0/32, 3/38 and
3/48 C3H/HeJ mice, respectively. The incidences of hyperplastic alveolar
nodules were also increased (0, 3, 5 and 14%). Adenocarcinomas of the
uterine horns were seen in 2 C3H/HeJ mice fed 100 and 10 µg/kg diet DES
for 74 and 78 weeks; and a tumour attached to the outer, upper portion
of the uterine horn was seen in another C3H/HeJ mouse fed 500 µg/kg diet
DES for 52 weeks. This tumour might have been an atypical endometrial
adenocarcinoma, but the possibility that it may have arisen in some
urogenital rest or have represented a mesothelioma could not be excluded.
Seven adenocarcinomas of the cervix (5 in the 500 µg/kg group and 2 in
the 100 µg/kg group) and 2 osteosarcomas, one of the cranium (in the 10
µg/kg group) and one of the sternum (in the 500 µg/kg group), were seen

---

[1]MTV[-]: mammary tumour virus not expressed (see p. 62)

in C3H/HeJ mice after feeding periods of 52-102 weeks. In C3HeB/FeJ
mice fed 500 μg/kg diet DES for 52-78 weeks, 2 adenocarcinomas of the
cervix, 1 squamous-cell carcinoma of the vagina and 1 osteosarcoma of
the cranium were observed; in those fed 100 μg/kg diet DES for 93 weeks,
1 adenocarcinoma of the cervix was seen (Highman *et al.*, 1977).

Rat: Groups of 20 male and 20 female weanling Sprague-Dawley rats
were fed diets containing DES at concentrations providing intakes of 0
(control), 0.02 or 0.2 mg/kg bw per day for 2 years. At that time 9
male and 12 female controls and 16 male and 14 female rats treated with
the low dose were still alive. All rats given the high dose that were
still alive at 18 months (9 males and 6 females) were killed because of
debilitation. At 18 months, mammary tumours had developed in 0 (controls),
0 (low dose) and 4 (high dose) male rats, and in 1, 0 and 4 females in
the corresponding groups. In rats that survived 18 months to 2 years,
mammary tumours developed in 0 (controls) and 1 (low dose) male rats,
and in 7 and 1 females. Most of the mammary tumours were fibroadenomas.
Pituitary tumours occurred in 4, 5 and 17 males and in 4, 9 and 18
females in the respective groups. Two hepatomas and 1 haemangioendothelioma
of the liver occurred in females given the low dose; no such tumours
were observed in controls (Gibson *et al.*, 1967).

(b) Subcutaneous and/or intramuscular administration

Mouse: Lacassagne (1938) first demonstrated the induction of
mammary tumours in 2 male R3 mice following the injection of 25 μg DES
twice weekly for 12-16 weeks. Shimkin & Andervont (1942) also studied
the effects of DES in mice: male C3H mice (MTV$^+$) were injected subcutaneously with DES in sesame oil once a week for 20 weeks (total, 4
mg). In a group suckled by MTV$^+$ C3H females, the breast tumour incidence
was 9/13 at an average induction time of 9.4 months. C3H males suckled
by MTV$^-$ C57 black females had a breast cancer incidence of 2/22, with a
latent period of 10.5 months [Although the MTV was absent in the latter
group, the probable presence of the nodule-inducing virus (NIV) must be
taken into account in assessing the factors involved in the emergence of
mammary tumours (Nandi, 1965)].

Gardner (1959) found neoplastic lesions of the cervix or vagina in
3/14 BC mice injected subcutaneously weekly with 250 μg DES in sesame
oil during 25-41 weeks [Evaluation of these data is difficult, since the
ages of the mice at start of treatment ranged from 26 to 59 weeks].

Murphy & Sturm (1949) reported 28 leukaemias in 40 untreated female
RIL mice and 37 leukaemias in untreated males; this incidence was
significantly increased in males (83/116) by weekly injections of 50 μg
DES in oil during 7 months.

Thirty male and 30 female 21-day old ICR Jcl mice received single
s.c. injections of 10 mg/kg bw DES, and a further group of 20 male and
20 female mice received 100 mg/kg bw DES. All mice were killed at 12
months of age. The incidence of ovarian cystadenomas was increased in
female mice treated with the higher dose (4/17 *versus* 1/77 in controls)
(Nomura & Kanzaki, 1977).

Rat: A group of 43 male Sprague-Dawley rats, 6-9 months of age,
received single s.c. injections of 20 mg/animal DES dipropionate in
ethyl oleate and were killed after 406 days; 13 rats were used as untreated
controls. In 6 treated rats, grossly enlarged pituitaries (>30 mg) were
observed; these were considered to be tumours. Hyperplasia of the
pituitary was seen in 24 rats (Jacobi *et al.*, 1975).

Hamster: When 0.6 mg DES in 0.2 ml of 0.9% saline was injected
subcutaneously every other day for 36 weeks or longer, 11/11 intact male
golden hamsters developed kidney tumours, compared with 0/17 in untreated
and 0/5 in saline-treated controls (Kirkman & Bacon, 1952b) [See also
'Subcutaneous implantation', p. 189].

Fifty-four 15-day-old male Syrian golden hamsters were given thrice
weekly s.c. injections of 0.2 ml of an 11.2 mM suspension of DES (6 mg/
animal) in carboxymethyl cellulose/saline. Of animals killed after 6-7,
7-8, 8-9 or 9-10 months, 0/5, 8/13, 22/25 and 11/11 developed renal
tumours. No such tumours occurred in 62 controls injected with carboxymethyl
cellulose/saline alone (Lacomba & Gabaldón, 1971). The morphological,
histochemical and ultrastructural characteristics of these tumours were
described by Llombart-Bosch & Peydro (1975).

Of 12 male Syrian hamsters given thrice weekly s.c. injections of
0.6 mg DES suspended in water plus daily s.c. injections of 500 μg 2-
bromo-α-ergocryptine methanesulphonate for 9 months, only 7 animals
developed kidney tumours (3 animals with bilateral tumours), compared
with 10 animals treated with DES alone (all bilateral) (Hamilton *et al.*,
1975).

In groups of 15-day old male Syrian golden hamsters given thrice-
weekly s.c. injections of 0.2 ml of a 0.3% suspension of DES in carboxymethyl
cellulose/saline [dose, 6 mg/animal], the incidences of gross renal
tumours (no histology) after 1-6, 6-7, 7-8 and 8-9 months were 0/6,
10/23, 10/16 and 3/4. No renal tumours occurred in the controls. When
the s.c. injections were alternated daily with 1 mg/animal nafoxidine (a
non-steroidal anti-oestrogen), the incidences of renal tumours were 0/5,
0/25, 0/14 and 0/7 at the respective time intervals. Renal tumours were
also produced by s.c. injection of polydiethylstilboestrol phosphate, a
water-soluble, high molecular weight polyester (Antonio *et al.*, 1974).

Thrice-weekly injections of 0.6 mg/animal DES for 9 months to 27 male hamsters resulted in renal tumours, classified as carcinomas, in 24/24 survivors. Histological examination of the pituitary glands showed hyperplastic and 'neoplastic changes' in the intermediate lobes (Hamilton *et al*., 1977).

Dog: Ovarian lesions (6 papillary carcinomas, 1 papillary adenoma and 1 hyperplasia) were found in all of 8 female dogs given s.c. injections of 15-60 mg DES in paraffin oil at 7-8 week intervals over 19 months (total dose, 90-495 mg) (Jabara, 1959).

In a further study, 10 female dogs received total s.c. doses of 60-495 mg/animal DES for up to 455 days: 9 developed ovarian tumours described as papillary carcinomas, and 1 had 'papillary dysplasia'; 3 carcinomas (diagnosed by biopsy) were found at the time of DES withdrawal (Jabara, 1962).

Frog: DES dipropionate in vegetable oil was injected subcutaneously into 46 female and 52 male frogs (*Rana temporaria*), aged 1-1.5 years, at doses of 40-200 μg per week. Neoplasms of the haematopoietic tissue (7) and liver (2) were observed in 6/21 females and 2/17 males that lived more than 9.5 weeks (Khudolei & Ermoshchenkov, 1976).

(c) Subcutaneous implantation

Mouse: Groups of 20-55 male and female strain C mice received implants of 4-6 mg pellets made from a mixture of cholesterol and amounts of DES ranging from 5-50% in the right axilla. Scrotal hernias developed in about 10% of males given 10-50% DES pellets; and interstitial-cell tumours of the testis were detected between 6 and 11 months in 1/10 mice given 5%, in 3/30 given 10%, in 4/14 given 25% and in 5/8 given 50% DES. Three of the tumours metastasized. Mammary tumours occurred in only 1/34 female mice and in 0/20 male mice observed up to 13 months. However, when strain C mice were cross-suckled on C3H mice (MTV[+]), mammary tumours occurred at between 8 and 11 months in 14/20 females and in 5/13 males implanted with pellets containing 10% DES. Foster nursing did not influence the incidence of testicular tumours, and 2 males had both mammary and testicular tumours. Lymphoid tumours were seen in 4/50 males and in 3/11 females aged 8-14 months. No lymphoid tumours appeared in 143 controls killed between 8 and 16 months of age (Shimkin *et al*., 1941).

Of 76 male BALB/c mice implanted with 5 mg pellets of 20% DES in cholesterol when they were 3-6-months old, 61 developed interstitial-cell tumours of the testis at 8-11 months of age. Tumour induction was found to be dependent on genetic factors, since BALB/c mice were far more susceptible than those of RIII, C57BL, C3H, DBA/2, Y and I strains implanted with 10 or 20% DES pellets. Hybridization of males of insusceptible strains with BALB/c females usually, but not invariably, yielded

susceptible offspring (interstitital-cell tumours occurred in 0/37
BALB/c x RIII hybrids and in 16/24 BALB/c x DBA/2 hybrids) (Andervont *et
al*., 1960).

In experiments to determine whether the susceptibility to interstitial-
cell tumours was determined by the genetic constitution of the testis or
by some other factor, testes from susceptible A strain or from resistant
C3H mice were transplanted into suceptible Fl hybrid males, which were
then implanted with 7 mg pellets containing 25% DES in cholesterol.
Tumours arose in a much higher incidence in the transplanted testes from
the susceptible A strain, indicating that the site of genetic susceptibility
was in the testis itself (Trentin & Gardner, 1958).

In a complex series of experiments, Andervont *et al*. (1957) showed
that interruption of exposure to DES for various periods did not affect
the induction of testicular tumours. Canter & Shimkin (1968) showed
that unilateral orchiectomy significantly reduced the incidence of
interstitial-cell tumours, presumably due to reduction of the amount of
target tissue. Many DES-induced tumours are dependent on oestrogenic
stimulation for continued growth in transplantation (Klein & Hellström,
1962).

When 1.8-2.2 mg pellets of 0.5-30% DES in cholesterol were implanted
into male C3H mice (MTV^+), mammary tumours arose in 1/40 mice bearing
pellets containing 0.01 mg DES, and the incidence rose progressively to
26/30 mice implanted with pellets containing 0.6 mg DES. The incidence
of spontaneous hepatomas was reduced from 88/341 (26%) in untreated
males (Andervont, 1941) to 6/44 (9%) in males with pellets containing
0.04-0.1 mg DES; there were no hepatomas in mice implanted with 0.2 mg
or more DES (Shimkin & Wyman, 1946).

In virgin Fl hybrid female RIII x C57L mice (MTV^+), implantation of
7-8 mg pellets of 20% DES in cholesterol resulted in an increased incidence
and decreased latent period for mammary carcinomas. In untreated female
mice, the incidence was 30/48 at an average age of 21.3 months; but
when the oestrogen pellet was present from 8 weeks of age until death,
the incidence of mammary carcinomas rose to 151/174, with a mean induction
time of 11.1 months. Exposure to DES pellets for periods of 4 or 8
weeks resulted in incidences of 30/40 and 46/52 and in latent periods of
19.6 and 16.9 months, respectively (Richardson, 1957).

Experiments intended to determine the carcinogenicity of DES in
MTV^- mice were carried out using mice which had been freed of the virus
by various means. Andervont *et al*. (1958) reported incidences of mammary
cancer varying between 4/32 and 21/25 in MTV^- intact or castrated hybrid
male or virgin or breeding female mice of the C3H strain and hybrids
with BALB/c, RIII and DBA/2 strains. Virgin C3H females, hybrids of C3H
with I and C57 mice or crosses between BALB/c, RIII and I and C57 strains

treated with DES had less than 10% incidences of mammary tumours. The number of mice involved altogether was greater than 2800. These results are qualified by the fact that, although MTV was excluded, other viruses not transmitted by suckling, such as nodule-inducing virus (Nandi, 1965), may have been present. The differences in tumour incidences in various strains were not, therefore, necessarily due to their differing susceptibilities to DES. The induction of mammary tumours in MTV$^-$ male C3H mice was also reported by Heston & Deringer (1953) and by Andervont (1950).

After cholesterol pellets of approximately 1.6 mg containing 25% DES were implanted into virgin female C3H mice (MTV$^+$), about 0.4 mg of the pellet (equivalent to 0.1 mg DES) had been absorbed after 1 year. When given a normal diet, 23/27 of the mice developed mammary cancer; however, this incidence was reduced to 17/40 when the animals were fed a diet deficient in cystine (White & White, 1944).

S.c. implants of DES in cholesterol pellets (amounts not clear) resulted in increased incidences of lymphoid tumours in mice of the C3H strain (13 lymphoid tumours in 51 treated mice *versus* 4 in 412 intact controls) (Gardner *et al.*, 1944).

Rat: Initial observations by Geschickter & Byrnes (1942) on the induction of mammary tumours by DES in rats were amplified by Dunning *et al.* (1947). They reported strain differences in susceptibility to mammary tumour induction after the s.c. implantation of pellets of DES: cholesterol (1:3; 4-15 mg DES) into 3-4 month-old rats of both sexes (average amount, 5.4-9 mg/rat). A x C rats had the highest incidences (17/29 males had a total of 39 tumours; 22/29 females had a total of 89 tumours); Fischer rats had lower incidences (5/30 males had 5 tumours; 1/22 females had a tumour); and Copenhagen rats developed no mammary tumours. Pituitary hypertrophy was least in those of the Copenhagen strain and greatest in A x C rats, in which the gland reached weights of 116-155 mg in both females and males. Adrenal cortical tumours occurred in 2 Fischer rats and in 1 A x C rat. Bladder cancers occurred in 22/58 Copenhagen rats and in 3/58 A x C rats, but there were none in Fischer rats. The development of bladder carcinoma was associated with the presence of bladder calculi.

The incidence of mammary cancer following DES treatment was increased by a high-fat diet but not with an isocaloric low-fat diet (Dunning *et al.*, 1949). Changes in the tryptophane content of the diet altered the mammary cancer incidence (Dunning *et al.*, 1950).

Groups of 42 female A x C rats were hysterectomized at 43-45 days of age and received either a s.c. implant of DES, a s.c. implant of DES following ovariectomy, a s.c. implant of DES following ovariectomy plus weekly s.c. injections of progesterone, or a s.c. implant of DES following ovariectomy plus a s.c. implant of progesterone. The incidences of mammary carcinomas were 23/39, 21/38, 18/39 and 17/33; there were 138, 29, 35 and 45 gross tumours. The median latent periods to appearance of the first tumour were 43.5, 51.5, 48 and 43.5 weeks. No mammary tumours were seen in untreated rats up to 116 weeks of age (Segaloff, 1974). In similar groups, A x C rats were given s.c. implants of DES and 2 days later received X-irradiation; the incidence of mammary carcinomas was increased and the latent period for tumour appearance decreased (Segaloff & Maxfield, 1971).

Continuous treatment of A x C female rats with 7,12-dimethylbenz[a]-anthracene and DES resulted in additive effects on the production of mammary adenocarcinomas (Shellabarger *et al.*, 1976a).

Groups of young female A x C rats were given 9.6 rads of 0.43-MeV neutrons (33 animals), implantation of a 20 mg pellet containing 5 mg DES and 15 mg cholesterol (25 animals) or implantation followed 2 days later by irradiation (25 animals). Of 32/33 irradiated rats that survived 50 weeks, 2 developed a total of 3 mammary adenocarcinomas and 3 a total of 4 mammary fibroadenomas. Average survival of rats that received DES implants was 284 days; 22 rats developed a total of 182 mammary adeno-carcinomas, and 21 developed pituitary tumours. In animals given DES plus irradiation, average survival was 239 days; 32 rats developed a total of 842 mammary adenocarcinomas, 1 rat developed a single mammary fibroadenoma, and 34 rats developed pituitary tumours. All of the 31 control rats survived the 50-week study period, and none developed tumours (Shellabarger *et al.*, 1976b).

Hamster: The induction of malignant adenomatous renal tumours following treatment with DES was first described by Kirkman & Bacon (1950) in intact male hamsters implanted with 20 mg pellets of DES for 200 days or longer. In a later study, s.c. implantations of 20 mg pellets of DES (repeated after 200 days) resulted in renal tumours in 52/53 intact male hamsters; metastases were seen in 33/53 animals. Castrated males were also susceptible (11/11), and metastases occurred within the abdominal cavity in 3/11 animals. The effective daily dose of DES liberated from the pellets was calculated to be 0.09 mg. Intact females treated with DES after ovulation were insusceptible to kidney tumour formation (Kirkman & Bacon, 1952a,b). Confirmation and expansion of these results (Horning, 1954, 1956a,b) showed that transplants could be made to hamsters of either sex treated with DES pellets, but that both the primary lesions and the grafts regressed on removal of the oestrogenic stimuli.

Monkey: Ten adult female squirrel monkeys were implanted subcutaneously with four 60 mg pellets of DES. Malignant uterine mesotheliomas occurred in 7/10 animals; and in the 3 remaining animals early proliferative lesions of the uterine serosa were observed. Malignant lesions were observed in one animal killed 5 months after implantation of DES; other animals were killed between 11 and 14 months after the initial implantation. No tumours occurred in 4 control animals implanted with cholesterol pellets (McClure & Graham, 1973).

In a report of a study in progress, 19 pregnant *Macaca mulatta* monkeys received 1 mg/day DES from day 21 to delvery, from day 100 to delivery or from day 130 to delivery. Regardless of the treatment period, female offspring showed teratogenic abnormalities (see section 3.2); but no vaginal or cervical adenocarcinomas had been observed by the 6th year of observation (Hendrickx *et al.*, 1979).

(d) Perinatal exposure

Prenatal exposure: Groups of 20 CD-1 timed-pregnant mice were given daily s.c. injections of 0 (control), 0.01, 1, 2.5, 5, 10 or 100 µg/kg bw DES on days 9-16 of pregnancy. The numbers of surviving offspring were 74 (control), 55, 54, 18, 16, 61 and 39, respectively. Adenocarcinomas of the uterine endometrium and epidermoid tumours of the cervix and vagina were observed at 6-15 months in 10% or less of female offspring in all treated groups (McLachlan, 1977). In male offspring of treated mothers, 1 preneoplastic growth was observed in the area of the seminal colliculus (McLachlan, 1977; McLachlan *et al.*, 1975a) [The Working Group noted the incomplete reporting regarding the females].

Groups of pregnant ICR/Jcl mice were given single s.c. injections of 10 mg/kg bw DES on day 7, 9, 11, 13, 15, 17 or 19 of pregnancy. The offspring were weaned at 4 weeks and observed until 12 months of age. The incidence of tumours of the lung (papillary adenomas) was significantly increased in mice of both sexes whose mothers had been treated on day 15 of pregnancy (7/29 *versus* 0/14 in controls). Tumours of the ovary (cystadenomas and granulosa-cell) were significantly increased in female offspring of mice treated on day 15, 17 or 19 of pregnancy (3/17, 6/15, 4/33 *versus* 0/8 controls). No tumours of the genital tract were observed (Nomura & Kanzaki, 1977).

Pregnant Syrian golden hamsters received DES suspended in distilled water containing 0.1% gelatin and administered by intragastric tube, either as a single dose of 20 or 40 mg/kg bw DES on day 15 of gestation, or as two consecutive daily doses of 20 or 40 mg/kg bw on days 14 and 15 of pregnancy. A total of 70 siblings were weaned, of 115 newborns from 11 litters. Both female and male progeny developed high incidences of metaplastic, dysplastic and neoplastic lesions in the various segments of the genital tract. Reproductive tract neoplasms (2 cervical polyps, 2 squamous-cell papillomas of the cervix and vagina, 1 myosarcoma) were seen in 28% (4/14) of female progeny exposed to a single 40 mg/kg bw dose of DES; 50% (4/8) of those exposed to two doses of 40 mg/kg bw had 5 genital-tract tumours (2 cervical polyps, 1 adenocarcinoma of the uterus, 2 squamous-cell papillomas of the cervix and vagina). Male progeny developed granulomas in the epididymis (70%) and testis (40%) and epididymal cystic formations (20%); 1 adenoma of the Cowper gland was seen in 1 animal given a single dose of 40 mg/kg bw, and 1 leiomyo-sarcoma of the seminal vesicle was seen in 1 animal given a single dose of 20 mg/kg bw DES (Rustia, 1979; Rustia & Shubik, 1976).

In a report of a study in progress, 19 pregnant *Macaca mulatta* (rhesus) monkeys received 1 mg DES daily from day 21 to delivery, from day 100 to delivery or from day 130 to delivery. Regardless of the treatment period, female offspring showed teratogenic abnormalities (see section 3.2); but no vaginal or cervical adenocarcinomas had been observed by the 6th year of observation (Hendrickx *et al.*, 1979).

Neonatal exposure: Newborn male and female mice were injected subcutaneously with 2 mg DES in saline suspension within the first 24 hrs after birth; cancers of the cervix and/or vagina occurred in 6/17 female BALB/c mice aged 13-26 months, in 3/10 C3Hf females at 20-26 months and in 1/4 controls. Precancerous lesions were found in 3 BALB/c mice at 13-21 months and in 4 female C3Hf mice at 24-26 months. Granular-cell myoblastomas occurred in 1/6 BALB/c females aged 24-26 months and in 1/9 C3Hf females at 24-26 months; however, one of these tumours also occurred in 1/2 controls at 26 months. Male mice showed no unusual tumours in any organ; however, 5/10 BALB/c and 7/10 C3HF mice showed single or multiple, often bilateral, epididymal cysts (Dunn & Green, 1963).

Male and female ICR/Jcl mice received a single s.c. injection of 50 mg/kg bw DES within 12 hrs after birth and were killed at 12 months of age. The incidence of tumours was not increased in the surviving 7 males and 11 females when compared with that in controls (Nomura & Kanzaki, 1977).

Random-bred male Wistar rats, either intact or castrated within 24 hrs after birth, were injected subcutaneously with 1 then 2 then 4 µg DES daily from 1-30 days of age (total, 70 µg). Two of 11 castrated rats developed invasive squamous-cell carcinomas by 21 months of age, which were confined to the coagulatory gland and the ejaculatory duct (Arai *et al.*, 1978). In an earlier study, which terminated when the animals were 9 months of age, hyperplastic epithelial alterations with squamous metaplasia were observed in the same organs in similarly treated male rats (Arai *et al.*, 1977).

(e) Other experimental systems

Local application: Epidermoid carcinomas of the vagina and/or cervix were observed in 3/21 mice of the BC and C57 strains given 1-4 µg DES in oil intravaginally 3 times weekly. Similar lesions occurred in 8/40 BC mice in which pellets of DES: cholesterol (1:3) were fixed in the upper vagina for periods averaging 37 weeks. Vaginal cancers occurred

in 1/43 untreated BC mice and in 1/30 BC mice given pellets containing
cholesterol only. No vaginal cancers were seen in 11 C57 control mice
(Gardner, 1959) [These data are difficult to evaluate because of the
advanced age of many of the mice at the start of treatment].

3.2 Other relevant biological data

The toxicity and metabolism of DES have been reviewed (McMartin *et
al.*, 1978).

(a) Experimental systems

Its relative biological activity in mice is 1/3 that of oestradiol-
17β after s.c. administration and 3 times that of oestradiol-17β after
oral administration (Emmeus & Martin, 1962). In the uterine growth
test (Rubin's test) in mice, it is about 1.2 times more active than
oestradiol-17β (Brotherton, 1976).

Toxic effects

The LD_{50} of DES by i.p. injection in mice is 67 mg/kg bw (Klaassen,
1973a) and that in rats 34 mg/kg bw (in ethanol) (Klaassen, 1973b).
High doses have been shown to be hepatotoxic in rats (Noller & Fish,
1974; Richards & Kueter, 1941).

Changes in thymus, spleen and blood-cell counts (Kalland *et al.*,
1978) and a reduction in the delayed hypersensitivity response to oxazolone
(Kalland & Forsberg, 1978) have been observed in mice exposed neonatally
to DES.

In female mice given daily s.c. injections of 5 μg DES for the first
5 days after birth and killed 13 months later, extensive adenosis was
observed, comprising most of the cervical wall; further epithelial
changes included hyperplasia and squamous metaplasia (Forsberg, 1975,
1979).

Embryotoxicity and teratogenicity

Doses of DES ranging from 0.01-100 μg/kg bw were injected subcutaneously into CD-1 mice on days 9-16 of gestation. In mature female
offspring, a dose-dependent decrease in reproductive capacity was observed;
at doses of 10 and 100 μg/kg bw complete sterility occurred. Abnormalities
of the genital tract in male and female offspring included cystic endometrial hyperplasia, inflammatory disease of the oviduct, persistent
cornification of the vaginal epithelium, oedema and stromal hyperplasia
of the cervix, ovarian cysts and hypospadias. Of mature male offspring
exposed prenatally to 100 μg/kg bw, 60% were sterile; 80% of these had
alterations of the reproductive tract, including metaplastic and neoplastic
tissue. Intraabdominal or fibrotic testes also occurred. Lower doses

had no effect in males. This study was considered to show that mice are useful animal models for lesions of the human male reproductive tract due to DES (McLachlan, 1976, 1977; McLachlan & Dixon, 1973; McLachlan *et al.*, 1975a,b, 1977).

ICR/Jcl mice received a single s.c. injection of 10 mg/kg bw DES disodium salt on day 7, 9, 11, 13, 15, 17 or 19 of gestation. Treatment on days 15-19 resulted in persistent urogenital sinus and hypertrophy of the portio vaginalis in female offspring. In male offspring exposed to DES *in utero* on days 17 and 19 of gestation, undescended testes and hypogenesis were noted in 70.4-73.3% of animals (Nomura & Kanzaki, 1977).

Swiss mice received 10 µg DES on days 11-13 of gestation together with 100-600 µg progesterone on days 11-16 of gestation and were delivered by caesarian section on the 17th day. Mortality was 50%, and cleft palate occurred in 20-32% of surviving foetuses when the dose of DES was kept constant (10 µg) and the doses of progesterone varied from 100-600 µg. When the dose of progesterone was kept constant (200 µg) and doses of 2.5-10 µg DES were administered, mortality and the occurrence of cleft palate were shown to be dependent on the dosage of DES (Gabriel-Robez *et al.*, 1972).

S.c. injection of total doses of 10-42 mg DES into rats from day 12 or 13 to day 18-21 of gestation led to reduced litter size, and 30% of 40 injected rats carried to term. Only 28 female and 18 male newborns were examined: due to these small numbers, no significant teratological data were obtained. However, feminization of the genitalia was noted in male offspring (Greene *et al.*, 1940).

Pregnant, random-bred rats were injected (site not specified) with 0.003 mg DES and 0.03 mg progesterone daily for 3 successive days. Treatment between days 16-19 led to a decrease in the number of erythrocytes and leucocytes in the peripheral blood and an increase in haemoglobin and reticulocytes. Haematopoiesis was stimulated in the bone marrow and spleen but inhibited in the liver. Injections made between days 9-11 of gestation had less effect on offspring examined 5 days postnatally (Balika *et al.*, 1976).

S.c. doses of 0.015-0.6 mg/kg bw DES were given to rats on days 13, 16, 18 and 20 of pregnancy and/or 0.2-10 mg/kg bw were given for 3 weeks *post partum*. In female offspring, hypospadia and urethrovaginal cloaca formation were seen. In male offspring, hypospadia, phallic hypoplasia, inhibition of the growth and descent of testes, as well as abnormalities of Wolffian derivatives were observed (Vorherr *et al.*, 1979).

Oral administration of 100 µg/kg bw DES to random-bred albino rats on day 15 of gestation resulted in lowered hepatic histidase activity in adult female offspring when compared with controls (Lamartiniere & Lucier, 1978).

Injection (site not specified) of 0.5-5.0 mg DES into rabbits on days 4-5 of gestation did not prevent blastocyst implantation, but administration before day 12-14 terminated pregnancy (Adams *et al.*, 1961).

Daily oral administration of 1 mg DES to pregnant *Macaca mulatta* (rhesus) monkeys during 3 different periods of gestation (day 21 to delivery, day 100 to delivery, day 130 to delivery) resulted in vaginal ridging and/or cervical hooding in offspring. In some cases, vaginal adenosis was also observed (Hendrickx *et al.*, 1979).

Absorption, distribution and excretion

The enterohepatic circulation of DES has been studied in rats: DES glucuronide, which is secreted into bile after DES administration, is split by intestinal bacteria, and the DES is reabsorbed from the gut (Fischer *et al.*, 1973, 1976).

Studies of the transfer of DES across the placenta in mice showed that accumulation of DES and its metabolites in the foetal genital tract was 3 times greater than that in foetal plasma (Shah & McLachlan, 1976).

Metabolism

Metabolic studies have been reported in rats, hamsters, mice, guinea-pigs, cattle and primates. The various pathways of DES metabolism are shown in Figure 1.

A possible pathway of DES metabolism in rats is *ortho*-hydroxylation to the catechol metabolite, followed by methylation, due to the catechol-O-methyltransferase (Engel *et al.*, 1976). Major metabolites of DES in several species (rat, mouse, hamster, primates) are dienoestrol and ω-hydroxydienoestrol (Metzler, 1975, 1976; Metzler & McLachlan, 1978; Metzler *et al.*, 1977), which are thought to originate from DES *via* a (possibly peroxidase-catalysed) oxidation of DES to the quinone inter-mediate (Metzler, 1977). Another possible pathway of DES metabolism in rats is epoxidation at the stilbene double-bond, possibly resulting in the ultimate formation of 4'-hydroxypropiophenone, which is excreted in rat urine after DES administration (Metzler, 1976). Both the epoxide (Metzler, 1976) and the quinone intermediate (Metzler, 1977) have been suggested as reactive metabolites of DES. It has been reported that metabolites of DES, produced either by rat liver microsomes or by primary

Figure 1

Metabolism of DES

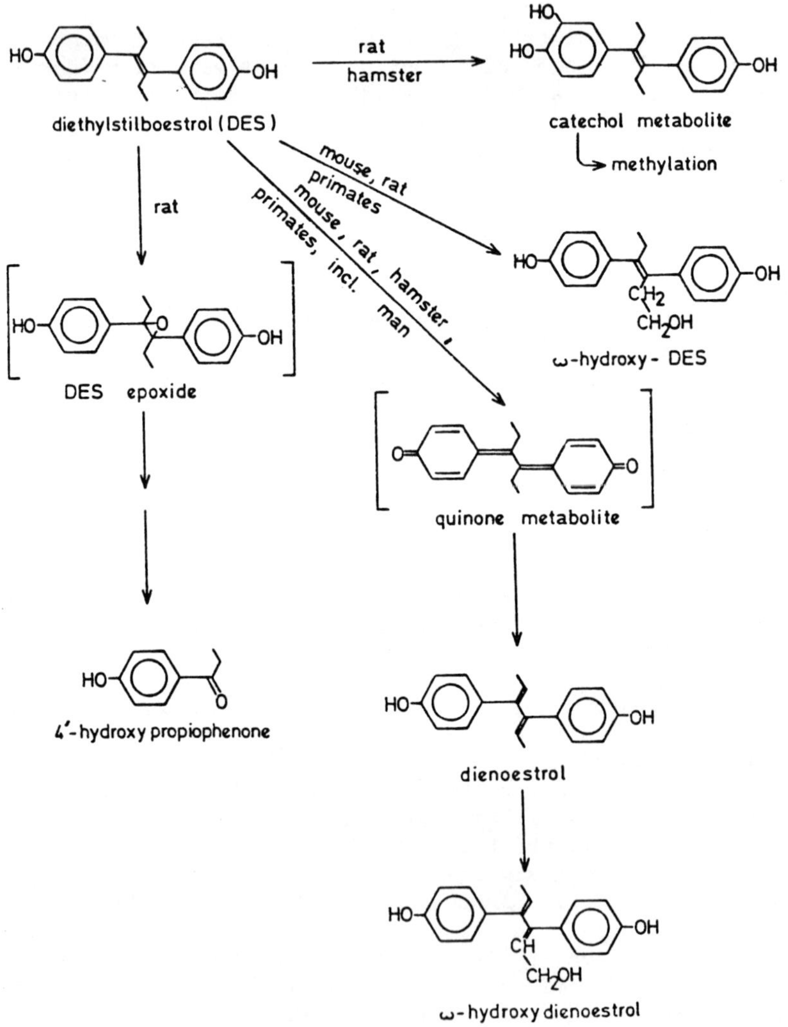
HO
OH
diethylstilboestrol (DES)
rat
hamster
catechol metabolite
methylation
mouse, rat
primates
mouse, rat, hamster,
primates, incl. man
rat
DES epoxide
ω-hydroxy- DES
CH_2
CH_2OH
quinone metabolite
O
4'-hydroxy propiophenone
dienoestrol
CH
ω-hydroxy dienoestrol

mouse foetal cells in culture, bind covalently to DNA (Blackburn et al., 1976). Oxidative metabolism of DES in vitro is enhanced by pretreatment with phenobarbitone (Levin et al., 1968).

Metabolic studies carried out in mice have shown extensive glucuronidation of DES and its metabolites in maternal and foetal mouse liver (Metzler & McLachlan, 1978; Shah & McLachlan, 1976). Excretion of DES metabolites in mice occurs mainly via the faeces (Helton et al., 1978a).

In contrast to rats, sulphate conjugation of DES is important in guinea-pigs (Barford et al., 1977). In cattle, DES is metabolized slowly and the metabolites excreted predominantly in the faeces (Aschbacher & Thacker, 1974).

The metabolism of DES has been investigated in Macaca mulatta (rhesus) monkeys and in chimpanzees: principal excretion occurs via the urine (Helton et al., 1978b; Metzler et al., 1977). Enterohepatic circulation plays a major role in the distribution of DES in rhesus monkeys, the major biliary compound after i.v. administration being DES monoglucuronide (Mroszczak & Riegelman, 1975). Metabolism of DES in these monkeys appears to be similar to that in humans, since the major glucuronide metabolites are dienoestrol, ω-hydroxydienoestrol and ω-hydroxydiethyl-stilboestrol (see Fig. 1) (Metzler et al., 1977).

Mutagenicity and other short-term tests

DES did not induce reverse mutations in Salmonella typhimurium strains TA1535, TA1537, TA1538, TA100 and TA98; and it gave no indication of a mutagenic effect in his⁻ S. typhimurium strains under 10 different metabolic situations (no exogenous metabolizing system; 9000 x g supernatant from liver homogenate of Aroclor 1254-induced rats with or without inhibition of epoxide hydratase; liver and/or kidney 9000 x g supernatant from control or Aroclor 1254-treated hamsters; horseradish peroxidase + H_2O_2). Furthermore, 11 metabolites and other derivatives of DES, two of which (diethylstilboestrol-3,4-oxide and β-dienoestrol; see monograph on dienoestrol, p.161) are potent inducers of sister chromatid exchanges in cultured human fibroblasts (Rüdiger et al., 1979), were not mutagenic in S. typhimurium TA100, TA98, TA1537 and TA1535 in the presence or absence of 9000 x g supernatant from liver homogenate of Aroclor 1254-induced rats (Glatt et al., 1979; McCann & Ames, 1976; McCann et al., 1975). The compound was also reported to be negative in several other systems using Escherichia coli and bacterial auxotrophs derived from S. typhimurium LT-2 (Cline & McMahon, 1977; Fluck et al., 1976; Hemmerly & Demerec, 1955).

It does not significantly increase sister chromatid exchanges in a pseudodiploid Chinese hamster cell line (Don) (Abe & Sasaki, 1977).

DES was positive in chromosomal aberration tests carried out *in vitro* with Chinese hamster fibroblasts (Ishidate & Odashima, 1977). Concentrations of 5, 15 and 20 µg/ml produced no chromosomal damage in human peripheral blood leucocytes in culture (Bishun *et al.*, 1977).

DES (concentration not given) induced mutations in the mouse lymphoma system L5178Y/TK$^{+/-}$ (Clive, 1977). A concentration of 10^{-6} M induced unscheduled DNA synthesis in HeLa cells in the presence of a liver activation system (Martin *et al.*, 1978).

Male mice exposed to a single i.p. injection of 1, 10 or 100 mg/kg bw diethylstilbestrol diphosphate had an increased number of aneuploid cells in their bone marrow after 6, 24 and 48 hrs. The effect was not dose-dependent (Chrisman & Hinkle, 1974).

Single doses of 1.0, 0.1, or 0.01 µg diethylstilboestrol diphosphate dissolved in 0.85% sodium chloride were injected intraperitoneally 6, 24 or 48 hrs before day 8.5 of gestation into 45 mice of strains LP/J, SJL/J, BALB/cJ and C57BL/6J; 307 embryos were collected on day 8.5 for chromosome preparation. Aneuploidy was significantly increased, depending on dose and time (Chrisman, 1974).

(b) Humans

Women exposed to diethylstilboestrol occupationally showed signs of hyperoestrogenism. Enlargement of the breast was noticed in a man with such exposure. Pigmentation of the nipples and breast enlargement were observed in children born to exposed women (Pacyn'ski *et al.*, 1971).

Sulphobromophthalein retention was significantly altered in women who received 120 mg DES over 6 days to suppress post-partum lactation (Clinch & Tindall, 1969). In contrast, it has been claimed that administration of diethylstilbestrol diphosphate to patients with prostatic carcinoma at daily doses of 500 mg for 3 weeks, then 60 mg per day oestradiol benzoate for 1 year, led to no marked changes in various liver function tests (Ishibe, 1975).

The metabolism of DES in humans is similar to that in other species, especially non-human primates (Metzler, 1976). About 40% of ^{14}C-DES injected into human volunteers is recovered from the first day's urine, glucuronides representing 90% of the activity; 70% of the glucuronides are conjugated with DES, about 10% with dienoestrol and about 20% with ω-hydroxydienoestrol (see Fig. 1).

Data on the teratogenic effects of DES in humans are given in the following section.

3.3 Case reports and epidemiological studies (of carcinogenicity and teratogenicity)

(a) Prenatal exposure

Vagina and cervix: Herbst & Scully (1970) first described 7 cases of adenocarcinoma (6 of the clear-cell type) of the vagina in females between the ages of 15 and 22 years. The 7 cases exceeded the total number of these cancers in this age group previously reported in the world literature. An epidemiological study the following year, which included an eighth additional case (Herbst *et al.*, 1971), related the occurrence of these tumours in 7 of the 8 patients to the fact that their mothers had received DES during the relevant pregnancy for threatened abortion or for prior pregnancy loss. None of the 8 matched control mothers had had a similar exposure. Within a few months, a confirmatory report of 4 cases with exposure to DES was published (Greenwald *et al.*, 1971). Later, clear-cell adenocarcinoma of the cervix was also shown to be related to prenatal exposure to DES (Herbst *et al.*, 1972a; Noller *et al.*, 1972). Within approximately one year, a number of additional reports dealing with individual cases of clear-cell adenocarcinoma of the vagina and cervix in the US were published (Greenwald *et al.*, 1973; Henderson *et al.*, 1973; Hill, 1973; Nissen & Goldstein, 1973; Tsukada *et al.*, 1972; Williams & Schweitzer, 1973).

Studies of the clinical, pathological and epidemiological aspects of these cancers have been made possible by centralizing pertinent data in a confidential file in the Registry for Research on Hormonal Transplacental Carcinogenesis (formerly the Registry for Clear-Cell Adenocarcinoma in the Genital Tract In Young Females). Although most cases in the Registry are from the US, DES-associated tumours have also been identified in Australia, Belgium, Canada, Czechoslovakia, France, Israel, the Ivory Coast, Mexico and The Netherlands (Alvarez Bravo *et al.*, 1970; Barrat *et al.*, 1975; De Graaff *et al.*, 1976; Herbst & Cole, 1978; Krupa & Pelikan, 1977; Verhoeven, 1972).

Detailed analyses have been published of the first 91 cases of clear-cell adenocarcinoma of the vaginal tract in the US (Herbst *et al.*, 1972a) and of 170 subsequent cases (Herbst *et al.*, 1974). Currently, approximately 350 cases have been made accessible and studied (Herbst & Cole, 1978; Herbst *et al.*, 1977a). Not all, however, are related to prenatal exposure to DES: clear-cell adenocarcinoma of the cervix and, to a lesser extent, clear-cell adenocarcinoma of the vagina in women under 25 years had been reported previous to the introduction of DES (Fawcett *et al.*, 1966; Hameed, 1968; Studdiford, 1957).

Among the cases for which a maternal history was available, 65% of mothers had been treated with DES or with the chemically similar substances, dienoestrol or hexoestrol, usually but not always for high-risk pregnancy.

In about 10% of the cases, the mother had received an unidentifiable drug for the treatment of a pregnancy complication; and in about 25% of the cases there was no evidence that the mother had received any hormonal medication during the relevant pregnancy. In all cases for which accurate dates were available, the mother began therapy during the first half of pregnancy. Dosages varied widely: maximum daily doses ranged from 1.5-150 mg; total doses throughout pregnancy varied from 135-18,200 mg (Herbst & Cole, 1978).

An analysis of incidence by age of diagnosis of the patients with clear-cell adenocarcinoma whose mothers had been treated with DES (Herbst *et al.*, 1977a) showed that the tumour occurred primarily after menarche, although prepubertal cases have been reported. The youngest exposed patient was aged 7 and the eldest 29. There is a sharp peak in the age incidence curve at 19 years; its shape beyond age 24 years is uncertain at present due to the young age of the population at risk (Herbst *et al.*, 1977b, 1979).

A recent analysis of five-year survival curves (Herbst *et al.*, 1979) shows excellent therapeutic results: over 90% for early, stage I carcinoma. Poor results are obtained for patients with advanced tumours. Metastases to the lung, parenchyma and supraclavicular nodal areas are more frequent in cases of clear-cell adenocarcinoma of the vagina and cervix than in cases of squamous-cell carcinoma at those sites (Robboy *et al.*, 1974). Currently, 68 patients reported to the Registry are known to be dead (Herbst *et al.*, 1979).

A Boston Collaborative Drug Surveillance Program study, reported by Heinonen (1973), analysed data regarding exposure to DES during pregnancy over the period 1959-1965 in the 12 centres participating in the US Collaborative Perinatal Study. A total of 217 women were found to have been exposed to DES among the 57,071 pregnancies included in the study; almost all of these occurred at 2 of the centres. The dose received varied widely, from 2.5-150 mg per day, with total doses of 0.175-46.6 g; and the duration of treatment varied from less than 1 week to 252 days. On the basis of market research data, it was estimated that the total number of live female offspring in the US who were exposed to DES *in utero* during the period 1960-1970 was likely to be between 10,000 and 16,000 *per annum*. The exposure rates for the 1950s are believed to be much higher. On the basis of cumulative incidence data on clear-cell adenocarcinoma from the Registry and of data on sales of 25-mg DES tablets from one of the many drug houses that sold them, it has been estimated (Herbst & Cole, 1978; Herbst *et al.*, 1977a) that peak exposure in the US occurred during the years 1951-1953. In the UK, Kinlen *et al.* (1974) estimated the number of exposed mothers to be about 7500 between 1940-1971 (mostly during the 1950s). No accurate statistics concerning the size of the exposed population are available from any country.

Lanier *et al.* (1973), reviewing case records at the Mayo Clinic, Rochester, Minn., identified 818 female infants born during the interval 1943-1959 whose mothers had received some form of oestrogen therapy during pregnancy (93% received DES). Follow-up by physical examination or mailed questionnaire was completed up to 1970 or later in 99% of the cases. No adenocarcinomas of the vagina or cervix were found. Herbst *et al.* (1977b) estimated that the risk among these exposed children of developing clear-cell adenocarcinoma of the vagina or cervix was 0.14-1.4 per 1000 through age 24. These estimates are consistent with the reports of Carstens & Clemmesen (1972), who found no cases in women under 25 in Denmark in 1943-1967, and of Ulfelder *et al.* (1971), who reported that there were no cases among thousands of gynaecological cancers treated in Basel and Frankfurt. It should be noted that use of DES during pregnancy has been very infrequent in those areas. Cases are rarely found in areas of limited use, such as the UK (Kinlen *et al.*, 1974), where only one DES-associated case has been identified (Monaghan & Sirisena, 1978).

Gross and microscopic abnormalities of the tissues of the vagina and cervix have frequently been reported and extensively described in females exposed prenatally to DES. The most common changes are vaginal adenosis (columnar epithelium or its mucinous products in the vagina), cervical ectropion (eversion or erosion, columnar epithelium or its mucinous products in the cervix) and transverse fibrous ridges in the vagina or on the cervix (transverse septum, cocks-comb cervix, vaginal hood) (Herbst *et al.*, 1972b; Pomerance, 1973; Sandberg, 1976; Scully *et al.*, 1974, 1978). Cervical ectropion is common among females of reproductive age in the absence of DES exposure, while adenosis and transverse ridges occur only rarely in the general population.

Case-control studies have confirmed the association of vaginal adenosis with prenatal exposure to DES. The rate of adenosis among the exposed daughters appears to be related linearly to the time during pregnancy at which the mother began medication: it was highest in early pregnancy and was not detected when treatment was initiated in the 18th week or later (Bibbo *et al.*, 1975a, 1977; Herbst *et al.*, 1975a).

A large, multi-institutional cooperative study (DESAD, DES adenosis) to evaluate the changes in 2000 DES-exposed offspring has been initiated (Sestili, 1977). Initial clinical findings have been reported for 3339 young women enrolled in the DESAD project. Vaginal epithelial changes, detected by colposcopy or iodine staining, occurred in 34% of 1275 participants identified by review of prenatal records; these changes are most closely associated with the timing of the onset of intrauterine exposure to DES, total dose and length of exposure. No severe dysplasia, carcinoma *in situ*, invasive squamous-cell carcinoma or clear-cell carcinoma were observed (O'Brien *et al.*, 1979).

Many non-controlled studies have described in detail the gross and microscopic genital changes in females exposed to DES prenatally (Burke *et al.*, 1974; Herbst *et al.*, 1975a; Sandberg, 1976; Sherman *et al.*, 1974; Stafl *et al.*, 1974; Townsend, 1978). The incidence of adenosis varied from 35-90%. Much of this discrepancy is due to the heterogeneity of the subjects examined, i.e., variations in maternal history of the exposed patients: one study was limited to patients whose exposure occurred during the first trimester, while others had random exposures, some as late as the 20th week of pregnancy. Differences in the definition of adenosis by various investigators also contribute to the variation in the reported prevalence of adenosis (Herbst *et al.*, 1975b). Older patients are reported to have a lower frequency of adenosis than younger subjects, presumably due to replacement of the columnar epithelium of adenosis by squamous metaplastic epithelium (Ng *et al.*, 1975, 1977; Scully *et al.*, 1974, 1978).

Stafl & Mattingly (1974) and Mattingly & Stafl (1976) have suggested that the large areas of squamous metaplasia found in the elongated transformation zone of females exposed prenatally to DES increase the risk of developing squamous-cell cancer. However, it appears that some cases diagnosed as neoplasia (dysplasia or carcinoma *in situ*) may actually be cases of active, immature squamous metaplasia; diagnosis of the changes in squamous epithelium thus poses a serious problem. The use of microspectrophotometric determination of nuclear DNA to estimate aneuploidy has been suggested to try to separate neoplastic from metaplastic squamous epithelial changes in females exposed prenatally to DES. At present, no increased risk of squamous-cell carcinoma of the vagina or cervix among such exposed persons has been established (Fu *et al.*, 1978a,b; Richart *et al.*, 1978; Robboy *et al.*, 1978).

There have been numerous reviews of the histopathological changes observed in females exposed prenatally to DES, including clear-cell adenocarcinoma, vaginal adenosis, cervical ectropion and transverse ridges (Antonioli & Burke, 1975; Robboy *et al.*, 1975; Scully *et al.*, 1974, 1978). Cytological features observed in the epithelium of such exposed females have also been reviewed extensively (Bibbo *et al.*, 1975b; Fu *et al.*, 1978a; Hart *et al.*, 1976; Ng *et al.*, 1975, 1977; Taft *et al.*, 1974). Benign atypical changes, such as microglandular hyperplasia ('the pill lesion'), which can be confused with clear-cell adenocarcinoma, have also been observed (Robboy & Welch, 1977).

Ultrastructural studies have been reported on clear-cell adenocarcinoma (Puri *et al.*, 1977; Silverberg & DeGiorgi, 1972) and on adenosis and cervical ectropion (Fenoglio *et al.*, 1976). These studies indicate that the observed changes are compatible with a Müllerian origin for the abnormal epithelium in females exposed to DES prenatally; this is consistent with the histogenesis suggested by light microscope studies (Haney *et al.*, 1979; Kurman & Scully, 1974; Scully *et al.*, 1974, 1978).

Uterine corpus: Structural changes, detected by hysterosalpingo-
graphy, were reported by Kaufman *et al.* (1977) in the uterus and Fallopian
tube of 40 of 60 females exposed prenatally to DES. Small endometrial
cavities, 'T'-shaped uteri and dilated cornual areas were noted. They
found no similar changes in hysterosalpingograms from unexposed females
of the same age. The effect, if any, of these changes on future fertility
is not known.

Kidney and ureter: Herbst & Cole (1978) reported that i.v. pyelo-
graphic examinations of females exposed prenatally to DES with clear-
cell adenocarcinoma of the vagina or cervix showed that approximately 5%
had some congenital abnormality of the kidney or ureter. This incidence
does not differ from that previously reported in the general population
(Smith & Orkin, 1945).

Male genital tract: Bibbo *et al.* (1977) and Gill *et al.* (1977,
1978) reported a greater frequency of abnormalities in the reproductive
tracts of males exposed prenatally to DES, in comparison with unexposed
controls. The most common genital lesions were epididymal cysts, hypotropic
testes, capsular induration of the testes and cryptorchidism. These
were observed in 30% of 289 exposed subjects, in comparison with 8% of 290
unexposed males. Analysis of single semen specimens from 88 DES-exposed
males revealed severe pathological changes in 23% and less severe changes
in 39%, whereas such changes were found in 5 and 14% of specimens from 55
males exposed to a placebo. No malignancies were observed, and the
effects of these findings on fertility rates are not known.

(b) Postnatal exposure:

Uterus and endometrium: Among 24 female patients with gonadal
dysgenesis (Turner's syndrome) treated for 5 or more years with DES,
endometrial carcinoma developed in 2 and possibly a third (Cutler *et
al.*, 1972). Three other cases that had previously been reported by
other authors were also reviewed. Of the total of 5 definite cases, 3
were of an unusual mixed or adeno-squamous type. It should be noted
that the risk of endometrial carcinoma in untreated gonadal dysgenesis
is unknown; however, the authors state that the only spontaneous endometrial carcinoma ever reported occurred in a 79-year-old woman.
Wilkinson *et al.* (1973) described a case of endometrial adenocarcinoma
which occurred after 9 years of DES therapy; no change was noted after
$4\frac{1}{2}$ months of progestational treatment, during which time the DES treatment
was discontinued.

In a recent literature review, Louka *et al.* (1978) identified a
total of 11 cases of endometrial carcinoma (including those reported and
reviewed by Cutler *et al.* and Wilkinson *et al.*) in patients with Turner's
syndrome. The average age of the patients was 31 years; 8 had been
given DES, 1 had been given DES and ethisterone, and 2 had received

oestrogens other than DES. McCarty *et al.* (1978) reported a 12th case
in a 49-year old patient treated intermittently for 30 years with oestrone
sulphate who had received DES for 12 months at the beginning of treatment.
Reid & Shirley (1974) reported a case of endometrial adenocarcinoma in a
42-year-old patient with Sheehan's syndrome who had been treated with DES
for 17 years. Khandekar *et al.* (1978) reported endometrial carcinoma in
3 patients treated with DES for metastatic breast cancer.

Breast: Bibbo *et al.* (1978) conducted a health survey by mail
questionnaire of mothers who had taken DES during pregnancy, and of a
group of unexposed controls. These women had participated in a study
to evaluate the effectiveness of DES in pregnancy treatment 25 years
earlier; 693 of 840 exposed mothers were located and agreed to participate,
in comparison with 668 of 806 unexposed. Most categories of health
characteristics in the women were highly comparable; these included
mean number of pregnancies, parity, age at menopause, history of reserpine
medication, history of oral contraceptive use, a history of surgery for
benign disease, frequency of hysterectomy and family history of breast
cancer. A history of breast biopsy was found for 97 (14%) of the exposed
and 80 (12%) of the unexposed, and most showed fibrocystic disease.
Breast cancers occurred in 32 (4.6%) exposed women, compared with 21
(3.1%) unexposed; the excess was not statistically significant (P = 0.16).
There was also an excess of deaths (38 exposed *versus* 28 unexposed),
which was accounted for almost entirely by the difference in breast
cancer deaths (12 exposed *versus* 4 unexposed); this difference was not
significant and was due to the appearance of breast cancer at a younger
age among the exposed. There was no difference in breast cancer experience
among the mothers who had started DES prior to the 11th week of pregnancy
in comparison with those who had started after the 11th week. The risk
of breast cancer among both exposed and unexposed women was higher than
that in the general population, on the basis of comparisons with population-
based tumour registries such as the Connecticut Cancer Registry. The
increase was particularly marked for those 50 years of age or over, and
the reason for this increased risk is not known. The existence of
some unknown selection factor for mothers entering the randomized clinical
trial 25 years ago was suggested by the authors.

It was reported in an abstract that there was no increased risk of
breast cancer in DES-exposed mothers enrolled in the national DESAD project at the Mayo Clinic Center (Brian *et al.*, 1978).

According to Campbell & Cummins (1951) and Benson (1957), the great
majority of cases of breast cancer reported in men treated with oestrogens
for cancer of the prostate are in fact metastases of the prostatic
tumour. The report of O'Grady & McDivitt (1969), however, describes a
case of primary carcinoma of the breast with Paget's disease of the

nipple in a man who had received long-term treatment with DES for carcinoma of the prostate. Bülow *et al.* (1973) reviewed 30 cases reported in the world literature between 1946 and 1972: among 16 men who had been treated with DES alone, with total doses varying from 200-44,200 mg, the breast tumour appeared from 1-57 months after the start of treatment. On the basis of histological and biochemical investigations, 6 of the tumours were considered to be new primaries and 10 to be metastases.

Liver: Galanaud *et al.* (1976) reported a hepatoma in a 74-year-old male treated with 10 mg DES daily for 15 years for metastatic prostatic carcinoma. Hoch-Ligeti (1978) reported a hepatic angiosarcoma in a 76-year-old male treated with 3 mg DES daily for 13 years for a well-differentiated adenocarcinoma of the liver.

Ovary: A recent study has raised the suspicion that an excess risk of ovarian cancer is associated with the use of DES in conjunction with Premarin (conjugated equine oestrogens) for symptoms of the climacteric; 3 ovarian cancers were observed in 21 patients, whereas 0.1 was expected (Hoover *et al.* 1977).

Skin: Two cases of melanoma have been reported in men receiving DES for treatment of prostatic cancer (Sadoff *et al.*, 1973).

4. Summary of Data Reported and Evaluation[1,2]

4.1 Experimental data

Diethylstilboestrol was tested in mice and rats by oral administration; in mice by local application; in mice, rats, hamsters and monkeys by subcutaneous implantation; and in mice, hamsters and dogs by subcutaneous injection. It was also tested by prenatal exposure in mice and hamsters and by neonatal exposure in mice and rats. Its administration to mice resulted in an increased incidence of mammary and lymphoid tumours in both males and females, and of interstitial-cell tumours of the testis in males and ovarian tumours in females; cervical and vaginal tumours were observed in females, including those exposed prenatally and on the first day of life. In rats, increased incidences of pituitary, mammary and bladder tumours (in conjunction with calculi) were observed. In hamsters, a high incidence of renal tumours was observed in castrated males and females and in intact males, but not in intact females. Following prenatal exposure of hamsters, tumours of the uterus, cervix and vagina were observed in female offspring, and tumours of the accessory sex organs occurred in males. In squirrel monkeys, malignant mesotheliomas of the uterine serosa were observed.

---

[1]This section should be read in conjunction with pp. 62-64 in the 'General Remarks on Sex Hormones' and with the 'General Conclusions on Sex Hormones,' p. 131.

[2]Subsequent to the meeting of the Working Group, the Secretariat became aware of a study in which rats were given a single s.c. injection of 1 mg/kg bw diethylstilboestrol propionate on day 19 of pregnancy. Tumours developed in 14/18 progeny and in 9/34 intact controls. Tumours of the ovary (2) and uterus (4) were seen only in treated animals (Napalkov & Anisimov, 1979).

In another study, rats were given s.c. injections of 0.015-0.6 mg/kg bw DES on days 13, 16, 18 and 20 of pregnancy and/or 0.2-10 mg/kg bw DES for 3 weeks *post partum*. Genital tumours (2 vaginal squamous-cell carcinomas, 1 endometrial adenocarcinoma, 1 ovarian adenocarcinoma) were observed among 10 female offspring. None of the controls developed such tumours (Vorherr *et al.*, 1979).

Another study has been reported in which male Syrian golden and European hamsters were implanted subcutaneously with a 25-mg DES pellet. The animals developed adenomas and adenocarcinomas of the kidney and adenohypophysis and adenomas of the testes and adrenal glands. European hamsters, which are more sensitive, also developed liver tumours (adenomas, cholangiocellular carcinomas and hepatocellular carcinomas) (Reznik-Schüller, 1979).

In most studies by pellet implantation, an accurate assessment of the effective carcinogenic dose could not be made. After oral administration, the lowest statistically significant dose that produced mammary carcinomas in mice was about 6 µg/kg bw per day. This dose is similar to that of diethylstilboestrol used in humans in the control of symptoms of the climacteric (10 µg/kg bw per day) and 30 times less than the dose given for the control of mammary or prostatic cancer (300 µg/kg bw per day).

Diethylstilboestrol dipropionate was tested by subcutaneous injection in rats and frogs, producing pituitary tumours in rats and tumours of the haematopoietic tissue in frogs.

Subcutaneous injection of polydiethylstilboestrol phosphate in hamsters produced renal tumours.

Diethylstilboestrol is embryolethal for pre- and postimplantation embryos in some species and causes teratogenic effects on the genital tract, which may be of significance for the carcinogenicity observed in these tissues.

4.2 Human data

Diethylstilboestrol taken during pregnancy has been shown to be causally associated with an increase in vaginal and cervical clear-cell adenocarcinoma in daughters, primarily in those between the ages of 10 and 30 years. The risk appears to be in the order of 0.14-1.4/1000 exposed daughters up to the age of 24 years. Because of the young age of the population at risk, further estimates of cancer risk cannot be made at this time.

Non-neoplastic epithelial and structural changes of the female genital tract have frequently been observed in the daughters of women exposed to diethylstilboestrol during pregnancy; these changes include transverse fibrous cervical and vaginal septa, vaginal adenosis and cervical ectropion. Non-malignant structural changes have been reported in the reproductive tracts of male children of exposed women; but the effect of diethylstilboestrol on fertility, if any, is uncertain. Cryptorchidism and hypoplastic testes observed in one study have been shown to be related to exposure to diethylstilboestrol; these conditions can predispose to malignant changes, but an increased risk of malignancy in males has not been demonstrated.

There appears to be an increased risk of endometrial carcinoma in young women with Turner's syndrome who were treated with diethylstilboestrol.

A few cases have been reported of breast cancer in men treated with diethylstilboestrol for metastatic prostatic carcinoma. Although a modest excess of breast cancer was observed in one study of mothers exposed to diethylstilboestrol, the difference from that in controls was not statistically significant.

Evidence strongly suggests that the administration of oestrogens for the control of symptoms of the climacteric is causally related to an increased incidence of endometrial carcinoma; diethylstilboestrol is no different from other oestrogens in this respect.

4.3 Evaluation

Diethylstilboestrol is causally associated with the occurrence of cancer in humans. There is also *sufficient evidence* for its carcinogenicity in experimental animals.

5. References

Abe, S. & Sasaki, M. (1977) Chromosome aberrations and sister chromatid exchanges in Chinese hamster cells exposed to various chemicals. J. natl Cancer Inst., 58, 1635-1641

Adams, C.E., Hay, M.F. & Lutwak-Mann, C. (1961) The action of various agents upon the rabbit embryo. J. Embryol. exp. Morphol., 9, 468-491

Alvarez Bravo, A., Andrade Sánchez, A. & Quiroz, R. (1970) A case of primary adenocarcinoma of the vagina and pregnancy (Sp.) Ginecol. Obstet. Méx., 28, 379-386

Andervont, H.B. (1941) Spontaneous tumours in a subline of strain C_3H mice. J. natl Cancer Inst., 1, 737-744

Andervont, H.B. (1950) Attempt to detect a mammary tumor-agent in strain C mice by estrogenic stimulation. J. natl Cancer Inst., 11, 73-81

Andervont, H.B., Shimkin, M.B. & Canter, H.Y. (1957) Effect of discontinued estrogenic stimulation upon the development and growth of testicular tumors in mice. J. natl Cancer Inst., 18, 1-25

Andervont, H.B., Dunn, T.B. & Canter, H.Y. (1958) Susceptibility of agent-free inbred mice and their F1 hybrids to estrogen-induced mammary tumors. J. natl Cancer Inst., 21, 783-804

Andervont, H.B., Shimkin, M.B. & Canter, H.Y. (1960) Susceptibility of seven inbred strains and the F1 hybrids to estrogen-induced testicular tumors and occurrence of spontaneous testicular tumors in strain BALB/c mice. J. natl Cancer Inst., 25, 1069-1081

Anon. (1977) Groups says DES safe, hits Delaney clause. Chemical & Engineering News, 31 January, p. 5

Anon. (1978) Consideration of labeling alternative for DES suggested. Food Chemical News, 13 March, pp. 37-38

Antonio, P., Gabaldón, M., Lacomba, T. & Juan, A. (1974) Effect of the antiestrogen nafoxidine on the occurrence of estrogen-dependent renal tumors in hamster. Horm. Metab. Res., 6, 522-524

Antonioli, D.A. & Burke, L. (1975) Vaginal adenosis. Analysis of 325 biopsy specimens from 100 patients. Am. J. clin. Pathol., 64, 625-638

Arai, Y., Suzuki, Y. & Nishizuka, Y. (1977) Hyperplastic and metaplastic lesions in the reproductive tract of male rats induced by neonatal treatment with diethylstilbestrol. Virch. Arch. A. Pathol. Histol., 376, 21-28

Arai, Y., Chen, C.-Y. & Nishizuka, Y. (1978) Cancer development in male reproductive tract in rats given diethylstilbestrol at neonatal age. Gann, 69, 861-862

Aschbacher, P.W. & Thacker, E.J. (1974) Metabolic fate of oral diethyl-stilbestrol in steers. J. Anim. Sci., 39, 1185-1192

Balika, Y.D., Kartasheva, V.E. & Fursova, Z.K. (1976) Effect of antenatal administration of diethylstilbestrol and progesterone on the blood system of the newborn progeny (Russ.). Byull. ekxp. Biol. Med., 82, 1250-1251 (Translation in Bull. exp. Biol. Med., 82, 1561-1563)

Ball, Z.B., Huseby, R.A. & Visscher, M.B. (1946) The effect of dietary pseudo-hypophysectomy upon the development of the mammary glands and mammary tumors in mice receiving diethylstilbestrol. Cancer Res., 6, 493

Barford, P.A., Olavesen, A.H., Curtis, C.G. & Powell, G.M. (1977) Biliary excretion of some anionic derivatives of diethylstilbestrol and phenolphthalein in the guinea pig. Biochem. J., 168, 373-377

Barrat, J., Brocheriou, C., Maria, B., Darbois, Y., Faguer, C. & Hervet, E. (1975) Clear-cell vaginal adenocarcinoma in young girls. A personal observation (Fr.). J. Gynecol. Obstet. Biol. Reprod., 4, 1093-1102

Benson, W.R. (1957) Carcinoma of the prostate with metastases to breasts and testis. Critical review of the literature and report of a case. Cancer, 10, 1235-1245

Bibbo, M. Al-Naqeeb, M., Baccarini, I., Gill, W., Newton, M., Sleeper, K.M., Sonek, M. & Wied, G.L. (1975a) Follow-up study of male and female offspring of DES-treated mothers. A preliminary report. J. reprod. Med., 15, 29-32

Bibbo, M., Ali, I., Al-Naqeeb, M., Baccarini, I., Climaco, L.A, Gill, W., Sonek, M. & Wied, G.L. (1975b) Cytologic findings in female and male offspring of DES treated mothers. Acta cytol., 19, 568-572

Bibbo, M., Gill, W.B., Azizi, F., Blough, R., Fang, V.S., Rosenfield, R.L., Schumacher, G.F.B., Sleeper, K., Sonek, M.G. & Wied, G.L. (1977) Follow-up study of male and female offspring of DES-exposed mothers. Obstet. Gynecol., 49, 1-8

Bibbo, M., Haenszel, W.M., Wied, G.L., Hubby, M. & Herbst, A.L. (1978) A twenty-five-year follow-up study of women exposed to diethylstilbestrol during pregnancy. New Engl. J. Med., 298, 763-767

Bishun, N.P., Smith, N., Eddie, H. & Williams, D.C. (1977) Cytogenetic studies and diethyl stilboestrol (Abstract no. 32). Mutat. Res., 46, 211-212

Blackburn, G.M., Thompson, M.H. & King, H.W.S. (1976) Binding of diethylstilbestrol to deoxyribonucleic acid by rat liver microsomal fractions in vitro and in mouse foetal cells in culture. Biochem. J., 158, 643-646

Brian, D., Tilley, B., Labarthe, D., O'Fallon, W. & Noller, K. (1978) Evidence against the association of breast cancer and DES exposure (Abstract). Am. J. Epidemiol., 108, 230

British Pharmacopoeia Commission (1973) British Pharmacopoeia, London, HMSO, p. 443

Brotherton, J. (1976) Sex Hormone Pharmacology, London, Academic Press, p. 49

Bülow, H., Wullstein, H.-K., Böttger, G. & Schröder, F.H. (1973) Carcinoma of the breast under estrogen treatment for prostatic carcinoma (Ger.). Urologe, A12, 249-253

Burke, L., Antonioli, D., Knapp, R.C. & Friedman, E.A. (1974) Vaginal adenosis. Correlation of colposcopic and pathologic findings. Obstet. Gynecol., 44, 257-264

Campbell, J.H. & Cummins, S.D. (1951) Metastases, simulating mammary cancer, in prostatic carcinoma under estrogenic therapy. Cancer, 4, 303-311

Canter, H.Y. & Shimkin, M.B. (1968) Effect of unilateral orchiectomy on induction of interstitial-cell tumors in BALB/c mice. Cancer Res., 28, 386-387

Carstens, P.H.B. & Clemmesen, J. (1972) Genital-tract cancer in Danish adolescents. New Engl. J. Med., 286, 198

Chrisman, C.L. (1974) Aneuploidy in mouse embryos induced by diethylstilbestrol diphosphate. Teratology, 9, 229-232

Chrisman, C.L. & Hinkle, L.L. (1974) Induction of aneuploidy in mouse bone marrow cells with diethylstilbestrol-diphosphate. Can. J. Genet. Cytol., 16, 831-835

Clinch, J. & Tindall, V.R. (1969) Effect of oestrogens and progestogens on liver function in the puerperium. Br. med. J., i, 602-605

Cline, J.C. & McMahon, R.E. (1977) Detection of chemical mutagens. Use of concentration gradient plates in a high capacity screen. Res. Commun. chem. Pathol. Pharmacol., 16, 523-533

Clive, D. (1977) A linear relationship between tumorigenic potency in vivo and mutagenic potency at the heterozygous thymidine kinase (TK+/-) locus of L5178Y mouse lymphoma cells coupled with mammalian metabolism. In: Scott, D., Bridges, B.A. & Sobels, F.H., eds, Progress in Genetic Toxicology, Amsterdam, Elsevier/North Holland, pp. 241-247

Council of Europe (1975) European Pharmacopoeia, Vol. 3, Sainte-Ruffine, France, pp. 205-206

Cutler, B.S., Forbes, A.P., Ingersoll, F.M. & Scully, R.E. (1972) Endometrial carcinoma after stilbestrol therapy in gonadal dysgenesis. New Engl. J. Med., 287, 628-631

Day, E.W., Jr, Vanatta, L.E. & Sieck, R.F. (1975) The confirmation of diethylstilbestrol residues in beef liver by gas chromatography-mass spectrometry. J. Assoc. off. analyt. Chem., 58, 520-524

De Graaff, J., Siregar-Emck, M.T.W. & Visser, G. (1976) Vaginal carcinoma in a young woman (Dutch). Ned. T. Geneesk., 120, 1569-1571

Dodds, E.C., Golberg, L., Lawson, W. & Robinson, R. (1938) Estrogenic activity of certain synthetic compounds. Nature, 141, 247-248 [Chem. Abstr., 32, 3369-8]

Dodds, E.C., Golberg, L., Lawson, W. & Robinson, R. (1939) Synthetic oestrogenic compounds related to stilbene and diphenylethane. I. Proc. R. Soc. (Lond.)., B127, 140-167

Donoho, A.L., Johnson, W.S., Sieck, R.F. & Sullivan, W.L. (1973) Gas chromatographic determination of diethylstilbestrol and its glucuronide in cattle tissues. J. Assoc. off. Analyt. Chem., 56, 785-792

Dorfman, R.I. (1966) Hormones (nonsteroidal estrogens). In: Kirk, R.E. & Othmer, D.F., eds, Encyclopedia of Chemical Technology, 2nd ed., Vol. 2, New York, Interscience, p. 132

Dunn, T.B. & Green, A.W. (1963) Cysts of the epididymis, cancer of the cervix, granular cell myoblastoma and other lesions after estrogen injection in newborn mice. J. natl Cancer Inst., 31, 425-438

Dunning, W.F., Curtis, M.R. & Segaloff, A. (1947) Strain differences in response to diethylstilbestrol and the induction of mammary gland and bladder cancer in the rat. Cancer Res., 7, 511-521

Dunning, W.F., Curtis, M.R. & Maun, M.E. (1949) The effect of dietary fat and carbohydrate on diethylstilbestrol-induced mammary cancer in rats. Cancer Res., 9, 354-361

Dunning, W.F., Curtis, M.R. & Maun, M.E. (1950) The effect of added dietary tryptophane on the occurrence of diethylstilbestrol-induced mammary cancer in rats. Cancer Res., 10, 319-323

Emmeus, C.W. & Martin, L. (1962) Estrogens. In: Dorfman, R.I., ed., Methods in Hormone Research, Vol. III, London, Academic Press, pp. 1-75

Engel, L.L., Weidenfeld, J. & Merriam, G.R. (1976) Metabolism of diethyl-stilbestrol by rat liver: a preliminary report. J. Toxicol. environ. Health, Suppl. 1, 37-44

Fawcett, K.J., Dockerty, M.B. & Hunt, A.B. (1966) Mesonephric carcinoma of the cervix uteri: a clinical and pathologic study. Am. J. Obstet. Gynecol., 95, 1068-1079

Fenoglio, C.M., Ferenczy, A., Richart, R.M. & Townsend, D. (1976) Scanning and transmission electron microscopic studies of vaginal adenosis and the cervical transformation zone in progeny exposed in utero to diethylstilbestrol. Am. J. Obstet. Gynecol., 126, 170-180

Fischer, L.J., Kent, T.H. & Weissinger, J.L. (1973) Absorption of diethyl-stilbestrol and its glucuronide conjugate from the intestines of five- and twenty-five-day-old rats. J. Pharmacol. exp. Ther., 185, 163-170

Fischer, L.J., Weissinger, J.L., Rickert, D.E. & Hintze, K.L. (1976) Studies on the biological disposition of diethylstilbestrol in rats and humans. J. Toxicol. environ. Health, 1, 587-605

Fluck, E.R., Poirier, L.A. & Ruelius, H.W. (1976) Evaluation of a DNA polymerase-deficient mutant of E. coli for the rapid detection of carcinogens. Chem. -biol. Interactions, 15, 219-231

Forsberg, J.-G. (1975) Late effects in the vaginal and cervical epithelia after injections of diethylstilbestrol into neonatal mice. Am. J. Obstet. Gynecol., 121, 101-104

Forsberg, J.-G. (1979) Developmental mechanism of estrogen-induced irreversible changes in the mouse-cervicovaginal epithelium. Natl Cancer Inst. Monogr., 51, 41-56

Fu, Y.S., Reagan, J.W., Hawliczek, S. & Wentz, W.B. (1978a) The use of cellular studies in the investigation of the DES-exposed woman. In: Herbst, A.L., ed., Intrauterine Exposure to Diethylstilbestrol in the Human, Chicago, American College of Obstetricians & Gynecologists, pp. 34-44

Fu, Y.S., Robboy, S.J. & Prat, J. (1978b) Nuclear DNA study of vaginal and cervical squamous cell abnormalities in DES exposed progeny. Obstet. Gynecol., 52, 129-137

Gabriel-Robez, O., Rhomer, A., Clavert, J. & Schneegans, E. (1972) Teratogenic and lethal actions of diethylstilbestrol on the mouse embryo (Fr.). Arch. fr. Pédiatr., 29, 149-154

Galanaud, P., Chaput, J.-C., Buffet, C. & Rain, B. (1976) Hepatoma after prolonged oestrogen therapy (Fr.). Nouv. Presse Méd., 5, 209

Gardner, W.U. (1959) Carcinoma of the uterine cervix and upper vagina: induction under experimental conditions in mice. Ann. N.Y. Acad. Sci., 75, 543-564

Gardner, W.U., Dougherty, T.F. & Williams, W.L. (1944) Lymphoid tumors in mice receiving steroid hormones. Cancer Res., 4, 73-87

Gass, G.H., Coats, D. & Graham, N. (1964) Carcinogenic dose-response curve to oral diethylstilbestrol. J. natl Cancer Inst., 33, 971-977

Gass, G.H., Brown, J. & Okey, A.B. (1974) Carcinogenic effects of oral diethylstilbestrol on C3H male mice with and without the mammary tumor virus. J. natl Cancer Inst., 53, 1369-1370

Geschickter, C.F. & Byrnes, E.W. (1942) Factors influencing the developme and time of appearance of mammary cancer in the rat in response to estrogen. Arch. Pathol., 33, 334-356

Gibson, J.P., Newberne, J.W., Kuhn, W.L. & Elsea, J.R. (1967) Comparative chronic toxicity of three oral estrogens in rats. Toxicol. appl. Pharmacol., 11, 489-510

Gill, W.B., Schumacher, G.F.B. & Bibbo, M. (1977) Pathological semen and anatomical abnormalities of the genital tract in human male subjects exposed to diethylstilbestrol in utero. J. Urol., 117, 477-480

Gill, W.B., Schumacher, G.F.B. & Bibbo, M. (1978) Genital and semen abnormalities in adult males two and one-half decades after in utero exposure to diethylstilbestrol. In: Herbst, A.L., ed., Intrauterine Exposure to Diethylstilbestrol in the Human, Chicago, American College of Obstetricians & Gynecologists, pp. 53-57

Glatt, H.R., Metzler, M. & Oesch, F. (1979) Diethylstilbestrol and 11 derivatives. A mutagenicity study with Salmonella typhimurium. Mutat. Res. 67, 113-121

Grasselli, J.G. & Ritchey, W.M., eds (1975) CRC Atlas of Spectral Data and Physical Constants for Organic Compounds, 2nd ed., Vol. 3, Cleveland, OH, Chemical Rubber Company, p. 458

Greene, R.R., Burrill, M.W. & Ivy, A.C. (1940)   Experimental intersexuality. The effects of estrogens on the antenatal sexual development of the rat. Am. J. Anat., 67, 305-345

Greenwald, P., Barlow, J.J., Nasca, P.C. & Burnett, W.S. (1971)   Vaginal cancer after maternal treatment with synthetic estrogens. New Engl. J. Med., 285, 390-392

Greenwald, P., Nasca, P.C., Burnett, W.S. & Polan, A. (1973)   Prenatal stilbestrol experience in mothers of young cancer patients. Cancer, 31, 568-572

Gutierrez-Cernosek, R.M. & Cernosek, S.F., Jr (1977)   Radioimmunoassays for monitoring exposure to potential carcinogens. Ann. clin. Lab. Sci., 7, 35-41

Hameed, K. (1968)   Clear cell 'mesonephric' carcinoma of uterine cervix. Obstet. Gynecol., 32, 564-575

Hamilton, J.M., Flaks, A., Saluja, P.G. & Maguire, S. (1975)   Hormonally induced renal neoplasia in the male Syrian hamster and the inhibitory effect of 2-bromo-α-ergocryptine methanesulfonate. J. natl Cancer Inst., 54, 1385-1400

Hamilton, J.M., Saluja, P.G., Thody, A.J. & Flaks, A. (1977)   The pars intermedia and renal carcinogenesis in hamsters. Eur. J. Cancer, 13, 29-32

Harvey, A.F., Hammond, C.B., Soules, M.R. & Creasman, W.T. (1979) Diethylstilbestrol-induced upper genital tract abnormalities. Fertil. Steril., 31, 142-146

Hart, W.R., Zaharov, I. Kaplan, B.J., Townsend, D.E, Aldrich, J.O., Henderson, B.E., Roy, M. & Benton, B. (1976)   Cytologic findings in stilbestrol exposed females with emphasis on detection of vaginal adenosis. Acta cytol., 20, 7-14

Harvey, S.C. (1975) Hormones. In: Osol, A. et al., eds, Remington's Pharmaceutical Sciences, 15th ed., Easton, PA, Mack, pp. 918-919

Heinonen, O.P. (1973) Diethylstilbestrol in pregnancy. Frequency of exposure and usage pattern. Cancer, 31, 573-577

Helton, E.D., Gough, B.J., King, J.W., Jr, Thenot, J.P. & Horning, E.C. (1978a) Metabolism of diethylstilbestrol in the C3H mouse: chromatographic systems for the quantitative analysis of DES metabolic products. Steroids, 31, 471-484

Helton, E.D., Hill, D.E., Gough, B.J., Lipe, G.W., King, J.W., Jr,
    Horning, E.C. & Thenot, J.P. (1978b) Comparative metabolism of
    diethylstilbestrol in the mouse, rhesus monkey, and chimpanzee.
    J. Toxicol. environ. Health, 4, 482-483

Hemmerly, J. & Demerec, M. (1955) Tests of chemicals for mutagenicity.
    Cancer Res., 15 (Suppl. 3), 69-75

Henderson, B.E., Benton, B.D.A., Weaver, P.T., Linden, G. & Nolan, J.F.
    (1973) Stilbestrol and urogenital-tract cancer in adolescents and
    young adults. New Engl. J. Med., 288, 354

Hendrickx, A.G., Benirschke, K., Thompson, R.S., Ahern, J., Lucas, W.E.
    & Oi, R.H. (1979) The effects of prenatal diethylstilbestrol (DES)
    exposure on the genitalia of pubertal Macaca mulatta. J. reprod.
    Med. (in press)

Herbst, A.L. & Cole, P. (1978) Epidemiologic and clinical aspects of
    clear cell adenocarcinoma in young women. In: Herbst, A.L., ed.,
    Intrauterine Exposure to Diethylstilbestrol in the Human, Chicago,
    American College of Obstetricians & Gynecologists, pp. 2-7

Herbst, A.L. & Scully, R E. (1970) Adenocarcinoma of the vagina in
    adolescence. A report of 7 cases including 6 clear-cell carcinomas
    (so-called mesonephromas). Cancer, 25, 745-757

Herbst, A.L., Ulfelder, H. & Poskanzer, D.C. (1971) Adenocarcinoma of
    the vagina. Association of maternal stilbestrol therapy with tumor
    appearance in young women. New Engl. J. Med., 284, 878-881

Herbst, A.L., Kurman, R.J., Scully, R.E. & Poskanzer, D.C. (1972a) Clear-
    cell adenocarcinoma of the genital tract in young females. Registry
    report. New Engl. J. Med., 287, 1259-1264

Herbst, A.L., Kurman, R.J. & Scully, R.E. (1972b) Vaginal and cervical
    abnormalities after exposure to stilbestrol in utero. Obstet.
    Gynecol., 40, 287-298

Herbst, A.L., Robboy, S.J., Scully, R.E. & Poskanzer, D.C. (1974) Clear-
    cell adenocarcinoma of the vagina and cervix in girls: analysis of
    170 Registry cases. Am. J. Obstet. Gynecol., 119, 713-724

Herbst, A.L., Poskanzer, D.C., Robboy, S.J., Friedlander, L. & Scully,
    R.E. (1975a) Prenatal exposure to stilbestrol. A prospective
    comparison of exposed female offspring with unexposed controls.
    New Engl. J. Med., 292, 334-339

Herbst, A.L., Scully, R.E. & Robboy, S.J. (1975b) Problems in the
    examination of the DES-exposed female. Obstet. Gynecol., 46, 353-355

Herbst, A.L., Cole, P., Colton, T., Robboy, S.J. & Scully, R.E. (1977a) Age-incidence and risk of diethylstilbestrol-related clear cell adenocarcinoma of the vagina and cervix. Am. J. Obstet. Gynecol., 128, 43-50

Herbst, A.L., Scully, R.E., Robboy, S.J., Welch, W.R. & Cole, P. (1977b) Abnormal development of the human genital tract following prenatal exposure to diethylstilbestrol. In: Hiatt, H.H., Watson, J.D. & Winsten, J.A., eds, Origins of Human Cancer, Cold Spring Harbor, NY, Cold Spring Harbor Laboratory, pp. 399-412

Herbst, A.L., Norusis, M.J., Rosenow, P.J., Welch, W.R. & Scully, R.E. (1979) An analysis of 346 cases of clear cell adenocarcinoma of the vagina and cervix with emphasis on recurrence and survival. Gynecol. Oncol., 7, 111-122

Heston, W.E. & Deringer, M.K. (1953) Occurrence of tumors in agent-free strain C3H$_f$ male mice implanted with estrogen-cholesterol pellets. Proc. Soc. exp. Biol. (N.Y.), 82, 731-734

Highman, B., Norvell, M.J. & Shellenberger, T.E. (1977) Pathological changes in female C3H mice continuously fed diets containing diethylstilbestrol or 17β-estradiol. J. environ. Pathol. Toxicol., 1, 1-30

Hill, E.C. (1973) Clear cell carcinoma of the cervix and vagina in young women. Am. J. Obstet. Gynecol., 116, 470-484

Hoch-Ligeti, C. (1978) Angiosarcoma of the liver associated with diethylstilbestrol. J. Am. med. Assoc., 240, 1510-1511

Hoover, R., Gray, L.A., Sr & Fraumeni, J.F., Jr (1977) Stilbestrol (diethylstilbestrol) and the risk of ovarian cancer. Lancet, ii, 533-534

Horning, E.S. (1954) The influence of unilateral nephrectomy on the development of stilboestrol-induced renal tumours in the male hamsters. Br. J. Cancer, 8, 627-634

Horning, E.S. (1956a) Observations on hormone-dependent renal tumours in the golden hamster. Br. J. Cancer, 10, 678-687

Horning, E.S. (1956b) Endocrine factors involved in the induction, prevention and transplantation of kidney tumours in the male golden hamster. Z. Krebsforsch., 61, 1-21

Horwitz, W., ed. (1975) Official Methods of Analysis of the Association of Official Analytical Chemists, 12th ed, Washington DC, Association of Official Analytical Chemists, pp. 745-746

Huseby, R.A. (1953) The effect of testicular function upon stilbestrol-induced mammary and pituitary tumors in mice. Proc. Am. Assoc. Cancer Res., 1, 25-26

IARC (1974) IARC Monographs on the Carcinogenic Risk of Chemicals to Man, 6, Sex Hormones, Lyon, pp. 55-76

Ishibe, T. (1975) Effect of long-term estrogen treatment on liver function in patients with prostatic carcinoma. J. Urol., 113, 829-833

Ishidate, M., Jr & Odashima, S. (1977) Chromosome tests with 134 compounds on Chinese hamster cells in vitro - a screening for chemical carcinogens. Mutat. Res., 48, 337-354

Jabara, A.G. (1959) Canine ovarian tumours following stilboestrol administration. Aust. J. exp. Biol. med. Sci., 37, 549-566

Jabara, A.G. (1962) Induction of canine ovarian tumours by diethylstilboestrol and progesterone. Aust. J. exp. Biol. med. Sci., 40, 139-152

Jacobi, J., Lloyd, H.M. & Meares, J.D. (1975) Induction of pituitary tumors in male rats by a single dose of estrogen. Horm. Metab. Res., 7, 228-230

Jarc, H., Ruttner, O. & Krocza, W. (1977) The quantatitive detection of estrogens and antithyroid drugs by thin-layer and high-performance thin-layer chromatography in animal tissue (Ger.). J. Chromatogr., 134, 351-358

Jeffus, M.T. & Kennert, C.T. (1972) Quantitative determination and confirmation of low levels of diethylstilbestrol in feeds. J. Assoc. off. analyt. Chem., 55, 1345-1353

Jeffus, M.T. & Kenner, C.T. (1973) Spectrophotofluorometric estimation of low levels of diethylstilbestrol in feedstuffs. J. Assoc. off. analyt. Chem., 56, 1483-1488

Jukes, T.H. (1974) Estrogens in beefsteaks. J. Am. med. Assoc., 229, 1920-1921

Jukes, T.H. (1976) Diethylstilbestrol in beef production: what is the risk to consumers? Prev. Med., 5, 438-453

Kalland, T. & Forsberg, J.-G., (1978) Delayed hypersensitivity response to oxazolone in neonatally estrogenized mice. Cancer Lett., 4, 141-146

Kalland, T., Fossberg, T.M. & Forsberg, J.-G. (1978) Effect of estrogen and corticosterone on the lymphoid system in neonatal mice. Exp. mol. Pathol., 28, 76-95

Kastrup, E.K., ed. (1976) Facts and Comparisons, St Louis, MO, Facts & Comparisons Inc., p. 101a

Kastrup, E.K., ed. (1977) Facts and Comparisons, St Louis, MO, Facts & Comparisons Inc., p. 114

Kastrup, E.K., ed. (1978) Facts and Comparisons, St Louis, MO, Facts & Comparisons Inc., p. 103

Kaufman, R.H., Binder, G.L., Gray, P.M., Jr & Adam, E. (1977) Upper genital tract changes associated with exposure in utero to diethylstilbestrol. Am. J. Obstet. Gynecol., 128, 51-59

Khandekar, J.D., Victor, T.A. & Mukhopadhyaya, P. (1978) Endometrial carcinoma following estrogen therapy for breast cancer. Report of three cases. J. Am. med. Assoc., 138, 539-541

Khudolei, V.V. & Ermoshchenkov, V.S. (1976) Carcinogenic action of diethylstilbestrol on frogs (Russ.). Byull. eksp. Biol. Med., 81, 723-724 (Translation in Bull. exp. Biol. Med., 1976, 81, 898-900)

King, J.R., Nony, C.R. & Bowman, M.C. (1977) Trace analysis of diethylstilbestrol [DES] in animal chow by parallel high-speed liquid chromatography, electron-capture gas chromatography, and radioassays. J. chromatogr. Sci., 15, 14-21

Kinlen, L.J., Badaracco, M.A., Moffett, J. & Vessey, M.P. (1974) A survey of the use of oestrogens during pregnancy in the United Kingdom and of the genito-urinary cancer mortality and incidence rates in young people in England and Wales. J. Obstet. Gynaecol. Br. Commonw., 81, 849-855

Kirkman, H. & Bacon, R.L. (1950) Malignant renal tumours in male hamsters (Cricetus auratus) treated with estrogen. Cancer Res., 10, 122-123

Kirkman, H. & Bacon, R.L. (1952a) Estrogen-induced tumors of the kidney. I. Incidence of renal tumors in intact and gonadectomized male golden hamsters treated with diethylstilbestrol. J. natl Cancer Inst., 13, 745-752

Kirkman, H. & Bacon, R.L. (1952b) Estrogen-induced tumors of the kidney. II. Effect of dose, administration, type of estrogen and age on the induction of renal tumors in intact male golden hamsters. J.. natl Cancer Inst., 13, 757-765

Klaassen, C.D. (1973a) Comparison of the toxicity of chemicals in newborn rats to bile duct-ligated and sham-operated rats and mice. Toxicol. appl. Pharmacol., 24, 37-44

Klaassen, C.D. (1973b) The effect of altered hepatic function on the
    toxicity, plasma disappearance and biliary excretion of diethylstil-
    bestrol. Toxicol. appl. Pharmacol., 24, 142-149

Klein, G. & Hellström, K.E. (1962) Transplantation studies on estrogen-
    induced interstitial-cell tumors of testis in mice. J. natl Cancer
    Inst., 28, 99-113

Kohrman, K.A. & MacGee, J. (1977) Simple and rapid gas-liquid
    chromatographic determination of diethylstilbestrol in biological
    specimens. J. Assoc. off. analyt. Chem., 60, 5-8

Kraybill, H.F., Helmes, C.T. & Sigman, C.C. (1977) Biomedical aspects
    of biorefractories in water. In: Hutzinger, O., ed., 2nd
    International Symposium on Aquatic Pollutants, Amsterdam,
    Noordwijkerhorit

Krupa, J. & Pelikán, K. (1977) Vaginal cancer composed of clear cells
    found in a girl age 18 years whose mother was treated during pregnancy
    by diethylstilbestrol (Agostilban) (Cz.). Cesk. Gynekol., 42, 264-
    268

Kurman, R.J. & Scully, R.E. (1974) The incidence and histogenesis of vaginal
    adenosis. An autopsy study. Hum. Pathol., 5, 265-276

Lacassagne, A. (1938) Appearance of mammary adenocarcinomas in male
    mice treated with a synthetic oestrogenic substance (Fr.). C.R. Soc.
    Biol. (Paris), 129, 641-643

Lacomba, T. & Gabaldón, M. (1971) Biochemical studies of diethylstilbes-
    trol-induced kidney tumors in the golden Syrian hamster. Cancer Res.,
    31, 1251-1256

Lamartiniere, C.A. & Lucier, G.W. (1978) Programming of hepatic histidase
    following prenatal administration of diethylstilbestrol. J. Steroid
    Biochem., 9, 595-598

Lanier, A.P., Noller, K.L., Decker, D.G., Elveback, L.R. & Kurland, L.T.
    (1973) Cancer and stilbestrol. A follow-up of 1,719 persons
    exposed to estrogens in utero and born 1943-1959. Mayo Clin. Proc.,
    48, 793-799

Lawrence, J.F. & Ryan, J.J. (1977) Comparison of electron-capture and
    electrolytic-conductivity detection for the gas-liquid chromato-
    graphic analysis of heptafluorobutyryl derivatives of some
    agricultural chemicals. J. Chromatogr., 130, 97-102

Levin, W., Welch, R.M. & Conney, A.H. (1968) Decreased uterotropic potency of oral contraceptives in rats pretreated with phenobarbital. Endocrinology, 83, 149-156

Llombart-Bosch, A. & Peydro, A. (1975) Morphological, histochemical and ultrastructural observations of diethylstilbestrol-induced kidney tumors in the Syrian golden hamster. Eur. J. Cancer, 11, 403-412

Louka, M.H., Ross, R.D., Lee, J.H., Jr & Lewis, G.C., Jr (1978) Endometrial carcinoma in Turner's syndrome. Gynecol. Oncol., 6, 294-304

Madan, D.K. & Cadwallader, D.E. (1973) Solubility of cholesterol and hormone drugs in water. J. pharm. Sci., 62, 1567-1569

Martin, C.N., McDermid, A.C. & Garner, R.C. (1978) Testing of known carcinogens and noncarcinogens for their ability to induce unscheduled DNA synthesis in HeLa cells. Cancer Res., 38, 2621-2627

Mattingly, R.F. & Stafl, A. (1976) Cancer risk in diethylstilbestrol-exposed offspring. Am. J. Obstet. Gynecol., 126, 543-548

Maugh, T.H., II (1976) The fatted calf: more weight gain with less feed. Science, 191, 453-454

McCann, J. & Ames, B.N. (1976) Detection of carcinogens as mutagens in the Salmonella/microsome test: assay of 300 chemicals: discussion. Proc. natl Acad. Sci. (Wash.), 73, 950-954

McCann, J., Choi, E., Yamasaki, E. & Ames, B.N. (1975) Detection of carcinogens as mutagens in the Salmonella/microsome test: assay of 300 chemicals. Proc. natl Acad. Sci. (Wash.), 72, 5135-5139

McCarty, K.S., Jr, Barton, T.K., Peete, C.H., Jr & Creasman, W.T. (1978) Gonadal dysgenesis with adenocarcinoma of the endometrium. An electron microscopic and steroid-receptor analyses with a review of the literature. Cancer, 42, 512-520

McClure, H.M. & Graham, C.E. (1973) Malignant uterine mesotheliomas in squirrel monkeys following diethylstilbestrol administration. Lab. Anim. Sci., 23, 493-498

McLachlan, J.A. (1976) Lesions in the genital tract of male mice following prenatal exposure to deithylstilbestrol. Proc. Eur. Soc. Toxicol., 17, 413-418

McLachlan, J.A. (1977) Prenatal exposure to diethylstilbestrol in mice. Toxicological studies. J. Toxicol. environ. Health, 2, 527-537

McLachlan, J.A. & Dixon, R.L. (1973) Effect of gestational exposure to DDT or diethylstilbestrol on the reproductive capacity of offspring (Abstract no. 238). Pharmacologist, 2, 199

McLachlan, J.A., Newbold, R.R. & Bullock, B. (1975a) Reproductive tract lesions in male mice exposed prenatally to diethylstilbestrol. Science, 190, 991-992

McLachlan, J.A., Shah, H.C., Newbold, R.R. & Bullock, B.C. (1975b) Effect of prenatal exposure of mice of diethylstilbestrol on reproductive tract function in the offspring (Abstract no. 173). Toxicol. appl. Pharmacol., 33, 190

McLachlan, J.A., Newbold, R.R. & Lamb, J.C. (1977) Genital tract abnormalities in mice following gestational exposure to DES. Environ. Health Perspect., 20, 240

McMartin, K.E., Kennedy, K.A., Greenspan, P., Alam, S.N., Greiner, P. & Jam, J. (1978) Diethylstilbestrol: a review of its toxicity and use as a growth promotant in food-producing animals. J. environ. Pathol. Toxicol., 1, 279-313

Metzler, M. (1975) Metabolic activation of diethylstilbestrol: indirect evidence for the formation of a stilbene oxide intermediate in hamster and rat. Biochem. Pharmacol., 24, 1449-1453

Metzler, M. (1976) Metabolic activation of carcinogenic diethylstilbestrol in rodents and humans. J. Toxicol. environ. Health, Suppl. 1, 21-35

Metzler, M. (1977) Peroxidase-mediated oxidation, a possible pathway for metabolic activation of the fetotoxic hormone diethylstilbestrol (Abstract no. P5). In: 4th Meeting of the European Association for Cancer Research, Lyon, Centre Léon Bérard, p. 28

Metzler, M. & McLachlan, J.A. (1978) Oxidative metabolites of diethyl-stilbestrol in the fetal, neonatal and adult mouse. Biochem. Pharmacol., 27, 1087-1094

Metzler, M., Müller, W. & Hobson, W.C. (1977) Biotransformation of diethylstilbestrol in the rhesus monkey and the chimpanzee. J. Toxicol. environ. Health, 3, 439-450

Monaghan, J.M. & Sirisena, L.A.W. (1978) Stilboestrol and vaginal clear-cell adenocarcinoma syndrome. Br. med. J., i, 1588-1590

Mroszczak, E.J. & Riegelman, S. (1975) Disposition of diethylstilboestrol in the rhesus monkey. J. Pharmacokinetics Biopharm., 3, 303-327

Murphy, J.B. & Sturm, E. (1949) The effect of diethylstilbestrol on
    the incidence of leukemia in male mice of the Rockefeller Institute
    Leukemia strain (R.I.L.). Cancer Res., 9, 88-89

Mussman, H.C. (1975) Drug and chemical residues in domestic animals.
    Fed. Proc., 34, 197-201

Nandi, S. (1965) Interactions among hormonal, viral and genetic factors
    in mouse mammary tumorigenesis. Can. Cancer Conf., 6, 69-81

Napalkov, N.P. & Anisimov, V.N. (1979) Transplacental effect of
    diethylstilbestrol in female rats. Cancer Lett., 6, 107-114

National Formulary Board (1975) National Formulary, 14th ed.,
    Washington DC, American Pharmaceutical Association, pp. 205-207

Ng, A.B.P., Reagan, J.W., Hawliczek, S. & Wentz, W.B. (1975) Cellular
    detection of vaginal adenosis. Obstet. Gynecol., 46, 323-328

Ng, A.B.P., Reagan, J.W., Nadji, M. & Greening, S. (1977) Natural history
    of vaginal adenosis in women exposed to diethylstilbestrol in
    utero. J. reprod. Med., 18, 1-13

Nissen, E.D. & Goldstein, A.I. (1973) Stilboestrol therapy in pregnancy.
    Relationship to vaginal neoplasia in offspring. Int. J. Gynecol.
    Obstet., 11, 138-142

Noller, K.L. & Fish, C.R. (1974) Diethylstilbestrol usage: its interesting
    past, important present, and questionable future. Med. Clin. N. Am.,
    58, 793-810

Noller, K.L., Decker, D.G., Lanier, A.P. & Kurland, L.T. (1972) Clear-cell
    adenocarcinoma of the cervix after maternal treatment with synthetic
    estrogens. Mayo Clin. Proc., 47, 629-630

Nomura, T. & Kanzaki, T. (1977) Introduction of urogenital anomalies
    and some tumors in the progeny of mice receiving diethylstilbestrol
    during pregnancy. Cancer Res., 37, 1099-1104

O'Brien, P.C., Noller, K.L., Robboy, S.J., Barnes, A.B., Kaufman, R.H.,
    Tilley, B.C. & Townsend, D.E. (1979) Vaginal epithelial changes in
    young women enrolled in the National Cooperative Diethylstilbestrol
    Adenosis (DESAD) project. Obstet. Gynecol., 53, 300-308

O'Grady, W.P. & McDivitt, R.W. (1969) Breast cancer in a man treated with
    diethylstilbestrol. Arch. Pathol., 88, 162-165

Okey, A.B. & Gass, G.H. (1968) Continuous versus cyclic estrogen
    administration: mammary carcinoma in C3H mice. J. natl Cancer
    Inst., 40, 225-230

Pacyn'ski, A., Budzyńska, A., Przytecki, S. & Robaczyn'ski, J. (1971)
    Hyperestrogenism in workers in a pharmaceutical establishment
    and their children as occupational disease. Pol. Endocrinol., 22,
    125-129

Pomerance, W. (1973) Post-stilbestrol secondary syndrome. Obstet.
    Gynecol., 42, 12-18

Ponder, C. (1974) Fluorometric determination and thin layer chromatographic
    identification of diethylstilbestrol in beef liver. J. Assoc. off.
    analyt. Chem., 57, 919-923

Puri, S., Fenoglio, C.M., Richart, R.M. & Townsend, D. (1977) Clear cell
    carcinoma of cervix and vagina in progeny of women who received
    diethylstilbestrol: three cases with scanning and transmission
    electron microscopy. Am. J. Obstet. Gynecol., 128, 550-555

Reid, D.E. & Shirley, R.L. (1974) Endometrial carcinoma associated with
    Sheehan's syndrome and stilbestrol therapy. Am. J. Obstet. Gynecol.,
    119, 264-266

Reznik-Schüller, H. (1979) Carcinogenic effects of diethylstilbestrol
    in male Syrian golden hamsters and European hamsters. J. natl Cancer
    Inst., 62, 1083-1088

Richards, R.K. & Kueter, K. (1941) Effect of stilbestrol upon liver
    and body growth in rats. Endocrinology, 29, 990-994

Richardson, F.L. (1957) Incidence of mammary and pituitary tumors in
    hybrid mice treated with stilbestrol for varying periods.
    J. natl Cancer Inst., 18, 813-829

Richart, R.M., Fu, Y.S., Reagan, J.W. & Barron, B.A. (1978) The
    problem squamous neoplasia in female DES progeny. In: Herbst, A.L.,
    ed., Intrauterine Exposure to Diethylstilbestrol in the Human,
    Chicago, Amercan College of Obstetricians & Gynecologists, pp. 45-52

Robboy, S.J. & Welch, W.R. (1977) Microglandular hyperplasia in vaginal
    adenosis associated with oral contraceptives and prenatal
    diethylstilbestrol exposure. Obstet. Gynecol., 49, 430-434

Robboy, S.J., Herbst, A.L. & Scully, R.E. (1974) Clear-cell adenocarcinoma
    of the vagina and cervix in young females: analysis of 37 tumors
    that persisted or recurred after primary therapy. Cancer, 34,
    606-614

Robboy, S.J., Scully, R.E. & Herbst, A.L. (1975) Pathology of vaginal and
    cervical abnormalities associated with prenatal exposure to
    diethylstilbestrol (DES). J. reprod. Med., 15, 13-18

Robboy, S.J., Keh, P.C., Nickerson, R.J., Helmanis, E.K., Prat, J. Szyfelbein, W.M., Taft, P.D., Barnes, A.B., Scully, R.E. & Welch, W.R. (1978) Squamous cell dysplasia and carcinoma *in situ* of the cervix and vagina after prenatal exposure to diethylstilbestrol. Obstet. Gynecol., 51, 528-535

Roos, R.W. (1974) Identification and determination of synthetic estrogens in pharmaceuticals by high-speed, reversed-phase partition chromatography. J. pharm. Sci., 63, 594-599

Rüdiger, H.W., Haenisch, F., Metzler, M., Glatt, H.R. & Oesch, F. (1979) Activation of diethylstilbestrol to metabolites which induce sister chromatid exchanges in human cultured fibroblasts. Science (in press)

Rurainski, R.D., Theiss, H.J. & Zimmermann, W. (1977) Occurrence of natural and synthetic oestrogens in drinking-water (Ger.). Gas-Wasserfach-Wasser Abwasser, 118, 288-291

Rustia, M. (1979) Role of hormone imbalance in transplacental carcinogenesis induced in Syrian golden hamsters by sex hormones. Natl Cancer Inst. Monogr., 51, 77-87

Rustia, M. & Shubik, P. (1976) Transplacental effects of diethyl-stilbestrol on the genital tract of hamster offspring. Cancer Lett., 1, 139-146

Sadolf, L., Winkley, J. & Tyson, S. (1973) Is malignant melanoma an endocrine-dependent tumor? The possible adverse effect of estrogen. Oncology, 27, 244-257

Sandberg, E.C. (1976) Benign cervical and vaginal changes associated with exposure to stilbestrol *in utero*. Am. J. Obstet. Gynecol., 125, 777-789

Scully, R.E., Robboy, S.J. & Herbst, A.L. (1974) Vaginal and cervical abnormalities, including clear-cell adenocarcinoma, related to prenatal exposure to stilbestrol. Ann. clin. Lab. Sci., 4, 222-233

Scully, R.E., Robboy, S.J. & Welch, W.B. (1978) Pathology and pathogenesis of diethylstilbestrol-related disorders of the female genital tract. In: Herbst, A.L., ed., Intrauterine Exposure to Diethylstilbestrol in the Human, Chicago, American College of Obstetricians & Gynecologists, pp. 8-22

Segaloff, A. (1974) The role of the ovary in estrogen production of mammary cancer in the rat. Cancer Res., 34, 2708-2710

Segaloff, A. & Maxfield, W.S. (1971) The synergism between radiation and estrogen in the production of mammary cancer in the rat. Cancer Res., 31, 166-168

Sestili, M.A. (1977) Genital tract anomalies and cancer in females exposed *in utero* to diethylstilbestrol. Brief report on the DESAD Project. Publ. Health Rep., 92, 481-484

Shah, H.C. & McLachlan, J.A. (1976) The fate of diethylstilbestrol in the pregnant mouse. J. Pharmacol. exp. Ther., 197, 687-696

Shellabarger, C.J., Stone, J.P. & Holtzman, S. (1976a) Interaction of DES and DMBA on mammary carcinogenesis in A X C female rats (Abstract no. 354). Proc. Am. Assoc. Cancer Res., 17, 89

Shellabarger, C.J., Stone, J.P. & Holtzman, S. (1976b) Synergism between neutron radiation and diethylstilbestrol in the production of mammary adenocarcinomas in the rat. Cancer Res., 36, 1019-1022

Sherman, A.I., Goldrath, M., Berlin, A., Vakhariya, V., Banooni, F., Michaels, W., Goodman, P. & Brown, S. (1974) Cervical-vaginal adenosis after *in utero* exposure to synthetic estrogens. Obstet. Gynecol., 44, 531-545

Shimkin, M.B. & Andervont, H.B. (1942) Effect of foster nursing on the induction of mammary and testicular tumors in mice injected with stilbestrol. J. natl Cancer Inst., 2, 611-622

Shimkin, M.B. & Grady, H.G. (1941) Toxic and carcinogenic effects of stilbestrol in strain C3H male mice. J. natl Cancer Inst., 2, 55-60

Shimkin, M.B. & Wyman, R.S. (1946) Mammary tumors in male mice implanted with estrogen-cholesterol pellets. J. natl Cancer Inst., 7, 71-75

Shimkin, M.B., Grady, H.G. & Andervont, H.B. (1941) Induction of testicular tumors and other effects of stilbestrol-cholesterol pellets in strain C mice. J. natl Cancer Inst., 2, 65-80

Silverberg, S.G. & DeGiorgi, L.S. (1972) Clear cell carcinoma of the vagina. A clinical, pathologic and electron microscopic study. Cancer, 29, 1680-1690

Smith, E.C. & Orkin, L.A. (1945) A clinical and statistical study of 471 congenital anomalies of the kidney and ureter. J. Urol., 53, 11-26

Stafl, A., Mattingly, R.F., Foley, D.V. & Fetherston, W.C. (1974) Clinical diagnosis of vaginal adenosis. Obstet. Gynecol., 43, 118-128

Stafl, A. & Mattingly, R.F. (1974) Vaginal adenosis: a precancerous lesion? Am. J. Obstet. Gynecol., 120, 666-677

Stecher, P.G., ed. (1968) The Merck Index, 8th ed. Rahway, NJ,
    Merck & Co., pp. 360-361

Stöckl, W., Bamberg, E., Choi, H.S. & Götzin, N. (1978) Radioimmunologic
    determination of diethylstilboestrol in blood of fatted cattle (Ger.).
    Wien. Tierärztl. Monats., 65, 329-331

Studdiford, W.E. (1957) Vaginal lesions of adenomatous origin.
    Am. J. Obstet. Gynecol., 73, 641-656

Taft, P.D., Robboy, S.J., Herbst, A.L. & Scully, R.E. (1974) Cytology
    of clear-cell adenocarcinoma of genital tract in young females:
    review of 95 cases from the Registry. Acta cytol., 18, 279-290

Townsend, D.E. (1978) Techniques of examination and screening of the
    DES-exposed female. In: Herbst, A.L, ed., Intrauterine Exposure
    to Diethylstilbestrol in the Human, Chicago, American College of
    Obstetricians & Gynecologists, pp. 23-29

Trentin, J.J. & Gardner, W.U. (1958) Site of gene action in susceptibility
    to estrogen-induced testicular interstitial-cell tumors of mice.
    Cancer Res., 18, 110-112

Tsukada, Y., Hewett, W.J., Barlow, J.J. & Pickren, J.W. (1972) Clear-cell
    adenocarcinoma ('mesonephroma') of the vagina. Three cases
    associated with maternal synthetic nonsteroid estrogen therapy.
    Cancer, 29, 1208-1214

Ulfelder, H., Poskanzer, D. & Herbst, A.L. (1971) Stilbestrol-adenosis-
    carcinoma syndrome: geographic distribution. New Engl. J. Med.,
    285, 691

Umberger, E. J. (1975) Products marketed to promote growth in food-
    producing animals: steroid and hormone products. Toxicology, 3,
    3-21

US Food & Drug Administration (1977) Patient labeling for estrogens
    for general use. Drugs for human use; drug efficacy study
    implementation. Fed. Regist., 42, 37645-37646

US Food & Drug Administration (1978) Food and drugs. US Code Fed. Regul.,
    Title 21, part 556.190, pp. 399-400

US International Trade Commission (1976) Imports of Benzenoid Chemicals
    and Products, 1974, USITC Publication 762, Washington DC,
    US Government Printing Office, p. 82

US International Trade Commission (1977a) Synthetic Organic Chemicals,
    US Production and Sales, 1975, USITC Publication 804, Washington
    DC, US Government Printing Office, pp. 90, 102

US International Trade Commission (1977b) Synthetic Organic Chemicals,
    US Production and Sales, 1976, USITC Publication 833, Washington
    DC, US Government Printing Office, p. 148

US International Trade Commission (1977c) Imports of Benzenoid
    Chemicals and Products, 1975, USITC Publication 806, Washington DC,
    US Government Printing Office, p. 83

US International Trade Commission (1977d) Imports of Benzenoid
    Chemicals and Products, 1976, USITC Publication 828, Washington DC,
    US Government Printing Office, p. 88

US Pharmacopeial Convention Inc. (1975) The US Pharmacopeia, 19th
    rev., Rockville, MD, pp. 142-143

US Tariff Commission (1945) Synthetic Organic Chemicals, US Production
    and Sales, 1941-43, Report No. 153, Second Series, Washington DC,
    US Government Printing Office, p. 101

US Tariff Commission (1968) Synthetic Organic Chemicals, US Production
    and Sales, 1966, TC Publication 248, Washington DC, US Government
    Printing Office, p. 126

US Tariff Commission (1969) Synthetic Organic Chemicals, US Production
    and Sales, 1967, TC Publication 295, Washington DC, US Government
    Printing Office, p. 123

Verhoeven, A.T.M. (1972) Mesonephric carcinoma of the cervix uteri
    in a 8-year-old girl treated by hysterectomy. Eur. J. Obstet.
    Gynecol., 5, 145-151

Vorherr, H., Messer, R.H., Vorherr, U.F., Jordan, S.W. & Kornfeld, M.
    (1979) Teratogenesis and carcinogenesis in rat offspring after
    transplacental and transmammary exposure to diethylstilbestrol.
    Biochem. Pharmacol., 28, 1865-1877

Wade, A., ed (1977) Martindale, The Extra Pharmacopoeia, 27th ed.,
    London, The Pharmaceutical Press, pp. 1426-1428

White, F.R. & White, J. (1944) Effect of diethylstilbestrol on mammary
    tumor formation in strain C3H mice fed a low cystine diet.
    J. natl Cancer Inst., 4, 413-415

Wilkinson, E.J., Friedrich, E.G., Jr, Mattingly, R.F., Regali, J.A. &
    Garancis, J.C. (1973) Turner's syndrome with endometrial
    adenocarcinoma and stilbestrol therapy. Obstet. Gynecol., 42,
    193-200

Williams, R.R. & Schweitzer, R.J. (1973) Clear-cell adenocarcinoma of the vagina in a girl whose mother had taken diethylstilbestrol. California Med., 118, 53-55

Windholz, M., ed. (1976) The Merck Index, 9th ed., Rahway, NJ, Merck & Co., p. 414

Young, C.L. (1978) Cancer Control Monograph, Diethylstilbestrol, project 4418, Stanford, CA, SRI International

ETHINYLOESTRADIOL

A monograph on this substance was published previously (IARC, 1974). Relevant data that have appeared since that time have been evaluated in the present monograph.

1. Chemical and Physical Data

1.1 Synonyms and trade names

Chem. Abstr. Services Reg. No.: 57-63-6

Chem. Abstr. Name: (17α)-19-Norpregna-1,3,5(10)-trien-20-yne-3,17-diol

Synonyms: EE; EE$_2$; EED; ethinylestradiol; 17-ethinylestradiol; 17α-ethinylestradiol; 17α-ethinyl-17β-estradiol; 17-ethinyl-3,17-estradiol; ethinylestriol; 17-ethinyloestradiol; 17α-ethinyl-oestradiol; 17α-ethinyl-17β-oestradiol; 17-ethinyl-3,17-oestradiol; ethinyloestriol; ethynylestradiol; 17-ethynylestradiol; 17α-ethynylestradiol; 17α-ethynyl-1,3,5(10)-estratriene-3,17β-diol; ethynyloestradiol; 17-ethynyloestradiol; 17α-ethynyloestradiol; 17α-ethynyl-1,3,5(10)-oestratriene-3,17β-diol; 19-nor-17α-pregna-1,3,5(10)-trien-20-yne-3,17-diol

Trade names[1]: Amenoron; [Amenorone]; [Anovlar]; [Anovlar 21]; [Anovlar Mite]; Brevicon; Brevicon 28-Day; Cavomen-F; Chee-O-Gen; Chee-O-Genf; [Ciclo Complex]; Climatone; [Controvlar]; Declimone; [Delpregnin]; Demulen; Demulen 28; [Demulen 50]; [Dimenoral]; [Diognat-E]; Diogyn-E; [Dipro]; [Duogynon]; [Duogynon Oral]; [Duoluton]; Dyloform; Edrol; Ertonyl; [Estandron]; Esteed; Estigyn; Estinyl; Eston-E; Estoral; Estorals; [Estrovister]; [Etalontin]; [Etalontin 28]; Ethidol; Ethinoral; Ethy; Ethy 11; [Ethinyl-oestranol]; Eticyclin; Eticyclol; Etifollin; Etinestrol; Etinestryl;

---

[1]Those in square brackets are preparations that are no longer produced commercially.

[Etinilestrad]; Etinoestryl; Etistradiol; Etivex;
[Eugynon]; [Eugynon 21]; [Eugynon 28]; [Eugynon ED]; [Evanor];
Feminone; Follicoral; Follikoral; [Folinett]; [Follinyl];
[Gestovex]; [Gineserpina]; Ginestrene; Gynetone; Gynolett;
Gynostat; [Gynovlane]; [Gynovlar]; [Gynovlar 21]; Halodrin;
[Hormoduvadilan]; Inestra; Kolpolyn; [Kombikwens]; [Kombiquens];
Linoral; Loestrin; Loestrin 21; Lo/Ovral; Lo/Ovral-28;
[Lutestral]; [Lutogynoestryl]; [Lutogynoestryl Fort];
Lynoral; [Menokwens]; Menolet Sublets; Menolyn; Menopax;
Menopax Forte; [Menoquens]; [Menstrogen]; [Menstrogon];
Mepilin; Metroval; [Metrulen]; [Milli-Anovlar]; [Minilyn];
[Minovlar]; [Minovlar ED]; Mixogen; Modicon; Modicon 28;
[Neo-Delpregnin]; Neo-Estrone; [Neogentrol]; [Neogynon];
[Neogynon 21]; [Neogynon 28]; [Neogynon ED]; [Neovlar 21];
[Neovulen]; [N Gestakliman]; Nogest-S; [Nordiol 21]; [Nordiol
28]; [Norlestrin]; Norlestrin 21; Norlestrin 28; Norlestrin
Fe; Normaoestren; Norma-ostren; [Norquentiel]; Novestrol;
[Novokwens]; [Nuvacon]; Oestradin; [Oracon]; [Oraconal];
Oradiol; Orestralyn; [Orlest]; [Orlest 28]; Os-cal Mone;
Ovcon 35; Ovcon 50; [Ovin]; [Ovisec]; Ovral; Ovral 28; [Ovran];
[Ovulen]; [Ovulen 1/50]; [Ovulen 50]; [Ovulene 50]; Palonyl;
Perovex; [Piloval]; [Planor]; [Planovin]; [Primodian];
[Primodos]; Primogyn; Primogyn C; Primogyn M; [Primosiston];
[Primovlar 21]; [Primovlar 28]; [Prociclo]; [Profinix];
[Progylut]; Progynon C; Progynon M; [Protex]; [Reglovis];
Roldiol; [Salvacal]; [Secrodyl]; [Secrovin]; [Serial];
[Serial 4x7]; [Serial 28]; [Serial C]; Spanestrin; [Stediril];
[Stediril D]; [Synchron]; Test-Estrin; [Tova]; Trimone
Sublets; [Verafem]; [Volidan]; [Volidan 21]; [Volidan V];
[Volplan]; [Voplan]; Ylestrol; Zorane

1.2   Structural and molecular formulae and molecular weight

C$_{20}$H$_{24}$O$_2$ Mol. wt: 296.4

1.3   Chemical and physical properties of the pure substance

From Windholz (1976), unless otherwise specified

(<u>a</u>)   Description: Fine white needles (from methanol and water)

(<u>b</u>)   Melting-point: 141-146°C for hemihydrate; dehydrates after melting and further heating, then melts at 182-184°C

(<u>c</u>)   Spectroscopy data: λ_{max} 281 nm (E$_1^1$ 76) in ethanol

(<u>d</u>)   Optical rotation: $[\alpha]_D^{24}$ +3.5° ± 0.5° (2% w/v in dioxane)
                                        -29.5° ± 1.0° (2% w/v in pyridine)

(<u>e</u>)   Solubility: Practically insoluble in water; soluble in ethanol (1 in 6), diethyl ether (1 in 4), acetone (1 in 5), dioxane (1 in 4) and chloroform (1 in 20). Soluble in vegetable oils and in solutions of fixed alkaline hydroxides

(<u>f</u>)   Stability: It should be stored in air-tight, non-metallic, light-resistant containers (US Pharmacopeial Convention Inc., 1975).

1.4   Technical products and impurities

Various national and international pharmacopoeias give specifications for the purity of ethinyloestradiol in pharmaceutical products. For example, ethinyloestradiol is available in the US as a USP grade containing 97-102% active ingredient on a dried basis. Tablets in 0.01, 0.02, 0.05 and 0.5 mg doses contain 90-115% of the stated amount of ethinyloestradiol (US Pharmacopeial Convention Inc., 1975). It is also available in 0.02-0.05 mg doses in combination with norethisterone acetate, ethynodiol

diacetate or norgestrel, for use as oral contraceptives, and in 0.005-
0.04 mg doses in combination with 2.67-10 mg methyltestosterone (Kastrup,
1977; US Pharmacopeial Convention Inc., 1975, 1978).

In the UK, ethinyloestradiol is available in tablets in 0.01, 0.05,
0.1 and 1 mg doses and in combination with a variety of drugs, including
papaverine hydrochloride and amylobarbitone, methyltestosterone, carbromal
and bromvaletone, ethisterone, ethynodiol diacetate, lynoestrenol,
norethisterone acetate and norgestrel. It is also available in an
elixir containing 0.005 mg ethinyloestriol, 8 mg phenobarbitone sodium,
60 mg sodium bromide, 8 mg sodium nitrite and 0.15 ml gelsemium tincture
in each 5 ml of elixir (Wade, 1977).

In Japan, ethinyloestradiol is available in 0.02 and 0.05 mg tablets.
It is also available in combinations with norethisterone acetate, methyl
testosterone and methylestrenolone.

2. Production, Use, Occurrence and Analysis

2.1 Production and use

(a) Production

The synthesis of ethinyloestradiol was first reported in 1938
(Inhoffen *et al.*, 1938), by treatment of oestrone with potassium acetylide
in liquid ammonia. It is believed to be produced commercially by the
same method.

Commercial production of ethinyloestradiol in the US was first
reported in 1945 (US Tariff Commission, 1947) and last reported (by a
single company) in 1955 (US Tariff Commission, 1956). Separate data on
US imports and exports are not available.

Ethinyloestradiol is believed to be produced commercially in France,
The Netherlands and the UK, but no information was available on the
quantities produced.

Ethinyloestradiol was first marketed commercially in Japan in 1953.
It is not produced in Japan; imports are estimated to have been 3 kg
in 1976 and 2 kg in 1977.

(b) Use

Ethinyloestradiol is one of the most active steroidal oestrogens
known when administered orally. It is used in human medicine (1) for
the treatment of symptoms of the climacteric and in replacement therapy
in hypogonadal women, in an oral dose of 0.01-0.15 mg per day adjusted

to the lowest maintenance dose; (2) for such functional disorders as primary and secondary amenorrhoea, in cyclic regimens, e.g., 0.025-0.15 mg per day continuously through the cycle, complemented by a progestin for 7 consecutive days; or 0.02-0.05 mg per day for 14 days and a progestin for the next 14 days and repeated; or 0.05 mg 1 to 3 times per day for 20 days each month with a progestin during the last two weeks; (3) for post-partum breast engorgement, in an initial dose of 0.5-1 mg per day for 3 days followed by 0.05-0.1 mg per day for 7 days; (4) for dysfunctional uterine bleeding, in an initial dose of 0.5 mg once or twice per day until bleeding stops, then 0.05 mg per day for 3 days followed by a rest to see if a normal cycle will commence; (5) for prostatic carcinoma, in a dose of 0.05 mg 1 to 3 times per day; and (6) for advanced breast cancer in postmenopausal women, in an initial dose of 0.05 mg 1 to 3 times per day, which is gradually increased as tolerated (Harvey, 1975). Ethinyloestradiol is used in combination with an androgen such as methyltestosterone in patients with symptoms of the climacteric that are difficult to control with ethinyloestradiol alone (Wade, 1977).

The largest use for ethinyloestradiol is in oral contraceptives, where it is administered in combination with a progestin, such as dimethisterone, ethynodiol diacetate, lynoestrenol, megestrol acetate, norethisterone acetate or norgestrel. In combination therapy, it is administered in conjunction with a progestin from the 5th to the 25th day of the cycle. In sequential therapy, it is given alone from the 5th to the 20th day and in conjunction with a progestin from the 21st to the 25th day of the cycle (Wade, 1977).

In 1972, it was estimated that 41-48 million women were exposed to ethinyloestradiol through regular use of contraceptive agents (Piotrow & Lee, 1974); in 1977, over 80 million women were using contraceptive agents (WHO, 1978).

In Japan, an oral dose of 0.02-0.05 mg is given 1 to 3 times per day for treatment of functional sterility and endometriosis. Less than 1000 kg ethinyloestradiol are used in France annually.

Veterinary use of ethinyloestradiol has been reported to be similar to that of oestradiol, e.g., as replacement therapy in underdeveloped females, for incontinence and vaginitis of spayed bitches and for reproductive disorders (Stecher, 1968).

The US Food & Drug Administration (1977) has ruled that with effect from 20 September 1977 oestrogens for general use must carry patient and physician warning labels concerning use, risks and contraindications. The same ruling was extended to all oral contraceptives with effect from 31 May 1978 (US Food & Drug Administration, 1978).

2.2 Occurrence

Ethinyloestradiol has not been reported to occur naturally.

Residues of ethinyloestradiol have been found in foliage, soil and water samples (Okuno & Higgins, 1977) and in some samples of drinking-water (Rurainski *et al.*, 1977). However, it did not occur in a list of carcinogens and mutagens found in water supplies of the US and Europe in which 1728 contaminants were identified (Kraybill *et al.*, 1977).

In the 1974 National Occupational Hazard Survey conducted by the US National Institute for Occupational Safety & Health, exposure to ethinyl-oestradiol was found to occur in industries manufacturing pharmaceutical preparations. On the basis of these data, it is estimated that 1230 US workers were exposed to ethinyloestradiol in 1974 (US National Institute for Occupational Safety & Health, 1977).

2.3 Analysis

Typical analytical methods for the determination of ethinyloestradiol are summarized in Table 1. Abbreviations used are: GC/FID, gas chroma-tography/flame-ionization detection; GC/MS, gas chromatography/mass spectrometry; TLC, thin-layer chromatography; UV, ultra-violet spectro-metry; RIA, radioimmunoassay; CC, column chromatography; and CPB, competitive protein binding radioassay. See also 'General Remarks on Sex Hormones', p. 60.

TABLE 1

Analytical methods for ethinyloestradiol

Sample matrix	Sample preparation	Assay procedure	Sensitivity or limit of detection	Reference
Bulk chemical	Add nitric acid; heat; cool; basify; dilute with ethanol	UV (430 nm)	10 µg/ml (10 ml cell)	Hassan & Zaki (1976)
Bulk chemical	Dissolve (chloroform:methanol, 1:1) to 0.1% concentration	TLC (UV, acid spray)	–	Cavina et al. (1975)
Bulk chemical	Dissolve (methanol); dilute (isooctane)	Treat with sulphuric acid-methanol; colorimetry (533 nm)	–	US Pharmacopeial Convention Inc. (1975)
Bulk chemical	Dissolve (tetrahydrofuran); add aqueous silver nitrate	Titration	–	Council of Europe (1971)
Tablets	Add dilute aqueous hydrochloric acid; extract (dichloromethane); add hydroquinone in sulphuric acid-ethanol	Fluorescence (560 nm)	–	Miller & Duguid (1976)
Tablets	Extract (ethanol); centrifuge; filter; evaporate; dissolve (alkali); treat with diazotized 5-chloro-2,4-dinitroaniline solution	Colorimetry (450 nm)	1 µg/ml (10 ml cell)	Eldawy et al. (1975)
Tablets	Extract (aqueous dilute sulphuric acid-chloroform); separate; evaporate; dissolve (acetone); treat with dansyl chloride	Fluorescence (502 nm)	0.05 mg	Fishman (1975)

Table 1 (continued)

Sample matrix	Sample preparation	Assay procedure	Sensitivity or limit of detection	Reference
Tablets	Separate from other components by a complex series of extrac- tions & washings	Add benzene solution of ethinyloestradiol to iron-phenol solution; then add sulphuric acid; measure absorbances at 529 & 420 nm	–	National Formulary Board (1975)
Tablets	Extract (acetone); centrifuge; reduce volume	TLC (UV, acid spray)	10 µg by UV; 1 µg by acid spray	Simard & Lodge (1970)
Tablets	Extract (aqueous methanol); separate; evaporate; re- dissolve (chloroform-isooc- tane)	Treat with sulphuric acid-methanol; colo- rimetry (538 nm)	–	US Pharmacopeial Con- vention Inc. (1975)
Drinking-water	Extract, TLC separation	TLC; radiometry	–	Rurainski et al. (1977)
Water	Extract (diethyl ether, chloroform & hydrochloric acid)	GC/FID	0.01 mg/l (200 ml sample)	Okuno & Higgins (1977)
Feeds	Extract (chloroform)	TLC & GC/FID	–	Wal et al. (1977)
Urine	Isolate by a series of extractions, hydrolysis & chromatographic separations	GC/MS	–	Braselton et al. (1977)
Urine	Isolate by a series of chroma- tographic, hydrolytic & extraction procedures; derivatize (trimethylsilyl ether)	GC/MS	–	Williams et al. (1975)
Plasma	Add acetone, centrifuge, decant & evaporate; dissolve residue (buffer solution); add tracer solution & antibody solution; incubate at 4° ; centrifuge	RIA	18 pg/ml (0.1 or 0.2 ml sample)	de la Peña et al. (1975)

Sample matrix	Sample preparation	Assay procedure	Sensitivity or limit of detection	Reference
Plasma	Add internal standard solution; incubate; extract (diethyl ether); evaporate; redissolve in benzene:methanol (9:1); CC; add tracer solution; incubate; centrifuge; decant	CPB	25 pg (1 ml sample)	Verma et al. (1975)
Human milk	Extract (diethyl ether); evaporate; redissolve (methanol); centrifuge; evaporate	RIA	50 pg/ml (0.2 ml sample)	Nilsson et al. (1978)
Foliage	Extract (acetonitrile-hydrochloric acid); CC (Florisil & gel permeation)	GC/FID	0.05 mg/kg (10 g sample)	Okuno & Higgins (1977)
Soil	Extract (acetone-hydrochloric acid); concentrate; extract (diethyl ether & chloroform); CC (Florisil & gel permeation)	GC/FID	0.1 mg/kg (10 g sample)	Okuno & Higgins (1977)
	(Matrix determines method of preparation)	TLC (acid spray & UV)	100 ng	Okuno & Higgins (1977)

3. Biological Data Relevant to the Evaluation
of Carcinogenic Risk to Humans

3.1 Carcinogenicity studies in animals

Most studies have been made with combinations of ethinyloestradiol with progestins. These experimental data have therefore been summarized both in this monograph and in those on the other compounds used in such combinations. It is important to note that the effects reported may reflect the action either of an individual constituent or of the combination.

(a) Oral administration

Mouse: Groups of 24 virgin female C57L mice received 7 or 70 µg of a mixture of norethisterone:ethinyloestradiol (50:1) in oil by gavage, 5 times per week, commencing when the animals were 13 weeks of age. Pituitary tumours were found at autopsy after 84-89 weeks of treatment in 7/15 surviving mice given the lower dose and in 5/8 mice given the higher dose, compared with 2/15 controls. Hepatomas were found in 10/96 mice treated with norethisterone:ethinyloestradiol and in a concurrent experiment with norethynodrel plus mestranol, but the report does not specify in which group or groups they arose. No hepatomas occurred in 48 controls (Poel, 1966).

Ethinyloestradiol alone or in combination with ethynodiol diacetate, norethisterone acetate, norgestrel or megestrol acetate was incorporated into the diet of groups of 120 male and 120 female CF-LP (MTV[+])[1] or BDH (MTV[-])[1] mice for 80 weeks. The doses were identified only as low (2-5 times the human contraceptive dose), medium (50-150 times) or high (200-400 times); the amounts administered were not specified. Ethinyloestradiol administered alone resulted in an increased incidence of pituitary tumours in both male (26 tumours) and female (38 tumours) CF-LP mice (MTV[+]) in one of two experiments, versus 2 and 8 tumours in male and female control groups of 120 animals. Similar increases were found after administration of ethinyloestradiol in combination with ethynodiol diacetate or norethisterone acetate but not with norgestrel [The negative findings in one group given ethinyloestradiol alone and in one group administered ethinyloestradiol plus norgestrel may have been due to undetected differences in the conduct of the trial]. Malignant tumours

---

[1]MTV[+]: mammary tumour virus expressed.; MTV[-]: mammary tumour virus not expressed (see p. 62)

of the connective tissue of the uterus (unspecified) were found in 6/120 female mice fed ethinyloestradiol plus ethynodiol diacetate, compared with 0-1/120 controls. In groups of 71-87 mice of the BDH-SPF Carshalton stock, administration of ethinyloestradiol alone or in combination with megestrol acetate was associated with a small increase in the incidence of pituitary tumours in treated males and females (4-10% in treated groups compared with 2% and 0% in 57 male and 65 female controls); benign gonadal tumours (unspecified) were found in males (8-10% compared with 0% in controls); incidences of malignant mammary tumours were increased in both males and females (9-32% compared with 0% and 3% in controls); malignant tumours of the uterine fundus and of the cervix were found in 4-11% and in 4%, respectively, of treated females, compared with 0 in female controls (Committee on Safety of Medicines, 1972).

Intact female RIII, C3H and (C3H x RIII)F1 mice (MTV$^+$) were fed Lutestral (97.5% chlormadinone acetate and 2.5% ethinyloestradiol) in the diet at 8 mg/kg (daily intake, 20-30 µg/mouse); neither the mammary tumour incidence nor latent period were altered. In intact male (C3H x RIII)F1 mice, the mammary tumour incidence was increased from 0/76 to 10/32, and in castrated male (C3H x RIII)F1 mice it was increased from 10/61 to 23/28, with a decrease in the latent period (Rudali, 1975).

Rat: Groups of 30 female Mead-Johnson rats administered ethinyl-oestradiol in the diet, either alone   at an average dose of 53 µg/kg bw per day or at the same dose level with megestrol acetate (average, 2.63 mg/kg bw per day), for 105 weeks had no increase in incidence of tumours in any tissue. When ethinyloestradiol (30 µg/kg bw per day) was given for 16 days followed by a mixture of ethinyloestradiol (30 µg/kg bw per day) plus megestrol acetate (1.5 mg/kg bw per day) for 5 days and then a period of no steroid treatment for 7 days, for a total of 26 cycles (104 weeks), there was a significant reduction in the incidence of mammary tumours compared with that in controls (McKinney *et al.*, 1968).

Groups of 73-120 rats were given ethinyloestradiol alone or in combination with ethynodiol diacetate, norethisterone acetate, norgestrel or megestrol acetate at low (2-5 times the human dose), medium (50-150 times) and high (200-400 times) doses for 104 weeks. Control groups consisted of 24-100 rats. Benign mammary tumours were found more frequently in males given the combination with norethisterone acetate (28% compared with 2% in controls), and malignant mammary tumours were found more frequently in males given the combination with ethynodiol diacetate (10% compared with 0% in controls). The incidence of benign liver-cell tumours was higher in males and females given ethinyloestradiol alone (15 and 23%) or in combination with megestrol acetate (11 and 14%) than in male (0) and female (8%) controls. In females, the incidence of malignant liver-cell tumours in groups treated with ethinyloestradiol alone or in combinations ranged from 4% for ethinyloestradiol plus megestrol acetate (1:5) to 7.5% for ethinyloestradiol alone, a significant finding compared with the virtual absence of such lesions in 12 separate control groups of female rats (Committee on Safety of Medicines, 1972).

Dog: In a preliminary report, it was stated that groups of 12-16
female dogs were given a combination of ethinyloestradiol and norgestrel
at dose levels of 0, 10 and 25 times the projected human dose levels.
After 5 years, 2/12, 3/12 and 5/12 animals, respectively, showed mammary
nodules (Finkel & Berliner, 1973).

Groups of 16 female beagles, 6-12 months of age at the start of the
experiment, were given combinations of norethisterone and dimethisterone
with ethinyloestradiol at dose levels of 1, 10 and 25 times the projected
human dose levels for 7 years. Dogs were killed after 2 and 4 years.
The combination with norethisterone resulted in a dose-related development
of cystic endometrial hyperplasia, pyometra and alopecia. None of the
controls showed mammary nodules, whereas one dog given the intermediate
dose had a single nodule in the fifth year. Dimethisterone and ethinyloestradiol were given sequentially, as oestrogen alone, and as oestrogen
combined with the progestin, followed by a steroid-free period. Again,
alopecia, cystic endometrial hyperplasia and pyometra were noted. Many
acne-like lesions were found in the group given the high dose and some
in the intermediate dose group. Four hyperplastic mammary nodules were
found by palpation in the group given the low dose, compared with 2 in
controls (Weikel & Nelson, 1977) [The Working Group noted the lack of
information concerning the number of tumour-bearing animals].

Monkey: In a preliminary report of a study in progress, a combination
of 20:1 ethynodiol diacetate:ethinyloestradiol (Demulen) was administered
orally at 1, 10 and 50 times the human contraceptive dose (0.021, 0.21
and 1.05 mg/kg bw) cyclically (3 weeks on and 1 week off) to 3 groups
of 16 mature (3-8-yr-old) female *Macaca mulatta* (rhesus) monkeys for 5
years. Clinical examination during 65 cycles revealed the presence and
subsequent disappearance of a nodule in one control animal and in one
monkey in the highest dose group (Drill & Golway, 1978).

(b) Subcutaneous and/or intramuscular administration

Rat: Groups of 10 female Wistar rats were injected subcutaneously
with 5, 10 or 15 mg/kg bw of a mixture of ethinyloestradiol:megestrol
acetate (1:8) in olive oil once every other day for 30 days. Mammary
fibroadenomas occurred in 2/10, 4/8 and 2/9 survivors at between 29 and
59 weeks, compared with none in 10 surviving controls (Hisamatsu, 1972)
[The Working Group noted the small numbers in each group].

3.2 Other relevant biological data

(a) Experimental systems

The relative activity of ethinyloestradiol in the Allen-Doisy test
in mice is about 1.2 times greater than that of oestradiol-17β after
s.c. administration and more than 10 times greater by oral administration
(Emmeus & Martin, 1962). In the uterine-growth test (Rubin's test) in
mice, it is about 1.2 times more active than oestradiol-17β (Brotherton
1976).

Toxic effects

The acute and chronic toxicity of this compound have been reviewed by Plotz & Haller (1971). The oral LD_{50}s in rats and mice are >5000 and >2500 mg/kg bw, respectively (Brotherton, 1976).

Embryotoxicity and teratogenicity

Oral administration of 0.1-3.0 mg ethinyloestradiol/animal on day 1 of gestation or 0.1-0.3 mg on days 2, 3 or 4 of gestation to Swiss albino mice terminated pregnancy in 100% of animals; administration of 0.003-0.03 mg terminated pregnancy in 20-60%. Four days after administration of 0.1-3.0 mg ethinyloestradiol on day 1 of gestation, 60% of embryos were found to have abnormalities, such as fragmental vacuolization. Simultaneous s.c. injections of progesterone (5 mg in a single dose or 20 mg in 4 injections) and ethinyloestradiol (0.1-0.3 mg on day 1 or on days 1, 2, 3 and 4 of gestation) did not prevent termination of all pregnancies induced by ethinyloestradiol (Yanagimachi & Sato, 1968).

Groups of 10 ICR/JCL mice were given 0.01 or 0.02 mg/kg bw ethinyloestradiol orally on days 11-17 of gestation. Female offspring were killed at 10-14 weeks of age; in 8/13 exposed *in utero* to the high dose and in 2/11 exposed to the low dose, cystic glandular hyperplasia was observed, suggested by the authors to be a precursor lesion of uterine cancer (Yasuda *et al.*, 1977).

Rats received 5-500 µg/kg bw ethinyloestradiol by gavage on the first 2 days of gestation; the highest dose terminated pregnancy in 50% of animals. Normally implanted foetuses were found on day 9; no abnormalities were reported (Blye, 1970).

Hamsters were fed ethinyloestradiol at various doses: a single dose of 2.5 mg on day 3 before mating decreased pregnancy rates by 50% without affecting oestrus. Treatment over three oestrus cycles with 0.21 mg per day on days 14-3 before mating delayed oestrus but did not reduce pregnancy rates. Treatment during one cycle with 0.63 mg per day on days 6-3 before mating impaired oestrus and pregnancy rates by 67% and induced 15.6% of foetuses to be resorbed (Davis *et al.*, 1972).

Absorption, distribution, excretion and metabolism

Studies on the metabolism of ethinyloestradiol have been carried out in rats, rabbits, guinea-pigs, dogs and monkeys. It is very rapidly and effectively absorbed from rat intestine; no appreciable metabolic transformation is reported to take place during the absorption process (Reed & Fotherby, 1976). The main metabolic pathway of ethinyloestradiol in rats is by aromatic 2-hydroxylation (Ball *et al.*, 1973; Bolt *et al.*, 1973); hydroxylations at ring B (C-6/C-7) are of only minor importance.

Rat liver forms 2-hydroxyethinyloestradiol and the methyl ethers thereof, 2-methoxyethinyloestradiol and 2-hydroxyethinyloestradiol-3-methyl ether, as its major metabolic products (see Fig. 1). This pathway is also important in humans (Bolt *et al.*, 1974a). Metabolites of ethinyl-oestradiol in rats are excreted almost exclusively in the faeces (Bolt & Remmer, 1972).

Rabbits excrete ethinyloestradiol metabolites mainly *via* the urine (Higashi, 1969). A peculiarity of the rabbit's metabolism of ethinyl-oestradiol is the large amount of 'ring-D-homoannulated' metabolites (D-homo-oestrone-17α and D-homo-oestradiol-17aα) that results from metabolic attack at the 17α-ethinyl group of ethinyloestradiol (Abdel-Aziz & Williams, 1969). This metabolic pathway is much less important in humans (Abdel-Aziz & Williams, 1970).

The pattern of urinary and faecal excretion of ethinyloestradiol metabolites in guinea-pigs (Reed & Fotherby, 1975) and in beagle dogs (Keeley *et al.*, 1975) is similar to that of humans, in that more than half of the ethinyloestradiol metabolites are excreted in the faeces.

In baboons, 2-hydroxylation and de-ethinylation of ethinyloestradiol to the 'natural' oestrogens, oestradiol, oestrone, etc., are important pathways (Helton *et al.*, 1977). This situation appears to be similar to that in humans (Williams *et al.*, 1975), although differences in quanti-tative metabolic patterns have been observed (Goldzieher & Kraemer, 1972).

Mutagenicity and other short-term tests
====================================

In a study reported as an abstract, no mutagenic activity was reported in *Salmonella typhimurium* G46 or *Escherichia coli* K12 in the presence of a liver microsomal system (Kraemer *et al.*, 1974).

No dominant lethal mutations were observed in female mice treated for 3 days with 8.5 μg ethinyloestradiol and 170 μg norethisterone (Badr & Badr, 1974).

(b) Humans

In humans, ethinyloestradiol is about 40 times more active than oestradiol-17β when administered orally (Brotherton, 1976; Kupperman *et al.*, 1953).

The metabolic fate of ethinyloestradiol in humans has been reviewed extensively (Helton & Goldzieher, 1977a). Comparisons with its metabolism in mammals are described in section 3.2 (a). The major pathways are 2-hydroxylation (Bolt *et al.*, 1974a; Williams *et al.*, 1975) and 16β-hydroxylation (Williams *et al.*, 1975) (see Fig. 1); only trace amounts

Figure 1

Major metabolic pathways of ethinyloestradiol in mammals[1]

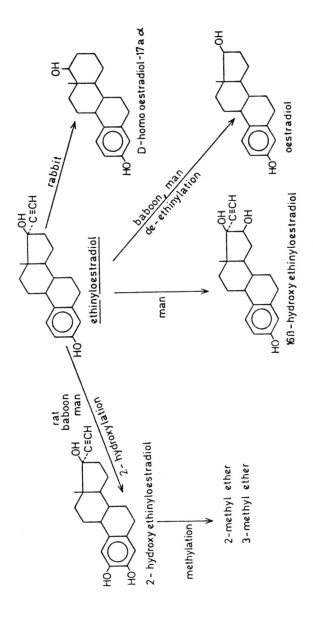

[1]From Abdel-Aziz & Williams (1969) and Bolt (1979)

of D-homo-annulated metabolites are detected (Abdel-Aziz & Williams, 1970). It has been reported that the ethinyl group is removed by oxidative mechanisms, giving rise to the metabolites oestrone, oestradiol-17β, oestriol and 2-methoxy-oestradiol (Williams *et al.*, 1975). A major portion of ethinyloestradiol is conjugated directly with glucuronic acid and excreted (Fotherby, 1973).

Quantitative evaluation of the metabolic breakdown of ethinyloestradiol is difficult, due to substantial interindividual variation (Goldzieher, 1976; Helton & Goldzieher, 1977b). The extent of 2-hydroxylation in humans averages 29% of the ethinyloestradiol dose given (Bolt *et al.*, 1977), but in some individuals it may be as high as 64% (Bolt *et al.*, 1974b). Recently, remarkable geographic differences in the pharmacokinetics of ethinyloestradiol have been reported (Helton & Goldzieher, 1977b).

In contrast to the metabolites of natural oestrogens, a significant proportion of the metabolites of ethinyloestradiol in humans are excreted by the faecal route; ethinyloestradiol itself is excreted in urine and faeces in a ratio of about 4:6. About 90% of the metabolites of tritiated ethinyloestradiol are recovered in both faeces and urine (Speck *et al.*, 1976).

No chromosomal effects were observed when 0.1-100 µg/ml ethinyl-oestradiol were added to cultures of lymphocytes grown from the blood of healthy women (Stenchever *et al.*, 1969).

3.3 Case reports and epidemiological studies

See the section, 'Oestrogens and Progestins in Relation to Human Cancer', p. 83.

4. Summary of Data Reported and Evaluation[1]

4.1 Experimental data

Ethinyloestradiol was tested in mice, rats, dogs and monkeys by oral administration and in rats by subcutaneous injection; in most studies it was administered in combination with progestins.

---

[1]This section should be read in conjunction with pp. 62-64 in the 'General Remarks on Sex Hormones' and with the 'General Conclusions on Sex Hormones', p. 131.

When administered alone to mice, it increased the incidence of pituitary tumours and malignant mammary tumours in both males and females and produced malignant tumours of the uterus and its cervix in females. In rats, it increased the incidence of benign liver-cell tumours in both males and females and produced malignant liver-cell tumours in females.

When ethinyloestradiol was given in combination with certain progestins, excess incidences of malignant tumours of the uterine fundus were observed in female mice and of benign and/or malignant mammary tumours in male rats; in female rats, the combinations reduced but did not prevent the incidence of malignant liver-cell tumours when compared with that produced by ethinyloestradiol alone. In dogs, no tumours that could be attributed to the treatment were found. The study in monkeys was still in progress at the time of reporting: no tumours had been found after 5 years of observation.

Mammary fibroadenomas were produced in female rats following subcutaneous injection of a combination of ethinyloestradiol with megestrol acetate.

Ethinyloestradiol is embryolethal for preimplantation embryos in some species.

4.2 Human data

No case reports or epidemiological studies on ethinyloestradiol alone were available to the Working Group. Epidemiological studies on steroid hormones used in oestrogen-progestin contraceptive preparations have been summarized in the section, 'Oestrogens and Progestins in Relation to Human Cancer', p. 83.

4.3 Evaluation

There is *sufficient evidence* for the carcinogenicity of ethinyloestradiol in experimental animals. In the absence of adequate data in humans, it is reasonable, for practical purposes, to regard ethinyloestradiol as if it presented a carcinogenic risk to humans. The use of oral contraceptives containing ethinyloestradiol in combination with progestins has been related causally to an increased incidence of benign liver adenomas and a decreased incidence of benign breast disease. Studies also strongly suggest that the administration of oestrogens is causally related to an increased incidence of endometrial carcinoma; there is no evidence that ethinyloestradiol is different from other oestrogens in this respect.

5. References

Abdel-Aziz, M.T. & Williams, K.I.H. (1969) Metabolism of 17α-ethyn-ylestradiol and its 3-methyl ether by the rabbit; an *in vivo* D-homoannulation. Steroids, 13, 809-820

Abdel-Aziz, M.T. & Williams, K.I.H. (1970) Metabolism of radioactive 17α-ethynylestradiol by women. Steroids, 15, 695-710

Badr, F.M. & Badr, R.S. (1974) Studies on the mutagenic effect of contraceptive drugs. I. Induction of dominant lethal mutations in female mice. Mutat. Res., 26, 529-534

Ball, P., Gelbke, H.P., Haupt, O. & Knuppen, R. (1973) Metabolism of 17α-ethynyl-[4-^{14}C]oestradiol and [4-^{14}C]mestranol in rat liver slices and interaction between 17α-ethynyl-2-hydroxyoestradiol and adrenalin. Hoppe-Seyler's Z. physiol. Chem., 354, 1567-1575

Blye, R.P. (1970) The effect of estrogens and related substances on embryonic viability. Adv. Biosci., 4, 323-343

Bolt, H.M. (1979) Metabolism of oestrogens - natural and synthetic. Pharm. Ther., 4, 155-181

Bolt, H.M. & Remmer, H. (1972) The accumulation of mestranol and ethynyloestradiol metabolites in the organism. Xenobiotica, 2, 489-498

Bolt, H.M., Kappus, H. & Remmer, H. (1973) Studies on the metabolism of ethynylestradiol *in vitro* and *in vivo*: the significance of 2-hydroxylation and the formation of polar products. Xenobiotica, 3, 773-785

Bolt, H.M., Kappus, H. & Käsbohrer, R. (1974a) Metabolism of 17α-ethinyl-estradiol by human liver microsomes *in vitro*: aromatic hydro-xylation and irreversible protein binding of metabolites. J. clin. Endocrinol. Metab., 39, 1072-1080

Bolt, H.M., Bolt, M. & Kappus, H. (1974b) Ring A oxidation of 17α-ethinylestradiol in man (Abstract). Horm. Metab. Res., 6, 432

Bolt, H.M., Bolt, M. & Kappus, H. (1977) Interaction of rifampicin treatment with pharmacokinetics and metabolism of ethinyl-oestradiol in man. Acta endocrinol., 85, 189-197

Braselton, W.E., Lin, T.J., Mills, T.M., Ellegood, J.O. & Mahesh, V.B. (1977) Identification and measurement by gas chromatography-gas spectrometry of norethindrone and metabolites in human urine and blood. J. Steroid Biochem., 8, 9-18

Brotherton, J. (1976) Sex Hormone Pharmacology, London, Academic Press,
    pp. 49, 65, 203

Cavina, G., Moretti, G. & Petrella, M. (1975) A solvent system for
    the separation of steroids with estrogenic and progestational
    activity by two-dimensional thin-layer chromatography. J. Chromatogr.,
    103, 368-371

Committee on Safety of Medicines (1972) Carcinogenicity Tests of
    Oral Contraceptives, London, HMSO

Council of Europe (1971) European Pharmacopoeia, Vol. II, Sainte
    Ruffine, France, pp. 150-152

Davis, B.K., Noske, I. & Chang, M.C. (1972) Effect of feeding
    ethinyloestradiol for various periods before mating on
    reproduction in the hamster. Acta endocrinol., 70, 582-590

Drill, V.A. & Golway, P.L. (1978) Effect of ethynodiol diacetate with
    ethinylestradiol on the mammary glands of rhesus monkeys: a
    preliminary report. J. natl Cancer Inst., 60, 1169-1170

Eldawy, M.A., Tawfik, A.S. & Elshabouri, S.R. (1975) Rapid, sensitive
    colorimetric method for determination of ethinylestradiol.
    J. pharm. Sci., 64, 1221-1223

Emmeus, C.W. & Martin, L. (1962) Estrogens. In: Dorfman, R.I., ed.,
    Methods in Hormone Research, Vol. III, London, Academic Press,
    pp. 1-75

Finkel, M.J. & Berliner, V.R. (1973) The extrapolation of experimental
    findings (animal to man): The dilemma of the systemically
    administered contraceptives. Bull. Soc. Pharmacol. environ.
    Pathol., 4, 13-18

Fishman, S. (1975) Determination of estrogens in dosage forms by
    fluorescence using dansyl chloride. J. pharm. Sci., 64, 674-680

Fotherby, K. (1973) Metabolism of synthetic steroids by animals and
    man. Acta. endocrinol., Suppl. 185, 119-147

Goldzieher, J.W. (1976) Discussion remark. J. Toxicol. environ. Health,
    Suppl. 1, 73

Goldzieher, J.W. & Kraemer, D.C. (1972) The metabolism and effects
    of contraceptive steroids in primates. Acta endocrinol.,
    Suppl. 166, 389-421

Harvey, S.C. (1975) Hormones. In: Osol, A. *et al*., eds, Remington's
  Pharmaceutical Sciences, 15th ed., Easton, PA, Mack, pp. 916,
  927-928

Hassan, S.S.M. & Zaki, M.T.M. (1976) New spectrophotometric method
  for the determination of phenolic hormones. Talanta, 23, 546-
  549

Helton, E.D. & Goldzieher, J.W. (1977a) The pharmacokinetics of
  ethynyl estrogens. A review. Contraception, 15, 255-284

Helton, E.D. & Goldzieher, J.W. (1977b) Metabolism of ethynyl estrogens.
  J. Toxicol. environ. Health, 3, 231-241

Helton, E.D., Williams, M.C. & Goldzieher, J.W. (1977) Oxidative
  metabolism and de-ethynylation of 17α-ethynylestradiol by baboon
  liver microsomes. Steroids, 30, 71-83

Higashi, Y. (1969) Metabolism of 17β-estradiol and 17α-ethynyl-
  estradiol in rabbits (Jpn.). Folia endocrinol. Jpn., 44, 1153-
  1167

Hisamatsu, T. (1972) Mammary tumorigenesis by subcutaneous administration
  of a mixture of megestrol acetate and ethynylestradiol in Wistar
  rats. Gann, 63, 483-485

IARC (1974) IARC Monographs on the Evaluation of Carcinogenic Risk
  of Chemicals to Man, 6, Sex Hormones, Lyon, pp. 77-85

Inhoffen, H.H., Logemann, W., Hohlweg, W. & Serini, A. (1938)
  Sex hormone series (Ger.). Ber. dtsch chem. Ges., 71, 1024-1032

Kastrup, E.K., ed. (1977) Facts and Comparisons, St Louis, MO, Facts &
  Comparisons Inc., pp. 108c, 108d, 114

Keeley, F.J., Okerholm, R.A., Peterson, F.E. & Glazko, A.J. (1975)
  The metabolic disposition of ethynyl estradiol (EE) in laboratory
  animals (Abstract no. 2915). Fed. Proc., 34, 734

Kraemer, M., Bimboes, D. & Greim, H. (1974) *S. typhimurium* and *E. coli*
  to detect chemical mutagens (Abstract). Naunyn Schmiedebergs'
  Arch. Pharmacol., 284, R46

Kraybill, H.F., Helmes, C.T. & Sigman, C.C. (1977) Biomedical aspects
  of biorefractories in water. In: Hutzinger, O., ed., Second
  International Symposium on Aquatic Pollutants, Amsterdam,
  Noordwijkerhorit, pp. 1-41

Kupperman, H.S., Blatt, M.H.G., Wiesbader, H. & Filler, W. (1953)
    Comparative clinical evaluation of estrogenic preparations by the
    menopausal and amenorrheal indices. J. clin. Endocrinol. Metab.,
    13, 688-703

McKinney, G.R., Weikel, J.H., Jr, Webb, W.K. & Dick, R.G. (1968) Use
    of the life-table technique to estimate effects of certain
    steroids on probability of tumor formation in a long-term study
    in rats. Toxicol. appl. Pharmacol., 12, 68-79

Miller, J.H.M. & Duguid, P. (1976) The fluorimetric analysis of
    oestrogen in oral contraceptive preparations. Proc. anal. Div.
    chem. Soc., 13, 9-13

National Formulary Board (1975) National Formulary, 14th ed.,
    Washington DC, American Pharmaceutical Association, pp. 223-224

Nilsson, S., Nygren, K.-G. & Johansson, E.D.B. (1978) Ethinyl estradiol
    in human milk and plasma after oral administration. Contraception,
    17, 131-139

Okuno, I. & Higgins, W.H. (1977) Method for determining residues of
    mestranol and ethynylestradiol in foliage, soil and water samples.
    Bull. environ. Contam. Toxicol., 18, 428-435

de la Peña, A., Chenault, C.B. & Goldzieher, J.W. (1975) Radioimmunoassay
    of unconjugated plasma ethynylestradiol in women given a single
    oral dose of ethynylestradiol or mestranol. Steroids, 25, 773-780

Piotrow, P.T. & Lee, C.M. (1974) Oral contraceptives - 50 million users.
    Population Reports, Series A, No. 1, Washington DC, George Washington
    University Medical Center, Department of Medical and Public Affairs,
    pp. A-1-A-26

Plotz, E.J. & Haller, J., eds (1971) Methoden der Steroid-Toxikologie,
    Stuttgart, Thieme

Poel, W.E. (1966) Pituitary tumors in mice after prolonged feeding
    of synthetic progestins. Science, 154, 402-403

Reed, M.J. & Fotherby, K. (1975) Metabolism of ethynyloestradiol
    and oestradiol in the guinea-pig. J. Steroid Biochem., 6, 121-125

Reed, M.J. & Fotherby, K. (1976) Intestinal absorption of two synthetic
    steroids. J. Endocrinol., 68, 16P

Rudali, G. (1975) Induction of tumors in mice with synthetic sex
    hormones. Gann Monogr., 17, 243-252

Rurainski, R.D., Theiss, H.J. & Zimmermann, W. (1977) Occurrence of natural and synthetic oestrogens in drinking-water (Ger.). Gas-Wasserfach. Wasser-Abwasser, 118, 288-291

Simard, M.B. & Lodge, B.A. (1970) Thin-layer chromatographic identification of estrogens and progestogens in oral contraceptives. J. Chromatogr., 51, 517-524

Speck, U., Wendt, H., Schulze, P.E. & Jentsch, D. (1976) Bio-availability and pharmacokinetics of cyproterone acetate-^{14}C and ethinyloestradiol-^{3}H after oral administration as a coated tablet. Contraception, 14, 151-163

Stecher, P.G., ed. (1968) The Merck Index, 8th ed., Rahway, NJ, Merck & Co., p. 443

Stenchever, M.A., Jarvis, J.A. & Kreger, N.K. (1969) Effect of selected estrogens and progestins on human chromosomes in vitro. Obstet. Gynecol., 34, 249-251

US Food & Drug Administration (1977) Patient labeling for estrogens for general use. Drugs for human use; drug efficacy study implementation. Fed. Regist., 42, 37645-37646

US Food & Drug Administration (1978) Oral contraceptive drug products. Physician and patient labeling; extension of effective date for physician labeling. Fed. Regist., 43, 9863-9864

US National Institute for Occupational Safety and Health (1977) 1974 National Occupational Hazard Survey, Cincinnati, OH, p. 4,893

US Pharmacopeial Convention Inc. (1975) The US Pharmacopeia, 19th rev., Rockville, MD, pp. 185-187, 192-193

US Pharmacopeial Convention Inc. (1978) The US Pharmacopeia, 19th rev., 4th suppl., Rockville, MD, pp. 347-348

US Tariff Commission (1947) Synthetic Organic Chemicals, US Production and Sales, 1945, TC Publication 157, Second Series, Washington DC, US Government Printing Office, p. 141

US Tariff Commission (1956) Synthetic Organic Chemicals, US Production and Sales, 1955, TC Publication 198, Second Series, Washington DC, US Government Printing Office, p. 112

Verma, P., Curry, C., Crocker, C., Titus-Dillon, P. & Ahluwalia, B. (1975) A competitive protein binding radioassay for 17α-ethynylestradiol in human plasma. Clin. chim. acta, 63, 363-368

Wade, A., ed. (1977) Martindale, The Extra Pharmacopoeia, 27th ed.,
    London, The Pharmaceutical Press, pp. 1396-1397

Wal, J.M., Peleran, J.C. & Bories, G. (1977) Simultaneous determination
    of ethynyloestradiol and trenbolone acetate in animal feeds using
    thin-layer chromatography-gas phase chromatography coupling
    (Fr.). J. Chromatogr., 136, 165-169

Weikel, J.H., Jr & Nelson, L.W. (1977) Problems in evaluating chronic
    toxicity of contraceptive steroids in dogs. J. Toxicol. environ.
    Health, 3, 167-177

WHO (1978) Steroid contraception and the risk of neoplasia. World
    Health Org. tech. Rep. Ser., No. 619

Williams, M.C., Helton, E.D. & Goldzieher, J.W. (1975) The urinary
    metabolites of 17α-ethynylestradiol-9α,11ζ-^{3}H in women.
    Chromatographic profiling and identification of ethynyl and non-
    ethynyl compounds. Steroids, 25, 229-246

Windholz, M., ed. (1976) The Merck Index, 9th ed., Rahway, NJ, Merck
    & Co., p. 507

Yanagimachi, R. & Sato, A. (1968) Effects of a single oral
    administration of ethinyl estradiol on early pregnancy in the
    mouse. Fertil. Steril., 19, 787-801

Yasuda, Y., Kihara, T. & Nishimura, H. (1977) Effect of prenatal
    treatment with ethinylestradiol on the mouse uterus and
    ovary. Am. J. Obstet. Gynecol., 127, 832-836

MESTRANOL

A monograph on this substance was published previously (IARC, 1974). Relevant data that have appeared since that time have been evaluated in the present monograph.

1. Chemical and Physical Data

1.1 Synonyms and trade names

Chem. Abstr. Services Reg. No.: 72-33-3

Chem. Abstr. Name: (17α)-3-Methoxy-19-norpregna-1,3,5(10)-trien-20-yn-17-ol

Synonyms: EE3ME; ethinylestradiol 3-methyl ether; 17α-ethinyl-estradiol 3-methyl ether; ethinyloestradiol 3-methyl ether; 17α-ethinyloestradiol 3-methyl ether; ethynylestradiol methyl ether; ethynylestradiol 3-methyl ether; 17-ethynylestradiol 3-methyl ether; 17α-ethynylestradiol methyl ether; 17α-ethynyl-estradiol 3-methyl ether; 17α-ethynyl-3-methoxy-1,3,5(10)-estratrien-17β-ol; ethynyloestradiol methyl ether; ethynyloestradiol 3-methyl ether; 17-ethynyloestradiol 3-methyl ether; 17α-ethynyloestradiol methyl ether; 17α-ethynyloestradiol 3-methyl ether; 17α-ethynyl-3-methoxy-1,3,5(10)-oestratrien-17β-ol; 3-methoxy-17α-ethinylestradiol; 3-methoxy-17α-ethinyloestradiol; 3-methoxyethynylestradiol; 3-methoxy-17α-ethynylestradiol; 3-methoxyethynyloestradiol; 3-methoxy-17α-ethynyloestradiol; 3-methoxy-19-nor-17α-pregna-1,3,5(10)-trien-20-yn-17-ol; 3-methylethynylestradiol; 3-methyl-ethynyloestradiol; Δ-MVE

Trade names[1]: [Aconcen]; [Anacyclin]; [Anconcene]; 8027 C.B., Compound 33355; [Conlunett]; [Conlunett 21]; [Conluten]; Conovid; [Conovid E]; [Consan]; C-Quens; [C-Quens-21]; [Cyclovul];

---

[1]Those in square brackets are preparations that are no longer produced commercially.

[Delpregnin]; Demulen; Devocin; Emetin; Enavid; Enavid E; Enovid; Enovid-E; Enovid-E21; [Estirona]; [Estirona 21]; [Eunomin]; [Feminor 21]: [Feminor Seq.]; [Gestakliman]; [Gynovin]; [Hestranol]; Inostral; [Luteolas]; [Lynacyclan]; [Lyndiol]; Lyndiol 2.5; [Lyndiol-22]; [Lyndiol Mite]; Menophase; [Mestrenol]; Metrulen; [Metrulene]; [Metrulen M]; [Neonovum]; [Nocon]; [Nonovul]; [Nor 50]; [Noracyclin]; [Noracyclin 22]; [Noracycline 22]; Norinyl; Norinyl 1; [Norinyl 1/28]; Norinyl 2; [Nuriphasic]; [Norolen]; Norquen; [Orgaluton]; [Ortho-Novin]; Ortho-Novin 2; Ortho-Novin 1/50; Ortho-Novin 1/80; [Ortho-Novin Mite]; [Ortho-Novin Sq.]; Ortho-Novum; [Orthonovum]; [Ortho-Novum 1/50]; [Ortho-Novum 1/80]; [Ortho-Novum 2]; [Orthonovum N]; [Ortho-Novum Sq.]; [OV 28]; Ovanon; [Ovariostat]; Ovastol; [Ovastat]; Ovulen; [Ovulen 0.5]; [Ovulen 1]; Ovulen-21; Ovulen-28; [Ovulen Mite]; [Plan]; [Previsan]; [Previsana]; Previson; SC 4725; Sequens; [Singestol]; [Singestrol]; [Sistometril]; Sophia; Syntex menophase; [Volenyl]

1.2 Structural and molecular formulae and molecular weight

C$_{21}$H$_{26}$O$_2$ Mol. wt: 310.4

1.3 Chemical and physical properties

From Wade (1977) and Windholz (1976), unless otherwise specified

(a) Description: White crystals (from methanol or acetone)

(b) Melting-point: 150–151°C

(c) Optical rotation: $[\alpha]_D$ +2 to +8° (2% w/v in dioxane) (US
Pharmacopeial Convention Inc., 1975)

(d) Solubility: Practically insoluble in water; soluble in
ethanol (1 in 44), acetone (1 in 23), diethyl ether (1 in
23), chloroform (1 in 4.5) and dioxane (1 in 12); slightly
soluble in methanol

(e) Stability: Unstable to air and light (US Pharmacopeial Convention Inc., 1975)

1.4 Technical products and impurities

Various national and international pharmacopoeias give specifications
for the purity of mestranol in pharmaceutical products. For example,
it is available in the US as a USP grade containing 97-102% mestranol,
calculated on a dried basis (US Pharmacopeial Convention Inc., 1975).
It is marketed in the US only in combination with progestins. Tablets
containing mestranol are available in 0.05, 0.06, 0.075, 0.08, 0.1 and
0.15 mg doses, in combination with norethisterone, norethynodrel and
ethynodiol diacetate (Kastrup, 1977, 1978; US Pharmacopeial Convention
Inc., 1978). In Japan, mestranol alone is available in tablets.

2. Production, Use, Occurrence and Analysis

2.1 Production and use

(a) Production

The first synthesis of mestranol was reported in 1954 (Colton,
1954), by the reaction of 3-methoxy-1,3,5-oestratrien-17-one with potassium
acetylide (formed by reacting the potassium salt of *tert*-amyl alcohol
with acetylene). Mestranol is believed to be produced commercially by
conversion of oestrone to its 3-methyl ether and introduction of the 17-
ethinyl group, either by reaction with sodium acetylide in liquid ammonia
or by the Grignard reaction with ethinyl magnesium bromide (Colton *et
al.*, 1957).

Mestranol is not produced commercially in the US, and separate data
on imports are not available.

Commercial production of mestranol in the UK was first reported in 1955. Annual production of mestranol in western Europe is estimated to be in the range of 100 thousand-1 million kg; Belgium, France, the Federal Republic of Germany, Luxembourg, The Netherlands and the UK are the major producing countries. It is also believed to be produced commercially in eastern Europe, but no information was available on the quantity produced. In 1977, imports by Spain and Italy were 10-100 thousand kg each; and imports by eastern European countries were 100 thousand-1 million kg. Exports from western Europe in 1977 amounted to 10-100 thousand kg.

It was first marketed in Japan around 1960. It is not produced there, and imports amounted to about 3-4 kg annually in 1975-1977.

(b) Use

The most widespread use of mestranol is in oral contraceptives, as the oestrogen in combination therapy (Murad & Gilman, 1975); it is also used in combination with a progestin for such conditions as endometriosis and amenorrhoea (Wade, 1977).

In Japan, mestranol is used mostly in combination with lynoestrenol, norethisterone and chlormadinone acetate.

The US Food & Drug Administration (1977) has ruled that with effect from 20 September 1977 oestrogens for general use must carry patient and physician warning labels concerning use, risks, and contraindications. The same ruling was extended to all oral contraceptives with effect from 31 May 1978 (US Food & Drug Administration, 1978).

2.2 Occurrence

Mestranol is not known to occur naturally. Residues have been found in foliage, soil and water samples (Okuno & Higgins, 1977). Up to 1% mestranol occurs in norethynodrel (B.P.) as normally manufactured (see monograph, p. 461) (Wade, 1977).

In a study carried out in a plant producing oral contraceptives, mestranol was found in various sectors of the working environment, at levels ranging from 0.06-8.61 $\mu g/m^3$, and on wipe samples, at levels of 0.003-2.05 $\mu g/cm^2$ (Harrington $et\ al.$, 1978).

2.3 Analysis

Typical analytical methods for the determination of mestranol are summarized in Table 1. Abbreviations used are: FL, fluorescence; GC, gas chromatography; GC/FID, gas chromatography/flame-ionization detection; HPLC, high-pressure liquid chromatography; CC, column chromatography; TLC, thin-layer chromatography; and UV, ultra-violet spectrometry. See also 'General Remarks on Sex Hormones', p. 60 .

TABLE 1

Analytical methods for mestranol

Sample matrix	Sample preparation	Assay procedure	Sensitivity or limit of detection	Reference
Bulk chemical	Dissolve (tetrahydrofuran); add silver nitrate solution	Titration (sodium hydroxide)	-	British Pharmacopoeia Commission (1973)
Bulk chemical	Dissolve (chloroform:methanol, 1:1)	Two-dimensional TLC (UV, acid spray)	-	Cavina et al. (1975)
Bulk chemical	Dissolve (acetonitrile-heptane); CC (diatomaceous earth-acetonitrile); elute (heptane); evaporate; dissolve (ethanol)	UV	-	Graham & Kenner (1973)
Bulk chemical	Dissolve	HPLC; UV (254 nm)	-	Hara & Hayashi (1977)
Bulk chemical	Dissolve (t-butanol:cyclo-hexane, 9:1); add sodium t-butoxide reagent, diethyl oxalate reagent & hydro-chloric acid	UV (294 nm)	-	Szepesi & Görög (1974)
Bulk chemical	Dissolve (chloroform); evaporate; dissolve (methanol-sulphuric acid)	Colorimetry (~545 nm)	-	US Pharmacopeial Convention Inc. (1975)
Tablets	Powder; dissolve (dimethyl-formamide:formamide, 1:1); CC (diatomaceous earth-sodium sulphate); elute (heptane); evaporate; dissolve (heptane:chloroform, 8:1)	UV (287 nm)	-	Horwitz (1975a,b)

Table 1 (continued)

Sample matrix	Sample preparation	Assay procedure	Sensitivity or limit of detection	Reference
Tablets (with ethynodiol diacetate)	Powder; dissolve (formamide); CC (diatomaceous earth-dimethyl sulphoxide-formamide); elute (heptane); extract (sulphuric acid-methanol)	Colorimetry (≈540 nm)	-	Horwitz (1975b)
Tablets	Powder & extract (ethyl acetate)	GC	-	Moretti *et al.* (1977)
Tablets	Extract (dichloromethane-hydrochloric acid); add hydroquinone in sulphuric acid-ethanol)	FL (560 nm)	-	Miller & Duguid (1976)
Tablets	Extract (chloroform-sodium hydroxide solution); evaporate; dissolve (sulphuric acid-methanol)	Colorimetry (~545 nm)	-	National Formulary Board (1975)
Tablets	Dissolve (water); extract (methylene chloride)	TLC (selenious acid spray); densitometry		Shroff & Shaw (1972)
Contraceptive preparations	Dissolve (ethanol); add silver nitrate solution; filter; add dithizone solution	Colorimetry (472 nm)	1 mg	Rizk *et al.* (1973)
Mestranol added to water & waste-water	Extract	TLC (FL)	-	Kirchner *et al.* (1973)
Water	Extract (diethyl ether, chloroform & hydrochloric acid)	GC/FID	0.01 mg/l (200 ml sample)	Okuno & Higgins (1977)
Foliage	Extract (acetonitrile-hydrochloric acid); CC (Florisil & gel permeation)	GC/FID	0.05 mg/kg (10 g sample)	Okuno & Higgins (1977)
Soil	Extract (acetone-hydrochloric acid); concentrate; extract (diethyl ether & chloroform); CC (Florisil & gel permeation)	GC/FID	0.1 mg/kg (10 g sample)	Okuno & Higgins (1977)
	(Matrix determines method of preparation)	TLC (acid spray & UV)	100 ng	Okuno & Higgins (1977)

3. Biological Data Relevant to the Evaluation
    of Carcinogenic Risk to Humans

3.1 Carcinogenicity studies in animals

In several of the following investigations, mestranol was administered
as the commercial product Enovid (1.5% mestranol and 98.5% norethynodrel),
or in combination with other progestins. The experimental data have
therefore been summarized both in this monograph and in that on norethynodrel (see p. 461). It should be noted that the effects reported may
reflect the action either of an individual constituent or of the combination.

(a) Oral administration

Mouse: Groups of 24 virgin female C57L mice (MTV$^-$)[1] received 7 or
70 µg of a mixture of mestranol:norethynodrel (1:50) in oil by gavage, 5
times per week, commencing when the animals were 13 weeks of age.
Pituitary tumours were found at autopsy in 7/7 mice given the higher
dose that lived 84-89 weeks and in 6/11 mice given the lower dose,
compared with 2/15 controls that lived 90 weeks. In this, and in a
concurrent experiment with norethisterone:ethinyloestradiol (50:1),
hepatomas were found in 10/96 treated mice, but the distribution within
the different treatment groups was not reported. No hepatomas occurred
among 48 control mice (Poel, 1966).

Female BALB/c mice (MTV$^-$) were fed a liquid diet (Metrecal) containing
Enovid such that each mouse consumed 10-12.5 µg per day. All of the 8
mice that survived more than 74 weeks of treatment had early or infiltrating
carcinomas of the cervix. No carcinomas of the uterine corpus or cervix
or of the vagina were found in 42 untreated females that lived 103-130
weeks nor in 8 females given Metrecal for 79-102 weeks (Dunn, 1969).

Castrated male (C3H x RIII)F1 mice (MTV$^+$) that received 15 mg/kg
(ppm) Enovid in the diet (average intake, 30-40 µg/mouse per day) had an
increased incidence of mammary tumours, from 10/61 to 20/23. The latent
period for tumour development was decreased in both castrated males and
ovariectomized females, but the incidence in ovariectomized females
was not significantly increased. In intact female RIII mice, Enovid had
no effect on incidence or on latent period (Rudali, 1975).

---

[1]MTV$^-$: mammary tumour virus not expressed; MTV$^+$: mammary tumour
virus expressed (see p. 62)

Intact male (C3H x RIII)Fl mice (MTV$^+$) given 3 mg/kg (ppm) Ovulen (90% ethynodiol diacetate and 10% mestranol) mixed into the diet (intake, 7.5-10.0 µg/mouse per day) showed an increased incidence of mammary tumours, from 0/76 to 14/25; in castrated males, the incidence was increased from 10/61 to 21/28. The high spontaneous incidence (161/167) and short latent period of tumour induction (30-33 weeks) in intact females were not altered (37/38). In ovariectomized females the tumour incidence was not altered by Ovulen (28/34 in controls as compared with 20/26), but the latent period was reduced in both ovariectomized females (from 49 to 26 weeks) and castrated males (from 82 to 43 weeks) (Rudali, 1975).

In C57BL females (MTV$^-$) given 20 mg/kg of diet Enovid for lifespan, chromophobe adenomas were seen in 36/49, compared with 15/51 in controls. In BALB/c females (MTV$^+$) treated similarly, an increased incidence of non-metastasizing epithelial tumorous lesions of the cervix and vagina was reported in excess over that in controls (32/55 *versus* 18/55). The incidence of ovarian tumours in treated C3H (MTV$^+$) and C$_3$HfB (MTV$^-$) females was unchanged, and the incidence of mammary tumours in treated C3H females was decreased (39/53 *versus* 55/55) (Heston *et al.*, 1973).

Twenty female BALB/c mice (MTV$^-$) were fed a liquid diet (Metrecal) containing an estimated dose of 10-12.5 µg Enovid/mouse per day for an average of 15 months. Among 16 mice that lived for 10 months or more, 3 developed precancerous lesions and 2, squamous-cell carcinomas of the cervix and/or vagina. Of a group of 40 mice treated with Enovid and with intravaginal inoculations of herpesvirus type 2, 31 survived 10 months or more; of these, 1 developed a precancerous lesion and 6, squamous-cell carcinomas of the cervix and/or vagina. In 15/20 control mice that lived for 10 months or more, 1 precancerous lesion of the cervix was detected (Muñoz, 1973).

Administration of mestranol alone at a level of 0.1 mg/kg of diet, giving an estimated daily intake of 0.25 µg/mouse per day, resulted in an increased incidence of mammary tumours (to 11/13) in castrated male RIII mice (MTV$^+$) within 8 months, compared with an incidence of 8/19 in intact male RIII (MTV$^+$) mice within 14 months. Of castrated male (C3H x RIII)Fl mice (MTV$^+$) fed 1 mg/kg of diet (2.5 µg/mouse per day), 24/26 developed mammary tumours within 28 weeks, compared with 7/41 controls within 69 weeks. No effects on the latent period or on the high spontaneous mammary tumour incidence were observed in females (Rudali *et al.*, 1971).

In castrated male (C3H x RIII)Fl mice (MTV$^+$), administration of mestranol in the diet at an estimated intake of 75 µg/kg bw per day resulted in an increased incidence of mammary tumours (26/32), with an average latent period of 30 weeks, as compared with an incidence of 10/61 at 82 weeks in untreated control castrates (Rudali *et al.*, 1972).

Mestranol alone or in combination with norethynodrel, ethynodiol diacetate, norethisterone, chlormadinone acetate or lynoestrenol was incorporated into the diet of CF-LP and Swiss mice for 80 weeks. The doses were identified only as low (2-5 times the human contraceptive dose), medium (50-150 times) and high (200-400 times); the amounts administered were not specified. Mestranol administered alone resulted in an increased incidence of pituitary tumours: 12 in 120 male and 17 in 120 female CF-LP mice, compared with 4 in 240 male and 12 in 240 female controls. Larger increases were found in both males and females given mestranol in combination with progestins, incidences ranging from 15-47 in males and from 27-42 in females per group of 120 animals. In groups of 47-123 Swiss mice administered mestranol alone, about 4% of malignant mammary tumours were found in males and females, compared with 0 in controls. When given in combination with lynoestrenol (1:33), the incidence in females increased to 6%, but no such tumours occurred in males (Committee on Safety of Medicines, 1972).

Administration of 5, 30, 60 and 200 μg/kg bw per day mestranol (2.5, 15, 30 and 100 times the human dose, respectively) to groups of 39-40 male and female Swiss-Webster mice and CF-LP mice did not influence the spontaneous incidence of hepatocellular tumours (Barrows *et al.*, 1977).

Rat: In a group of 21 female Wistar rats given daily gastric instillations of 3 mg Enovid 6 times per week for 50 weeks, no mammary tumours were observed, compared with 1/54 in a group of untreated controls. In a further group of 47 female rats given a similar dose of Enovid together with 2-5 mg 3-methylcholanthrene 6 times per week for 52 weeks, the incidence of mammary tumours was neither increased nor decreased when compared with that produced by the administration of 3-methylcholanthrene alone (Gruenstein *et al.*, 1964). Some inhibition of the induction of mammary tumours following a single dose of 15 or 20 mg 7,12-dimethylbenz[*a*]anthracence was observed after Enovid administration (Stern & Mickey, 1969; Weisburger *et al.*, 1968).

A group of 100 female rats were given mestranol alone for 104 weeks. Twenty-two % of malignant mammary tumours were found in 100 treated animals and 5% in 50 controls. When mestranol was administered to male and female rats in combination with norethynodrel or norethisterone, the incidence of malignant mammary tumours in males was 12-20%, compared with 0 in controls, and 6-30% in females, compared with 5-7% in controls; the increase was significant. In male rats, the incidences of benign liver-cell tumours were 8-29% in groups of 120 rats administered mestranol with norethynodrel and 23% in 120 rats administered mestranol with norethisterone, compared with 2.5 and 4.0% in groups of 120 and 40 controls (Committee on Safety of Medicines, 1972) [The Working Group noted that the effective number of animals was not given].

Wistar rats of both sexes were fed 0.01% for 2 years and 0.02% for 1 year of the oral contraceptive Sophia (norethisterone:mestranol, 100:1) in food pellets, resulting in daily doses of 1.53 mg norethisterone and 0.015 mg mestranol in the 0.01% group and in 3.74 mg and 0.037 mg for females and 4.28 and 0.43 mg for males in the 0.02% group. In those fed 0.01%, 6 mammary fibroadenomas and 1 pituitary tumour developed in 39 effective females, as compared with 0/6 female controls. No tumours were seen in 18 males treated with 0.01%, whereas 4/9 male controls developed mammary fibroadenomas. Considerable losses of animals occurred due to intercurrent deaths. Animals fed 0.02% lived for only one year. No tumours were observed within that time in animals of either group (Takahashi, 1974).

Three groups of female Wistar rats received 40 mg/kg bw N-nitroso-methylurea (NMU) on 3 subsequent days. One group received an oral contraceptive (0.25 mg lynoestrenol + 0.075 mg mestranol) daily for 30 days before NMU treatment, whereas the other group received the contraceptive after the treatment. The third group served as a control. Tumour induction (especially of nephroblastomas) was changed only in the group that received the oral contraceptive before the carcinogen: a significant decrease was observed (Thomas *et al.*, 1972).

Dog: Groups of 13-20 female dogs were given mestranol alone (at 10 and 25 times the human dose, i.e., 0.02 and 0.05 mg/kg bw per day) or combinations of mestranol with chloroethinylnorgestrel or ethynerone (1:20) (at 2, 10 and 25 times the human dose, i.e., 0.084, 0.42 and 1.05 mg/kg bw per day) or mestranol:anagestone acetate (1:10) (at 10 and 25 times the human dose, i.e., 0.44 and 1.10 mg/kg bw per day). At the time of sacrifice, animals had received the combinations for 4.5-5 years and for 6.25 yrs. In the mestranol-treated dogs, one mammary adenoma was found in the highest dose group, whereas two benign mixed mammary tumours were found in controls. Dogs given progestin:mestranol developed more hyper- and neoplastic mammary nodules than did control dogs. Of animals given ethynerone plus mestranol, 2/16, 5/16 and 15/17 dogs, respectively, showed such nodules; whereas 7/16, 16/17 and 16/16 of the chloroethinylnorgestrel plus mestranol-treated dogs and 13/13 and 12/13 of the anagestone acetate plus mestranol-treated dogs showed nodules. Since pyometra occurred in some animals, all dogs, including the controls, were hysterectomized after 2 years of treatment (Geil & Lamar, 1977; Giles *et al.*, 1978).

Monkey: In a study still in progress at the time of reporting, an adenocarcinoma of the mammary gland was observed after 18 months in 1/6 female *Macaca mulatta* (rhesus) monkeys administered 1 mg Enovid per day. Widespread metastases were associated with the tumour (Kirchstein *et al.*, 1972) [The Working Group noted the incomplete reporting of this experiment].

In a preliminary report of a study in progress, oral administration of Enovid-E (2.5 mg norethynodrel and 0.1 mg mestranol per human dose) and Ovulen (1.0 mg ethynodiol diacetate and 0.1 mg mestranol) in dosages 1, 10 and 50 times the average human contraceptive dose to mature female rhesus monkeys (16 per group) resulted in no clinical evidence of mammary gland lesions or tumours after 5 years (Drill *et al.*, 1974).

Groups of 16-20 female monkeys were given mestranol alone or in combination with chloroethinylnorgestrel, ethynerone or anagestone acetate orally in dosages of 2, 10 and 50 times the human dose level. At the time of publication, after 7 years of observation, some palpable mammary nodules had been found distributed randomly in all groups, including the controls. Biopsies of mammary tissue revealed a slight ductal epithelial hyperplasia in some of the treated animals, also evenly distributed among the groups (Geil & Lamar, 1977).

(b)   Subcutaneous and/or intramuscular administration

Mouse: Nulliparous C3H/HeJ female mice (MTV$^+$) were administered 0.1 mg Enovid subcutaneously twice weekly from 1 month of age for 21 months. A significantly increased incidence of mammary tumours was observed (30/100, as compared with 14/100 in controls) [$P<0.01$] (Welsch *et al.*, 1977).

Rat: Repeated s.c. injections of 10 or 100 µg Enovid per day into 2 groups of 25 female Sprague-Dawley rats for 40 days reduced the number of mammary tumours/rat produced by a single i.v. injection of 5 mg 7,12-dimethylbenz[*a*]anthracence (DMBA) given on day 25 of treatment. The average numbers of tumours/rat were 10.9 in 37 controls given DMBA alone, compared with 7.6 and 3.9 in rats given 10 or 100 µg Enovid per day, respectively (Welsch & Meites, 1969).

Hamster: Thrice weekly s.c. injections to 46 male Syrian golden hamsters of 34 mg/kg bw Enovid in sesame oil, reduced to 17 mg/kg bw at 94 weeks and to 8.5 mg/kg bw at 104 weeks, did not affect the incidence of any tumour type (Sichuk *et al.*, 1967) [The Working Group noted that the average age of the animals at the start of the experiment was 76 weeks and that 50% of the animals had died by 103 weeks].

3.2   Other relevant biological data

(a)   Experimental systems

In animals, as in humans, the oestrogenic activity of mestranol is equal to or slightly less than that of ethynyloestradiol, depending on species and route of administration (Haller, 1971). See also 'General Remarks on Sex Hormones', pp. 42 & 43.

Toxic effects

The LD$_{50}$ of mestranol by i.p. administration in mice is 3500 mg/kg bw (Gosselin, 1968).

Geil & Lamar (1977) found a dose-dependent, non-progressive decrease in haemoglobin and haematocyte levels in dogs treated with mestranol or a combination of mestranol with ethynerone, chloroethinylnorgestrel or anagestone acetate. Diabetes mellitus developed in 10 dogs, all in groups that had received the medium or high dose of the chloroethinyl-norgestrel/mestranol or anagestone acetate/mestranol combinations. In addition, 3 monkeys (2 anagestone acetate + mestranol-treated and one ethynerone + mestranol-treated) developed diabetes mellitus.

Embryotoxicity and teratogenicity

Daily oral administration of 0.05 or 0.2 mg/kg bw mestranol to NMRI x ABAF$_1$ hybrid mice daily from day 4-8 after mating inhibited implantation and increased the number of resorptions. Foetuses of mice of the NMRI strain had accessory ribs. Treatment from day 7-11 with doses of 0.1-0.2 mg/kg bw induced abortions but had no teratogenic effects (Heinecke & Klaus, 1975).

In rats, s.c. injection of 0.002-0.02 mg/kg bw mestranol 5 days before and 30 days after mating prevented implantation in a dose-dependent manner. S.c. injection of 0.02 mg/kg bw or oral administration of 0.1 mg/kg bw on days 2-4 of gestation terminated pregnancy (Saunders & Elton, 1967).

Charles River rats received daily oral doses of 0.05-0.2 mg/kg bw Enovid (2.5 mg norethynodrel + 0.1 mg mestranol) or 0.01-0.1 mg/kg bw mestranol throughout pregnancy and for 21 days after parturition. The highest dose of mestranol terminated a significant percentage of pregnancies. No genital defects were observed in surviving male offpsring, but female offspring showed an enlarged genital papilla and a prematurely open vagina, even with lower doses. In female offspring of rats treated with 0.1 mg Enovid, fertility was impaired by 55%. Higher doses of Enovid and a dose of 0.02 mg mestranol induced complete sterility in female offspring; examination of the ovary showed no corpora lutea and follicles of reduced size (Saunders, 1967).

Sixty female Wistar rats were given oral doses of 1 mg/kg bw Enidrel (0.075 mg mestranol + 9.2 mg norethynodrel) daily for 2 months, at which time they were mated. In 30 animals in which treatment was continued, complete foetal resorption occurred rapidly; however, after 2 weeks without treatment, fertility rates and litter sizes were normal. In the 30 animals in which treatment was discontinued, fertility and pre- and postnatal development of the offspring were also normal. No teratogenic effects were observed (Tuchmann-Duplessis & Mercier-Parot, 1972).

In rabbits, pregnancy was terminated by daily oral doses of more than 0.02 mg/kg bw mestranol from day 1-28 or 0.05 mg/kg bw from day 10-28 of pregnancy and by s.c. doses of 0.005 mg/kg bw from day 1-28 or more than 0.002 mg/kg bw from day 10-28. Doses that did not terminate pregnancy had no effects on litter size or weights of the offspring (Saunders & Elton, 1967).

In female Syrian golden hamsters that received a contraceptive steroid containing 18.7 µg mestranol and 0.6 mg lynoestrenol (route unspecified) daily for 4.5-8 months, fertility was found to be normal; no effects were seen on the sexual behaviour or fecundity of offspring of the following two generations (Cottinet *et al.*, 1974).

Adult female beagle dogs received 5 mg/kg bw mestranol orally on day 6 or 21 of pregnancy. Embryonic losses, based on corpora lutea counts, were 95.5 and 67.3%, respectively, as compared with 34.5% in controls. Surviving offspring appeared normal (Kennelly, 1969).

Absorption, distribution and excretion

Studies in rats indicate that enterohepatic circulation of metabolites of mestranol is an important factor in the excretion of this compound and may be impaired by administration of antibiotics like neomycin (Brewster *et al.*, 1977).

Metabolism

Mestranol, the 3-methyl ether of ethinyloestradiol, is more lipophilic than ethinyloestradiol and has a greater affinity for adipose tissues, as shown by experiments in rats (Appelgren & Karlsson, 1971). Mestranol itself does not bind significantly to oestrogen receptors at the sites of their antifertility action; its hormonal effectiveness relies on transformation to ethinyloestradiol (Eisenfeld, 1974). About 35% of a mestranol dose is transformed into ethinyloestradiol in rats (Kappus *et al.*, 1972), 61% in mice (Bolt & Remmer, 1972), 56% in rabbits and 54% in man (Bolt & Bolt, 1974). The demethylated portion then follows the pathways for ethinyloestradiol that are typical for the particular species, e.g., 2-hydroxylation in rats (Ball *et al.*, 1973) and D-homoannulation in rabbits and guinea-pigs (Abdel-Aziz & Williams, 1969, 1974, 1975). Mestranol is also demethylated to ethinyloestradiol in non-human primates (Kulkarni *et al.*, 1977).

Mutagenicity and other short-term tests

Dominant lethal mutations were observed in female mice treated for 3 days prior to mating with doses of 12.5 µg mestranol and 420 µg lynoestrenol/kg bw (Badr & Badr, 1974) [For a consideration of the possible mutagenicity of this compound, see 'General Remarks on Sex Hormones', p. 64].

Female Holtzman rats treated orally for 5 days with 0.02 or 0.2 mg/kg bw mestranol were sacrificed on day 6. No damage to bone-marrow chromosomes, as compared with corn-oil-treated controls, was observed (Edwards *et al.*, 1971).

(b) Humans

The metabolism of mestranol in humans is closely related to that of ethinyloestradiol (see monograph, p.233). Mestranol is transformed to ethinyloestradiol by demethylation (Warren & Fotherby, 1973): after i.v. administration of ^{14}C-mestranol to human volunteers, about 50% of the dose is demethylated to ethinyloestradiol (Bolt & Bolt, 1974). The main compound found in plasma is ethinyloestradiol-3-sulphate (Bird & Clark, 1973).

The excretion of metabolites in urine ranged from 10-27%; that of ethinyloestradiol metabolites ranges from 36-54% (Kulkarni & Goldzieher, 1970). When position 2 or 4 of the mestranol molecule is tritiated or marked with ^{14}C, between 14-45% of the radioactivity is released into the body water. Metabolites identified were ethinyloestradiol, 2-hydroxyethinyloestradiol, 2-methoxyethinyloestradiol and 2-hydroxy-ethinyloestradiol 3-methyl ether (Williams & Williams, 1975; Williams *et al.*, 1975).

No cytogenetic changes were detected in cultured human lymphocytes exposed *in vitro* to mestranol or derived from women exposed *in vivo* to mestranol in oestrogen/progestin contraceptive preparations (de Gutiérrez & Lisker, 1973; Shapiro *et al.*, 1972; Singh & Carr, 1970).

3.3 Case reports and epidemiological studies

See the section, 'Oestrogens and Progestins in Relation to Human Cancer', p. 83.

4. Summary of Data Reported and Evaluation[1]

4.1 Experimental data

Mestranol was tested in mice, rats, dogs and monkeys by oral administration; in most studies it was administered in combination with progestins. When administered alone, it increased the incidences of pituitary tumours in both sexes of one strain of mice and increased the incidence of malignant mammary tumours in castrated males of two further strains and in males and females of another strain. It also produced an increased incidence of malignant mammary tumours in female rats.

_____

[1]This section should be read in conjunction with pp. 62-64 of the 'General Remarks on Sex Hormones' and with the 'General Conclusions on Sex Hormones', p. 131.

Studies in dogs and monkeys are still in progress. Although no
tumours have been observed in either species after 7 years, no conclusive
evaluation can yet be made.

In experiments in which mestranol was administered to female mice
in combination with norethynodrel, pituitary tumours and vaginal and
cervical squamous-cell carcinomas were produced; in male mice, an
increased incidence of mammary tumours was observed following administration of mestranol in combination with norethynodrel or ethynodiol
diacetate. Combinations with norethynodrel or norethisterone resulted
in an excess of benign liver-cell tumours in male rats and increased the
incidence of malignant mammary tumours in rats of both sexes.

In dogs, administration of combinations with various synthetic
progestins led to the formation of mammary tumours. In monkeys given
these combinations as well as combinations with norethynodrel or ethynodiol
diacetate, no mammary nodules were observed after 5 and 7 years of
experimentation, respectively. These experiments are still in progress.

It was also tested in combination with norethynodrel by subcutaneous
administration in mice, rats and hamsters; it produced an increased
incidence of mammary tumours in female mice.

Mestranol is embryolethal for pre- and postimplantation embryos in
some species.

4.2 Human data

No case reports or epidemiological studies on mestranol alone were
available to the Working Group. Epidemiological studies on steroid
hormones used in oestrogen-progestin contraceptive preparations have
been summarized in the section, 'Oestrogens and Progestins in Relation
to Human Cancer', p. 83.

4.3 Evaluation

There is *sufficient evidence* for the carcinogenicity of mestranol
in experimental animals. In the absence of adequate data in humans, it
is reasonable, for practical purposes, to regard mestranol as if it
presented a carcinogenic risk to humans. The use of oral contraceptives
containing mestranol in combination with progestins has been related
causally to an increased incidence of benign liver adenomas and a decreased
incidence of benign breast disease. Studies also strongly suggest that
the administration of oestrogens is causally related to an increased
incidence of endometrial carcinoma; there is no evidence that mestranol
is different from other oestrogens in this respect.

5. References

Abdel-Aziz, M.T. & Williams, K.I.H. (1969) Metabolism of 17α-ethynyl-
    estradiol and its 3-methyl ether by the rabbit; an *in vivo*
    D-homoannulation. Steroids, 13, 809-820

Abdel-Aziz, M.T. & Williams, K.I.H. (1974) Urinary metabolites of
    mestranol by guinea pigs. J. Drug Res. (Cairo), 6, 195-201

Abdel-Aziz, M.T. & Williams, K.I.H. (1975) Fecal metabolites of
    mestranol by guinea pigs. J. Drug Res. (Cairo), 7, 89-94

Appelgren, L.-E. & Karlsson, R. (1971) The distribution of
    ^{14}C-4-mestranol in mice. Acta pharmacol. toxicol., 29, 65-74

Badr, F.M. & Badr,, R.S. (1974) Studies on the mutagenic effect
    of contraceptive drugs. I. Induction of dominant lethal
    mutations in female mice. Mutat. Res., 26, 529-534

Ball, P., Gelbke, H.P., Haupt, O. & Knuppen, R. (1973) Metabolism of
    17α-ethynyl-[4-^{14}C]oestradiol and [4-^{14}C]mestranol in rat liver
    slices and interaction between 17α-ethynyl-2-hydroxyoestradiol and
    adrenalin. Hoppe-Seyler's Z. physiol. Chem., 354, 1567-1575

Barrows, G.H., Christopherson, W.M. & Drill, V.A. (1977) Liver lesions
    and oral contraceptive steroids. J. Toxicol. environ. Health,
    3, 219-230

Bird, C.E. & Clark, A.F. (1973) Metabolic clearance rates and
    metabolism of mestranol and ethynylestradiol in normal young
    women. J. clin. Endocrinol. Metab., 36, 296-302

Bolt, H.M. & Bolt, W.H. (1974) Pharmacokinetics of mestranol in man in
    relation to its oestrogenic activity. Eur. J. clin. Pharmacol.,
    7, 295-305

Bolt, H.M. & Remmer, H. (1972) The accumulation of mestranol and
    ethynyloestradiol metabolites in the organism. Xenobiotica, 2,
    489-498

Brewster, D., Jones, R.S. & Symons, A.M. (1977) Effects of neomycin
    on the biliary excretion and enterohepatic circulation of
    mestranol and 17β-oestradiol. Biochem. Pharmacol., 26, 943-946

British Pharmacopoeia Commission (1973) British Pharmacopoeia, London,
    HMSO, p. 291

Cavina, G., Moretti, G. & Petrella, M. (1975) A solvent system for the preparation of steroids with estrogenic and progestational activity by two-dimensional thin-layer chromatography. J. Chromatogr., 103, 368-371

Colton, F.B. (1954) 17-Glycolylestradiols. US Patent 2,666,769, 19 January, to G.D. Searle & Co. [Chem. Abstr., 49, 1827c]

Colton, F.B., Nysted, L.N., Riegel, B. & Raymond, A.L. (1957) 17-Alkyl-19-nortestosterones. J. Am. chem. Soc., 79, 1123-1127

Committee on Safety of Medicines (1972) Carcinogenicity Tests of Oral Contraceptives, London, HMSO

Cottinet, D., Czyba, J.C., Dams, R. & Laurent, J.L. (1974) Effect of long-term administration of anti-ovulatory steroids on the fertility of female golden hamsters and their offspring (Fr.). C.R. Soc. Biol. (Paris), 168, 517-520

Drill, V.A., Martin, D.P., Hart, E.R. & McConnell, R.G. (1974) Effect of oral contraceptives on the mammary glands of rhesus monkeys: a preliminary report. J. natl Cancer Inst., 52, 1655-1657

Dunn, T.B. (1969) Cancer of the uterine cervix in mice fed a liquid diet containing an antifertility drug. J. natl Cancer Inst., 43, 671-692

Edwards, C.W., Calhoun, F.J. & Green, S. (1971) The effects of mestranol and several progestins on chromosomes and fertility in the rat (Abstract no. 157). Toxicol. appl. Pharmacol., 19, 421

Eisenfeld, A. (1974) Oral contraceptives: ethinyl estradiol binds with higher affinity than mestranol to macromolecules from the sites of anti-fertility action. Endocrinology, 94, 803-807

Geil, R.G. & Lamar, J.K. (1977) FDA studies of estrogen, progestogens and estrogen/progestogen combinations in the dog and monkey. J. Toxicol. environ. Health, 3, 179-193

Giles, R.C., Kwapien, R.P., Geil, R.G. & Casey, H.W. (1978) Mammary nodules in beagle dogs administered investigational oral contraceptive steroids. J. natl Cancer Inst., 60, 1351-1364

Gosselin, R., ed. (1968) Clinical Toxicology of Commercial Products -
Acute Poisoning, 3rd ed., Baltimore, Williams & Wilkins

Graham, R.E. & Kenner, C.T. (1973) Acetonitrile-diatomaceous earth
column for separation of steroids and other compounds. J. pharm. Sci.,
62, 1845-1849

Gruenstein, M., Shay, H. & Shimkin, M.B. (1964) Lack of effect of
norethynodrel (Enovid) on methylcholanthrene-induced mammary
carcinogenesis in female rats. Cancer Res., 24, 1656-1658

de Gutiérrez, A.C. & Lisker, R. (1973) Longitudinal study of the effects
of oral contraceptives on human chromosomes. Ann. Génét., 16,
259-262

Haller, J. (1971) Ovulationshemmung durch Hormone, 3rd ed., Stuttgart,
Thieme

Hara, S. & Hayashi, S. (1977) Correlation of retention behaviour of
steroidal pharmaceuticals in polar and bonded reversed-phase liquid
column chromatography. J. Chromatogr., 142, 689-703

Harrington, J.M., Rivera, R.O. & Lowry, L.K. (1978) Occupational
exposure to synthetic estrogens - the need to establish safety
standards. Am. ind. Hyg. Assoc. J., 39, 139-143

Heinecke, H. & Klaus, S. (1975) Effect of mestranol on the gestation
of mice (Ger.). Pharmazie, 30, 53-56

Heston, W.E., Vlahakis, G. & Desmukes, B. (1973) Effects of the
antifertility drug Enovid in five strains of mice with particular
regard to carcinogenesis. J. natl Cancer Inst., 51, 209-224

Horwitz, W., ed. (1975a) Official Methods of Analysis of the
Association of Official Analytical Chemists, 12th ed., Washington
DC, Association of Official Analytial Chemists, p. 748

Horwitz, W. (1975b) Official methods of analysis of the Association
of Official Analytical Chemists. J. Assoc. off. anal. Chem.,
58, 403-404

IARC (1974) IARC Monographs on the Evaluation of Carcinogenic Risk
of Chemicals to Man, 6, Sex Hormones, pp. 87-97

Kappus, H., Bolt, H.M. & Remmer, H. (1972) Demethylation of mestranol
to ethinyloestradiol in vitro and in vivo. Acta endocrinol., 71,
374-384

Kastrup, E.K., ed. (1977) Facts and Comparisons, St Louis, MO, Facts &
    Comparisons Inc., pp. 107b, 108b, 108c

Kastrup, E.K., ed. (1978) Facts and Comparisons, St Louis, MO,
    Facts & Comparisons Inc., p. 107a

Kennelly, J.J. (1969) Effect of mestranol on canine reproduction.
    Biol. Reprod., 1, 282-288

Kirchner, M., Holsen, H. & Norpoth, K. (1973) Fluorescence spectroscopic
    determination of anti-ovulatory steroids in water and waste water
    on the thin layer chromatography plate (Ger.). Zbl. Bakteriol. Hyg.,
    Abt. I Orig. B, 157, 44-52

Kirchstein, R.L., Rabson, A.S. & Rusten, G.W. (1972) Infiltrating
    duct carcinoma of the mammary gland of a rhesus monkey after
    administration of an oral contraceptive: a preliminary report.
    J. natl Cancer Inst., 48, 551-556

Kulkarni, B.D. & Goldzieher, J.W. (1970) Urinary excretion pattern and
    fractionation of radioactivity after injection of $4-^{14}C$-mestranol
    (17α-ethynylestradiol-3-methyl ether) in women. A preliminary
    report. Contraception, 1, 131-136

Kulkarni, B.D., Avila, T.D. & O'Leary, J.A. (1977) Steroid contra-
    ceptives in non-human primates. II. Metabolic fate of synthetic
    estrogens in the baboon after exposure to oral contraceptives.
    Contraception, 15, 307-317

Miller, J.H.M. & Duguid, P. (1976) The fluorimetric analysis of
    oestrogen in oral contraceptive preparations. Proc. anal.
    Div. chem. Soc., 13, 9-13

Moretti, G., Cavina, G., Chiapetta, G., Fattori, I., Petrella, M.
    & Pompi, V. (1977) Simultaneous gas-chromatographic determination
    of mestranol and norethisterone in oral estrogen-progestin
    combinations. Boll. Chim. Farmacol., 116, 463-472 [Chem. Abstr.,
    88, 94887m]

Muñoz, N. (1973) Effect of herpesvirus type 2 and hormonal imbalance
    on the uterine cervix of the mouse. Cancer Res., 33, 1504-1508

Murad, F. & Gilman, A.G. (1975) Estrogens and progestins. In:
    Goodman, L.S. & Gilman, A., eds, The Pharmacological Basis of
    Therapeutics, 5th ed., New York, Macmillan, pp. 1423-1450

National Formulary Board (1975) National Formulary, 14th ed.,
    Washington DC, American Pharmaceutical Association, pp. 419-420

Okuno, I. & Higgins, W.H. (1977) Method for determining residues of
    mestranol and ethynylestradiol in foliage, soil and water samples.
    Bull. environ. Contam. Toxicol., 18, 428-435

Poel, W.E. (1966) Pituitary tumors in mice after prolonged feeding
    of synthetic progestins. Science, 154, 402-403

Rizk, M., Vallon, J.J. & Badinand, A. (1973) Colorimetric measurement
    of acetylenic steroids using Ag+ ions (Fr.). Anal. chem. acta,
    65, 220-222

Rudali, G. (1975) Induction of tumors in mice with synthetic sex
    hormones. Gann Monogr., 17, 243-252

Rudali, G., Coezy, E., Frederic, F. & Apiou, F. (1971) Susceptibility
    of mice of different strains to the mammary carcinogenic action
    of natural and synthetic oestrogens. Rev. eur. Etudes clin.
    biol., 16, 425-429

Rudali, G., Coezy, E. & Chemama, R. (1972) Mammary carcinogenesis in
    female and male mice receiving contraceptives or gestagens.
    J. natl Cancer Inst., 49, 813-819

Saunders, F.J. (1967) Effects of norethynodrel combined with mestranol
    on the offspring when administered during pregnancy and
    lactation in rats. Endocrinology, 80, 447-452

Saunders, F.J. & Elton, R.L. (1967) Effects of ethynodiol diacetate
    and mestranol in rats and rabbits on conception, on the outcome of
    pregnancy and on the offspring. Toxicol. appl. Pharmacol., 11,
    229-244

Shapiro, L.R., Graves, Z.R. & Hirschhorn, K. (1972) Oral contraceptives
    and in vivo cytogenetic studies. Obstet. Gynecol., 39, 190-192

Shroff, A.P. & Shaw, C.J. (1972) In situ quantitation of norethindrone
    and mestranol by spectrodensitometry of thin layer chromatograms.
    J. chromatogr. Sci., 10, 509-512

Sichuk, G., Fortner, J.G. & Der, B.K. (1967) Evaluation of the influence
    of norethynodrel with mestranol (Enovid) in middle-aged male
    Syrian (golden) hamsters, with particular reference to spontaneous
    tumours. Acta endocrinol., 55, 97-107

Singh, O.S. & Carr, D.H. (1970) A study of the effects of certain
    hormones on human cells in culture. Can. med. Assoc. J., 103,
    349-350

Stern, E. & Mickey, M.R. (1969) Effects of a cyclic steroid contraceptive regimen on mammary gland tumor induction in rats. Br. J. Cancer, 23, 391-400

Szepesi, G. & Görög, S. (1974) Analysis of steroids. XXIV. A specific method for the spectrophotometric determination of 17-ethynyl steroids. Analyst (Lond.), 99, 218-221

Takahashi, A. (1974) Chronic toxicity and effects of an oral contraceptive (Sophia) on reproductive organs and blood coagulation in Wistar rats. J. Nara med. Assoc., 25, 684-724

Thomas, C., Rogg, H. & Bücheler, J. (1972) Cancer inducing effect of N-nitrosomethylurea after administration of hormonal contraceptives (Ger.). Beitr. Path., 147, 332-338

Tuchmann-Duplessis, H. & Mercier-Parot, L. (1972) Effect of a contraceptive steroid on progeny (Fr.). J. Gynécol. Obstét. Biol. Reprod., 1, 141-159

US Food & Drug Administration (1977) Patient labeling for estrogens in general use. Drugs for human use; drug efficacy study implementation. Fed. Regist., 42, 37645-37646

US Food & Drug Administration (1978) Oral contraceptive drug products. Physician and patient labeling; extension of effective date for physician labeling. Fed. Regist., 43, 9863-9864

US Pharmacopeial Convention Inc. (1975) The US Pharmacopeia, 19th rev., Rockville, MD, p. 308

US Pharmacopeial Convention Inc. (1978) The US Pharmacopeia, 19th rev., 4th suppl., Rockville, MD, pp. 123-124

Wade, A., ed. (1977) Martindale, The Extra Pharmacopoeia, 27th ed., London, The Pharmaceutical Press, pp. 1398, 1405-1406, 1413

Warren, R.J. & Fotherby, K. (1973) Plasma levels of ethynyloestradiol after administration of ethynyloestradiol or mestranol to human subjects. J. Endocrinol., 59, 369-370

Weisburger, J.H., Weisburger, E.K., Griswold, D.P., Jr & Casey, A.E. (1968) Reduction of carcinogen-induced breast cancer in rats by an anti-fertility drug. Life Sci., 7, 259-266

Welsch, C.W. & Meites, J. (1969) Effects of norethynodrel-mestranol combination (Enovid) on development and growth of carcinogen-induced mammary tumors in female rats. Cancer, 23, 601-607

Welsch, C.W., Adams, C., Lambrecht, L.K., Hassett, C.C. & Brooks, C.L. (1977) 17β-Oestradiol and Enovid mammary tumorigenesis in C3H/HeJ female mice: counteraction by concurrent 2-bromo-α-ergocryptine. Br. J. Cancer, 35, 322-328

Williams, J.G. & Williams, K.I.H. (1975) Metabolism of 2-^{3}H- and 4-^{14}C-17α-ethynylestradiol 3-methyl ether (mestranol) by women. Steroids, 26, 707-720

Williams, M.C., Helton, E.D. & Goldzieher, J.W. (1975) The urinary metabolites of 17α-ethynylestradiol-9α,11ζ-^{3}H in women. Chromatographic profiling and identification of ethynyl and non-ethynyl compounds. Steroids, 25, 229-246

Windholz, M., ed. (1976) The Merck Index, 9th ed., Rahway, NJ, Merck & Co., p. 770

OESTRADIOL-17β, OESTRADIOL 3-BENZOATE, OESTRADIOL DIPROPIONATE,

OESTRADIOL-17β-VALERATE and POLYOESTRADIOL PHOSPHATE

A monograph on oestradiol-17β was published previously (IARC, 1974). Relevant data that have appeared since that time have been evaluated in the present monograph.

1. Chemical and Physical Data

Oestradiol-17β

1.1 Synonyms and trade names

Chem. Abstr. Services Reg. No.: 50-28-2

Chem. Abstr. Name: (17β)-Estra-1,3,5(10)-triene-3,17-diol

Synonyms: E_2; Dihydrofollicular hormone; dihydrofolliculin; dihydrotheelin; 3,17β-dihydroxyestra-1,3,5-triene; 3,17β-dihydroxyestra-1,3,5(10)-triene; dihydroxyestrin; 3,17β-dihydroxyoestra-1,3,5-triene; 3,17β-dihydroxyoestra-1,3,5(10)-triene; dihydroxyoestrin; 3,17-epidihydroxyestratriene; estradiol; β-estradiol; 17β-estradiol; estradiol-17β; 3,17β-estradiol; d-3,17β-estradiol; *cis*-estradiol; estra-1,3,5(10)-triene-3,17β-diol; oestradiol; β-oestradiol; 17β-oestradiol; 3,17β-oestradiol; d-3,17β-oestradiol; *cis*-oestradiol; oestra-1,3,5(10)-triene-3,17β-diol

Trade names[1]: [Ablacton]; Altrad; [Androtardyl-Oestr.]; Aquadiol; Aquagen; Bardiol; [Benzogynoestryl]; [Benzo-Gynoestryl 5]; [Ciclo Complex]; [Climastat]; [Clivion]; [Combidurin]; Corpagen; C-Progynova; [Depofemin]; Dihydromenformon; Dimenformon; [Dimenformon Prolong.]; Diogyn; Diogynets; [Duogynon]; [Emmenovis]; [Emonovister]; Estrace; [Estradurin]; [Estradurine]; Estraldine; [Estrandon]; [Estrandron Prolong]; Estrobe; Estrovite; Femestral;

---

[1]Those in square brackets are preparations that are no longer produced commercially.

Femogen; [Folicular]; [Folicular Depot]; [Foliteston Retard];
Follicyclin; Ginosedol; [Gravibinan]; [Gravibinon];
[Gynecormone]; Gynergon; [Gynoestrel]; Gynoestryl; [Heptylate
de Test.]; [Hormonin]; Lamdiol; Lip-Oid; [Luteo Folicular];
[Lutestron]; [Lutestron Dep.]; [Lut Ovociclina]; [Lutrogen];
Macrodiol; Macrol; Microdiol; Nordicol; Oestergon; [Oestradiol
R]; Oestroglandol; [Oestrogynal]; Ormogamma; Ovahormon; [Ova
Repos]; Ovasterol; Ovastevol; [Ovestin]; [Ovex]; [Ovex Prolong.];
[Ovociclina]; Ovocyclin; [Ovocycline]; Ovocylin; [Ovolacer];
Perlatanol; [Primodian D]; [Primodian Depot]; Primofol;
[Primogyn Depot]; [Primosiston]; Profoliol; Progynon; [Progynon
B Oleoso]; [Progynon D]; [Progynon Depot]; Progynon-DH;
[Progynon Pomada]; [Progynon Retard]; [Progynon S]; [Progynova];
[Proluton-Oestradiol]; [Proluton Z]; Propagon-E; [Stroluten];
Syndiol; Test-Estrin; [Test.-Oestr. R]; [Testo Folicular];
[Trioestrine]; [Trioestrine R]; [Trioestrin Vitam]

1.2 Structural and molecular formulae and molecular weight

$C_{18}H_{24}O_2$ Mol. wt: 272.4

1.3 Chemical and physical properties

From Wade (1977) and Windholz (1976), unless otherwise specified

(a) Description: White or creamy-white prisms

(b) Melting-point: 178-179°C (Weast, 1977)

(c) <u>Spectroscopy data</u>: λ_{max} 225 and 280 nm (E_1^1 = 78.5 in ethanol); infra-red data have been tabulated (Grasselli & Ritchey, 1975).

(d) <u>Optical rotation</u>: $[\alpha]_D^{25}$ +76 to +83° (dioxane)

(e) <u>Solubility</u>: Practically insoluble in water; soluble in ethanol (1 in 28), acetone (1 in 17), chloroform (1 in 435) and diethyl ether (1 in 150). Also soluble in dioxane and solutions of alkaline hydroxides; sparingly soluble in fixed oils

(f) <u>Stability</u>: Unstable to air and light

1.4 Technical products and impurities

Various national and international pharmacopoeias give specifications for the purity of oestradiol-17β in pharmaceutical products. For example, oestradiol-17β is available in the US as a NF grade containing 97-103% active ingredient on a dried basis and not more than 3% foreign steroids and other impurities. Pellets in 25 mg doses contain 97-103% of the stated amount of oestradiol-17β; sterile aqueous suspensions in 0.25 and 1 mg/ml, 2.2, 2.5, 4.4 and 11 mg/10 ml, and 5.5 mg/25 ml contain 90-110% of the stated amount (National Formulary Board, 1975). Oestradiol-17β is also available in the US in tablets in 1 and 2 mg doses and in oil injections in 0.1, 0.2, 0.5, 1 and 1.25 mg/ml doses. Combinations of oestradiol-17β with testosterone are also available in tablets, aqueous injections and suppositories (Kastrup, 1976, 1977, 1978).

In Japan, oestradiol-17β is available in injections containing 4.76 mg testosterone and 0.24 mg oestradiol.

Oestradiol 3-benzoate

1.1 Synonyms and trade names

Chem. Abstr. Services Reg. No.: 50-50-0

Chem. Abstr. Name: Estra-1,3,5(10)-triene-3,17-diol(17β)-3-benzoate

Synonyms: Estradiol benzoate; β-estradiol benzoate; β-estradiol 3-benzoate; 17β-estradiol 3-benzoate; estradiol monobenzoate; 1,3,5(10)-estratriene-3,17β-diol 3-benzoate; oestradiol benzoate;

β-oestradiol benzoate;   β-oestradiol 3-benzoate;   17β-oestradiol 3-benzoate;   oestradiol monobenzoate;   1,3,5(10)-oestratriene-3, 17β-diol 3-benzoate

Trade names: Benovocylin; Benzhormovarine; Benzoestrofol; Benzofoline; Benzo-Gynoestryl; De Graafina; Diffollisterol; Difolliculine; Dimenformon benzoate; Diogyn B; Eston-B; Femestrone; Follicormon; Follidrin; Graafina; Gynécormone; Gynformone; Hidroestron; Hormogynon; Oestroform (BDH); Ovahormon benzoate; Ovasterol-B; Ovex; Ovocyclin benzoate; Ovocyclin M; Ovocyclin-MB; Primogyn B; Primogyn Boleosum; Primogyn I; Progynon B; Progynon-B; Progynon benzoate; Recthormone Oestradiol; Solestro; Unistradiol

1.2   Structural and molecular formulae and molecular weight

$C_{25}H_{28}O_3$ Mol. wt: 376.5

1.3   Chemical and physical properties

From Wade (1977) and Windholz (1976)

(a) Description: Colourless, odourless crystals or white crystalline powder

(b) Melting-point: 190–198°C

(c) Optical rotation: $[\alpha]_d^{25}$ +58 to +63° (2 in dioxane)

(d) Solubility: Practically insoluble in water; soluble in ethanol (1 in 150), acetone (1 in 50), arachis oil (1 in 500), chloroform (1 in 5), diethyl ether (1 in 150), ethyl oleate (1 in 200); also soluble in dioxane; slightly soluble in fixed oils; insoluble in solutions of alkaline hydroxides

1.4 Technical products and impurities

Oestradiol 3-benzoate is available in the US as a NF grade containing 97-103% active ingredient on a dried basis. Injections in doses of 10 and 33.3 mg in 10 ml contain 90-115% of the stated amount (National Formulary Board, 1975). It is also available in the UK as nasal drops, in a dose of 8 mg in 100 ml of light liquid paraffin (Wade, 1977). It is available in Japan in injections.

Oestradiol dipropionate

1.1 Synonyms and trade names

Chem. Abstr. Services Reg. No.: 113-38-2

Chem. Abstr. Name: Estral,3,5(10)-triene-3,17-diol (17β)-dipropionate

Synonyms: Estradiol dipropionate; β-estradiol dipropionate; 17β-estradiol dipropionate; 3,17β-estradiol dipropionate; oestradiol 3,17-dipropionate; β-oestradiol dipropionate; 17β-oestradiol dipropionate; 3,17β-oestradiol dipropionate

Trade names: Agofollin; Dimenformon dipropionate; Diovocyclin; Diovocylin; Diprostron; Endofollicolina D.P.; Estroici; Estronex; Follicyclin P; Nacyclyl; Ovocyclin dipropionate; Ovocyclin P; Ovocyclin-P; Progynon-DP

1.2 Structural and molecular formulae and molecular weight

$C_{24}H_{32}O_4$ Mol. wt: 384.5

1.3 Chemical and physical properties

From Wade (1977)

(a) Description: Small, white or slightly off-white crystals, or crystalline powder

(b) Melting-point: 104-109°C

(c) Solubility: Practically insoluble in water; soluble in ethanol (1 in 55); also soluble in acetone, dioxane and diethyl ether; sparingly soluble in fixed oils; insoluble in solutions of alkaline hydroxides

1.4 Technical products and impurities

Oestradiol dipropionate is available in the US as a NF grade containing 97-103% active ingredient on a dried basis. It is available in injections containing 2.5 mg in 1 ml oil and 10 and 50 mg in 10 ml of oil, each containing 90-115% of the stated amount (National Formulary Board, 1975). It is available in Japan in injections.

Oestradiol-17β-valerate

1.1 Synonyms and trade names

Chem. Abstr. Services Reg. No.: 979-32-8

Chem. Abstr. Name: (17β)-Estra-1,3,5-triene-3,17-diol 17-pentanoate

Synonyms: Estradiol valerate; estradiol 17-valerate; estradiol 17β-valerate; estradiol valerianate; oestradiol valerate; oestradiol 17-valerate; oestradiol 17β-valerate; oestradiol valerianate; 17β-valeryl-oxyoestra-1,3,5(10)-trien-3-ol

Trade names: Ardefem; Atladiol; Bimone-L.A.; Cyclo-Progynova; Deladiol; Deladumone; Delahormone unimatic; Delestrogen; Delestrogen 4X; Depogen; Diol-20; Dioval; Ditate; Ditate DS; Duoval-P.A.; Dura-Estradiol; Duragen; Duratrad; Estate; Estradiol-L.A.; Estra-L; Estratab; Estraval; Estraval-P.A.; Estroval-10; Eval; Femogen; Femogen-L.A.; Femogex; Lastrogen;

Mal-O-Fem LA; Neofollin; Oestradiol retard Pharlon;

Oestragynol sine; Pharlon; Primogyn-Depot; Progynon-Depot;

Progynova; Rep-Estra; Repestrogen; Rep-Estro Med; Retestrin;

Span-Est; Teev; Testadiate; Valergen; Valertest No. 1;

Valertest No. 2

1.2 Structural and molecular formulae and molecular weight

$C_{23}H_{32}O_3$ Mol. wt: 356.5

1.3 Chemical and physical properties

From Wade (1977) and Windholz (1976)

(a) Description: White crystals

(b) Melting-point: 144-145°C

(c) Solubility: Practically insoluble in water; soluble in
     benzyl benzoate, dioxane, methanol and castor oil;
     sparingly soluble in arachis oil and sesame oil

(d) Stability: Unstable to air and light

1.4 Technical products and impurities

Oestradiol-17β-valerate is available in the US as a USP grade
containing 97-101% active ingredient and not more than 1% free oestradiol,
0.5% free valeric acid and 0.1% water. Injections in 10, 20 and 40
mg/ml doses in vegetable oil contain 90-115% of the stated amount of
oestradiol-17β-valerate and not more than 3% free oestradiol (US Pharmacopeial Convention Inc., 1975).

In the UK, oestradiol-17β-valerate is available in injections in 10 mg/ml doses in sesame oil, in tablets in 1 and 2 mg doses and in packets of 11 white tablets containing 2 mg oestradiol-17β-valerate and 10 orange tablets containing 2 mg oestradiol-17β-valerate with 0.5 mg norgestrel (Wade, 1977).

It is available in Japan in injections.

Polyoestradiol phosphate

1.1   Synonyms and trade names

Chem. Abstr. Services Reg. No.:   28014-46-2

Chem. Abstr. Name: (17β)-Estra-1,3,5(10)-triene-3,17-diol polymer with phosphoric acid

Synonyms: Estradiol phosphate polymer; estradiol polyester with phosphoric acid; oestradiol phosphate polymer; oestradiol polyester with phosphoric acid; PEP; poly(estradiol phosphate); poly(oestradiol phosphate)

Trade name: Estradurin

1.2   Structural and molecular formulae and molecular weight

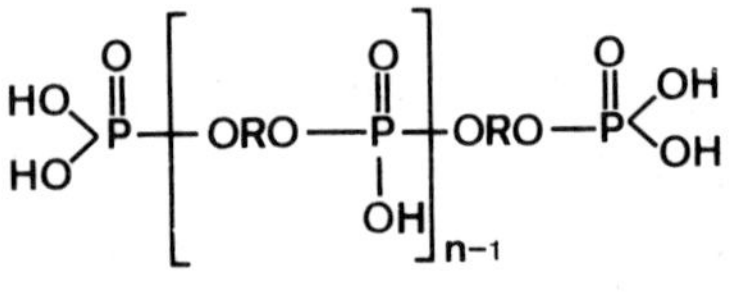

(where –ORO– is the oestradiol radical and n = about 80) Windholz (1976)

$$(C_{18}H_{24}O_2 \cdot H_3O_4P)_x$$

Mol. wt: ~ 26,000
Wade (1977)

1.3   Chemical and physical properties

From Windholz (1976)

(a) Description: White solid

(b) Melting-point: 195-202°C

(c) Solubility: Very slightly soluble in water, ethanol, acetone,

chloroform and dioxane; very soluble in aqueous pyridine;

soluble in aqueous alkali

1.4 Technical products and impurities

Polyoestradiol phosphate is available in the US in injection form;
each ampoule contains 40 mg polyoestradiol phosphate, 25 mg nicotinamide,
9.76 mg sodium phosphate, 4 mg propylene glycol and sodium hydroxide and
0.02 mg phenylmercuric nitrate to be combined with 2 ml of sterile
diluent (Kastrup, 1977).

Polyoestradiol phosphate is available in a powder, for preparation
in an injection, containing 40 or 80 mg polyoestradiol phosphate, 5 mg
mepivacaine [N-(2,6-dimethylphenyl)-1-methyl-2-piperidinecarboxamide]
hydrochloride, 25 or 40 mg nicotinamide and 0.02 mg phenylmercuric
nitrate (Wade, 1977).

2. Production, Use, Occurrence and Analysis

2.1 Production and use

(a) Production

The isolation of oestradiol-17β from the liquor folliculi of sow
ovaries as the di-α-naphthoate and *meta*-bromobenzoate derivatives was
first reported by MacCorquodale *et al*. (1936). Butenandt & Goergens
(1937) reported the preparation of oestradiol-17β by the hydrogenation
of oestrone over a nickel catalyst. Oestradiol-17β is produced
commercially by the reduction of oestrone using, for example, complex
metal hydrides, such as sodium borohydride and lithium aluminium hydride
(Dorfman, 1966). Oestradiol-17β-valerate can be prepared by the esterification of oestradiol-17β with valeryl chloride in pyridine (Harvey,
1975). Polyoestradiol phosphate was first prepared by Diczfalusy in
1954 (Windholz, 1976) by the condensation polymerization of oestradiol
dihydrogen phosphate with dilute hydrochloric acid at low temperature
(Harvey, 1975).

Preparation of oestradiol 3-benzoate was first reported in 1936
(Schwenk & Hildebrandt, 1936). It can be prepared by benzoylation of
the phenolic hydroxyl group of oestradiol-17β with benzoyl chloride.
Preparation of oestradiol dipropionate was first reported in 1939 (Miescher
& Scholz, 1939). It is prepared by esterification of both the 3 and
17 positions of oestradiol-17β with propionyl chloride in the presence
of pyridine.

Commercial production of oestradiol-17β in the US was first reported in 1939 (US Tariff Commission, 1940) and was last reported in 1955 (US Tariff Commission, 1956). No evidence was found that oestradiol 3-benzoate, oestradiol dipropionate, oestradiol-17β-valerate or polyoestradiol phosphate have ever been produced commercially in the US. It is believed that polyoestradiol phosphate is produced in Canada.

US imports of oestradiol 3-benzoate through principal customs districts amounted to 2.7 kg in 1975 (US International Trade Commission, 1977a) and 172 kg in 1975 (US International Trade Commission, 1977b). Data on US exports of oestradiol-17β and its derivatives are not available.

Oestradiol-17β and its esters are produced commercially in the Federal Republic of Germany, France, Italy, The Netherlands and the UK, but no information was available on the quantities produced.

Oestradiol-17β was first marketed commercially in Japan in the mid-1950s. The valerate and benzoate were also introduced at this time, and the propionate was first marketed there a few years later. Oestradiol-17β and its esters are not produced in Japan; and small amounts are imported annually.

(b) Use

Oestradiol-17β is the most active naturally occurring oestrogenic hormone. It is now seldom used, and ethinyloestradiol, quinoestradiol and diethylstilboestrol are generally preferred for oral administration; for i.m. administration, the esters of oestradiol-17β have more prolonged action and are often used in preference to oestradiol-17β itself. Oestradiol-17β is given in doses of up to 1.5 mg daily by mouth or twice or thrice weekly intramuscularly.

It is used in human medicine primarily for the treatment of symptoms of the climacteric, particularly for vasomotor and psychological disturbances. It is also used for local treatment of atrophic vaginitis, for the chemotherapy of advanced prostatic carcinoma and for the prevention of post-partum breast engorgement. Other uses for oestradiol-17β are in the treatment of primary amenorrhoea, delayed onset of puberty and chemotherapy of breast neoplasms in postmenopausal women (Harvey, 1975; Wade, 1977).

It is believed to be a component of hormones derived from pregnant mares' urine used in cosmetic skin preparations (Miller, 1976).

In Japan, oestradiol-17β is used for the treatment of symptoms of the climacteric.

It is used in veterinary medicine for oestrogenic hormone therapy, administered by injection to mares and cows (1-5 mg), ewes (0.3-2.5 mg) and bitches (0.1-1 mg) (Harvey, 1975).

Oestradiol 3-benzoate and oestradiol dipropionate are used in human medicine to treat the same conditions as oestradiol-17β. They are usually administered as an i.m. injection (for slow release) in an oil solution. The low level of oestrogen released in this way gives a more even effect than larger doses of oestrogens that are destroyed more rapidly, such as oestradiol-17β. Oestradiol 3-benzoate is given as an initial dose of 1-1.66 mg 2 or 3 times a week for 2 or 3 weeks, and then the dose is gradually decreased to the lowest maintenance dose (Harvey, 1975). It can also be used in the form of nasal drops (Wade, 1977). Oestradiol dipropionate gives a more sustained depot-action than oestradiol 3-benzoate, and although it is only half as active, it is more potent with respect to cumulative maintenance dosage. It is given in a dose of 1-5 mg every 1-2 weeks; the maintenance dose is usually 1-2.5 mg every 10-14 days (Harvey, 1975).

Oestradiol-17β-valerate has the same uses as oestradiol-17β. It is usually administered as an i.m. injection of 10-40 mg/ml in oil suspension to provide a depot from which the drug is liberated slowly. For symptoms of the climacteric, it is given orally in doses of 1-2 mg per day in a cyclic regimen. It is also used for the treatment of prostatic carcinoma, in a dose of 30-40 mg every 1 or 2 weeks. For the prevention of post-partum breast engorgement and suppression of lactation, it has been given in a dose of 10-25 mg at the end of the first stage of labour, sometimes in combination with testosterone enanthate. Oestradiol-17β-valerate has also been used in the treatment of primary and secondary amenorrhoea and dysfunctional uterine bleeding, when it may be given in combination with a progestational agent (Harvey, 1975). It has also been used to treat type II hyperlipoproteinaemia in postmenopausal women (Tikkanen et al., 1978).

Oestradiol 3-benzoate has also been used in hormonal skin preparations for cosmetic use at levels of 0.1% or less. It has been used in veterinary medicine for oestrogenic hormone therapy (Windholz, 1976).

In Japan, the various esters are used for treatment of symptoms of the climacteric, hypertrophy of the prostatic gland and menstrual disorders.

Polyoestradiol phosphate is used in human medicine for the treatment of prostatic carcinoma. It is administered as a deep i.m. injection, in doses of 80-160 mg every 4 weeks; doses of 40-80 mg may be used for maintenance (Wade, 1977). Polyoestradiol phosphate is gradually depolymerized in the body to release oestradiol-17β.

The US Food & Drug Administration (1977a) requires that residues of oestradiol 3-benzoate should not be found in the uncooked edible tissue of heifers, lambs or steers. The US Food & Drug Administration (1977b) has ruled that with effect from 20 September 1977, oestrogens for general use must carry patient and physician warning labels concerning use, risks and contraindications.

2.2 Occurrence

Oestradiol-17β is a widely occurring natural oestrogen (see the section 'General Remarks on Sex Hormones', pp. 42-56). It has been found in certain drinking-water samples at levels of 0.12-0.42 ng/l (Rurainski *et al.*, 1977); however, it did not appear on a list of carcinogens and mutagens identified in water supplies in the US and Europe in which 1728 contaminants were identified (Kraybill *et al.*, 1977).

Oestradiol 3-benzoate, oestradiol dipropionate, oestradiol-17β-valerate, and polyoestradiol phosphate are not known to occur naturally.

2.3 Analysis

(a) Oestradiol-17β

Analytical methods for the determination of oestradiol-17β in urine and plasma, based on gas chromatography, spectrophotometry and radio-immunoassay, have been reviewed by Chattoraj & Wotiz (1975). Radioimmuno-assay techniques for the determination of oestradiol-17β in plasma or serum have been reviewed by Abraham *et al.* (1977) and Edqvist *et al.* (1976).

Typical analytical methods for the determination of oestradiol-17β are summarized in Table 1. Abbreviations used are: GC/ECD, gas chroma-tography/electron-capture detection; GC/MS, gas chromatography/mass spectrometry; GC/FID, gas chromatography/flame-ionization detection; MS, mass spectrometry; HPLC, high-pressure liquid chromatography; CC, column chromatography; TLC, thin-layer chromatography; UV, ultra-violet spectrometry; RIA, radioimmunoassay; and FL, fluorimetry. See also 'General Remarks on Sex Hormones', p. 60 .

(b) Esters of oestradiol-17β

Analytical methods for the determination of oestradiol-17β-valerate based on gas, thin-layer and paper chromatography, ultra-violet spectro-metry, fluorescence and colorimetry have been reviewed (Florey, 1975). Typical analytical methods for the esters of oestradiol-17β are summarized in Tables 2-4. Abbreviations used are: GC/FID, gas chromatography/flame-ionization detection; HPLC, high-pressure liquid chromatography; CC, column chromatography; TLC, thin-layer chromatography; UV, ultra-violet spectrometry; and FL, fluorimetry. See also 'General Remarks on Sex Hormones', p. 60 .

TABLE 1

Analytical methods for oestradiol-17β

Sample matrix	Sample preparation	Assay procedure	Sensitivity or limit of detection	Reference
Bulk chemical	Add antiserum & incubate; add steroid-mediated bacteriophage T4 & incubate; plate with *Escherichia coli* & incubate	Viroimmunoassay	15 pg	Dray *et al.* (1975)
Bulk chemical	Dissolve (absolute ethanol)	UV (230 nm)	-	Khayam-Bashi & Boroumand (1975)
Bulk chemical	Dissolve & derivatize (hepta-fluoributyryl)	GC/ECD	<10 pg	Lawrence & Ryan (1977)
Bulk chemical	Dissolve	TLC (iodine vapour)	-	Ruh (1976)
Bulk chemical	Dissolve	HPLC (UV, 280 nm)	-	Sataswaroop *et al.* (1977)
Bulk chemical	Dissolve (chloroform)	TLC (molybdovana-dophosphoric acid spray)	0.1 ng	Scott & Sawyer (1975)
Bulk chemical & pellets	Dissolve (methanol); evaporate; add iron-phenol reagent & sulphuric acid	Colorimetry (520 nm)	-	National Formulary Board (1975)
Tablets (sodium sulphate salt)	Hydrolyse (hydrochloric acid); neutralize (sodium bicarbonate solution); extract (chloroform); multiple TLC; elute (sodium hydroxide solution)	UV (296 nm)	-	Schroeder *et al.* (1975)

Table 1 (continued)

Sample matrix	Sample preparation	Assay procedure	Sensitivity or limit of detection	Reference
Sesame oil formulation	Dissolve (petroleum ether); perform a series of extractions & washings; add dansyl chloride reagent; extract; evaporate; dissolve (chloroform)	FL (502 nm)	0.5 μg/ml	Fishman (1975)
Water suspension	CC; elute (diethyl ether); evaporate; dissolve (methanol); evaporate; add iron-phenol reagent & sulphuric acid	Colorimetry (520 nm)	–	National Formulary Board (1975)
Drinking-water	Extract, TLC	RIA	–	Rurainski et al. (1977)
Animal chow	Extract (methanol); CC (Sephadex LH-20); extract; wash; CC (silica gel); derivatize (pentafluoropropionyl); CC	GC/ECD	3 μg/kg (20 g sample)	Bowman & Nony (1977)
Animal tissue	Homogenize (aqueous acetonitrile); hydrolyse (hydrochloric acid); perform a series of extractions & washings	High-performance TLC; UV-densitometry (287 nm)	10 ng	Jarc et al. (1977)
Plasma	Extract (diethyl ether); evaporate; CC; evaporate; dissolve (ethanol); add enzyme reagent & incubate; add base & neutralize; add cycling reagent & incubate; add 6-phosphogluconate reagent & incubate	FL	~ 7 pg	Härkönen et al. (1974)
Plasma	Add radioactive steroids; hydrolyse (hydrochloric acid); perform a series of extractions & washings; TLC; elute; add Ittrich reagent	FL	8 ng	Mathur et al. (1975)

Table 1 (continued)

Sample matrix	Sample preparation	Assay procedure	Sensitivity or limit of detection	Reference
Plasma	Extract (diethyl ether); CC (Sephadex LH-20); add immobilized antibody; incubate; add oestradiol-horse radish peroxidase conjugate, incubate, centrifuge & add fluorogenic substrate	Enzyme immunoassay, FL (420 nm)	~ 50 pg	Numazawa et al. (1977)
Serum	Extract	High-performance TLC; UV-densitometry (287 nm)	20 ng	Jarc et al. (1977)
Serum	Add tetradeuteriated oestradiol-17β internal standard; extract (diethyl ether); CC (Sephadex LH-20) & derivatize (trimethyl-silyl)	GC/MS	~ 10 pg	Zamecnik et al. (1978)
Serum	Add tracer solution, incubate & extract (diethyl ether); evaporate, dissolve (buffer), add antiserum & incubate; add dextran-coated charcoal & centrifuge	RIA	5-10 pg	Korenman et al. (1974)
Serum & urine	Extract (diethyl ether) & derivatize (trimethylsilyl)	GC/MS	2 pg	Heki et al. (1977)
Urine	Hydrolyse (enzyme); extract (ethyl acetate, hexane, ethanol); CC (ion exchange) & derivatize (trimethylsilyl)	GC/FID	~ 40 µg/l (50 ml sample)	Adessi et al. (1975)
Urine	Hydrolyse (hydrochloric acid); extract (diethyl ether)	HPLC (UV, 280 nm)	-	Dolphin & Pergande (1977)
Urine	Extract	High-performance TLC; UV-densitometry (287 nm)	10 ng	Jarc et al. (1977)

Table 1 (continued)

Sample matrix	Sample preparation	Assay procedure	Sensitivity or limit of detection	Reference
Urine (as the glucosi-duronate)	Add phosphate buffered saline, antiserum, tracer solution & incubate; add dextran-coated charcoal, incubate & centrifuge	RIA	~ 6 pg	Wright *et al.* (1978)
Bile, urine & plasma	Isolate by a series of chroma-tographic, hydrolytic & extrac-tion procedures; derivatize (trimethylsilyl)	GC/MS	–	Adlercreutz *et al.* (1974)
Ovarian tissue	Dissect, dry and homogenize	MS	~ 1 ng	Snedden & Parker (1976)

TABLE 2

Analytical methods for oestradiol 3-benzoate

Sample matrix	Sample preparation	Assay procedure	Sensitivity or limit of detection	Reference
Bulk chemical	Dissolve	HPLC, UV (254 nm)	–	Hara & Hayashi (1977)
Bulk chemical	Dissolve (chloroform:methanol, 1:1)	Two-dimensional TLC (UV, acid spray)	–	Cavina et al. (1975)
Bulk chemical	Dissolve (methanol-water); CC (diatomaceous earth-acetonitrile); elute (heptane); evaporate; dissolve (ethanol)	UV	–	Graham & Kenner (1973)
Bulk chemical	Dissolve	TLC	–	Hara & Mibe (1975)
Sesame oil formulations	Elute (heptane); evaporate; dissolve (acetone); add sodium carbonate; add dansyl chloride reagent; extract (diethyl ether); evaporate; dissolve (chloroform)	FL (502 nm)	0.5 μg	Fishman (1975)
Olive oil formulations	Dissolve (benzene); evaporate; extract (acetonitrile); centrifuge; extract (petroleum ether); add testosterone propionate; evaporate; derivatize (trimethylsilyl)	GC/FID	-	Youssef & Mestres (1973)

Table 3

Analytical methods for oestradiol dipropionate

Sample matrix	Sample preparation	Assay procedure	Reference
Bulk chemical	Dissolve (chloroform:methanol, 1:1)	Two-dimensional TLC (UV, acid spray)	Cavina et al. (1975)
Bulk chemical	Dissolve	HPLC, UV (254 nm)	Hara & Hayashi (1977)

TABLE 4

Analytical methods for oestradiol-17β-valerate

Sample matrix	Sample preparation	Assay procedure	Sensitivity or limit of detection	Reference
Bulk chemical	Dissolve	HPLC, UV (254 nm)	–	Hara & Hayashi (1977)
Bulk chemical	Dissolve (chloroform:methanol, 1:1)	Two-dimensional TLC (UV, acid spray)	–	Cavina et al. (1975)
Bulk chemical	Dissolve (methanol-water); CC (diatomaceous earth-acetonitrile); elute (heptane); evaporate; dissolve (ethanol)	UV	–	Graham & Kenner (1973)
Bulk chemical	Dissolve	TLC	–	Hara & Mibe (1975)
Bulk chemical	Dissolve (ethanol)	UV (281 nm)	–	US Pharmacopeial Convention Inc. (1975)
Vegetable oil formulations	Dissolve (methanol); add potassium hydroxide solutions	UV (300 nm)	–	US Pharmacopeial Convention Inc. (1975)
Vegetable oil formulations	Dissolve (heptane); CC (diatomaceous earth-nitromethane); elute (heptane); evaporate; dissolve (anhydrous ethanol)	FL (328 nm)	–	Horwitz (1975)
Castor oil & sesame oil formulations	Dissolve (heptane or petroleum ether); perform a series of extractions & washings; evaporate; dissolve (acetone); add dansyl chloride reagent; extract (diethyl ether); evaporate; dissolve (chloroform)	FL (502 nm)	0.5 μg	Fishman (1975)
Olive oil formulations	Dissolve (benzene); evaporate; extract (acetonitrile); centrifuge; extract (petroleum ether); add testosterone propionate; evaporate; derivatize (trimethylsilyl)	GC/FID	–	Youssef & Mestres (1973)

3. Biological Data Relevant to the Evaluation

of Carcinogenic Risk to Humans

3.1 Carcinogenicity studies in animals

(a) Oral administration

Mouse: Administration of 0.5 mg/1 oestradiol-17β in the drinking-
water for 19 months to C3H/HeJ (MTV$^+$)[1] female mice resulted in a significantly increased mammary tumour incidence (27/99, compared with 11/100
in controls); a combination of oestradiol-17β with a prolactin inhibitor,
2-bromo-α-ergocryptine (CB-154), prevented this increased tumour incidence
(9/100) (Welsch et al., 1977).

Groups of 48 C3H/HeJ (MTV$^+$) mice were fed 0, 100, 1000 and 5000
μg/kg of diet oestradiol-17β for 24 months starting at 6 weeks of age.
Mammary adenocarcinomas were found in 4/47, 0/35, 6/36 and 8/48 animals
in the respective groups after 52 weeks. Other malignant tumours occurred
in those given 100 μg/kg: 1 adenocarcinoma of the cervix and 1 osteosarcoma of the cranium; in the 5000 μg/kg group, 2 adenocarcinomas of
the uterus, 3 adenocarcinomas of the cervix and 1 adenoacanthoma of the
uterus were seen. No such tumours were described in the controls (Highman
et al., 1977).

(b) Subcutaneous and/or intramuscular administration

Mouse: Interstitial-cell tumours of the testis occurred in 10/24
male Strong A mice given weekly s.c. injections of 16.6 or 50 μg oestradiol 3-benzoate in sesame oil for 6 months (for the higher dose group)
or until death. Concurrent administration of 1.25 mg testosterone
propionate reduced the incidence of testicular tumours to 2/15 and
increased the time of induction (Hooker & Pfeiffer, 1942).

S.c. injections of 16.6 or 50 μg oestradiol 3-benzoate were given
weekly for lifespan to 4-8-week old hybrid mice derived from reciprocal
matings of the C57 strain [MTV⁻], which have a high incidence of oestrogen-
induced pituitary tumours (Gardner & Strong, 1940), and CBA (MTV$^+$)
mice. Pituitary tumours were found in 16/30 female and 19/23 male
hybrids of C57 mothers and in 9/28 female and 18/24 male hybrids of CBA
mothers. Mammary carcinomas (14/24 in males and 17/28 in females)
occurred only in hybrid mice with CBA mothers and in 17/20 female and 0/4
male controls and were presumed to be dependent on the presence of the

---

[1]MTV$^+$: mammary tumour virus expressed; MTV⁻: mammary tumour virus
not expressed (see p. 62)

mammary tumour virus. The incidence of lymphoid tumours was higher in treated groups (7/52 males and females with CBA mothers and 5/53 males and females with C57 mothers) than in controls (2/24 and 2/48), but the differences were not statistically significant (Gardner, 1941).

Of 31 male RIII mice (MTV$^+$) given weekly s.c. injections of 50 µg oestradiol dipropionate, 13 were still alive after 20 weeks; mammary carcinomas were seen in 9 animals between 20-40 weeks. The incidence of mammary cancer in untreated females was about 63%. No mammary tumours occurred in treated CBA (MTV$^-$) males (Bonser & Robson, 1940).

Twice-weekly s.c. or i.m. injections of 80 µg oestradiol-17β for 6 months (total dose, 3.3-4.2 mg) did not increase the incidence of mammary tumours in groups of 40 intact and 40 ovariectomized female Marsh-Buffalo mice [MTV$^+$] above that found in untreated controls. However, lymphosarcomas occurred earlier (between 3 and 10 months) and in a higher incidence (28% in intact, 47% in ovariectomized) than in controls (10%), the first tumour appearing at 12 months (Bischoff *et al.*, 1942a). With discontinuous treatment in groups of 36-43 intact and castrated males of the same strain, lymphoid tumours occurred in 34% of castrates, compared with 8% in intact treated males and 5% in controls; the tumours developed much earlier in castrates (at 6-14 months) than in the other groups (Bischoff *et al.*, 1942b).

Oestradiol-17β administered subcutaneously to mice of 7 strains resulted in a greater incidence of lymphoid tumours than other oestrogens tested, the nature of which was not clearly defined. Oestradiol dipropionate given subcutaneously once a week for 10 weeks increased the incidence of lymphoid tumours in C3H mice (sex not stated) to 10/54 with 10 µg doses, to 4/18 with 25 µg and to 18/78 with 50 µg. The incidence of tumours in untreated mice was low (5/481 in C$_3$H mice; total, 11/822 in all strains tested) (Gardner *et al.*, 1944).

BALB/c and CBA mice less than 57-weeks old were relatively resistant to the induction of lymphoid tumours by either X-rays, 3-methylcholanthrene or oestradiol dipropionate (5 µg in oil subcutaneously weekly for 14 weeks); however, in BALB/c mice, a combination of oestradiol dipropionate with 200-rad whole-body irradiation increased the incidence from 3/47 (with oestradiol dipropionate alone) to 16/71. Although 400 rads alone were no more effective than were 200 rads, the incidence of lymphomas was greater when 400-rad irradiation was combined with administration of 5 µg oestradiol dipropionate weekly for 14 weeks (12/30 by 43 weeks of age in BALB/c mice and 15/27 by 57 weeks in CBA mice). Thymectomy abolished the synergistic action of these two agents. The leukaemogenic action of 3-methylcholanthrene was not increased by combination with oestradiol-17β; however, in DBA mice, oestradiol dipropionate increased the leukaemogenic activity of both X-rays and 3-methylcholanthrene (Kirschbaum *et al.*, 1953).

Invasive cervical lesions or carcinomas occurred in 4/10 female
hybrid mice (C3H x PM strain) administered 16.6 µg oestradiol 3-benzoate
subcutaneously, once weekly, starting at 4-9 weeks of age. In 25 female
mice of the reciprocal hybrid (PM x C3H) strain receiving 16.6 or 25 µg
oestradiol 3-benzoate, carcinomas or invasive epithelial lesions arose in
the uterine cervix in 8 mice and in the vagina in 1 mouse after 29 weeks
or more of treatment. No carcinomas of the uterine corpus, cervix or
vagina were found in 82 controls (Pan & Gardner, 1948).

Four female BC mice and 1 female CBA mouse that were injected subcutaneously with 16.6 µg oestradiol 3-benzoate in sesame oil once weekly
commencing at ages ranging from 41-65 weeks had tumours of the uterine
corpus at 78-89 weeks. Two of the BC mice also had cervical tumours
(Gardner & Ferrigno, 1956) [The total incidence of these lesions in the
treated mice cannot be assessed from the data, nor is the incidence of
similar lesions in untreated mice known].

In an unspecified number of female mice of reciprocal crosses between
C57 and CBA strains injected subcutaneously with weekly doses of 16.6 or
50 µg oestradiol 3-benzoate (vehicle not stated) commencing at 4-8 weeks
of age, cervical lesions, ranging from invasion to gross tumours which
invaded adjacent tissues, were seen in 15/24 mice with C57 mothers and
in 10/20 with CBA mothers and surviving for more than 52 weeks. In the
latter group there was a high incidence of mammary cancer, which reduced
the lifespan. No lesions were seen before 59 weeks in either group. Of
10 mice in the two groups which survived more than 86 weeks, 6 had
lesions at death. Although none of the tumours metastasized, it was
concluded that the range of lesions seen probably represented various
stages of carcinoma development. No cervical tumours occurred among an
equal number of control mice (Allen & Gardner, 1941).

In a group of female CBA mice, 3 s.c. injections of 0.25 mg/animal
polyoestradiol phosphate (Estradurin), 7 days before and 30 and 60 days
after an i.p. injection of ^{90}Sr, led to an increased incidence of osteo-
genic tumours over that found with ^{90}Sr alone (from 36/50 to 44/49)
and a shorter latent period (403$\pm$9 *versus* 252$\pm$4 days) (Nilsson & Broomé-
Karlsson, 1976).

Rat: Female Sprague-Dawley rats were given 20 mg 7,12-dimethylbenz-
[*a*]anthracene (DMBA) in sesame oil by stomach tube at 50 days of age;
15 days later they were injected subcutaneously with oestradiol 3-benzoate
and progesterone, either alone or in combination, at low incremental
(0.01-1.6 µg), high incremental (1.0-7 µg) or constant (low, 0.1 µg;
high, 1 µg) doses, daily for 21 days. All rats were observed for more
than 5 months. All DMBA-treated control rats developed mammary tumours
(usually adenocarcinomas) within a short latent period (average, 69
days). Administration of low or high incremental doses of oestradiol
3-benzoate alone increased the latent period and depressed both the

number of tumour-bearing animals and the number of tumours per animal. High doses of the combination with progesterone resulted in an increased latent period and a decreased tumour incidence. The administration of incremental doses of progesterone alone or in combination with a constant dose of 0.1 μg oestradiol 3-benzoate stimulated the appearance of tumours (McCormick & Moon, 1973).

In a similar combination experiment, s.c. administration of 20 μg oestradiol 3-benzoate daily for 40 days, of 4 mg progesterone for 40 days or of a combination of 5 μg oestradiol 3-benzoate and 4 mg progesterone daily for 40 days significantly reduced the incidence of DMBA-induced mammary tumours in Sprague-Dawley rats (Kledzik *et al.*, 1974).

S.c. administration of 20 μg oestradiol 3-benzoate daily for 3 weeks to Sprague-Dawley rats 60 days after i.v. treatment with 5 mg DMBA at day 55, or of 20 μg oestradiol 3-benzoate with 2 mg/kg bw of a prolactin inhibitor, ergocornine methanesulphonate, led to a significant decrease in tumour size and in number of tumours per animal. The combination with the prolactin inhibitor was the most effective (Quadri *et al.*, 1974).

Guinea-pig: In 22/24 ovariectomized guinea-pigs given s.c. injections 3 times weekly of 20-80 μg oestradiol 3-benzoate in olive oil (Progynon B), multiple tumours, described as fibromas or fibromyomas, arose in the uterus and mesentery at several locations. No tumours occurred in the thorax (Lipschütz & Iglesias, 1938; Lipschütz *et al.*, 1938). Unesterified oestrogens that were tested concurrently were less active than the benzoate (Lipschütz & Vargas, 1939a).

Intact and castrated male guinea-pigs given 80 μg oestradiol 3-benzoate 3 times weekly were susceptible to induction of tumours in spleen, stomach and abdomen, but the size and extent of the abdominal lesions were less than in females (Koref *et al.*, 1939). The tumours regressed after cessation of the treatment (Lipschütz *et al.*, 1939). Histologically, these tumours had varying degrees of fibromyomatous and fibromatous proliferation, with some suggestion of transition to sarcoma. The tentative conclusion was that they were benign lesions peculiar to oestrogen-treated guinea-pigs (Lipschütz & Vargas, 1941).

(c) Subcutaneous implantation

Mouse: When castrated male (C3H x RIII)F₁ mice (MTV⁺) were given a s.c. implant of a pellet containing 0.5-1 mg oestradiol-17β in paraffin wax at the age of 10 or 70 days, 15/16 and 18/18, respectively, developed mammary cancer. Such tumours also occurred in 7/41 castrated controls, within a mean latent period of 69 weeks, compared with 25-27 weeks in treated mice. In C3H and RIII strains, the incidences of mammary cancer in groups of castrated males treated at 10 days of age with oestradiol-17β paraffin pellets were 14/18 and 14/17, respectively. Mammary tumours

occurred in only 3/19 male NLC mice and none of C57BL males (MTV⁻) given
similar implants (Rudali *et al.*, 1971).

Lymphoid tumours, almost all thymic lymphosarcomas, were seen in
27/84 male BALB/c mice before 57 weeks of age after the s.c. implantation
of a 1-2 mg pellet of oestradiol dipropionate at 18, 36 or 72 days of
age. No lymphosarcomas were observed in 240 control mice before 57
weeks of age (Kirschbaum *et al.*, 1953).

Of 20 BALB/c female mice treated every 3-4 months with 5 mg s.c.
implants of an oestradiol-17β-cholesterol mixture for 20 months, 17
survived 10 months or more; 2 developed precancerous lesions, and 5
developed squamous-cell carcinomas of the cervix and/or vagina. Of 40
mice treated with s.c. pellets of oestradiol-17β and with intravaginal
inoculations of herpesvirus type 2, 36 survived 10 months or more; 10
developed precancerous lesions, and 7 developed squamous-cell carcinomas
of the cervix and/or vagina. No cervical or vaginal lesions were seen
in 16/20 control mice that lived for 10 months or more (Muñoz, 1973).

Paraffin pellets containing 10% oestradiol-17β or 10% oestriol
(0.64-0.85 mg oestrogen) were implanted subcutaneously into (C3H x RIII)
F1 (MTV⁺) mice of both sexes, castrated on day 22-24 of life. Negative
controls received a pellet containing only paraffin. Pellets recovered
from mice at sacrifice contained 2-5% oestrogen; it was thus assumed
that most mice absorbed at least several hundred µg of oestrogen.
Mammary tumours (type not stated) occurred in 15/16 females and 15/16
males treated with oestradiol-17β, in 18/18 females and 25/30 males
treated with oestriol and in 28/34 female and 10/61 male controls. The
latent periods were 176 (+31), 133 (+10) and 446 (+28) days, respectively
in females and 137 (+15), 135 (+44) and 576 (+54) days, respectively, in
males (Rudali *et al.*, 1975).

In castrated male (C3H x RIII) F1 mice treated subcutaneously with
paraffin pellets containing 0, 1, 2.5, 5, 10 or 100 µg oestradiol-17β,
the incidences of mammary tumours were 11/33, 11/31, 23/27, 24/27, 27/27
and 23/24, with average latent periods of 515, 675, 270, 145, 185 and
175 days (Rudali *et al.*, 1978).

Rat: Rats of the Wistar albino (Glaxo) strain (WAG), albino rats
of the Royal Cancer Hospital (London) strain and hooded rats originally
derived from the MRC (London) strain were given two pellets of 5-6 mg
oestradiol-17β or oestradiol dipropionate, the initial implant at the
age of 4 weeks and a further implant after 1-3 months. Pituitary enlargement due to chromophobe adenomas (320 mg; range, 29-606 mg) was common
in all strains, occurring in 69/92 rats. Mammary cancers developed in
10/27 female WAG rats between 29 and 64 weeks of age; no such tumours
were seen in 5 males that lived longer than 64 weeks. Mammary cancers
occurred in 2/38 female Cancer Hospital rats and in 6/19 female rats of

the hooded MRC strain which lived longer than 29 weeks. The tumours were classified as adenocarcinomas, papillary carcinomas and anaplastic carcinomas. No carcinomas of the mammary gland occurred among equivalent numbers (not stated) of breeding or control rats of the strains used (Mackenzie, 1955).

Pituitary tumours occurred in adult Wistar albino rats (sex not stated) implanted with pellets of oestradiol 3-benzoate weighing 6-8 mg. The incidence of tumours is not clear from the data given, but an average pituitary weight of 217 mg was recorded in 8 rats 14-21 weeks after the start of the experiment; this average was maintained or increased to 50 weeks in 73 other rats. Thrice weekly injections of 20 μg thyroxine accelerated pituitary hypertrophy in a smaller group treated with oestradiol 3-benzoate pellets. Treatment with oestradiol 3-benzoate did not induce pituitary hypertrophy in groups of rats fed a diet containing 0.5% thiouracil (Gillman & Gilbert, 1955).

Oestradiol-17β, oestriol and oestrone were administered subcutaneously to intact female Sprague-Dawley rats, 48 hrs before treatment with DMBA or procarbazine, as 1-20% pellets weighing 5-7 mg each. DMBA and procarbazine were given by gavage at amounts of 20 and 50-70 mg, respectively. No mammary carcinomas occurred up to 370 days in untreated controls or in oestrogen-treated female rats. Higher doses of oestradiol-17β had an inhibitory effect on carcinogen-induced tumour development (Lemon, 1975).

Hamster: Malignant renal tumours were found in 15/15 intact and 12/12 castrated male hamsters and in 10/16 ovariectomized female hamsters given one or more 20 mg pellets of oestradiol-17β subcutaneously every 21 weeks. The age at autopsy varied between 45 and 81 weeks for males and between 24 and 58 weeks for the ovariectomized females. No kidney tumours were found in 6 treated intact females, nor among 145 intact or 72 castrated controls of either sex (Kirkman, 1959).

Guinea-pig: Fibromyomas in the uterine corpus, mesentery and other abdominal sites were found in female guinea-pigs that had been ovariectomized 3 months before the s.c. implantation of a 20 or 50 mg pellet of oestradiol-17β. Fibromyomas were detected as early as 19 days after the start of treatment in all animals. The pellets lost up to 10 mg in weight over 7 weeks (Lipschütz & Vargas, 1939b). Similar results were obtained by Woodruff (1941) with oestradiol 3-benzoate, and by Riesco (1947) with oestradiol dipropionate.

Monkey: Total doses of 575-825 mg oestradiol-17β were implanted subcutaneously at intervals of 5-6 weeks over a 24-28 month period in 5 female *Macaca mulatta* (rhesus) monkeys. Cystic hyperplasia of the mammary gland but no tumours were found (Engle *et al.*, 1943).

Five female Capuchin monkeys (*Cebus apella*) were given s.c. implants of oestradiol dipropionate and/or oestradiol-17β. In some cases the pellet consisted of pure oestrogen and in others of a mixture of 40% oestrogen and 60% cholesterol. The amount of oestrogen absorbed per day was about 250-700 µg/animal, and the total duration of treatment ranged from 29-145 weeks. In addition, 3 animals received s.c injections of other oestradiol esters (100-200 µg) twice weekly. A high degree of cystic and polypous glandular hyperplasia of the uterine mucosa developed in all animals. The only tumour observed (found in the longest survivor) was an adenocarcinoma or endothelioma of the pericardium, but it was considered not to be due to the treatment (Iglesias & Lipschütz, 1947).

(d) Neonatal exposure

Mouse: Data on vaginal lesions seen in female mice administered oestrogens neonatally have been summarized by Takasugi *et al.* (1970). Evidence that oestrogens given neonatally to mice 'select' special cell populations in the vagina and uterine cervix, which may give rise to abnormal lesions, has been presented by Forsberg (1972, 1973, 1975, 1979) and by Takasugi & Kamishima (1973). See also Takasugi (1976, 1979). It is apparent now that at least two different responses may occur in the genital tract of female mice given oestrogens neonatally: (1) retention of Müllerian-derived epithelium in the upper vagina (especially the fornix) and its proliferation in the fornical and cervical areas to give rise to adenosis (Forsberg, 1975, 1979), and (2) retention of a population of oestrogen-independent, cornifying cells in the vagina which proliferate, replace the original epithelium and give rise to irreversible, persistent vaginal cornification, hyperplastic downgrowths and squamous-cell carcinomas (Jones & Bern, 1977; Takasugi, 1976, 1979). The relation of adenosis to cervicovaginal adenocarcinomas is at present unknown (Scully *et al.*, 1978).

Increased mammary tumorigenesis has been reported in MTV[+] mice treated neonatally with oestradiol-17β (Bern *et al.*, 1975, 1976; Mori, 1968a,b); and hyperplastic nodules or metaplastic lesions have also been found in various accessory sex organs, including prostatic lobes, in male C3H/MS mice given oestrogens neonatally (Mori, 1967).

Female mice of 4 strains that received 5 µg oestradiol-17β daily for the first 5 days after birth showed hyperplastic and epidermoid vaginal lesions at 32-63 weeks of age: 16/23 of A/Crgl strain, 6/14 of BALB/cCrgl, 4/16 of C57BL/Crgl and 3/15 of RIII/Crgl. No lesions were found in 6 treated C3H/Crgl mice at 44 weeks of age, and 1 lesion occurred in 5 C57BL/Crgl controls, although most of these mice showed persistent vaginal cornification. Vaginal concretions ('stones') were found in almost all mice with vaginal lesions (Takasugi & Bern, 1964).

Female BALB/cCrgl mice were injected with 25, 5 or 0.1 µg oestradiol-
17β as an aqueous suspension daily for the first 5 days of life. Approximately half the animals in each group were ovariectomized at 16-17 weeks
of age. All mice that received the two higher doses and 37/42 mice that
received the lower dose developed persistent vaginal cornification;
this cornification was maintained after ovariectomy in all mice that had
received 25 or 5 µg oestradiol-17β but not in those that had received
0.1 µg. The mice were killed between 64 and 73 weeks of age. Vaginal
epithelial downgrowths were found in all of 16 and 11 intact mice that
had been given 25 and 5 µg and in 16/19 intact mice that had received
0.1 µg. In the corresponding ovariectomized groups, the incidences of
downgrowths were reduced to 15/16, 5/10 and 0/9, respectively. Hyperplastic vaginal lesions resembling epidermoid carcinoma were found at
termination of the experiment in 19/27 intact mice and in 8/26 ovariectomized mice given 25 or 5 µg oestradiol-17β, but in only 3/19 intact
mice and 0/9 ovariectomized mice that had been given 0.1 µg. The mean
ovarian weights of all the intact oestradiol-17β-treated mice were more
than twice those of the controls. Epithelial downgrowth was found in
the vaginas of 5/10 intact controls, but no hyperplastic lesions were
seen. Four ovariectomized controls had no vaginal dysplasias (Kimura &
Nandi, 1967).

Groups of 2-19 newborn BALB/cfC3H (MTV$^+$), BALB/c (MTV$^-$) and C57BL
(MTV$^-$) female mice were treated for 5 days with 5 or 20 µg/day oestradiol-
17β and with 5 or 20 µg/day testosterone alone or in combination with 5
or 20 µg/day prolactin. In two identical experiments, both steroids
resulted in higher mammary tumour incidences in BALB/cfC3H mice, as
compared with those in untreated (0/40) and prolactin-treated (9/43)
mice. Testosterone induced higher incidences (42/49 and 22/35) than
oestradiol-17β (8/35 and 32/64). The combination with prolactin did not
influence tumour incidence significantly. No mammary tumours occurred
in the MTV$^-$ strains (Mori et al., 1976).

Neonatal s.c. administration to newborn BALB/cfC3H mice (MTV$^+$) of 5
or 20 µg oestradiol-17β, alone or in combination with 100 µg progesterone,
daily for 5 days resulted in an increased incidence of mammary adenocarcinomas at an earlier age, except in those given the high dose of
oestradiol-17β. The number of animals with mammary adenocarcinomas was
17/19 in the low-oestradiol-17β, 20/32 in the low-oestradiol-17β-plus-
progesterone, 4/11 in the high-oestradiol-17β, 33/44 in the high-oestra-
diol-17β-plus-progesterone and 5/17 in the vehicle control groups
(Jones & Bern, 1977).

Female BALB/c mice (MTV$^-$) given s.c. injections of 40 µg oestradiol-
17β daily for the first 5 days of life showed more and different kinds
of mammary dysplasias than untreated controls when given DMBA by gavage
later in life (Warner & Warner, 1975).

Rat: Single s.c. injections of 0.1 mg oestradiol 3-benzoate in 0.05
ml sesame oil to 5-day-old female Sprague-Dawley rats reduced the incidence
of DMBA-induced mammary tumours at 190 days of age (10/31 *versus* 20/33,
P<0.05).   Treatment decreased mammary adenocarcinoma response to DMBA
(4/28 total tumours *versus* 27/30) and increased fibroadenoma response to
DMBA (24/28 total tumours *versus* 3/30, P<0.01).   No tumours occurred in
rats given oestradiol 3-benzoate only (Shellabarger & Soo, 1973).

In female Sprague-Dawley rats given s.c. injections of increasing
doses of oestradiol-17β (10-40 µg) for the first 30 days of life, DMBA-
induced mammary tumorigenesis was completely inhibited 120 days after
DMBA administration at 60 days of age (none *versus* 15/27 in DMBA controls).
The degree of normal mammary development was no different among treated
and untreated groups at 60 days of age;   however, at 160 days after DMBA
administration, mammary glands in oestrogenized rats had regressed
completely (Nagasawa *et al.*, 1974).

Neonatal treatment of Sprague-Dawley rats with 100 µg oestradiol-
17β did not influence the incidence of ear-duct tumours induced by 20 mg
DMBA given by stomach tube (Yoshida & Fukunishi, 1977).

Female Sprague-Dawley rats were given a single s.c. injection of
0.1 mg oestradiol-17β at 2 days of age and 20 mg DMBA by gavage at 50
days of age.   The induction of mammary dysplasia was significantly
accelerated in rats given oestradiol-17β, when compared with DMBA controls
(37/44 *versus* 26/40);   mammary carcinoma incidence was significantly
reduced (24/44 *versus* 34/40) after 300 days of observation (Yoshida &
Fukunishi, 1978).

3.2 Other relevant biological data

Oestradiol-17β is the most potent naturally-occurring steroidal
oestrogen (See also 'General Remarks on Sex Hormones', pp. 42 & 43).

(a) Experimental systems

No data were available on its toxic effects.

Embryotoxicity and teratogenicity

Swiss-Webster mice were injected subcutaneously with oestradiol
3-benzoate between days 11-16 of gestation at alternating doses of 0.1
and 0.2 mg.   A significant incidence of cleft palate occurred in offspring
(13.6% *versus* 1.1% in controls) (Nishihara, 1958).

ICR mouse foetuses from the 15th or 17th day of gestation were injected subcutaneously with 50 μg oestradiol-17β. Irreversible cornification or stratification of the vaginal epithelium was seen at birth in 85% of those treated on day 17 and in 66% of those treated on day 15. When examined at the age of 3 months, corpora lutea were absent in 4/12 treated on day 17 and in 5/6 mice treated on day 15. Administration of 50 μg oestradiol-17β on the day of birth or 3 days later to ICR mice resulted in absence of corpora lutea. The changes in their vaginal epithelium were less marked (Kimura, 1975).

Administration of 500 μg oestradiol-17β on day 15 of gestation to BALB/cfC3H/Crgl and C3H/Tw mice resulted in abnormal oestrus cycles in female offspring late in life and abnormalities of the cervicovaginal epithelium. Administration on day 12 had no such effects (Mori *et al.*, 1978).

Pregnant rats were given s.c. injections of 0.8-35 mg oestradiol-17β daily from day 12-13 until day 18-21 of gestation, or 0.375-100 mg oestradiol dipropionate every second or third day from day 12 or 13 of gestation until day 17-19; in some animals, the latter compound was given as a single dose on day 12 or 13. Only 12/28 oestradiol-17β-treated rats and 94/164 oestradiol dipropionate-treated rats carried to term; litter size was reduced and post-partum mortality was 66 and 81%. In female offspring (106 newborn, 11 adult) of the 2 groups combined, abnormalities of the reproductive tract and absence of corpora lutea were observed. In male offspring (98 newborn, 22 adult), 3-6 pairs of well developed nipples, undescended testes and impairment of Wolffian-derived tissues occurred (Greene *et al.*, 1940).

A single s.c. injection of 10 mg oestradiol dipropionate to rats on day 14 of gestation induced malformations of the mammary glands (missing mammary glands and hypertrophic nipples) in offspring of both sexes (Delost *et al.*, 1962, 1963).

Rabbits were injected intramuscularly with 15 or 30 μg oestradiol-17β for 3-5 consecutive days during different periods of gestation, starting on the 5th day. Administration of 15 μg terminated pregnancy when given before day 21 of gestation; later, 30 μg were required to terminate pregnancy (Schofield, 1962).

Metabolism[1]

The metabolism of oestradiol-17β and oestrone is similar in rats and in humans, in that both species transform these steroids mainly by

---

[1]The metabolism of oestradiol-17β, of oestrone and of oestriol are considered together, since there is interconversion between oestradiol-17β and oestrone, and the latter is converted to oestriol.

(aromatic) 2-hydroxylation (Bartke *et al.*, 1971; Keith & Williams, 1970), and also by 16α-hydroxylation (Bolt, 1979). Glucuronides of the various metabolites are excreted in the bile (Fig. 1). Differences in the metabolism of oestrogens by humans and rats lie mostly in the type of conjugation (Williams, 1970). A relatively large proportion of administered oestrone, oestradiol-17β and oestriol is transformed in rats to metabolites oxygenated both at C-2 and C-16 (Honma & Nambara, 1974; Menzies & Watanabe, 1976; Watanabe & Menzies, 1973). When oestriol is administered to rats, glucuronides and, to a lesser extent, sulphates of 16-ketooestradiol and of 2- and 3-methyl ethers of 2-hydroxyoestriol and 2-hydroxy-16-ketooestradiol are excreted in the bile (Nambara & Kawarada, 1975; Nambara *et al.*, 1974). In contrast, hydroxylations at C-6 or C-7 of ring B of oestradiol-17β and oestrone are a minor pathway in rats (Lehmann & Breuer, 1969). 2-Hydroxyoestrogens ('catechol oestrogens') are further transformed by various routes (see Gelbke *et al.*, 1978), including covalent binding to proteins.

Rabbit liver can form 2-hydroxylated oestriol (King, 1961). However, the presence of two enzymes unique to this organ leads to an oestrogen metabolite pattern that cannot be compared with the human situation: (1) in addition to glucuronyltransferase, rabbit liver microsomes also contain glucosyl and *N*-acetylglucosaminyl transferases, which transfer glucose from UDP-glucose to the 3-hydroxy group of oestrone and oestradiol or *N*-acetylglucosamine from the UDP form to the 17α-hydroxy group of oestradiol-17α (Collins *et al.*, 1970); (2) in addition to microsomal and cytoplasmic 17β-hydroxysteroid dehydrogenase, a 17α-hydroxysteroid dehydrogenase is found in rabbit liver cytosol (Breuer & Knuppen, 1968). Hence, the major metabolite of oestrone or oestradiol-17β in rabbits is oestradiol-17α, which is mainly conjugated to oestradiol-17α-*N*-acetylglucosaminide (Breuer & Knuppen, 1968) or to oestradiol-3-glucuronide-17α-*N*-acetylglucosaminide (Quamme *et al.*, 1972). These metabolic pathways do not occur in man.

Sulphates are the major conjugates of oestradiol-17β and oestrone in guinea-pigs, and metabolism by 16α-hydroxylation is thought to take place on the oestrone 3-sulphate (Hobkirk *et al.*, 1977). Glucuronidation, if any, plays only a minor role, in contrast to the human situation; 2-hydroxylation of oestrone also occurs. Only small amounts of labelled oestrone are converted to oestradiol in guinea-pigs (Yoshizawa *et al.*, 1977).

Canine metabolism of oestrogens differs greatly from that in humans. Only small amounts of labelled oestradiol-17β are converted to oestriol; the bulk of the radioactive dose is excreted in urine as conjugates of oestradiol-17β and oestrone (Beling *et al.*, 1975). After administration of labelled oestriol to dogs, a unique pattern of conjugates was found in bile and urine, probably including polyglucuronides (Kirdani & Sandberg, 1974). Furthermore, no significant enterohepatic circulation occurs, in contrast to the distribution of oestrogenic hormones in most other species.

Figure 1

Major pathways in metabolism of natural oestrogens in rats
(conjugation reactions are not shown)[1]

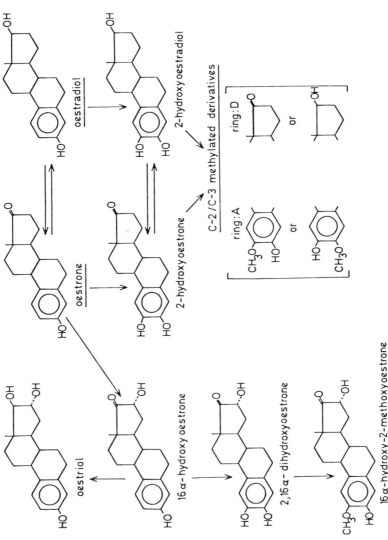

[1]From Bolt (1979)

Oestradiol-17α is also a major oestrogenic metabolite in some other species, including domestic fowl (Chan & Common, 1974; Common & Robinson, 1976), bulls (Leung et al., 1975) and sheep (Challis et al., 1973). Liver tissues of pigs contain significant amounts of 17β-hydroxysteroid dehydrogenase and glucuronyl transferase (Rao et al., 1974); in minipigs, oxidoreduction at C-17 is the predominant reaction; whereas, in contrast to humans, hydroxylation of oestrogens plays only a minor role (Beckmann & Breuer, 1975). The metabolism of oestrogens in these species thus differs markedly from that in humans.

On the basis of the urinary and faecal excretion of oestrogens, non-human primates resemble humans much more closely than do rodents or dogs (Goldzieher & Kraemer, 1972). The conjugates of oestrogens are similar in *Macaca mulatta* (rhesus) monkeys and in humans (Musey et al., 1977). Baboons also show some similarities to humans in oestrogen metabolism (Musey et al., 1973).

No data on oestradiol-17β-valerate were available, but it is known that similar oestradiol esters, such as the benzoate (Kaltenbach et al., 1976), are converted in the organism to the corresponding active oestrogens. The derivatives as such are almost devoid of oestrogenic activity (in terms of affinity for oestrogen receptors); oestrogenicity relies on metabolic transformation to the parent compounds. The extent and pharmacokinetics of this metabolic step are very much dependent on the particular compound in question.

Mutagenicity and other short-term tests

Twice weekly injections to male Wistar rats of 1 mg/animal oestradiol 3-benzoate significantly lowered the mitotic index of bone marrow but induced no detectable chromosome aberrations (Málková et al., 1977).

A two-fold increase in the number of chromosomal aberrations was observed in cultures of human embryonic fibroblasts and renal epithelial cells treated with 1 μg/ml oestradiol-17β (Serova & Kerkis, 1974).

When cultures of human diploid synovial cells were exposed to 2.5 x 10^{-6} - 10^{-9}M oestradiol-17β, high concentrations significantly increased the number of aneuploid cells in cultures from some individuals (Lycette et al., 1970).

No obvious chromosomal effects were observed when 0.1-100 μg/ml oestradiol-17β were added to cultures of lymphocytes grown from the blood of healthy women (Stenchever et al., 1969).

(b) Humans

The metabolic pathways of oestradiol-17β in humans have been reviewed extensively (Breuer *et al.*, 1968; Diczfalusy & Lauritzen, 1961). Comparisons with its metabolism in mammals are described in section 3.2(a). 16-Oxygenation is a major step in the conversion of natural oestrogens. After injection of [16α-³H]-oestradiol, 55% of the tritium is liberated into the body water, although only 8% of the dose is excreted as urinary oestriol (Fishman *et al.*, 1966); this indicates that 16α-hydroxylation is a quantitatively important pathway and that it may be followed by secondary routes of conversion. Another major pathway for the conversion of natural oestrogens in humans is 2-hydroxylation, since about 33% of the tritium of [2-³H]-oestradiol is released into the body water (Fishman *et al.*, 1970). The product of 2-hydroxylation, 2-hydroxyoestrone, is found in human plasma (Yoshizawa & Fishman, 1971).

The two main metabolic routes, 2- and 16α-hydroxylation, are competitive. With high levels of thyroid hormone, 2-hydroxylation is increased and 16α-hydroxylation decreased (Fishman *et al.*, 1965); whereas in liver cirrhosis, 2-hydroxylation is decreased and 16α-hydroxylation of oestrone enhanced (Zumoff *et al.*, 1968). Oestriol also undergoes 2-hydroxylation, since 2-hydroxyoestriol has been identified in late-pregnancy urine (Gelbke & Knuppen, 1974). The catechol oestrogens, 2-hydroxyoestrone, 2-hydroxyoestradiol and 2-hydroxyoestriol, undergo further metabolic alteration; this has been reviewed extensively by Gelbke *et al.* (1978).

Oestrogens may be conjugated at the phenolic hydroxyl group of ring A, either by sulphuric or glucuronic acid. Moreover, conjugation with glucuronic acid has been reported to occur at hydroxy groups of ring D (Hobkirk & Nilsen, 1971). The predominant conjugate in human plasma is oestrogen-3-sulphate: levels exceed those of oestradiol-17β by about 10 times (Longcope, 1972; Ruder *et al.*, 1972). Oestrone sulphate may be reconverted to oestrone and oestradiol in extrahepatic organs like the uterus (Trolp *et al.*, 1977).

3.3 Case reports and epidemiological studies

See the section, 'Oestrogens and Progestins in Relation to Human Cancer', p. 83.

4. Summary of Data Reported and Evaluation[1]

4.1 Experimental data

Oestradiol-17β and its esters were tested in mice, rats, hamsters, guinea-pigs and monkeys by subcutaneous injection or implantation and in mice by oral administration. Its subcutaneous administration resulted in increased incidences of mammary, pituitary, uterine, cervical, vaginal and lymphoid tumours and interstitial-cell tumours of the testis in mice. In rats, there was an increased incidence of mammary and/or pituitary tumours. In hamsters, a high incidence of malignant kidney tumours occurred in intact and castrated males and in ovariectomized females, but not in intact females. In guinea-pigs, diffuse fibromyomatous uterine and abdominal lesions were observed. Oral administration of oestradiol-17β in mice led to an increased mammary tumour incidence. Subcutaneous injections in neonatal mice resulted in precancerous and cancerous cervical and vaginal lesions in later life and an increased incidence of mammary tumours.

Oestradiol-17β has teratogenic actions on the genital tract and possibly on other organs and impairs fertility.

4.2 Human data

No case reports or epidemiological studies on oestradiol-17β alone were available to the Working Group. Case reports and epidemiological studies on steroid hormones used in oestrogen treatment have been summarized in the section, 'Oestrogens and Progestins in Relation to Human Cancer', p. 83.

4.3 Evaluation

There is *sufficient evidence* for the carcinogenicity of oestradiol-17β in experimental animals. In the absence of adequate data in humans, it is reasonable, for practical purposes, to regard oestradiol-17β as if it presented a carcinogenic risk to humans. Studies in humans strongly suggest that the administration of oestrogens is causally related to an increased incidence of endometrial carcinoma; there is no evidence that oestradiol-17β is different from other oestrogens in this respect.

---

[1]This section should be read in conjunction with pp. 62-64 in the 'General Remarks on Sex Hormones' and with the 'General Conclusions on Sex Hormones', p. 131

5. <u>References</u>

Abraham, G.E., Manlimos, F.S. & Garza, R. (1977) <u>Radioimmunoassay of steroids</u>. In: Abraham, G.E., ed., <u>Handbook of Radioimmunoassay</u>, New York, Marcel Dekker, pp. 591-656

Adessi, G.L., Eichenberger, D., Nhuan, T.Q. & Jayle, M.F. (1975) Gas chromatography profile of estrogens: application to pregnancy urine. <u>Steroids</u>, <u>25</u>, 553-564

Adlercreutz, H., Tikkanen, M.J. & Hunneman, D.H. (1974) Mass fragmentographic determination of eleven estrogens in the body fluids of pregnant and nonpregnant subjects. <u>J. Steroid Biochem.</u>, <u>5</u>, 211-217

Allen, E. & Gardner, W.U. (1941) Cancer of the cervix of the uterus in hybrid mice following long-continued administration of estrogen. <u>Cancer Res.</u>, <u>1</u>, 359-366

Bartke, A., Steel, R.E., Williams, J.G. & Williams, K.I.H. (1971) Biliary metabolites of ^{14}C-estrone and ^{14}C-estradiol from the rat. <u>Steroids</u>, <u>18</u>, 303-311

Beckmann, D. & Breuer, H. (1975) Studies on the metabolism of oestrone and oestradiol-17β in the liver of minipigs of different ages and sexes (Ger.). <u>Hoppe-Seyler's Z. physiol. Chem.</u>, <u>356</u>, 1743-1751

Beling, C.G., Gustafsson, P.-O. & Kasström, H. (1975) Metabolism of estradiol in greyhounds and German shepherd dogs. <u>Acta radiol.</u>, Suppl. 344, 109-120

Bern, H.A., Jones, L.A., Mori, T. & Young, P.N. (1975) Exposure of neonatal mice to steroids: longterm effect on the mammary gland and other reproductive structures. <u>J. Steroid Biochem.</u>, <u>6</u>, 673-676

Bern, H.A., Jones, L.A., Mills, K.T., Kohrman, A. & Mori, T. (1976) Use of the neonatal mouse in studying long-term effects of early exposure to hormones and other agents. <u>J. Toxicol. environ. Health</u>, Suppl. 1, 103-116

Bischoff, F., Long, M.L., Rupp, J.J. & Clarke, G.J. (1942a) Carcinogenic effect of estradiol and of theelin in Marsh-Buffalo mice. <u>Cancer Res.</u>, <u>2</u>, 52-55

Bischoff, F., Long, M.L., Rupp, J.J. & Clarke, G.J. (1942b) Influence of toxic amounts of estrin upon intact and castrated male Marsh-Buffalo mice. <u>Cancer Res.</u>, <u>2</u>, 198-199

Bolt, H.M. (1979) Metabolism of estrogens - natural and synthetic.
    Pharmac. Ther., 4, 155-181

Bonser, G.M. & Robson, J.M. (1940) The effects of prolonged oestrogen
    administration upon male mice of various strains: development of
    testicular tumours in the Strong A strain. J. Pathol. Bacteriol.,
    51, 9-22

Bowman, M.C. & Nony, C.R. (1977) Trace analysis of estradiol in
    animal chow by electron-capture gas chromatography.
    J. chromatogr. Sci., 15, 160-163

Breuer, H. & Knuppen, R. (1968) Comparative studies on the metabolism
    of estrogens in the rabbit under various experimental conditions:
    in vivo, during perfusion, in vitro. Adv. Biosci., 3, 71-79

Breuer, H., Breuer, J., Dahm, K., Knuppen, R. & Lehmann, W.D. (1968)
    Some newer aspects of oestrogen metabolism. Adv. Biosci., 2,
    113-144

Butenandt, A. & Goergens, C. (1937) α- and β-Estradiol. Z. physiol.
    Chem., 248, 129-141 [Chem. Abstr., 31, 7880-1]

Cavina, G., Moretti, G. & Petrella, M. (1975) A solvent system for
    the separation of steroids with estrogenic and progestational
    activity by two-dimensional thin-layer chromatography.
    J. Chromatogr., 103, 368-371

Challis, J.R.G., Harrison, F.A. & Heap, R.B. (1973) The metabolic
    clearance rate, production rate and conversion ratios of oestrone
    in the sheep. J. Endocrinol., 58, 435-446

Chan, A.H.-H. & Common, R.H. (1974) Identification of radioactive
    oestradiol-17α and oestradiol-17β in the plasma of the laying hen
    after injection of oestrone-4-[14]C. Comp. Biochem. Physiol., 49B,
    105-111

Chattoraj, S.C. & Wotiz, H.H. (1975) Estrogens. In: Dorfman, R.I.,
    ed., Steroid Hormones, Amsterdam, North-Holland, pp. 2-49

Collins, D.C., Williamson, D.G. & Layne, D.S. (1970) Steroid glucosides.
    Enzymatic synthesis by a partially purified transferase from
    rabbit liver microsomes. J. biol. Chem., 245, 873-876

Common, R.H. & Robinson, A.R. (1976) Identifications of radioactive
    steroid oestrogen conjugates in bile of laying hens after
    intramuscular injection of [4-^{14}C]-oestrone. Comp. Biochem.
    Physiol., 53B, 239-243

Delost, P., Jean, C. & Jean, C. (1962) Experimental production of mammary malformations in rat foetuses by injection of oestradiol to the mother on the 14th day of gestation (Fr.). C.R. Soc. Biol. (Paris), 156, 2048-2054

Delost, P., Jean, C. & Jean, C. (1963) Malformations of the mammary gland and the nipple in the fetus produced by oestradiol injected in the pregnant rat (Fr.). J. Physiol (Paris), 55, 237-238

Diczfalusy, E. & Lauritzen, C. (1961) Östrogene beim Menschen, Berlin, Springer

Dolphin, R.J. & Pergande, P.J. (1977) Improved method for the analysis of estrogenic steroids in pregnancy urine by high-performance liquid chromatography. J. Chromatogr., 143, 267-274

Dorfman, R.I. (1966) Hormones (sex). In: Kirk, R.E. & Othmer, D.F., eds, Encyclopedia of Chemical Technology, 2nd ed., Vol. II, New York, John Wiley & Sons, p. 117

Dray, F., Andrieu, J.M. & Mamas, S. (1975) A viroimmunological method of estradiol-17β. A quantitation with the help of estradiol bacteriophage conjugate. In: Radioimmunoassay of Steroid Hormones, pp. 197-207

Edqvist, L.-E., Häggström, A., Kindahl, H. & Stabenfeldt, G.H. (1976) Radioisotopic techniques for the study of reproductive physiology in domestic animals. 1. Assay procedures. In: Proceedings of an International Symposium on Nuclear Techniques in Animal Production and Health, IAEA-SM-205/3, Vienna, International Atomic Energy Agency, pp. 513-524

Engle, E.T., Krakower, C. & Haagensen, C.D. (1943) Estrogen administration to aged female monkeys with no resultant tumors. Cancer Res., 3, 858-866

Fishman, S. (1975) Determination of estrogens in dosage forms by fluorescence using dansyl chloride. J. pharm. Sci., 64, 674-680

Fishman, J., Hellman, L., Zumoff, B. & Gallagher, T.F. (1965) Effect of thyroid on hydroxylation of estrogen in man. J. clin. Endocrinol. Metab., 25, 365-368

Fishman, J., Hellman, L., Zumoff, B. & Cassouto, J. (1966) Pathway and stereochemistry of the formation of estriols in man. Biochemistry, 5, 1789-1794

Fishman, J., Guzik, H. & Hellman, L. (1970) Aromatic ring hydroxylation of estradiol in man. Biochemistry, 9, 1593-1598

Florey, K. (1975) Estradiol valerate. In: Florey, K., ed.,
    Analytical Profiles of Drug Substances, Vol. IV, New York,
    Academic Press, pp. 193-208

Forsberg, J.-G. (1972) Estrogen, vaginal cancer and vaginal
    development. Am. J. Obstet. Gynecol., 113, 83-87

Forsberg, J.-G. (1973) Cervicovaginal epithelium: its origin and
    development. Am. J. Obstet. Gynecol., 115, 1025-1043

Forsberg, J.-G. (1975) Late effects in the vaginal and cervical
    epithelia after injections of diethylstilbestrol into neonatal
    mice. Am. J. Obstet. Gynecol., 121, 101-104

Forsberg, J.-G. (1979) Developmental mechanism of estrogen-induced irrever-
    sible changes in the mouse cervicovaginal epithelium. Natl Cancer
    Inst. Monogr., 51, 41-56

Gardner, W.U. (1941) The effect of estrogen on the incidence of
    mammary and pituitary tumors in hybrid mice. Cancer Res., 1,
    345-358

Gardner, W.U. & Ferrigno, M. (1956) Unusual neoplastic lesions of
    the uterine horns of estrogen-treated mice. J. natl Cancer Inst.,
    17, 601-613

Gardner, W.U. & Strong, L.C M. (1940) Strain-limited development of
    tumors of the pituitary gland in mice receiving estrogens.
    Yale J. Biol. Med., 12, 543-549

Gardner, W.U., Dougherty, T.F. & Williams, W.L. (1944) Lymphoid
    tumors in mice receiving steroid hormones. Cancer Res., 4,
    73-87

Gelbke, H.P. & Knuppen, R. (1974) Identification and quantitative
    determination of 2-hydroxyoestriol in human late-pregnancy
    urine. J. Steroid Biochem., 5, 1-7

Gelbke, H.P., Ball, P. & Knuppen, R. (1978) 2-Hydroxyoestrogens.
    Chemistry, biogenesis, metabolism and physiological significance.
    In: Briggs, M.H. & Christie, G.A., eds, Advances in Steroid
    Biochemistry and Pharmacology, Vol. 6, New York, Academic Press,
    pp. 81-154

Gillman, J. & Gilbert, C. (1955) Modulating action of the thyroid on
    oestrogen-induced pituitary tumours in rats. Nature, 175, 724-725

Goldzieher, J.W. & Kraemer, D.C. (1972) The metabolism and effects of contraceptive steroids in primates. Acta endocrinol., Suppl. 166, 389-421

Graham, R.E. & Kenner, C.T. (1973) Acetonitrile-diatomaceous earth column for separation of steroids and other compounds. J. pharm. Sci., 62, 1845-1849

Grasselli, J.G. & Ritchey, W.M., eds (1975) CRC Atlas of Spectral Data and Physical Constants for Organic Compounds, 2nd ed., Vol. III, Cleveland, OH, Chemical Rubber Co., p. 231

Greene, R.R., Burrill, M.W. & Ivy, A.C. (1940) Experimental inter-sexuality. The effects of estrogens on the antenatal sexual development of the rat. Am. J. Anat., 67, 305-345

Hara, S. & Hayashi, S. (1977) Correlation of retention behaviour of steroidal pharmaceuticals in polar and bonded reversed-phase liquid column chromatography. J. Chromatogr., 142, 689-703

Hara, S. & Mibe, K. (1975) The solvent selectivity of the mobile phase in thin-layer chromatography in relation to the mobility and the structure of steroidal pharmaceuticals. Chem. pharm. Bull., 23, 2850-2859

Härkönen, M., Adlercreutz, H. & Groman, E.V. (1974) Enzymatic techniques in steroid assay. J. Steroid Biochem., 5, 717-725

Harvey, S.C. (1975) Hormones. In: Osol, A. et al., eds, Remington's Pharmaceutical Sciences, 15th ed., Easton, PA, Mack, pp. 914-915, 917

Heki, N., Noto, M. & Hosojima, H. (1977) Microanalysis of estrone, estradiol and estriol of serum and urine by mass fragmentography using gas chromatography-mass spectrometry (Jpn.). Nippon Naibumpi Gakkai Zasshi, 53, 167-174 [Chem. Abstr., 86, 152212j]

Highman, B., Norvell, M.J. & Shellenberger, T.E. (1977) Pathological changes in female C3H mice continuously fed diets containing diethylstilbestrol or 17β-estradiol. J. environ. Pathol. Toxicol., 1, 1-30

Hobkirk. R. & Nilsen, M. (1971) Metabolism of 17β-estradiol to 17β-estradiol-3-glucosiduronate and 17β-estradiol-17-glucosiduronate by the normal human female. J. clin. Endocrinol. Metab., 32, 779-785

Hobkirk, R., Freeman, D.J., Harvey, P.R.C., Nilsen, M. & Jennings, B. (1977) In vitro and in vivo studies on the metabolism of estrogens and their sulfates in guinea-pigs. Can. J. Biochem., 55, 390-397

Honma, S. & Nambara, T. (1974)   Isolation and characterization of
    biliary metabolites of estrone in the rat. Chem. pharm. Bull.,
    22, 687-695

Hooker, C.W. & Pfeiffer, C.A. (1942)   The morphology and development
    of testicular tumors in mice of the A strain receiving estrogens.
    Cancer Res., 2, 759-769

Horwitz, W., ed. (1975)   Official Methods of Analysis of the Association
    of Official Analytical Chemists, 12th ed., Washington DC,
    Association of Official Analytical Chemists, p. 745

IARC (1974)   IARC Monographs on the Evaluation of Carcinogenic Risk of
    Chemicals to Man, 6, Sex Hormones, Lyon, pp. 99-115

Iglesias, R. & Lipschütz, A. (1947)   Effects of prolonged oestrogen
    administration in female New World monkeys, with observations on
    a pericardial neoplasm. J. Endocrinol., 5, 88-98

Jarc, H., Ruttner, O. & Krocza, W. (1977)   The quantitative detection
    of estrogens and antithyroid drugs by thin-layer and high-performance
    thin-layer chromatography in animal tissue (Ger.). J. Chromatogr.,
    134, 351-358

Jones, L.A. & Bern, H.A. (1977)   Long-term effects of neonatal treatment
    with progesterone, alone and in combination with estrogen, on the
    mammary gland and reproductive tract of female BALB/cfC3H mice.
    Cancer Res., 37, 67-75

Kaltenbach, C.C., Dunn, T.G., Koritnik, D.R., Tucker, W.F., Batson,
    D.B., Staigmiller, R.B. & Niswender, G.D. (1976)   Isolation and
    identification of metabolites of ^{14}C-labeled estradiol in cattle.
    J. Toxicol. environ. Health, 1, 607-616

Kastrup, E.K., ed. (1976)   Facts and Comparisons, St Louis, MO,
    Facts & Comparisons Inc., p. 101

Kastrup, E.K., ed. (1977)   Facts and Comparisons, St Louis, MO,
    Facts & Comparisons Inc., pp. 113-114, 670

Kastrup, E.K., ed. (1978)   Facts and Comparisons, St Louis, MO,
    Facts & Comparisons Inc., pp. 98, 103

Keith, W.B. & Williams, K.I.H. (1970)   Metabolism of radioactive
    estrone in rats. Biochim. biophys. acta, 210, 328-332

Khayam-Bashi, H. & Boroumand, M. (1975)   Spectrophotometric estimation
    of estradiol-17β, progesterone, and testosterone. Biochem. Med.,
    14, 104-108

Kimura, T. (1975) Persistant vaginal cornification in mice treated with estrogen prenatally. Endocrinol. Jpn., 22, 497-502

Kimura, T. & Nandi, S. (1967) Nature of induced persistent vaginal cornification in mice. IV. Changes in the vaginal epithelium of old mice treated neonatally with estradiol or testosterone. J. natl Cancer Inst., 39, 75-83

King, R.J.B. (1961) Oestriol metabolism by rat- and rabbit-liver slices. Isolation of 2-methoxyoestriol and 2-hydroxyoestriol. Biochem. J., 79, 355-360

Kirdani, R.Y. & Sandberg, A.A. (1974) The fate of estriol in dogs. Steroids, 23, 667-686

Kirkman, H. (1959) Estrogen-induced tumors of the kidney. IV. Incidence in female Syrian hamsters. Natl Cancer Inst. Monogr., 1, 59-75

Kirschbaum, A., Shapiro, J.R. & Mixer, H.W. (1953) Synergistic action of leukemogenic agents. Cancer Res., 13, 262-268

Kledzik, G.S., Bradley, C.J. & Meites, J. (1974) Reduction of carcinogen-induced mammary cancer incidence in rats by early treatment with hormones or drugs. Cancer Res., 34, 2953-2956

Koref, O., Lipschütz, A. & Vargas, L., Jr (1939) Sexual and tumorigenic specificity (Fr.). C.R. Soc. Biol. (Paris), 103, 303-306

Korenman, S.G., Stevens, R.H., Carpenter, L.A., Robb, M., Niswender, G.D. & Sherman, B.M. (1974) Estradiol radioimmunoassay without chromatography: procedure, validation and normal values. J. clin. Endocrinol. Metab., 38, 718-720

Kraybill, H.F., Helmes, C.T. & Sigman, C.C. (1977) Biomedical aspects of biorefractories in water. In: Hotzinger, O., ed. Second International Symposium on Aquatic Pollutants, 1977, Amsterdam, Noordwijkerhorit, pp. 1-41

Lawrence, J.F. & Ryan, J.J. (1977) Comparison of electron-capture and electrolytic-conductivity detection for the gas-liquid chromatographic analysis of heptafluorobutyryl derivatives of some agricultural chemicals. J. Chromatogr., 130, 97-102

Lehmann, W.D. & Breuer, H. (1969) Metabolism of estrogens in rat liver before and after castration, and after administration of various steroid hormones (Ger.). Hoppe-Seyler's Z. physiol. Chem., 350, 191-200

Lemon, H.M. (1975) Estriol prevention of mammary carcinoma induced by 7,12-dimethylbenzanthracene and procarbazine. Cancer Res., 35, 1341-1353

Leung, B.S., Pearson, J.R. & Martin, R.P. (1975) Enterohepatic cycling of ^{3}H-estrone in the bull: identification of estrone-3-glucuronide. J. Steroid Biochem., 6, 1477-1481

Lipschütz, A. & Iglesias, R. (1938) Multiple uterine and extragenital tumours induced by oestradiol benzoate (Fr.). C.R. Soc. Biol. (Paris), 129, 519-524

Lipschütz, A. & Vargas, L., Jr (1939a) Comparative study on the tumorigenic action of different oestrogenic substances (Fr.). C.R. Soc. Biol. (Paris), 130, 9-11

Lipschütz, A. & Vargas, L., Jr (1939b) Experimental tumorigenesis with subcutaneous tablets of oestradiol. Lancet, i, 1313-1318

Lipschütz, A. & Vargas, L., Jr (1941) Structure and origin of uterine and extragenital fibroids induced experimentally in the guinea-pig by prolonged administration of estrogens. Cancer Res., 1, 236-248

Lipschütz, A., Vargas, L., Jr & Iglesias, R. (1938) Microscopic structure of uterine and abdominal tissues due to oestradiol benzoate (Fr.). C.R. Soc. Biol. (Paris), 129, 524-528

Lipschütz, A., Iglesias, R. & Vargas, L., Jr (1939) Regression of experimental fibromyomas and inhibition of epithelial tumour formation in the absence of follicular hormone (Fr.). C.R. Soc. Biol. (Paris), 130, 1536-1540

Longcope, C. (1972) The metabolism of estrone sulfate in normal males. J. clin. Endocrinol. Metab., 34, 113-122

Lycette, R.R., Whyte, S. & Chapman, C.J. (1970) Aneuploid effect of oestradiol on cultured human synovial cells. N.Z. med. J., 72, 114-117

MacCorquodale, D.W., Thayer, S.A & Doisy, E.A. (1936) The isolation of the principal estrogenic substance of liquor folliculi. J. biol. Chem., 115, 435-448 [Chem. Abstr., 30, 7653-8]

Mackenzie, I. (1955) The production of mammary cancer in rats using oestrogens. Br. J. Cancer, 9, 284-299

Málková, J., Michalová, K., Přibyl, T. & Schreiber, V. (1977) Chromosomal changes in rat pituitary and bone marrow induced by long-term estrogen administration. Neoplasma, 24, 277-284

Mathur, R.S., Leaming, A.B. & Williamson, H.O. (1975) An assessment of the total estrone, estradiol-17β and estriol in high risk pregnancy plasma. J. Steroid Biochem., 6, 1421-1427

McCormick, G.M. & Moon, R.C. (1973) Effect of increasing doses of estrogen and progesterone on mammary carcinogenesis in the rat. Eur. J. Cancer, 9, 483-486

Menzies, J.A. & Watanabe, H. (1976) Biliary metabolites of estriol in the rat. Steroids, 27, 595-601

Miescher, K. & Scholz, C. (1939) Therapeutic esters of unsaturated polyhydroxyestrane. US Patent, 2,205,627, 25 June to Society for Chemical Industry, Basel [Chem. Abstr., 34, 7542-3]

Miller, A. (1976) Cosmetic ingredients. Household and Personal Products Industry, October, pp. 57, 62, 64, 66, 68

Mori, T. (1967) Effects of early postnatal injections of estrogen on endocrine organs and sex accessories in male C3H/MS mice. J. Fac. Sci. Univ. Tokyo, Sect. IV, 11, 243-254

Mori, T. (1968a) Changes in reproductive organs and some other glands in old C3H/MS mice treated neonatally with low doses of estrogen. Annot. Zool. Jpn., 41, 43-52

Mori, T. (1968b) Changes in the reproductive and some other organs in old C3H/MS mice given high-dose estrogen injections during neonatal life. Annot. Zool. Jpn, 41, 85-94

Mori, T., Bern, H.A., Mills, K.T. & Young, P.N. (1976) Long-term effects of neonatal steroid exposure on mammary gland development and tumorigenesis in mice. J. natl Cancer Inst., 57, 1057-1062

Mori, T., Bern, H.A. & Mills, K.T. (1978) Exposure of pregnant mice to hormones: effects on the reproductive cycles and organs in their female offspring. Int. Res. Commun. med. Sci., 6, 275

Muñoz, N. (1973) Effect of herpesvirus type 2 and hormonal imbalance on the uterine cervix of the mouse. Cancer Res., 33, 1504-1508

Musey, P.I., Kirdani, R.Y., Bhanalaph, T. & Sandberg, A.A. (1973) Estriol metabolism in the baboon: analysis of urinary and biliary metabolites. Steroids, 22, 795-811

Musey, P.I., Collins, D.C. & Preedy, J.R. (1977) Estrogen metabolites in nonhuman primates. I. In vitro biosynthesis of estrogen glucosiduronates in rhesus monkey liver. Steroids, 29, 93-104

Nagasawa, H., Yanai, R., Shodono, M., Nakamura, T. & Tanabe, Y. (1974)
    Effect of neonatally administered estrogen or prolactin on normal
    and neoplastic mammary growth and serum estradiol-17β level in
    rats. Cancer Res., 34, 2643-2646

Nambara, T. & Kawarada, Y. (1975) Conjugated metabolites of estriol
    in rat bile. Chem. pharm. Bull., 23, 698-700

Nambara, T., Ishiguro, J., Kawarada, Y. & Tajima, H. (1974) Isolation
    and characterization of biliary metabolites of estriol in the
    rat. Chem. pharm. Bull., 22, 889-893

National Formulary Board (1975) National Formulary, 14th ed.,
    Washington DC, American Pharmaceutical Association, pp. 264-272

Nilsson, A. & Broomé-Karlsson, A. (1976) Influence of steroid
    hormones on the carcinogenicity of ^{90}Sr. Acta radiol. ther. phys.
    biol., 15, 417-426

Nishihara, G. (1958) Influence of female sex hormones in experimental
    teratogenesis. Proc. Soc. exp. Biol. (N.Y.), 97, 809-812

Numazawa, M., Haryu, A., Kurosaka, K. & Nambara, T. (1977) Picogram
    order enzyme immunoassay of oestradiol. Fed. eur. biochem. Soc.
    Lett., 79, 396-398

Pan, S.C. & Gardner, W.U. (1948) Carcinomas of the uterine cervix and
    vagina in estrogen- and androgen-treated hybrid mice. Cancer Res.,
    8, 337-341

Quadri, S.K., Kledzik, G.S. & Meites, J. (1974) Enhanced regression
    of DMBA-induced mammary cancers in rats by combination of
    ergocornine with ovariectomy or high doses of estrogen. Cancer
    Res., 34, 499-501

Quamme, G.A., Layne, D.S. & Williamson, D.G. (1972) The metabolism of
    ^{3}H-labelled estrone by the isolated perfused liver of the rabbit,
    chicken, and guinea-pig. Can. J. Physiol. Pharmacol., 50, 45-57

Rao, G.S., Rao, M.L., Haueter, G. & Breuer, H. (1974) Steroid
    glucuronyltransferases. V. Formation and hydrolysis of oestrogen
    glucuronides by the liver, kidney and intestine of the pig.
    Hoppe-Seyler's Z. physiol. Chem., 355, 881-890

Riesco, A. (1947) On the bearing of time on the neoplastic action of
    small quantities of α-oestradiol in the endometrium of guinea-pigs.
    Br. J. Cancer, 1, 166-172

Rudali, G., Coezy, E., Frederic, F. & Apiou, F. (1971) Susceptibility
    of mice of different strains to the mammary carcinogenic action of
    natural and synthetic oestrogens. Rev. eur. Etud. clin. Biol.,
    16, 425-429

Rudali, G., Apiou, F. & Muel, B. (1975) Mammary cancer produced in
    mice with estriol. Eur. J. Cancer, 11, 39-41

Rudali, G., Jullien, P., Vives, C. & Apiou, F. (1978) Dose-effect
    studies on estrogen induced mammary cancers in mice. Biomedicine,
    29, 45-46

Ruder, H.J., Loriaux, L. & Lipsett, M.B. (1972) Estrone sulfate:
    production rate and metabolism in man. J. clin. Invest., 51, 1020-
    1033

Ruh, T.S. (1976) Simultaneous separation of estrogens and androgens using
    thin-layer chromatography. J. Chromatogr., 121, 82-84

Rurainski, R.D., Theiss, H.J. & Zimmermann, W. (1977) Occurrence of
    natural and synthetic oestrogens in drinking-water (Ger.).
    Gas-Wasserfach. Wasser Abwasser, 118, 288-291

Satyaswaroop, P.G., Lopez de la Osa, E. & Gurpide, E. (1977) High
    pressure liquid chromatographic separation of C_{18} and C_{19} steroids.
    Steroids, 30, 139-145

Schofield, B.M. (1962) The effect of injected oestrogen on pregnancy
    in the rabbit. J. Endocrinol., 25, 95-100

Schroeder, I., López-Sánchez, G., Medina-Acevedo, J.C. & del Carmen
    Espinosa, M. (1975) Quantitative determination of conjugated or
    esterified estrogens in tablets by thin-layer chromatography.
    J. chromatogr. Sci., 13, 37-40

Schwenk, E. & Hildebrandt, F. (1936) Crystallized hormone esters.
    US Patent, 2,054,271, Sept. 15 to Schering-Kahlbaum A.-G.
    [Chem. Abstr., 30, 7788-5]

Scott, R.M. & Sawyer, R.T. (1975) Detection of steroids with molybdo-
    vanadophosphoric acids on thin-layer chromatograms. Microchem.
    J., 20, 309-312

Scully, R.E., Robboy, S.J. & Welch, W.R. (1978) Pathology and
    pathogenesis of diethylstilbestrol-related disorders of the
    female genital tract. In: Herbst, A.L., ed., Intrauterine Exposure
    to Diethylstilbestrol in the Human, Chicago, IL, American College of
    Obstetricians & Gynecologists, pp. 8-22

Serova, I.A. & Kerkis, Y.J. (1974) Cytogenetic effect of some steroid hormones and change in activity of lysosomal enzymes *in vitro*. Genetica, 10, 142-149

Shellabarger, C.J. & Soo, V.A. (1973) Effects of neonatally administered sex steroids on 7,12-dimethylbenz[*a*]anthracene-induced mammary neoplasia in rats. Cancer Res., 33, 1567-1569

Snedden, W. & Parker, R.B. (1976) The direct determination of oestrogen and progesterone in human ovarian tissue by quantitative high resolution mass spectrometry. Biomed. Mass Spectrom., 3, 295-298

Stenchever, M.A., Jarvis, J.A. & Kreger, N.K. (1969) Effect of selected estrogens and progestins on human chromosomes *in vitro*. Obstet. Gynecol., 34, 249-251

Takasugi, N. (1976) Cytological basis for permanent vaginal changes in mice treated neonatally with steroid hormones. Int. Rev. Cytol., 44, 193-224

Takasugi, N. (1979) Development of permanently proliferated and cornified vaginal epithelium in mice treated neonatally with steroid hormones and the implication in tumorigenesis. Natl Cancer Inst. Monogr., 51, 57-66

Takasugi, N. & Bern, H.A. (1964) Tissue changes in mice with persistent vaginal cornification induced in early post-natal treatment with estrogen. J. natl Cancer Inst., 33, 855-865

Takasugi, N. & Kamishima, Y. (1973) Development of vaginal epithelium showing irreversible proliferation and cornification in neonatally estrogenized mice: an electron microscope study. Dev. Growth Differ., 15, 127-140

Takasugi, N., Kimura, T. & Mori, T. (1970) Irreversible changes in mouse vaginal epithelium induced by early post-natal treatment with steroid hormones. In: Kazda, S. & Denenberg, V.H., eds, The Postnatal Development of Phenotype, Prague, Academia, pp. 229-251

Tikkanen, M.J., Nikkila, E.A. & Vartiainen, E. (1978) Natural oestrogens as an effective treatment for type II hyperlipoproteinaemia in postmenopausal women. Lancet, ii, 490-491

Trolp, R., Breckwoldt, M. & Hoff, A. (1977) Metabolism of ^{3}H-Oe$_1$-SO$_4$ in postmenopausal uterine tissue (Abstract no. 68). Acta endocrinol., Suppl. 208, 73

US Food & Drug Administration (1977a) Food and drugs. US Code Fed. Regul., Title 21, part 556.240, p. 353

US Food & Drug Administration (1977b) Patient labeling for estrogens for general use. Drugs for human use; drug efficacy study implementation. Fed. Regist., 42, 37645-37646

US International Trade Commission (1977a) Imports of Benzenoid Chemicals and Products, 1975, USITC Publication 806, Washington DC, US Government Printing Office, p. 83

US International Trade Commission (1977b) Imports of Benzenoid Chemicals and Products, 1976, USITC Publication 828, Washington DC, US Government Printing Office, p. 88

US Pharmacopeial Convention Inc. (1975) The US Pharmacopeia, 19th rev., Rockville, MD, pp. 180-181

US Tariff Commission (1940) Synthetic Organic Chemicals, US Production and Sales, 1939, Report No. 140, Second Series, Washington DC, US Government Printing Office, p. 37

US Tariff Commission (1956) Synthetic Organic Chemicals, US Production and Sales, 1955, Report No. 198, Second Series, Washington DC, US Government Printing Office, p. 111

Wade, A., ed. (1977) Martindale, The Extra Pharmacopoeia, 27th ed., London, The Pharmaceutical Press, pp. 1415-1419, 1422

Warner, M.R. & Warner, R.L. (1975) Effects of exposure of neonatal mice to 17β-estradiol on subsequent age-incidence and morphology of carcinogen-induced mammary dysplasia. J. natl Cancer Inst., 55, 289-298

Watanabe, H. & Menzies, J.A. (1973) Isolation of 16α-hydroxy-2-methoxyestrone from rat bile. Steroids, 21, 123-132

Weast, R.C., ed. (1977) CRC Handbook of Chemistry and Physics, 58th ed., Cleveland, OH, Chemical Rubber Co., p. C-290

Welsch, C.W., Adams, C., Lambrecht, L.K., Hassett, C.C. & Brooks, C.L. (1977) 17β-Oestradiol and Enovid mammary tumorigenesis in C3H/HeJ female mice: counteraction by concurrent 2-bromo-α-ergocryptine. Br. J. Cancer., 35, 322-328

Williams, K.I.H. (1970) Species difference in the structure of urinary 2-hydroxyestrone 'glucuronide'. Steroids, 15, 105-111

Windholz, M., ed. (1976) The Merck Index, 9th ed., Rahway, NJ, Merck
    & Co., pp. 485-486, 983

Woodruff, L.M. (1941) Tumors produced by estradiol benzoate in the
    guinea pig. Cancer Res., 1, 367-370

Wright, K., Collins, D.C., Musey, P.I. & Preedy, J.R.K. (1978) Direct
    radioimmunoassay of specific urinary estrogen glucosiduronates in
    normal men and nonpregnant women. Steroids, 31, 407-426

Yoshida, H. & Fukunishi, R. (1977) Effect of neonatal administration
    of sex steroids on 7,12-dimethylbenz(a)anthracene-induced
    auditory sebaceous gland tumor in female rats. Gann, 68, 851-
    852

Yoshida, H. & Fukunishi, R. (1978) Effect of neonatal administration of
    sex steroids on 7,12-dimethylbenz[a]anthracene-induced mammary
    carcinoma and dysplasia in female Sprague-Dawley rats. Gann, 69,
    627-631

Yoshizawa, I. & Fishman, J. (1971) Radioimmunoassay of 2-hydroxyestrone
    in human plasma. J. clin. Endocrinol. Metab., 32, 3-6

Yoshizawa, I., Ohuchi, R., Nakagawa, A. & Kimura, M. (1977) Metabolism
    of estrone-6,7-^{3}H in guinea pigs (Jpn.). Yakugaku Zasshi, 97, 197-201

Youssef, A.F. & Mestres, R. (1973) Gas chromatographic analysis of oil
    solutions and suppositories containing progesterone, testosterone
    oenanthate and oestradiol esters (Fr.). Trav. Soc. Pharm.
    Montpellier, 33, 35-46

Zamecnik, J., Armstrong, D.T. & Green, K. (1978) Serum estradiol-17β
    as determined by mass fragmentography and by radioimmunoassay.
    Clin. Chem., 24, 627-630

Zumoff, B., Fishman, J., Gallagher, T.F. & Hellman, L. (1968)
    Estradiol metabolism in cirrhosis. J. clin. Invest., 47, 20-25

OESTRIOL

A monograph on this substance was published previously (IARC, 1974). Relevant data that have appeared since that time have been evaluated in the present monograph.

1. Chemical and Physical Data

1.1 Synonyms and trade names

Chem. Abstr. Services Reg. No.: 50-27-1

Chem. Abstr. Name: (16α,17β)-Estra-1,3,5(10)-triene-3, 16,17-triol

Synonyms: 1,3,5-Estratriene-3β,16,17β-triol; estra-1,3,5(10)-triene-3,16α,17β-triol; estra-1,3,5(10)-triene-3,16α,17β-triol; estratriol; estriol; 16α,17β-estriol; 3,16α,17β-estriol; follicular hormone hydrate; 16α-hydroxy-estradiol; 1,3,5-oestratriene-3β,16,17β-triol; oestra-1,3,5(10)-triene-3,16α,17β-triol; oestra-1,3,5(10)-triene-3,16α,17β-triol; oestratriol; 16α,17β-oestriol; 3,16α,17β-oestriol; 16α-hydroxy-oestradiol; 3,16α,17β-trihydroxyestra-1,3,5(10)-triene; 3,16α-17β-trihydroxyoestra-1,3,5(10)-triene; 3,16α,17β-trihydroxy-Δ1,3,5-estratriene; trihydroxyestrin; 3,16α,17β-trihydroxy-Δ1,3,5-oestratriene; trihydroxyoestrin

Trade names[1]: Aacifemine; [Colpovister]; Destriol; Deuslon-A; [Gynaesan]; Hemostyptanon; Holin; Hormomed; Hormonin; Klimoral; NSC-12169; OE3; Orgastyptin; Ovesterin; Ovestin; [Ovestinon]; Ovestrion; Stiptanon; Synapause; Theelol; Tridestrin; Triodurin; Triovex

---

[1]Those in square brackets are preparations that are no longer produced commercially.

1.2 Structural and molecular formulae and molecular weight

$$C_{18}H_{24}O_3 \qquad\qquad\qquad Mol.\ wt:\ \ 288.4$$

1.3 Chemical and physical properties of the pure substance

From Wade (1977) and Windholz (1976), unless otherwise specified

(a) Description: Monoclinic crystals from dilute ethanol

(b) Melting-point: Rearrangement of the crystal structure takes place at $270^{\circ}C$ and $275^{\circ}C$; melts at $282^{\circ}C$

(c) Spectroscopic data: λ_{max} 280 nm; infra-red and nuclear magnetic resonance spectral data have been tabulated (Grasselli & Ritchey, 1975).

(d) Optical rotation: $[\alpha]_D^{25}$ $+58^{\circ} \pm 5^{\circ}$ (4% w/v dioxane)

(e) Solubility: Practically insoluble in water; sparingly soluble in ethanol (1 in 500); soluble in acetone, dioxane, chloroform, diethyl ether, pyridine, vegetable oils and aqueous solutions of alkaline hydroxides

1.4 Technical products and impurities

Various national and international pharmacopoeias give specifications for the purity of oestriol in pharmaceutical products. For example, oestriol is available in the US as a USP grade containing 97–102% active ingredient on a dried basis, and not more than 2% foreign steroids and other impurities. Residue on ignition must not exceed 0.1%. Tablets are available containing 0.135 mg and 0.27 mg oestriol in combination with 0.7 mg and 1.4 mg oestrone and 0.30 mg and 0.60 mg oestradiol, respectively (Litton Industries Inc., 1978; US Pharmacopeial Convention Inc., 1978, 1979)

In the UK, tablets are available containing 0.25 mg oestriol alone or 0.27 mg in combination with 1.4 mg oestrone or 0.60 mg oestradiol (Wade, 1977).

2.   Production, Use, Occurrence and Analysis

2.1 Production and use

(a)   Production

Isolation of oestriol from the urine of pregnant women was first reported by Marrian in 1929 (Windholz, 1976). An extraction and crystallization process was used commercially for the isolation of oestriol from pregnant mares' urine for several years. In a synthetic route reported in 1954, oestrone is converted to its enol acetate with isopropenyl acetate, which in turn is treated with perbenzoic acid to give the $16\alpha,17\alpha$-epoxide; this is treated with perchloric acid in acetic acid followed by lithium aluminium hydride reduction to produce oestriol (Leeds *et al*., 1954). It is not known whether this is the process used for commercial production.

Oestriol is not produced commercially in the US, and separate data on US imports are not available.

It is believed to be produced commercially in the Federal Republic of Germany, France, Italy, The Netherlands and the UK, but no information was available on the quantities produced.

It was first marketed in Japan in 1962. It is not produced there, and imports were about 40 kg in 1975 and 1976 and 30 kg in 1977.

(b)   Use

Oestriol is used alone or in combination with oestrone and oestradiol for treatment of symptoms of the climacteric at daily doses of 0.25-0.5 mg. It is also used locally in the treatment of atrophic or senile vaginitis and vulvovaginitis. The usual dose is 0.06-0.12 mg given 1-4 times daily. Doses of up to 1 mg daily have been given in the treatment of dysmenorrhoea (Harvey, 1975; Wade, 1977).

In Japan, oestriol is used in tablet and injection form for the treatment of vaginitis and climacteric symptoms.

Less than 1000 kg oestriol are used in France annually.

The US Food & Drug Administration (1977) has ruled that, with effect from 20 September 1977, oestrogens for general use must carry patient and physician warning labels concerning use, risks and contra-indications.

2.2 Occurrence

Oestriol is a widely-occurring natural oestrogen (see 'General Remarks on Sex Hormones', pp. 42-56). It has also been found in plant material, e.g., the flowers of *Salix* (pussy-willows) (Sharzyński, 1933).

In the 1974 National Occupational Hazard Survey conducted by the US National Institute for Occupational Safety & Health, exposure to oestriol was found to occur in industries manufacturing pharmaceutical preparations. On the basis of these data, it is estimated that 1230 US workers were exposed to oestriol in 1974 (US National Institute for Occupational Safety & Health, 1977).

2.3 Analysis

Analytical methods for the determination of oestriol in plasma and urine based on gas chromatography, spectrophotometry and radioimmunoassay have been reviewed (Abraham *et al.*, 1977; Chattoraj & Wotiz, 1975).

Typical analytical methods are summarized in Table 1. Abbreviations used are: GC, gas chromatography; GC/ECD, gas chromatography/electron-capture detection; GC/FID, gas chromatography/flame-ionization detection; GC/MS, gas chromatography/mass spectrometry; CC, column chromatography; HPLC, high-pressure liquid chromatography; MS, mass spectrometry; UV, ultra-violet spectrometry; RIA, radioimmunoassay; CPB, competitive protein binding; and FL, fluorimetry. See also the 'General Remarks on Sex Hormones', p. 60.

TABLE 1

Analytical methods for oestriol

Sample matrix	Sample preparation	Assay procedure	Sensitivity or limit of detection	Reference
Bulk chemical	Dissolve (ethanol)	UV (281 nm)	-	US Pharmacopeial Convention Inc. (1978)
Bulk chemical	Dissolve	HPLC	-	Hara & Hayashi (1977)
Bulk chemical	Dissolve	TLC	-	Ruh (1976)
Plasma	Add labelled oestriol; extract (dichloromethane); CC (Celite); add antiserum	RIA	-	Abraham et al. (1977)
Plasma	Dilute (buffer, pH 4.1); extract (diethyl ether); hydrolyse aqueous phase (enzyme); extract (diethyl ether); combine extracts; extract (sodium hydroxide); methylate; extract (benzene); CC (alumina); derivatize (trimethylsilyl)	GC/MS	10–30 pg	Adlercreutz et al. (1974)
Plasma	Hydrolyse (hydrochloric acid); add buffer; extract (diethyl ether); evaporate; partition (water/benzene:hexane, 1:1); extract aqueous phase (diethyl ether); dissolve (sulphuric acid)	FL	0.013 µg/ml	Mathur et al. (1972, 1975)
Plasma	Hydrolyse (hydrochloric acid); adjust to pH 10.5; extract (diethyl ether); evaporate; suspend (water); wash (benzene:hexane, 1:1); extract (diethyl ether); evaporate; dissolve (Kober reagent)	FL (537/563 nm)	> 300 pg	Miklosi et al. (1975)

Table 1 (continued)

Sample matrix	Sample preparation	Assay procedure	Sensitivity or limit of detection	Reference
Plasma	Add labelled oestriol; CC (Sephadex); add antiserum	RIA	0.2 µg/l	Miller & Fetter (1977)
Plasma	Extract (chloroform:methanol, 2:1); TLC	GC	-	Sharma & Subramanian (1974)
Plasma	Extract (dichloromethane); evaporate; add antiserum & labelled oestriol	RIA	0.2-0.6 ng/ml (0.1 ml sample)	Thompson & Haven (1977)
Plasma	Saturate (sodium chloride); extract (tetrahydrofuran); CC (Sephadex); derivatize (heptafluorobutyrate)	GC/ECD	50 pg/ml	Touchstone & Dobbins (1975)
Plasma	Add labelled oestriol; extract (diethyl ether); evaporate; dissolve (buffer); wash (benzene:petroleum ether, 1:1)	CPB	50 pg (0.5 ml sample)	Wilkinson et al. (1972)
Urine	Hydrolyse (hydrochloric acid); adjust to pH 6.8-7.0; dilute; add labelled oestriol; add antiserum	RIA	2.3 µg/l (25 µl sample)	Anderson & Goebelsmann (1976)
Urine	Hydrolyse; extract; CC (Sephadex)	GC/MS	-	Bègue et al. (1974)
Urine	Precipitate (ammonium sulphate); hydrolyse (β-glucuronidase); wash (benzene:petroleum ether, 1:1); extract (diethyl ether); wash (sodium carbonate)	FL (310 nm)	2 µg/ml	Bramhall & Britten (1976)

Table 1 (continued)

Sample matrix	Sample preparation	Assay procedure	Sensitivity or limit of detection	Reference
Urine	Hydrolyse (hydrochloric acid); extract (diethyl ether); wash (sodium carbonate)	HPLC	20 ng (40 ml sample)	Dolphin, 1973; Dolphin & Pergande (1977)
Urine	Hydrolyse (sulphuric acid); add equilin; extract (diethyl ether); wash (sodium bicarbonate); extract (sodium hydroxide); acidify (hydrochloric acid); extract (diethyl ether); derivatize (trimethylsilyl)	GC/FID	–	Gold & Mathew (1977)
Urine	Hydrolyse (sulphuric acid); extract; TLC	GC	–	Sharma & Subramanian (1974)
Urine	Add labelled oestriol; hydrolyse (hydrochloric acid); extract (diethyl ether); wash (sodium carbonate); extract (sodium hydroxide); extract (diethyl ether); derivatize (acetate)	GC	–	Thompson & Haven (1977)
Urine	Dilute (water); hydrolyse (hydrochloric acid); extract (diethyl ether); wash (sodium bicarbonate); extract (sodium hydroxide); adjust to pH 2-4 (hydrochloric acid); extract (diethyl ether); wash (sodium bicarbonate, water)	TLC	0.05 µg	Wortmann et al. (1974)
Tissue	Homogenize (acetonitrile:water, 9:1); filter; wash (hexane); add benzene; wash (sodium carbonate); extract (sodium hydroxide); acidify (hydrochloric acid); extract (benzene)	TLC; high-performance TLC	50-200 ng 10-200 ng	Jarc et al. (1977)

Table 1 (continued)

Sample matrix	Sample preparation	Assay procedure	Sensitivity or limit of detection	Reference
Breast tumour tissue	Homogenize (acetone); decant; evaporate; dissolve (80% aqueous methanol); wash (petroleum ether); evaporate; dissolve (diethyl ether); wash (water); derivatize (trimethylsilyl)	GC/MS	10 pg/µl	Millington et al. (1974)
Ovarian tissue	Dry	MS	1 ng	Snedden & Parker (1976)
Amniotic fluid	Wash (hexane); absorb (Amberlite XAD-2; elute (methanolic 0.75% hydro-quinone diacetate); evap-orate; dissolve (2% Quino in 65% sulphuric acid); extract (tetrachloroethane containing para-nitrophenol)	Colorimetry (510, 540 & 570 nm)	–	Ryu et al. (1974)
Amniotic fluid	Dilute (water); perform a series of extractions and washings	GC (argon-ion detection)	1 µg/100 ml (5 ml sample)	Touchstone et al. (1972)

3. Biological Data Relevant to the Evaluation
of Carcinogenic Risk to Humans

3.1 Carcinogenicity studies in animals

Subcutaneous implantation

Mouse: Paraffin pellets containing 10% oestradiol-17β or 10% oestriol (0.64-0.85 mg oestrogen) were implanted subcutaneously into castrated male and female (C3H x RIII)F1 (MTV$^+$)[1] mice and castrated male RIII (MTV$^+$) mice on day 22-24 of life. Controls received a pellet containing only paraffin. The RIII males received only oestriol or control pellets. Pellets recovered from mice at sacrifice 4-5 months after implantation contained 2-5% oestrogen; it was thus assumed that most mice absorbed at least several hundred µg of oestrogen. Mammary tumours (type not stated) occurred in 15/16 female and 15/16 male F1 hybrids treated with oestradiol-17β, in 18/18 female and 25/30 male F1 hybrids treated with oestriol and in 28/34 female and 10/61 male control hybrids. The latent periods were 176 (+31), 133 (+10) and 446 (+28) days, respectively, in females and 137 (+15), 135 (+44) and 567 (+54) days, respectively, in males. All castrated RIII males treated with oestriol developed mammary tumours in 137+6 days, compared with 0/22 controls (Rudali et al., 1975).

Rat: Oestradiol-17β, oestriol and oestrone were administered subcutaneously to intact female Sprague-Dawley rats 48 hrs before treatment with 7,12-dimethylbenz[a]anthracence (DMBA) or procarbazine as 1-20% pellets weighing 5-7 mg each. DMBA and procarbazine were given by gavage at amounts of 20 and 50-70 mg, respectively. No mammary cancers occurred up to 370 days in untreated controls or in oestrogen-treated female rats. Higher doses of oestriol (0.53-0.65 mg/pellet) had an inhibitory effect on carcinogen-induced tumour development (Lemon, 1975).

Hamster: Hamsters of heterogeneous origin were given s.c. implants of 20 mg pellets of oestriol, reimplanted every 150 days to ensure constant absorption, for 318-601 days. After latent periods of 396-593 days, 6/11 animals developed tumours in one or both kidneys. No data on controls were reported (Kirkman, 1959).

---

[1]MTV+: mammary tumour virus expressed (see p. 62)

3.2 Other relevant biological data

Oestriol has about 1/10 the activity of oestradiol-17β or oestrone after s.c. administration (Diczfalusy & Lauritzen, 1961).

Administration of 0.1 μmol oestriol to Wistar rats from day 16-19 of gestation induced partial feminization of male foetuses (Bruni *et al.*, 1975).

Treatment of female rats with 10 μg oestriol 7 days before mating led to a reduction of one-third of the litter size. Treatment on day of mating had only a slight effect on litter size; treatment during the early period of gestation (first 5-6 days) decreased litter size by two-thirds; and treatment on day of mating and on day 4 reduced litter size by one-third (Velardo *et al.*, 1956).

Oestriol is a common metabolite of oestrone and oestradiol-17β (see monograph on oestradiol-17β, p. 307) in animals and in humans. Oestriol is excreted in humans as conjugated and unconjugated 2-hydroxyoestriol after 2-hydroxylation (Gelbke & Knuppen, 1974).

No data on the mutagenicity of oestriol were available.

3.3 Case reports and epidemiological studies

See the section, 'Oestrogens and Progestins in Relation to Human Cancer', p. 83.

4. Summary of Data Reported and Evaluation[1]

4.1 Experimental data

Oestriol was tested by subcutaneous implantation in castrated mice and in rats and hamsters. It increased the incidence and accelerated the appearance of mammary tumours in both male and female mice and produced kidney tumours in hamsters.

Oestriol is embryolethal, especially for preimplantation embryos, in some species.

----

[1]This section should be read in conjunction with pp. 62-64 in the 'General Remarks on Sex Hormones' and with the 'General Conclusions on Sex Hormones', p. 131.

4.2 Human data

No case reports or epidemiological studies on oestriol alone were available to the Working Group. Case reports and epidemiological studies on steroid hormones used in oestrogen treatment have been summarized in the section, 'Oestrogens and Progestins in Relation to Human Cancer', p. 83.

4.3 Evaluation

There is *limited evidence* for the carcinogenicty of oestriol in experimental animals. Studies in humans strongly suggest that the administration of oestrogens is causally related to an increased incidence of endometrial carcinoma; there is no evidence that oestriol is different from other oestrogens in this respect.

5. References

Abraham, G.E., Manlimos, F.S. & Garza, R. (1977) Radioimmunoassay of steroids. In: Abraham, G.E., ed., Handbook of Radioimmunoassay, New York, Marcel Dekker, pp. 591-656

Adlercreutz, H., Nylander, P. & Hunneman, D.H. (1974) Studies on the mass fragmentographic determination of plasma estriol. Biomed. Mass Spectrom., 1, 332-339

Anderson, D.W. & Goebelsmann, U. (1976) A rapid radioimmunoassay of total urinary estriol. Clin. Chem., 22, 611-615

Bègue, R.J., Desgrès, J., Padieu, P. & Gustafsson, J.A. (1974) Method of analysis of urinary steroids of human pregnancy by GLC and GC-MS of Sephadex LH-20 chromatographic fractions. J. chromatogr. Sci., 12, 763-766

Bramhall, J. & Britten, A.Z. (1976) A new rapid assay of estrogens in pregnancy urine using the substrate native fluorescence. Clin. chim. acta, 68, 203-213

Bruni, G., Rossi, G.L., Celasco, G. & Falconi, G. (1975) Effects of estriol and quinestradol administered in pregnant rats on fetal sexual differentiation (Ital.). Ann. Obstet. Ginecol. Med. Perinatal., 96, 83-90

Chattoraj, S.C. & Wotiz, H.H. (1975) Estrogens. In: Dorfman, R.I., ed., Steroid Hormones, Amsterdam, North-Holland, pp. 3-49

Diczfalusy, E. & Lauritzen, C. (1961) Oestrogene beim Menschen, Berlin, Springer

Dolphin, R.J. (1973) The analysis of estrogenic steroids in urine by high-speed liquid chromatography. J. Chromatogr., 83, 421-429

Dolphin, R.J. & Pergande, P.J. (1977) Improved method for the analysis of estrogenic steroids in pregnancy urine by high-performance liquid chromatography. J. Chromatogr., 143, 267-274

Gelbke, H.P. & Knuppen, R. (1974) Identification and quantitative determination of 2-hydroxyoestriol in human late-pregnancy urine. J. Steroid Biochem., 5, 1-7

Gold, M. & Mathew, G. (1977) The use of equilin as an internal standard to quantitate estriol in pregnancy urine. Clin. Biochem., 10, 191-192

Grasselli, J.G. & Ritchey, W.M., eds (1975) CRC Atlas of Spectral Data
    and Physical Constants for Organic Compounds, 2nd ed., Vol. III,
    Cleveland, OH, Chemical Rubber Co., p. 234

Hara, S. & Hayashi, S. (1977) Correlation of retention behaviour of
    steroidal pharmaceuticals in polar and bonded reversed-phase
    liquid column chromatography. J. Chromatogr., 142, 689-703

Harvey, S.C. (1975) Hormones. In: Osol, A. et al., eds, Remington's
    Pharmaceutical Sciences, 15th ed., Easton, PA, Mack, pp. 912-
    913, 917

IARC (1974) IARC Monographs on the Evaluation of Carcinogenic Risk
    of Chemicals to Man, 6, Sex Hormones, Lyon, pp. 117-121

Jarc, H., Ruttner, O. & Krocza, W. (1977) The quantitative detection
    of estrogens and antithyroid drugs by thin-layer and high-performance
    thin-layer chromatography in animal tissue (Ger.). J. Chromatogr.,
    134, 351-358

Kirkman, H. (1959) Estrogen-induced tumors of the kidney. III. Growth
    characteristics in the Syrian hamster. Natl Cancer Inst. Monogr.,
    1, 1-57

Leeds, N.S., Fukushima, D.K. & Gallagher, T.F. (1954) Studies on steroid
    ring D epoxides of enol acetates; a new synthesis of estriol and of
    androstane-3β,16α,17β-triol. J. Am. chem. Soc., 76, 2943-2948

Lemon, H.M. (1975) Estriol prevention of mammary carcinoma induced by
    7,12-dimethylbenzanthracene and procarbazine. Cancer Res., 35,
    1341-1353

Litton Industries Inc. (1978) Supplement B - 1978 PDR (Physician's
    Desk Reference), Oradell, NJ, Medical Economics Co., p. 736

Mathur, R.S., Leaming, A.B. & Williamson, H.O. (1972) A simplified method
    for estimation of estriol in pregnancy plasma. Am. J. Obstet.
    Gynecol., 113, 1120-1129

Mathur, R.S., Leaming, A.B. & Williamson, H.O. (1975) An assessment of
    the total estrone, estradiol-17β and estriol in high risk pregnancy
    plasma. J. Steroid Biochem., 6, 1421-1427

Miklosi, S., Biggs, J.S.G., Selvage, N., Canning, J. & Lythal, G. (1975)
    A rapid method for the estimation of estriol in plasma during
    pregnancy. Steroids, 26, 671-681

Miller, C.A. & Fetter, M.C. (1977) A rapid radioimmunoassay for serum
    unconjugated estriol with a directly iodinated estriol radioligand.
    J. Lab. clin. Med., 89, 1125-1134

Millington, D., Jenner, D.A., Jones, T. & Griffiths, K. (1974) Endogenous steroid concentrations in human breast tumours determined by high-resolution mass fragmentography. Biochem. J., 139, 473-475

Rudali, G., Apiou, F. & Muel, B. (1975) Mammary cancer produced in mice with estriol. Eur. J. Cancer, 11, 39-41

Ruh, T.S. (1976) Simultaneous separation of estrogens and androgens using thin-layer chromatography. J. Chromatogr., 121, 82-84

Ryu, M., Hoshaku, K., Kosaka, J. & Fugiwara, Y. (1974) Measurement of estriol in amniotic fluid using Amberlite XAD-2. Horumon To Rinsho, 22, 1091-1094 [Chem. Abstr., 82, 1728y]

Sharma, D.P. & Subramanian, T.A.V. (1974) Simultaneous determination of adreno-ovarian steroids from a single aliquot. Biochem. Med., 11, 103-113

Sharzyński, B. (1933) An oestrogenic substance from plant material. Nature, 131, 766

Snedden, W. & Parker, R.B. (1976) The direct determination of oestrogen and progesterone in human ovarian tissue by quantitative high resolution mass spectrometry. Biomed. Mass Spectrom., 3, 295-298

Thompson, J. & Haven, G. (1977) Evaluation of a radioimmunoassay for serum unconjugated estriol using commercial reagents. Am. J. clin. Pathol., 68, 474-480

Touchstone, J.C. & Dobbins, M.F. (1975) Direct determination of steroidal sulfates. J. Steroid Biochem., 6, 1389-1392

Touchstone, J.C., Murawec, T. & Bolognese, R.J. (1972) Gas-chromaographic determination of total estriol in amniotic fluid. Clin. Chem., 18, 129-130

US Food & Drug Administration (1977) Patient labeling for estrogens for general use. Drugs for human use; drug efficacy study implementation. Fed. Regist., 42, 37645-37646

US National Institute for Occupational Safety & Health (1977) 1974 National Occupational Hazard Survey, Cincinnati, OH, p. 4,617

US Pharmacopeial Convention Inc. (1978) The US Pharmacopeia, 19th rev., 4th suppl., Rockville, MD, p. 73

US Pharmacopeial Convention Inc. (1979) The US Pharmacopeia, 19th rev., 5th suppl., Rockville, MD, pp. 79-80

Velardo, J.T., Raney, N.M., Smith, B.G. & Sturgis, S.H. (1956) Effect of various steroids on gestation and litter size in rats. *Fertil. Steril.*, 7, 301-311

Wade, A., ed. (1977) *Martindale, The Extra Pharmacopoeia*, 27th ed., London, The Pharmaceutical Press, p. 1419

Wilkinson, M., Effer, S.B., Younglai, E.V. & Gupta, K. (1972) Free estriol in human pregnancy plasma. *Am. J. Obstet. Gynecol.*, 114, 867-872

Windholz, M., ed. (1976) *The Merck Index*, 9th ed., Rahway, NJ, Merck & Co., p. 487

Wortmann, W., Wortmann, B., Schnabel, C. & Touchstone, J.C. (1974) Rapid determination of estriol of pregnancy by spectrodensitrometry of thin layer chromatograms. *J. chromatogr. Sci.*, 12, 377-379

OESTRONE and OESTRONE BENZOATE

A monograph on oestrone was published previously (IARC, 1974).
Relevant data that have appeared since that time have been evaluated in
the present monograph.

1. Chemical and Physical Data

Oestrone

1.1 Synonyms and trade names

Chem. Abstr. Services Reg. No.: 53-16-7

Chem. Abstr. Name: 3-Hydroxyestra-1,3,5(10)-trien-17-one

Synonyms: E_1; 1,3,5-estratrien-3-ol-17-one; estrone; follicular
hormone; folliculin; ketohydroxyestrin; ketohydroxyoestrin;
1,3,5-oestratrien-3-ol-17-one; theelin; thelykinin; tokokin

Trade names[1]: Andrestraq; Aquacrine; A.T.V.; Bestrone; Centro-
gen-20; Cormone; Crinovaryl; Cristallovar; Crystogen; Destrone;
Di-Est Modified; Di-Met; Disynformon; Duogen; Endofolliculina;
Esterone; Estrol; Estrolin; Estromone; Estron; [Estrone-A];
Estronol; Estrovag; Estrovarin; Estrugenone; Estrusol; Evagen;
Femestrone injection; Femidyn; Femogen; Femspan; Folikrin;
Folipex; Folisan; Follestrine; Follestrol; Follicormone;
Follicunodis; Follidrin; Follikulin; Foygen; Glandubolin;
Glyestrin; Gravigen; [Harmogen]; Hiestrone; Hormofollin;
[Hormonin]; Hormovarine; Kestrin; Kestrone; Ketodestrin;
[Klimkton]; Kolpon; Mal-O-Fem; Menagen; Menformon; Mer-Estrone;
Neo-Genic DA; Oestrilin; Oestrin; Oestroform; Oestroglandol;
Oestroperos; Ovex; Ovifollin; [Percutacrine Lut.]; [Percutacrine
Oest.]; Perlatan; [Proluton D]; Solestrin; Solliculin;

---

[1]Those in square brackets are preparations that are no longer
produced commercially.

Spanestrin; [Templodine]; Testagen; Thelestrin; Thynestron; Tri-Es; Tri-Estrin; [Trioestrine]; Unden; Urestrin; Wehgen; Wynestron

1.2 Structural and molecular formulae and molecular weight

$C_{18}H_{22}O_2$ Mol. wt: 270.4

1.3 Chemical and physical properties

From Wade (1977) and Windholz (1976), unless otherwise specified

(a) Description: White crystals (from acetone)

(b) Melting-point: d-form (natural), 254.5-256°C; dl-form, 251-254°C

(c) Spectroscopy data: λ_{max} 283-285 nm; infra-red spectra have been tabulated (Grasselli & Ritchey, 1975).

(d) Optical rotation: $[\alpha]_D^{25}$ +158 to +168°(dioxane)
$[\alpha]_D^{22}$ +152° (0.995% w/v in chloroform)

(e) Solubility: 3 mg in 100 ml water at 25°C; 1 g in 250 ml 96% ethanol at 15°C, in 50 ml boiling ethanol, in 50 ml acetone at 15°C, in 110 ml chloroform at 15°C and 145 ml boiling benzene; soluble in fixed oils (1 in 800), dioxane, pyridine and fixed alkaline hydroxide solutions; slightly soluble in absolute ethanol, diethyl ether and vegetable oils

1.4 Technical products and impurities

Various national and international pharmacopoeias give specifications for the purity of oestrone in pharmaceutical products. For example, oestrone is available in the US as a NF grade containing 97-103% active

ingredient on a dried basis and not more than 3% foreign steroids and
other impurities.   Injections in 0.2, 0.5 and 1 mg/ml doses in a suitable oil and aqueous suspensions in 1, 2, and 5 mg/ml doses contain 90-
115% of the stated amount of oestrone (National Formulary Board, 1975).
It is also available in the US in 2 mg/ml doses in aqueous suspensions
combined with potassium oestrone sulphate (1 mg) and/or oestradiol (0.2 mg)
or with testosterone (10 or 25 mg).   Suppositories containing 0.2 mg
oestrone in a glycerin-gelatin base or in combination with 50 mg lactose
in polyethylene glycols are also available (Kastrup, 1977, 1978).

In Japan, oestrone is available in tablets.

Oestrone benzoate

1.1   Synonyms and trade names

Chem. Abstr. Services Reg. No.:   2393-53-5

Chem. Abstr. Name: 3-(Benzoyloxy)estra-1,3,5(10)-trien-17-one

Synonym: Estrone benzoate

1.2   Structural and molecular formulae and molecular weight

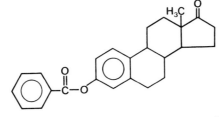

$C_{25}H_{26}O_3$ Mol. wt: 374

1.3   Chemical and physical properties

No data were available to the Working Group.

1.4   Technical products and impurities

No data were available to the Working Group.

2. Production, Use, Occurrence and Analysis

2.1 Production and use

(a) Production

The isolation of oestrone in crystalline form, from the urine of pregnant women, was first reported by Butenandt (1929) and by Doisy *et al.* (1929); the first total synthesis of oestrone from methyl-1-keto-2-methyl-7-methoxy-1,2,3,4,4a,9,10,10a-octahydro-2-phenanthrene-carboxylate was reported by Anner & Miescher (1948). Oestrone can be prepared by extraction from pregnant mares' urine and by various synthetic methods: (1) from diosgenin (extracted from the Mexican yam, *Dioscorea mexicana*) *via* 16-dehydropregnenolone acetate, which is obtained by acetolysis, chromic acid oxidation and cleavage of the ketoester di-acetate with boiling acetic acid; the 16-dehydropregnenolone acetate is converted to the 20-oxime followed by a Beckmann rearrangement with *para*-acetamidobenzenesulphonyl chloride to the 17-acetamido derivative, which is treated with dilute sulphuric acid to form the enamine acetate, and subsequent aromatization to oestrone (Harvey, 1975); (2) from sitosterol, a by-product of soya bean processing, by an oxidation step involving myco-bacterial fermentation to the steroid intermediate, androst-4-ene-3,17-dione (Anon., 1975); and (3) from cholesterol (extracted from wool grease) *via* a fermentation process yielding suitable steroid intermediates (Anon., 1977).

Oestrone benzoate can be prepared by benzoylation of the phenolic hydroxyl group of oestrone with benzoyl chloride.

Commercial production of oestrone in the US was first reported in 1941 (US Tariff Commission, 1945) and was last reported in 1955 (US Tariff Commission, 1956). Data on US imports and exports are not available.

Commercial production of oestrone in the UK was first reported in 1937. It is produced commercially in France, The Netherlands and the UK, but no information was available on the quantities produced. In 1977, European imports are estimated to have amounted to 2-20 million kg.

Oestrone was first marketed commercially in Japan in 1966. It is not produced there, and imports have been negligible in recent years.

No evidence was found that oestrone benzoate has ever been produced commercially in the US, Europe or Japan.

(b) Use

Oestrone is a metabolite of the most potent naturally occurring oestrogen, oestradiol-17β. It is used in human medicine: (1) for the treatment of symptoms occurring during or after the climacteric and following ovariectomy, in an initial i.m. dose of 0.1-1.5 mg per week in 2 or 3 divided doses, followed by gradual reductions to the lowest effective maintenance dose; (2) for dysfunctional uterine bleeding, in a daily dose of 2-5 mg until bleeding stops, followed by a cyclic regimen of 1 mg per day for 20 days with a progestin added during the 11th-20th day or 16th-20th day and a rest of 10 days; (3) for prostatic carcinoma, in a dose of 5-20 mg per week in 2-3 divided doses (Harvey, 1975); (4) for female hypogonadism and primary ovarian failure; and (5) for atrophic vaginitis (associated with the climacteric), administered in a vaginal suppository or intramuscularly (Kastrup, 1978).

Oestrone has also been used in hormonal skin preparations for cosmetic use at levels of less than 0.1%. Unspecified oestrogen and oestrogenic hormones, which are believed to consist mainly of oestrone (Miller, 1976), have been used in hormonal skin preparations (at levels of < 0.1%-5%), moisturizing lotions (1-5%), wrinkle-smoothing creams, hair conditioners, hair straighteners, shampoos and grooming aid tonics (< 0.1%).

In Japan, oestrone is used in women in the treatment of climacteric symptoms.

The US Food & Drug Administration (1977) has ruled that, with effect from 20 September 1977, oestrogens for general use must carry patient and physician warning labels concerning use, risks and contraindications.

2.2 Occurrence

Oestrone is a naturally occurring substance (see section 'General Remarks on Sex Hormones', pp. 42-56) found in the urine of pregnant women, mares, bulls and stallions, in the follicular liquor of many animals, in human placentas and in palm-kernel oil (Windholz, 1976). It has also been found in plant material, e.g., in the roots of moghat (*Clossostemon bruguieri*) and in the pollen grains of the date palm (*Phoenix dactylifera*) (Amin *et al.*, 1969).

Oestrone benzoate is not known to occur naturally.

2.3 Analysis

Analytical methods for determining oestrone in biological matrices based on radioisotopic (Abraham *et al.*, 1977; Doerr, 1976) and general techniques (Chattoraj & Wotiz, 1975) have been reviewed. Typical analytical methods are summarized in Table 1. Abbreviations used are:

GC, gas chromatography; MS, mass spectrometry; RIA, radioimmunoassay;
GC/FID, gas chromatography/flame-ionization detection; GC/MS, gas
chromatography/mass spectrometry; HPLC, high-pressure liquid chromatography; TLC, thin-layer chromatography; HPTLC, high-performance thin-
layer chromatography; CC, column-chromatography; FL, fluorimetry;
UV, ultra-violet spectrometry.   See also 'General Remarks on Sex
Hormones', p. 60.

TABLE 1

Analytical methods for oestrone

Sample matrix	Sample preparation	Assay procedure	Sensitivity or limit of detection	Reference
Bulk chemical	Dissolve	HPLC (UV, 254 nm)	-	Butterfield et al. (1973)
Bulk chemical	Dissolve (ethanol)	UV (280 nm)	-	Council of Europe (1971)
Bulk chemical	Dissolve (ethanol)	UV (280 nm)	-	National Formulary Board (1975)
Bulk chemical	Derivatize (dimethylphosphinyl); purify (TLC)	GC (alkaline flame-ionization detector)	10 pg	Vogt et al. (1974)
Tablet formulations (sulphate salt)	Hydrolyse (hydrochloric acid); neutralize (sodium bicarbonate); extract (chloroform); TLC; elute (sodium hydroxide)	UV (296 nm)	-	Schroeder et al. (1975)
Aqueous suspensions	Dissolve (acetone); filter; derivatize (dansyl)	FL (502 nm)	0.5 µg/ml	Fishman (1975)
Injection	Perform a series of extractions, washings & evaporations	Gravimetry	-	National Formulary Board (1975)
Sterile suspension	Filter; wash (water); dissolve (ethanol)	UV (280 nm)	-	National Formulary Board (1975)
Serum	Extract	TLC	20 ng	Jarc et al. (1977)
Plasma	Add radiolabelled oestrone; hydrolyse (hydrochloric acid); perform a series of extractions, washings & evaporations; TLC; elute (diethyl ether); add Ittich reagent	FL	50 ng (1 ml sample)	Mathur et al. (1975)

Table 1 (continued)

Sample matrix	Sample preparation	Assay procedure	Sensitivity or limit of detection	Reference
Urine	Hydrolyse (enzyme); extract (ethyl acetate-hexane-ethanol); CC (anion-exchange); derivatize (trimethylsilyl)	GC/FID	40 µg/l (50 ml sample)	Adessi et al. (1975)
Urine	Hydrolyse; perform a series of extractions, washings & evaporations; CC (Sephadex LH-20); derivatize (trimethylsilyl)	GC/MS	-	Bègue et al. (1974)
Urine	Hydrolyse (hydrochloric acid); extract (diethyl ether)	HPLC (UV, 230 nm)	-	Dolphin & Pergande (1977)
Urine	Extract; CC (Sephadex LH 20); derivatize (trimethylsilyl)	GC (open tubular column)	-	Fels et al. (1975)
Urine	Add antiserum and tracer; incubate; add dextran-coated charcoal; incubate & centrifuge	RIA	2.6 pg	Wright et al. (1978)
Serum and urine	Extract (diethyl ether); derivatize (trimethylsilyl)	GC/MS	2 pg	Heki et al. (1977)
Serum	Hydrolyse (enzyme); extract (diethyl ether); add antiserum and tracer (non-chromatographic RIA)	RIA	0.33 nM (200 µl sample)	Carlström & Sköldefors (1977)
Biological fluids	Perform a series of extractions, filtrations, hydrolysis & CC; derivatize (trimethylsilyl)	GC/MS	-	Adlercreutz et al. (1975)
Human breast tumour	Homogenize (acetone); perform a series of extractions, washings & evaporations; derivatize (trimethylsilyl)	GC/MS	1 ng/g wet wt	Millington et al. (1974)

Table 1 (continued)

Sample matrix	Sample preparation	Assay procedure	Sensitivity or limit of detection	Reference
Human ovarian tissue	Dissect; dry	MS	–	Snedden & Parker (1976)
Animal tissue	Homogenize (acetonitrile-water); perform a series of extractions, washings and evaporations; dissolve (anhydrous ethanol)	HPTLC (UV, 287 nm)	10 ng	Jarc et al. (1977)

3. Biological Data Relevant to the Evaluation
of Carcinogenic Risk to Humans

3.1 Carcinogenicity studies in animals

(a) Oral administration

Mouse: Administration of 125 µg/l oestrone in the drinking-water resulted in the appearance of mammary tumours in 33/68 gonadectomized male C3H and C3He mice (MTV⁻)[1].   With a concentration of 2000 µg/l, the incidence of these tumours increased to 119/169.   No data were given on controls (Boot & Muhlbock, 1956).

In castrated male (C3H × RIII)Fl mice (MTV⁺)[1] fed 0, 0.06, 0.6 or 6 µg oestrone per day in the diet, the incidences of mammary tumours were 12/33, 11/33, 15/30 and 33/34, respectively, with average latent periods of 540, 535, 475 and 190 days (Rudali et al., 1978).

(b) Skin application

Mouse: Mammary tumours were observed in 5/5 male RIII mice (MTV+) after skin application of oestrone as a 0.01% solution in chloroform twice weekly for 16 or more weeks.   Female RIII mice had no mammary tumours after receiving the same treatment for more than 6 months, although the incidence in untreated females was 60-70%.   Three pituitary tumours were observed among 12 mice of both sexes treated with oestrone.   In a mixed strain of mice with a low incidence of mammary tumours, none were induced by oestrone treatment after 44 weeks (Cramer & Horning, 1936).

(c) Subcutaneous and/or intramuscular administration

Mouse: Lacassagne (1932) first reported the induction of mammary tumours in 3/3 male RIII mice (MTV+) after weekly injections (not specified) of 0.6 mg oestrone benzoate for more than 5 months.   Lacassagne (1939) also demonstrated the role of the maternal influence (i.e., transmission of the milk-borne MTV), by crossing RIII strain mice, which have a high incidence in untreated females, with strain 39 mice, which have no spontaneous mammary tumour incidence.   Injection (not specified) of 50 µg oestrone benzoate weekly induced tumours of the mammary gland only in male hybrids whose mothers were of the high mammary tumour incidence strain (RIII).   Males with a strain 39 mother and an RIII father had no mammary tumours with this treatment.

---

[1]MTV⁻: mammary tumour virus not expressed;   MTV+:   mammary tumour virus expressed (see p. 62)

Bonser (1936) found mammary tumours in 3/21 male A strain mice
(MTV+) but in none of 40 CBA males (MTV⁻) after weekly s.c. injections
of 30-50 µg oestrone benzoate in oil for 43 weeks or more.   Shimkin
& Grady (1940) induced mammary tumours in 2/10 male C3H mice (MTV+) by
the s.c. injection of 50 µg oestrone in oil weekly for 24 weeks.   Similar
treatment of female C3H mice reduced the average age at the appearance of
mammary cancer from 46 weeks in untreated controls to 30 weeks in the
treated animals.   In both groups of females the incidence of tumours
was 100%.

Rat: Daily injection of 50-200 µg oestrone in oil (total dose,
30-40 mg) resulted in mammary cancers in 6/6 castrated male rats and in
4/5 ovariectomized females.   A lower incidence was found in intact
males (2/6) and in intact females (3/8).   The average induction time
ranged from 83 weeks with the lowest dose to 31 weeks with the highest
(Geschickter & Byrnes, 1942).   Mammary cancers were found in 1/2 male
and 5/8 female rats given twice-weekly s.c. injections of 50-100 µg
oestrone benzoate in oil for 20 months.   Pituitary tumours (140-271 mg
in weight) were present in all rats (Chamorro, 1943).

Hamster: Malignant kidney tumours of different structures were
found after 8 months in about 60% of 86 castrated male golden hamsters
injected with oestrone (dose not stated).   Pituitary adenomas also
occurred in about 25% of the animals (Dontenwill, 1958).

(d) Subcutaneous implantation

Mouse: Pellets of oestrone (2 mg) were implanted subcutaneously
in A and C3H mice (MTV+) when the animals were 4-6 weeks of age.
Mammary tumours arose in treated A males and in C3H and A females, but
not in mice fostered by C57BL females nor in MTV⁻ strains (Bittner,
1941).

Mice of various hybrids between the A, C3H, C57 and JK strains,
which were implanted with 1-7 mg pellets of oestrone, had an overall
incidence of lymphoid tumours of 19/105, compared with 21/391 in
corresponding control mice (Gardner & Dougherty, 1944).

Rat: Mammary tumours were observed in AxC rats (3/32 females,
4/30 males), Fischer rats (3/29 females, 2/29 males) and August rats
(5/12 females, 9/25 males) implanted with a single pellet of 8-12 mg
oestrone; average latent periods ranged from 50-97 weeks.   Mammary
cancer incidence was doubled in AxC rats by the implantation of two
such pellets, and the latent period was reduced by about 50%.   Adrenal
cortical tumours were found in small numbers of rats with one pellet,
but the incidence was greatly reduced with two pellets.   No mammary
tumours were seen in either sex of rats of the Copenhagen strain, but
6/10 males and 1/11 female had bladder cancer associated with bladder
stones.   The amount of oestrone absorbed was calculated to be between

3.2 and 9.6 mg per rat (Dunning *et al.*, 1953) [There was no control group. The occurrence of bladder cancer may have been related to the presence of stones].

Adrenal cortical tumours were found in 20% of female hooded rats implanted with pellets of oestrone (dose not stated). The tumours frequently metastasized and were transplantable, but they regressed if the oestrone treatment was withdrawn. Adrenal tumours occurred in about 5% of untreated rats in that colony (Noble, 1967).

Cutts (1966) summarized extensive experiments in rats involving s.c. implantation of pellets of oestrone (average, 10 mg). The number of females of different strains with mammary tumours after 43-57 weeks of treatment were: Fischer, 12/74; Wistar, 12/50; Lewis, 17/44; Sprague-Dawley, 16/38; and hooded, 182/212. The estimated absorption of oestrone was 6-7 μg/day. There was no control group.

Black hooded rats (Nb strain) were given subcutaneously implanted pellets containing 90% oestrone and 10% cholesterol, weighing approximately 10 mg each. Pellets were implanted for 10-53 weeks or more in small groups of animals 3, 8, 12 or 38 weeks of age. An increased incidence of tumours was observed in treated rats of both sexes, as compared with 32 controls; the incidences of adrenal carcinomas, mammary carcinomas and pituitary tumours were increased. The incidence of mammary adenomas was increased in treated males and females up to 1 yr but was lower than that in the controls thereafter. The duration of the experiment was not stated. Most of the tumours arising in the oestrogen-treated rats proved to be hormone-dependent upon transplantation into syngeneic hosts (Noble *et al.*, 1975).

Testosterone propionate (TPP) and oestrone were administered subcutaneously to intact male Nb rats as 10 mg pellets containing 90% hormone and 10% cholesterol, either alone or in combination; 2 or 3 pellets were implanted and replaced every 6-8 weeks. Adenocarcinomas of the prostate developed in 5/30 and 11/55 TPP-treated rats that received 18 and 27 mg, respectively, as compared with 2/409 in untreated historical controls. Oestrone shortened the latent period of induction of these tumours; however, alone, it did not result in the development of carcinomas of the prostate (Noble, 1977).

Oestradiol-17β, oestriol and oestrone were administered subcutaneously to intact female Sprague-Dawley rats 48 hrs before treatment with 7,12-dimethylbenz[*a*]anthracene (DMBA) or procarbazine as 1-20% pellets weighing 5-7 mg each. DMBA and procarbazine were given by gavage at amounts of 20 and 50-70 mg, respectively. Mammary tumours were observed in the groups given DMBA, procarbazine or a combination of DMBA and oestrogen or procarbazine and oestrogen; no such tumours occurred in untreated controls or in oestrogen-treated female rats. Pellets containing 10% oestrone had an inhibitory effect on carcinogen-induced tumour development. The total length of the study was 370 days (Lemon, 1975).

Hamster: Implantation of 20 mg pellets of oestrone resulted in malignant kidney tumours (not specified) in 7/8 intact male Syrian hamsters and in 10/10 castrates. No kidney tumours were seen in 61 intact or in 60 castrated untreated males (Kirkman, 1959).

3.2 Other relevant biological data

No data on the toxicity of oestrone or oestrone benzoate were available.

Embryotoxicity and teratogenicity

When mice were injected subcutaneously with oestrone between days 11-16 of gestation at alternating doses of 0.1 and 0.2 mg, 12.4% of the offspring had cleft palates, compared with 1.1% in controls (Nishihara, 1958).

Injection of 1 µg oestrone to rats on day 3 of gestation had no embryotoxic effects (Dickmann, 1973).

Single doses of 0.02 mg/kg bw oestrone injected into rats during the early phase of gestation (time of tubal transport) terminated pregnancy. Injection of a single dose of 0.4 mg/kg bw oestrone on day 8-11 of gestation resulted in a marked reduction in the number of sur- viving foetuses and delayed delivery but had no effect on surviving foetuses (Dreisbach, 1959).

Single s.c. injections of 1-140 µg/rat were given at different times of gestation between days 1-10. Termination of pregnancy (100%) was achieved by administration of 20 µg on days 1 and 2, by 40 µg on day 3, by 80 µg on day 4 and by 50 µg on day 5. An injection of 140 µg oestrone did not terminate pregnancy when given between days 6-10 but induced a decreased number of implantations, an increased number of dead foetuses and abnormal growth and spacing of the foetuses (Haddad & Ketchel, 1969).

S.c. injection of 0.002-0.05 mg/kg bw oestrone to rats on days 2-4 of gestation induced a dose-dependent reduction in fertility; significant effects were obtained with doses of 0.02 and 0.05 mg/kg bw (Saunders, 1965).

S.c. injection of 0.0175 mg/kg per day oestrone into rats during days 1-7 of gestation terminated 50% of pregnancies (Saunders & Elton, 1967).

S.c. administration of 0.5 µg-10 mg oestrone in combination with 1-4 mg progesterone to rats from day 3 after mating until term resulted in 100% resorptions (Cheng, 1959).

Metabolism

The 17β-hydroxy steroid dehydrogenase transforms oestrone to oestradiol reversibly. This enzyme occurred in all tissues of all species examined and is linked to either the cytosolic or microsomal subcellular compartment. In human liver, a NAD-linked 17β-hydroxy steroid 3-hydrogenase occurs in cytosol and in microsomes, and a further NADP-linked enzyme has been found in cytosol (Littmann *et al.*, 1971). Hence, oestrone and oestradiol are largely biologically equivalent; they are also metabolized *via* the same pathways (see monograph on oestradiol-17β, p. 307).

No data on the mutagenicity of oestrone or oestrone benzoate were available.

3.3 Case reports and epidemiological studies

See the section 'Oestrogens & Progestins in Relation to Human Cancer', p. 83 .

4. Summary of Data Reported and Evaluation[1]

4.1 Experimental data

Oestrone was tested in mice by oral administration; in mice, rats and hamsters by subcutaneous injection and implantation; and in mice by skin painting. Its administration resulted in an increased incidence of mammary tumours in mice; in pituitary, adrenal and mammary tumours, as well as bladder tumours in association with stones, in rats; and in renal tumours in both castrated and intact male hamsters.

Oestrone benzoate increased the incidence of mammary tumours in mice following its subcutaneous injection.

Oestrone is embryolethal for preimplantation embryos in some species.

4.2 Human data

No case reports or epidemiological studies on oestrone alone were available to the Working Group. Case reports and epidemiological studies on steroid hormones used in oestrogen treatment have been summarized in the section, 'Oestrogens and Progestins in Relation to Human Cancer', p. 83 .

---

[1]This section should be read in conjunction with pp. 62-64 in the 'General Remarks on Sex Hormones' and with the 'General Conclusions on Sex Hormones', p. 131.

4.3 Evaluation

There is *sufficient evidence* for the carcinogenicity of oestrone in experimental animals.   In the absence of adequate data in humans, it is reasonable, for practical purposes, to regard oestrone as if it presented a carcinogenic risk to humans.   Studies in humans strongly suggest that the administration of oestrogens is causally related to an increased incidence of endometrial carcinoma;   there is no evidence that oestrone is different from other oestrogens in this respect.

5. References

Abraham, G.E., Manlimos, F.S. & Garza, R. (1977)   Radioimmunoassay of steroids.   In: Abraham, G.E., ed., Handbook or Radioimmunoassay, New York, Marcel Dekker, pp. 591-656

Adessi, G.L., Eichenberger, D., Nhuan, T.Q. & Jayle, M.F. (1975) Gas chromatography profile of estrogens: application to pregnancy urine. Steroids, 25, 553-564

Adlercreutz, H., Martin, F., Wahlroos, Ö. & Soini, E. (1975)   Mass spectrometric and mass fragmentographic determination of natural and synthetic steroids in biological fluids.   J. Steroid Biochem., 6, 247-259

Amin, E.S., Awad, O., El Samad, M.A. & Iskander, M.N. (1969) Isolation of estrone from moghat roots and from pollen grains of Egyptian date palm.   Phytochemistry, 8, 295-297

Anner, G. & Miescher, K. (1948)   Synthesis of natural oestrone.   Total synthesis in the oestrone series. III. (Ger.).   Helv. chim. acta, 31, 2173-2183

Anon. (1975)   New processes and technology.   Organic chemicals. Chemical Engineering, 21 July, p. 100

Anon. (1977)   New steroid sources uproot Barbasco.   Chemical Week, 29 June, pp. 49-50

Bègue, R.J., Desgrès, J. & Padieu, P. (1974)   Method of analysis of urinary steroids of human pregnancy by GLC and GC-MS of Sephadex LH-20 chromatographic fractions.   J. chromatogr. Sci., 12, 763-766

Bittner, J.J. (1941)   The influence of estrogens on the incidence of tumors in foster nursed mice.   Cancer Res., 1, 290-292

Bonser, G.M. (1936)   The effect of oestrone administration on the mammary glands of male mice of two strains differing greatly in their susceptibility to spontaneous mammary carcinoma.   J. Pathol. Bacteriol., 42, 169-181

Boot, L.M. & Muhlbock, O. (1956)   The mammary tumour incidence in the C3H mouse strain with and without the agent (C3H, C3H$_f$, C3H$_e$). Acta unio int. cancrum, 12, 569-581

Butenandt, A. (1929)   Progynon, a crystalline female sex hormone (Ger.).   Naturwissenschaften, 17, 879

Butterfield, A.G., Lodge, B.A. & Pound, N.J. (1973)   High-speed liquid
    chromatographic separation of equine estrogens. J. chromatogr.
    Sci., 11, 401-405

Carlström, K. & Sköldefors, H. (1977)   Determination of total oestrone
    in peripheral serum from non pregnant humans. J. Steroid
    Biochem., 8, 1127-1128

Chamorro, A. (1943)   Production of mammary adenocarcinomas in rats by
    oestrone benzoate (Fr.). C.R. Soc. Biol. (Paris), 137, 325-326

Chattoraj, S.C. & Wotiz, H.H. (1975)   Estrogens. In: Dorfman, R.I.,
    ed., Steroid Hormones, Vol. 3, Amsterdam, North Holland, pp. 2-49

Cheng, D.W. (1959)   Effect of progesterone and estrone on the incidence
    of congenital malformations due to maternal vitamin E deficiency.
    Endocrinology, 64, 270-275

Council of Europe (1971)   European Pharmacopoeia, Vol. II, Sainte-
    Ruffine, France, pp. 326-327

Cramer, W. & Horning, E.S. (1936)   Experimental production by oestrin of
    pituitary tumours with hypopituitarism and of mammary cancer.
    Lancet, i, 247-249

Cutts, J.H. (1966)   Estrogen-induced breast cancer in the rat. Can.
    Cancer Conf., 6, 50-68

Dickmann, Z. (1973)   Postcoital contraceptive effects of medroxyprogeste-
    rone acetate and oestrone in rats. J. Reprod. Fertil., 32, 65-69

Doerr, P. (1976)   Radioimmunoassay of oestrone in plasma. A comparison
    of different methods with respect to the relation between assay
    specificity, sample purification and antibody specificity. Acta
    endocrinol., 81, 655-667

Doisy, E.A., Veler, C.D. & Thayer, S. (1929)   Folliculin from the
    urine of pregnant women. Am. J. Physiol., 90, 329-330

Dolphin, R.J. & Pergande, P.J. (1977)   Improved method for the analysis
    of estrogenic steroids in pregnancy urine by high-performance liquid
    chromatography. J. Chromatogr., 143, 267-274

Dontenwill, W. (1958)   Experimental production of kidney and liver
    tumours with follicular hormone (Ger.). Verh. dtsch. Ges. Path.,
    42, 458-461

Dreisbach, R.H. (1959)   The effects of steroid sex hormones on pregnant
    rats. J. Endocrinol., 18, 271-277

Dunning, W.F., Curtis, M.R. & Segaloff, A. (1953)   Strain differences in response to estrone and the induction of mammary gland, adrenal and bladder cancer in rats.   Cancer Res., 13, 147-152

Fels, J.P., Dehennin, L. & Scholler, R. (1975)   Determination of estrogens by gas-liquid chromatography with an open tubular column. J. Steroid Biochem., 6, 1201-1203

Fishman, S. (1975)   Determination of estrogens in dosage forms by fluorescence using dansyl chloride.   J. pharm. Sci., 64, 674-679

Gardner, W.U. & Dougherty, T.F. (1944)   The leukemogenic action of estrogens in hybrid mice.   Yale J. Biol. Med., 17, 75-90

Geschickter, C.F. & Byrnes, E.W. (1942)   Factors influencing the development and time of appearance of mammary cancer in the rat in response to estrogen.   Arch. Pathol., 33, 334-356

Grasselli, J.G. & Ritchey, W.M., eds (1975)   CRC Atlas of Spectral Data and Physical Constants for Organic Compounds, 2nd ed., Vol. 4, Cleveland, OH, Chemical Rubber Co., p. 234

Haddad, V. & Ketchel, M.M. (1969)   Termination of pregnancy and occurrence of abnormalities following estrone administration during early pregnancy.   Int. J. Fertil., 14, 56-63

Harvey, S.C. (1975)   Hormones.   In: Osol, A. et al., eds, Remington's Pharmaceutical Sciences, 15th ed., Easton, PA, Mack, pp. 915-917

Heki, N., Noto, M. & Hosojima, H. (1977)   Microanalysis of estrone, estradiol and estriol of serum and urine by mass fragmentography using gas chromatography-mass spectrometry (Jpn.).   Nippon Naibumpi Gakkai Zasshi, 53, 167-174 [Chem. Abstr., 86, 152212j]

IARC (1974)   IARC Monographs on the Evaluation of Carcinogenic Risk of Chemicals to Man, 6, Sex Hormones, Lyon, pp. 123-132

Jarc, H., Ruttner, O. & Krocza, W. (1977)   The quantitative determination of estrogens and antithyroid drugs by thin-layer and high-performance thin-layer chromatography in animal tissue (Ger.).   J. Chromatogr., 134, 351-358

Kastrup, E.K., ed. (1977)   Facts and Comparisons, St Louis, MO, Facts & Comparisons Inc., p. 113

Kastrup, E.K., ed. (1978)   Facts and Comparisons, St Louis, MO, Facts & Comparisons Inc., pp. 97, 97a, 103

Kirkman, H. (1959)   Estrogen-induced tumors of the kidney. IV.
    Incidence in female Syrian hamsters.   Natl Cancer Inst. Monogr., 1,
    59-75

Lacassagne, A. (1932)   Appearance of mammary cancers in male mice given
    injections of folliculine (Fr.).   C.R. Acad. Sci. (Paris), 195,
    630-632
Lacassagne, A. (1939)   Confirmation, by experiments with oestrone treat-
    ment, of the predominant role of the mother in the hereditary trans-
    mission of mammary carcinoma (Fr.).   C.R. Soc. Biol. (Paris), 132,
    222-224

Lemon, H.M. (1975)   Estriol prevention of mammary carcinoma induced by
    7,12-dimethylbenzanthracene and procarbazine.   Cancer Res., 35,
    1341-1353

Littmann, K.-P., Gerdes, H. & Winter, G. (1971)   Kinetics and
    characterization of 17β-hydroxy steroid dehydrogenases sensitive
    to oestradiol in human liver (Ger.).   Acta endocrinol., 67, 473-482

Mathur, R.S., Leaming, A.B. & Williamson, H.O. (1975)   An assessment of
    the total estrone, estradiol-17β and estriol in high risk pregnancy
    plasma.   J. Steroid Biochem., 6, 1421-1427

Miller, A. (1976)   Cosmetic ingredients.   Household and Personal Products
    Industry, October, pp. 57, 62, 64, 66, 68

Millington, D., Jenner, D.A., Jones, T. & Griffiths, K. (1974)   Endogenous
    steroid concentration in human breast tumours determined by high-
    resolution mass fragmentography.   Biochem. J., 139, 473-475

National Formulary Board (1975)   National Formulary, 14th ed.,
    Washington DC, American Pharmaceutical Association, pp. 272-275

Nishihara, G. (1958)   Influence of female sex hormones in experimental
    teratogenesis.   Proc. Soc. exp. Biol. (N.Y.)., 97, 809-812

Noble, R.L. (1967)   Induced transplantable estrogen-dependent carcinoma
    of the adrenal cortex in rats.   Proc. Am. Assoc. Cancer Res., 8, 51

Noble, R.L. (1977)   The development of prostatic adenocarcinoma in Nb
    rats following prolonged sex hormone administration.   Cancer Res.,
    37, 1929-1933

Noble, R.L., Hochachka, B.C. & King, D. (1975)   Spontaneous and estrogen-
    produced tumors in Nb rats and their behavior after transplantation.
    Cancer Res., 35, 766-780

Rudali, G., Jullien, P., Vives, C. & Apiou, F. (1978) Dose-effect studies on estrogen induced mammary cancers in mice. Biomedicine, 29, 45-46

Saunders, F.J. (1965) Effects on the course of pregnancy of norethynodrel with mestranol (Enovid) administered to rats during early pregnancy. Endocrinology, 77, 873-878

Saunders, F. & Elton, R.L. (1967) Effects of ethynodiol diacetate and mestranol in rats and rabbits, on conception, on the outcome of pregnancy and on the offspring. Toxicol. appl. Pharmacol., 11, 229-244

Schroeder, I., López-Sánchez, G., Medina-Acevedo, J.C. & Espinosa, M. del C. (1975) Quantitative determination of conjugated or esterified estrogens in tablets by thin layer chromatography. J. Chromatogr. Sci., 13, 37-40

Shimkin, M.B. & Grady, H.G. (1940) Carcinogenic potency of stilbestrol and estrone in strain C3H mice. J. natl Cancer Inst., 1, 119-128

Snedden, W. & Parker, R.B. (1976) The direct determination of oestrogen and progesterone in human ovarian tissues by quantitative high resolution mass spectrometry. Biomed. Mass Spectrom., 3, 295-298

US Food & Drug Administration (1977) Patient labeling for estrogens for general use. Drugs for human use; drug efficacy study implementation. Fed. Regist., 42, 37645-37646

US Tariff Commission (1945) Synthetic Organic Chemicals, US Production and Sales, 1941-1943, Report No. 153, Second Series, Washington DC, US Government Printing Office, p. 105

US Tariff Commission (1956) Synthetic Organic Chemicals, US Production and Sales, 1955, Report No. 198, Second Series, Washington DC, US Government Printing Office, p. 112

Vogt, W., Jacob, K. & Knedel, M. (1974) A high sensitive and selective gas chromatographic determination of monohydroxy steroids as phosphinic esters with the alkali flame detector. J. chromatogr. Sci., 12, 658-661

Wade, A., ed. (1977) Martindale, the Extra Pharmacopoeia, 27th ed., London, The Pharmaceutical Press, p. 1420

Windholz, M., ed. (1976) The Merck Index, 9th ed., Rahway, NJ, Merck & Co., pp. 487-488

Wright, K., Collins, D.C., Musey, P.I. & Preedy, J.R.K. (1978) Direct radioimmunoassay of specific urinary estrogen glucosiduronates in normal men and nonpregnant women. Steroids, 31, 407-426

PROGESTINS

CHLORMADINONE ACETATE

A monograph on this substance was published previously (IARC, 1974). Relevant data that have appeared since that time have been evaluated in the present monograph.

1.   Chemical and Physical Data

1.1   Synonyms and trade names

Chem. Abstr. Services Reg. No.:   302-22-7

Chem. Abstr. Name: 17-(Acetyloxy)-6-chloropregna-4,6-diene-3, 20-dione

Synonyms: 17α-Acetoxy-6-chloro-6,7-dehydroprogesterone;   17α-acetoxy-6-chloro-4,6-pregnadiene-3,20-dione;   chlormadinon acetate;   6-chloro-Δ^6-17-acetoxyprogesterone;   6-chloro-Δ^6-(17α)acetoxyprogesterone;   6-chloro-6-dehydro-17α-acetoxyprogesterone;   6-chloro-6-dehydro-17α-hydroxyprogesterone acetate;   6-chloro-17-hydroxypregna-4,6-diene-3, 20-dione acetate;   chloromadinone acetate

Trade names[1]:   [Aconcen];   Amenyl;   [Anconcene];   Ay 13390-6; Bovisynchron;   CAP;   Cero;   Chlordion;   Clordion;   [Consan]; C-Quens;   [C-Quens 21];   [Estirona];   [Estirona 21];   [Eunomin]; Gestafortin;   [Gestakliman];   Gestogan;   Lormin;   [Luteral]; Lutéran;   Lutestral;   Lutinyl;   Lutoral;   Matrol;   Menova; Menstridyl;   [Nocon];   Normenen;   Normenon;   Retex;   RS 1280; Sequens;   Skedule;   Skedule TM;   [St 155];   Synchrosyn;   Synchrosyn P;   Traslan;   Verton;   [Volenyl]

---

[1]Those in square brackets are preparations that are no longer produced commercially.

1.2 Structural and molecular formulae and molecular weight

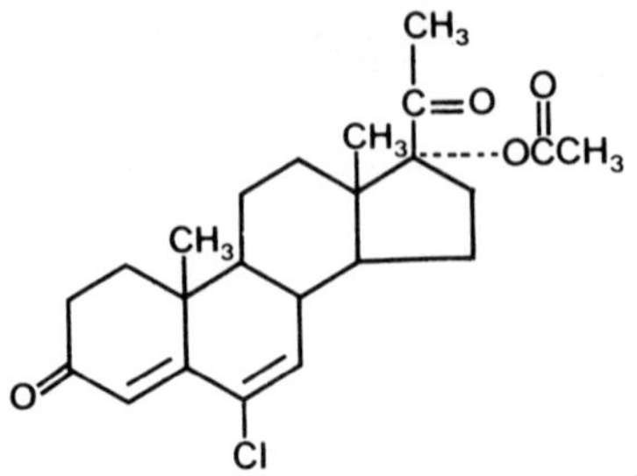

C$_{23}$H$_{29}$ClO$_4$ Mol. wt: 404.9

1.3 Chemical and physical properties

From Wade (1977) and Windholz (1976)

(a) Description: White, odourless, crystalline powder

(b) Melting point: 212-214°C

(c) Spectroscopy data: λ_{max} 283.5 nm and 286 (E_1^1 = 578 and 545.8)

(d) Optical rotation: $[\alpha]_D$ +6° (in 1% chloroform)

(e) Solubility: Practically insoluble in water; soluble in ethanol (1 in 160), chloroform (1 in 1.5), diethyl ether (1 in 210) and methanol (1 in 130)

(f) Stability: Unstable to light

1.4 Technical products and impurities

     No specifications for the purity of chlormadinone acetate were found in the available national pharmacopoeias or national formularies. In Japan, chlormadinone acetate is available as 2 mg tablets.

2. Production, Use, Occurrence and Analysis

2.1 Production and use

(a) Production

     Synthesis of chlormadinone acetate was first reported in 1960, by the treatment of 17-acetoxyprogesterone with ethyl orthoformate in the presence of an acid catalyst to produce the 3-enol ether of the corresponding 3,5-dione; conversion of this enol ether to 6-chloro-17α-acetoxyprogesterone with *N*-chlorosuccinimide is followed by dehydrogenation with chloranil (Brückner, 1960; Brückner *et al.*, 1961).

Chlormadinone acetate is believed to be produced in Italy, but no information was available on the quantity produced.

It was first marketed commercially in Japan in 1967. It is not produced there, and imports amounted to about 7 kg in 1975, 6 kg in 1976 and 5 kg in 1977.

(b) Use

Chlormadinone acetate has not been used in the US since 1970, when the only product (an oral contraceptive) was removed from the market by the US Food and Drug Administration. Its use in the UK was suspended in the same year. Before suspension, chlormadinone acetate was used in oral contraceptives either together with mestranol as a 'sequential' contraceptive or as a 'progestin only' oral contraceptive in a dose of 0.5 mg daily. In Japan, chlormadinone acetate is used (frequently in combination with mestranol) in a dose of 2 mg 1-6 times daily for treatment of threatened abortion and dysmenorrhoea. It is believed to be used as a contraceptive in the German Democratic Republic.

Chlormadinone acetate is approved, with certain restrictions, by the US Food and Drug Administration for use in cattle feed as an oestrus regulator (US Food & Drug Administration, 1969).

2.2 Occurrence

Chlormadinone acetate is not known to occur naturally. Residues have been found in cows' milk following its i.m. injection (Chemnitius *et al.*, 1972).

2.3 Analysis

Typical analytical procedures for the determination of chlormadinone acetate are summarized in Table 1. Abbreviations used are: GC/ECD, gas-liquid chromatography/electron capture detection; TLC, thin-layer chromatography; and HPLC, high-pressure liquid chromatography. See also 'General Remarks on Sex Hormones', p. 60.

TABLE 1

Analytical methods for chlormadinone acetate

Sample matrix	Sample preparation	Assay procedure	Sensitivity or limit of detection	Reference
Bulk chemical	Dissolve	HPLC	-	Hara & Hayashi (1977)
Bulk chemical	Spot; pyrolyse (110°, 18 hrs); develop	TLC	-	Martin et al. (1975)
Plasma	Add sodium carbonate; extract (hexane); wash (sodium hydroxide)	GC/ECD	0.5 ng	Bopp et al. (1972)
Cows' milk	Extract (chloroform); filter; dissolve (heptane); extract (methanol); wash (heptane); evaporate	TLC[a]	-	Chemnitius et al. (1972)

[a]Chemical detection; progestational activity measured by a modified McPhail test

3. Biological Data Relevant to the Evaluation

of Carcinogenic Risk to Humans

3.1 Carcinogenicity studies in animals

Oral administration

Mouse: Chlormadinone acetate alone or in combination with mestranol was incorporated into the diet of CF-LP [MTV⁻][1] mice for 80 weeks. The doses were identified only as low (2-5 times the human contraceptive dose), medium (50-150 times) and high (200-400 times); the amounts were not specified. There was no increase in the incidence of tumours in any tissues of male or female mice given chlormadinone acetate alone in the diet. When it was combined with mestranol (25:1), there was a 5- to 10-fold increase in the incidence of pituitary tumours, but no increase in tumours of other tissues (Committee on Safety of Medicines, 1972).

Groups of 19-46 mice of different strains were administered chlormadinone acetate at levels of 0.8 and 8 mg/kg of diet: daily intakes were estimated to be 60-80 and 600-800 µg, respectively. With an intake of 60 µg/day, the high incidences of mammary cancer in female RIII, C3H and (C3H × RIII)Fl mice (MTV⁺)[1] were not significantly affected, and they did not exhibit vaginal keratinization. Untreated, castrated male (C3H × RIII)Fl mice had an incidence of 10/61 mammary tumours, which was not significantly changed by administration of 60 µg chlormadinone acetate daily, although the development of post-castration adrenal adenomas was inhibited. With a daily dosage of 600 µg, the latent period for mammary tumour development in female mice was slightly increased, from 49 to 66 weeks in RIII females, from 55 to 65 weeks in C3H females and from 30 to 36 weeks in (C3H × RIII)Fl females; however, there was no significant change in the incidence or latent period of mammary tumours appearing in castrated male (C3H × RIII)Fl mice (Rudali *et al.*, 1972).

Intact female RIII, C3H or (C3H × RIII)Fl mice were fed Lutestral (97.5% chlormadinone acetate and 2.5% ethinyloestradiol) in the diet at 8 mg/kg (ppm) (daily intake, 20-30 µg/mouse); neither the mammary tumour incidence nor the latent period was altered. In intact male (C3H × RIII)Fl mice, the tumour incidence was increased from 0/76 to 10/32; and in castrated male (C3H × RIII)Fl mice it was increased from 10/61 to 23/28, with a decrease in the latent period (Rudali, 1975).

---

[1]MTV⁻: mammary tumour virus not expressed; MTV⁺: mammary tumour virus expressed (see p. 62)

Rat: In 75 male and 75 female rats fed chlormadinone acetate in the diet at dosages of 2-5 (low), 50-150 (medium) and 200-400 (high) times the human dose for 104 weeks, no differences in tumour incidence were observed (Committee on Safety of Medicines, 1972).

Dog: Twenty female beagle dogs were given 0.25 mg/kg bw chlormadinone acetate in lactose tablets (representing 25 times the human dose) daily, commencing at 26-52 weeks of age. After 104 weeks, 6/20 treated animals had small (< 1.0 cm) nodules in mammary tissue, and similar but transitory nodules were palpated in 4 untreated controls. Autopsy of 4 control dogs at this time revealed no abnormal mammary proliferation. A further treated dog had a mammary nodule measuring 2.5 × 2.0 × 2.0 cm, which at autopsy was found to be a well-encapsulated cystic tumour composed of connective tissue and some epithelial elements with proliferation of myoepithelial tissue. It was classified as a benign mixed mammary tumour and was reported to be similar to the nodules found by Vallance & Capel-Edwards (1971) in 2/5 dogs treated for 74 months with high doses of progesterone (Nelson et al., 1972).

Nelson et al. (1973) published a more detailed account of mammary nodules which appeared in 14 dogs after 4 years of treatment with chlormadinone acetate: of a total of 22 nodules studied, 12 were diagnosed as nodular hyperplasia, 4 as benign, mixed mammary tumours and 1 as a mammary adenocarcinoma; the 5 remaining nodules contained no mammary tissue. By the seventh year (Weikel & Nelson, 1977), there had been an increase in the total number of neoplastic lesions of the mammary glands from 5 to 14 (benign, mixed tumours from 4 to 9; ductal papillomas from 0 to 3; and adenocarcinomas from 1 to 2). One benign, mixed tumour was observed in the controls.

3.2 Other relevant biological data

For a review of the biological activities of the progestin compounds, see Tausk & de Visser (1972). Chlormadinone acetate has a high parenteral and oral progestational effectiveness in oestrogen-sensitized animals (Desaulles & Krähenbühl, 1959; Neumann, 1968).

No data on the toxicity of chlormadinone acetate were available.

Embryotoxicity and teratogenicity

Administration of chlormadinone acetate by gastric tube in doses of 1, 3, 10 and 50 mg/kg bw to ddS mice from day 8-15 or 14-17 of gestation resulted in malformations in the offspring, the most frequent of which was cleft palate. The highest doses (10 and 50 mg/kg bw from day 8-15) resulted in 33.1% foetal deaths and 68.9% resorptions. When CF-1 mice were given doses of 1 or 10 mg/kg bw, only the higher dose resulted in a significant rate of malformations. In rabbits treated between days 8-20 of gestation, doses of 1 or 3 mg/kg bw had no effect, while 10 mg/kg

bw resulted in malformations in 60% of offspring and 45% embryolethality
(Takano, 1964;   Takano *et al*., 1966).

Absorption, distribution and excretion

The compound is readily absorbed from rat intestine;   absorption
is modulated by biliary constituents (Pelzmann, 1973).   When rats were
administered radioactive chlormadinone acetate intraduodenally, about 34%
of that associated with biliary metabolites underwent enterohepatic
circulation (Hanasono & Fischer, 1974);   however, in baboons, no significant enterohepatic circulation of chlormadinone acetate metabolites was
found (Honjo *et al*., 1976).   No significant degree of deacetylation at
C-17 occurs in baboons (Honjo *et al*., 1976) or in rabbits (Abe & Kambegawa,
1974), the only species studied.

Metabolism

It has been inferred on the basis of pharmacokinetic data that some
similarities in chlormadinone acetate metabolism ought to exist between
Macaca mulatta (rhesus) monkeys and humans (Laumas *et al*., 1977).   There
are wide variations in its progestational activity among species, dogs
being especially highly sensitive (Gräf *et al*., 1975);   this might be
related to the very slow metabolic breakdown of chlormadinone acetate in
that species (Forchielli & Murthy, 1970).

Chlormadinone acetate is metabolized in rabbits by two main pathways,
2-hydroxylation and dechlorination at C-6, and, to some extent, by hydrogenation of one or both of the double bonds at rings A and B.   A small
amount of a metabolite oxidized at C-21 was detected (Abe & Kambegawa,
1974).

Incubation of chlormadinone acetate with rat and human liver microsomes produced the 3β-hydroxy product (17α-acetoxy-6-chloro-3β-hydroxy-
pregna-4,6-diene-20-one) as the major metabolite.   When chlormadinone
acetate was incubated with liver microsomes from phenobarbitone-pretreated
rats and rabbits, the major metabolite was the 2α-hydroxy derivative.
Although species differences have to be taken into account, the production
of the 2α-hydroxy metabolite is thus dependent on the induced state of the
hepatic monooxygenases (Handy *et al*., 1974).

Mutagenicity and other short-term tests

No chromosomal effects were observed when concentrations of 0.1-100
µg/ml chlormadinone acetate were added to cultures of lymphocytes grown
from the blood of healthy women (Stenchever *et al*., 1969).

3.3 Case reports and epidemiological studies

See the section, 'Oestrogens and Progestins in Relation to Human
Cancer', p. 83 .

4. Summary of Data Reported and Evaluation[1]

4.1 Experimental data

Chlormadinone acetate was tested in mice, rats and dogs by oral administration. When given alone to dogs, chlormadinone acetate produced mammary tumours. When given to mice in combination with mestranol, it increased the incidence of pituitary tumours in animals of both sexes; in combination with ethinyloestradiol, it increased the incidence of mammary tumours in intact and castrated male mice of one hybrid strain.

Chlormadinone acetate has been reported to be embryolethal and teratogenic when given during the organogenesis stage in some species.

4.2 Human data

No case reports or epidemiological studies on chlormadinone acetate alone were available to the Working Group. Epidemiological studies on steroid hormones used in oestrogen-progestin contraceptive preparations have been summarized in the section, 'Oestrogens and Progestins in Relation to Human Cancer', p. 83.

4.3 Evaluation

There is *limited evidence* for the carcinogenicity of chlormadinone acetate in dogs. In humans, oral contraceptives containing oestrogens in combination with progestins have been related causally to an increased incidence of benign liver adenomas and a decreased incidence of benign breast disease.

---

[1]This section should be read in conjunction with pp. 62-64 in the 'General Remarks on Sex Hormones' and with the 'General Conclusions on Sex Hormones', p. 131.

5. References

Abe, T. & Kambegawa, A. (1974)   Urinary and biliary metabolites of 17α-acetoxy-6-chloro-4,6-pregnadiene-3,20-dione in the rabbit. Chem. pharm. Bull., 22, 2824-2829

Bopp, R.J., Murphy, H.W., Nash, J.F. & Novotny, C.R. (1972)   GLC determination of chlormadinone acetate in plasma. J. pharm. Sci., 61, 1441-1444

Brückner, K. (1960)   6-Halo-3-oxo steroids, German Patent, 1,075, 114, 11 February to E. Merck Akt.-Ges [Chem. Abstr., 55, 12458a]

Brückner, K., Hampel, B. & Johnsen, U. (1961)   Synthesis and properties of monohalogenated 3-keto-Δ⁴,⁶-diene-steroids (Ger.). Ber. dtsch. chem. Ges., 94, 1225-1240

Chemnitius, K.-H., Oettel, M., Richter, J., Sachweh, H., Trolldenier, H. & Zwacka, G. (1972)   Testing for residues of chlormadinone acetate (Jenapharm) in the milk of ruminants (Ger.). Arch. exp. Veterinaermed., 26, 999-1012

Committee on Safety of Medicines (1972)   Carcinogenicity Tests of Oral Contraceptives, London, HMSO

Desaulles, P.A. & Krähenbühl, C. (1959)   Modern development in the field of gestagen therapy (Ger.). In: Nowakowski, H., ed., Modern Development in the Field of Gestagen Therapy. Hormones in Veterinary Medicine, Berlin, Springer, pp. 1-10

Forchielli, E. & Murthy, D.V.K. (1970)   Metabolism of chlormadinone acetate in the human and in laboratory animals (Abstract no. 123). Excerpta Medica Int. Congr. Ser., 210, 64-65

Gräf, K.-J., El Ettreby, M.F.A., Richter, K.-D., Günzel, P. & Neumann, F. (1975)   The progestogenic potencies of different progestogens in the beagle bitch. Contraception, 12, 529-540

Hanasono, G.K. & Fischer, L.J. (1974)   The excretion of tritium-labelled chlormadinone acetate, mestranol, norethindrone, and norethynodrel in rats and the enterohepatic circulation of metabolites. Drug Metab. Disposition, 2, 159-168

Handy, R.W., Palmer, K.H., Wall, M.E. & Piantadosi, C. (1974)   The metabolism of antifertility steroids. The *in vitro* metabolism of chlormadinone acetate. Drug Metab. Disposition, 2, 214-220

Hara, S. & Hayashi, S. (1977)   Correlation of retention behaviour of
    steroidal pharmaceuticals in polar and bonded reversed-phase liquid
    column chromatography.   J. Chromatogr., 142, 689-703

Honjo, H., Ishihara, M., Osawa, Y., Kirdani, R.Y. & Sandberg, A.A. (1976)
    The metabolic fate of chlormadinone acetate in the baboon.   Steroids,
    27, 79-98

IARC (1974)   IARC Monographs on the Evaluation of Carcinogenic Risk
    of Chemicals to Man, 6, Sex Hormones, Lyon, pp. 149-155

Laumas, V., Farooq, A. & Laumas, K.R. (1977)   Disappearance of [1α-³H]-
    chlormadinone acetate in the plasma and red cells of rhesus monkeys.
    J. Steroid Biochem., 8, 781-786

Martin, J.L., Duncombe, R.E. & Shaw, W.H.C. (1975)   Thin-layer chromato-
    graphic test for the identification of some drugs: its application
    to steroids, tetracyclines, penicillins, and cephalosporins.
    Analyst (Lond.), 100, 243-248

Nelson, L.W., Carlton, W.W. & Weikel, J.H., Jr (1972)   Canine mammary
    neoplasms and progestogens.   J. Am. med. Assoc., 219, 1601-1606

Nelson, L.W., Weikel, J.H., Jr & Reno, F.E. (1973)   Mammary nodules in
    dogs during four years' treatment with megestrol acetate or chlorma-
    dinone acetate.   J. natl Cancer Inst., 51, 1303-1311

Neumann, F. (1968)   Chemical constitution and pharmacologic action
    (Ger.).   In: Langecker, H., ed., Handbuch der Experimenteller
    Pharmakologie, Vol. 22, Die Gestagene, Berlin, Springer, pp. 680-1025

Pelzmann, K.S. (1973)   Absorption of chlormadinone acetate and nore-
    thisterone from in situ rat gut.   J. pharm. Sci., 62, 1609-1614

Rudali, G. (1975)   Induction of tumors in mice with synthetic sex
    hormones.   Gann Monogr., 17, 243-252

Rudali, G., Coezy, E. & Chemama, R. (1972)   Mammary carcinogenesis in
    female and male mice receiving contraceptives or gestagens.   J. natl
    Cancer Inst., 49, 813-819

Stenchever, M.A., Jarvis, J.A. & Kreger, N.K. (1969)   Effect of selected
    estrogens and progestins on human chromosomes in vitro.   Obstet.
    Gynecol., 34, 249-251

Takano, K. (1964)   The effect of several synthetic progestagens adminis-
    tered to pregnant animals upon their offspring.   Proc. Congenital
    Anomalies Res. Assoc. Jpn., 4, 3-4

Takano, K., Yamamura, H., Suzuki, M. & Nishimura, H. (1966)   Teratogenic effect of chlormadinone acetate in mice and rabbits.   Proc. Soc. Biol. Med. (N.Y.), 121, 455-457

Tausk, M. & de Visser, J. (1972)   International Encyclopedia of Pharmacology and Therapeutics, Vol. II, section 48, Elmsford, NY, Pergamon Press, pp. 35-194

US Food & Drug Administration (1969)   Subpart C - Food additives. Fed. Regist., 34, 25

Vallance, D.K. & Capel-Edwards, K. (1971)   Chlormadinone and mammary nodules.   Br. med. J., ii, 221-222

Wade, A., ed. (1977)   Martindale, The Extra Pharmacopoeia, 27th ed., London, The Pharmaceutical Press, pp. 1391-1392

Weikel, J.H., Jr & Nelson, L.W. (1977)   Problems in evaluating chronic toxicity of contraceptive steroids in dogs.   J. Toxicol. environ. Health, 3, 167-177

Windholz, M., ed. (1976)   The Merck Index, 9th ed., Rahway, NJ, Merck & Co., p. 267

DIMETHISTERONE

A monograph on this substance was published previously (IARC, 1974). Relevant data that have appeared since that time have been evaluated in the present monograph.

1. Chemical and Physical Data

1.1 Synonyms and trade names

Chem. Abstr. Services Reg. No.: 79-64-1

Chem. Abstr. Name: (6α,17β)-17-Hydroxy-6-methyl-17-(1-propynyl)-androst-4-en-3-one

Synonyms: Dimethesterone; dimethisteron; 6α,21-dimethyl-ethisterone; 6α,21-dimethyl-17β-hydroxy-17α-pregn-4-en-20-yn-3-one; 17α-ethynyl-6α,21-dimethyltestosterone; 17α-ethynyl-17-hydroxy-6α,-21-dimethylandrost-4-en-3-one; 17β-hydroxy-6α-methyl-17-(1-propynyl)-androst-4-en-3-one; 6α-methyl-17α-propynyltestosterone; 6α-methyl-17-(1-propynyl)testosterone

Trade names[1]: [Dimethasterone]; Lutogan; Oracon; Ovin; P-5048; [Secrodyl]; Secrosteron; [Secrovin]; Tova

---

[1]Those in square brackets are preparations that are no longer produced commercially.

1.2   Structural and molecular formulae and molecular weight

C$_{23}$H$_{32}$O$_2$ Mol. wt: 340.5

1.3   Chemical and physical properties

From Wade (1977) and Windholz (1976)

(a)   Description: White, odourless, tasteless, crystalline powder

(b)   Melting point: ~100°C (with decomposition)

(c)   Spectroscopy data: λ_{max} 240 nm (E_1^1 = 450)

(d)   Optical rotation: $[\alpha]_D^{20}$ +10° (1% w/v in chloroform)

(e)   Solubility: Practically insoluble in water; soluble in
      ethanol (1 in 3), arachis oil (1 in 80), chloroform (1 in 0.7)
      and pyridine (1 in 1); slightly soluble in acetone

(f)   Stability: Unstable to air and light

1.4 Technical products and impurities

   Dimethisterone is available in the US as the monohydrate, containing
97-103% active ingredient.   It was also available as a combination,
containing 25 mg dimethisterone and 0.1 mg ethinyloestradiol, with 90-
110% of the labelled amount of dimethisterone (National Formulary Board,
1975).

2. Production, Use, Occurrence and Analysis

2.1 Production and use

(a) Production

Synthesis of dimethisterone was first reported in 1959 (Barton *et al.*, 1959), by oxidation of 17α-prop-1'-ynylandrost-5-ene-3β:17β-diol with monoperphthalic acid to give the 5,6-epoxides. Treatment of the 5α,6α-epoxide with methylmagnesium iodide and oxidation of the resulting triol with chromium trioxide-pyridine produced the β-hydroxy-ketone, which was dehydrated catalytically and epimerized to dimethisterone. Patents were subsequently obtained for several routes; in one method, dehydroepiandrosterone is treated with potassium acetylide, and the 3- and 17-hydroxyl groups of the resulting 17-ethinyl derivative are then protected as tetrahydropyranyl ethers before introduction of the 21-methyl group with lithium and methyl iodide. After acid-catalysed removal of the protecting ether groups, the resulting diol is epoxidized at the 5,6-position with perbenzoic acid; treatment of the epoxide with methylmagnesium bromide followed by mild acid is used to open the epoxy ring and to methylate the 6-position. The resulting 5α-hydroxy-6β-methyl compound is dehydrated to introduce the 4,5-double bond. Equilibration with a base produces dimethisterone, which has the more stable 6α-methyl configuration. Whether this is the synthesis route used for commercial production is not known.

Dimethisterone has not been produced commercially in the US, and separate data on US imports are not available.

No data on its production in Europe were available.

Dimethisterone is not produced commercially in Japan; imports amounted to about 6 kg in 1975 and 1976 and 5 kg in 1977.

(b) Use

In the US, dimethisterone is used primarily as a progestin in sequence with a suitable oestrogen (such as ethinyloestradiol) for oral contraception (Harvey, 1975). In the UK, it is used in a dose of 5 mg 3 times daily in the treatment of menstrual disorders (Wade, 1977).

In Japan, dimethisterone is used in the treatment of dysfunctional uterine bleeding at a dosage of 5-15 mg daily.

The US Food & Drug Administration (1978) has ruled that with effect from 31 May 1978 all oral contraceptives for general use must carry patient and physician warning labels concerning use, risks and contraindications.

2.2 Occurrence

Dimethisterone is not known to occur naturally.

2.3 Analysis

Typical analytical methods for the determination of dimethisterone are summarized in Table 1.   Abbreviations used are: TLC, thin-layer chromatography; HPLC, high-pressure liquid chromatography; UV, ultra-violet spectrometry; and IR, infra-red spectrometry.   See also the section 'General Remarks on Sex Hormones', p. 60.

TABLE 1

Analytical methods for dimethisterone

Sample matrix	Sample preparation	Assay procedure	Reference
Bulk chemical	Dissolve (ethanol)	UV (240 nm)	British Pharmacopoeia Commission (1973)
Bulk chemical	–	IR	Chatten et al. (1976)
Bulk chemical	Dissolve	HPLC	Hara & Hayashi (1977)
Bulk chemical	Spot; pyrolyse (110°, 18 hrs); develop	TLC	Martin et al. (1975)
Bulk chemical	Dissolve (ethanol)	UV (242 nm)	National Formulary Board (1975)
Tablets	Powder; extract (hexane)	UV (232 nm)	National Formulary Board (1975)
Tablets	Extract (dimethylformamide); reduce volume; add buffer	Polarography	Chatten et al. (1977)
Tablets	Powder; suspend (water); extract (chloroform); derivatize (isonicotinic acid hydrazide)	UV (380 nm)	National Formulary Board (1975)

3. Biological Data Relevant to the Evaluation
of Carcinogenic Risk to Humans

3.1 Carcinogenicity studies in animals

Oral administration

Dog: Three groups of 16 female beagle dogs were given a cyclic regime of dimethisterone and ethinyloestradiol; ethinyloestradiol was given for 16 days and the combination for 5 days, followed by no drug for 7 days. The doses were equivalent to 1, 10 and 25 times the projected human dose: ethinyloestradiol, 2, 20 and 50 µg/kg bw, and dimethisterone 500, 5000 and 12,500 µg/kg bw. Over a 7-year period, one control animal, 2 given the low dose, 2 given the intermediate dose and 9 given the high dose died. Alopecia, cystic endometrial hyperplasia, pyometra and acne-like lesions were noted in dogs given the high and intermediate doses. Four hyperplastic nodules of the mammary gland were found by palpation among dogs treated with the low dose, whereas none occurred in dogs treated with the intermediate and high doses. Two mammary nodules were found in controls (Weikel & Nelson, 1977) [The Working Group noted the lack of information concerning the number of tumour-bearing animals].

3.2 Other relevant biological data

For a review of the biological activity of the progestin compounds, see Tausk & deVisser (1972). Dimethisterone is a weak progestational compound in humans (see 'General Remarks on Sex Hormones', p. 44).

The oral LD_{50} of dimethisterone in mice is 7.65 g/kg bw (Windholz, 1976). No other data on the toxicity, embryotoxicity or teratogenicity of this compound were available.

Dimethisterone, although not a 19-nortestosterone derivative, appears to be metabolized similarly to those progestins, by reductive pathways. The principal urinary metabolite in humans is the tetrahydro derivative, 6α-methyl-17α-(1-propynyl)-5β-androstane-3α,17β-diol (Stillwell et al., 1972). No other studies on the metabolism of this compound were available.

No chromosomal effects were observed when 0.1-100 µg/ml dimethisterone were added to cultures of lymphocytes grown from the blood of healthy women (Stenchever et al., 1969).

3.3 Case reports and epidemiological studies

See the section, 'Oestrogens and Progestins in Relation to Human Cancer', p. 83.

4. Summary of Data Reported and Evaluation[1]

4.1 Experimental data

Dimethisterone was tested in dogs in combination with ethinyl-oestradiol by oral administration. No increase in incidence of mammary tumours was found.

4.2 Human data

No case reports or epidemiological studies on dimethisterone alone were available to the Working Group. Epidemiological studies on steroid hormones used in oestrogen-progestin oral contraceptive preparations have been summarized in the section, 'Oestrogens and Progestins in Relation to Human Cancer', p. 83, and see in particular pp. 111-112.

4.3 Evaluation

Owing to the lack of experimental and human data on dimethisterone alone, no evaluation of the carcinogenicity of dimethisterone could be made. In humans, oral contraceptives containing oestrogens in combination with progestins have been related causally to an increased incidence of benign liver adenomas and a decreased incidence of benign breast disease.

---

[1]This section should be read in conjunction with pp. 62-64 in the 'General Remarks on Sex Hormones' and with the 'General Conclusions on Sex Hormones', p. 131.

5. References

Barton, S.P., Burn, D., Cooley, G., Ellis, B. & Petrow, V. (1959)
Modified steroid hormones. XI. Some ethisterone homologues.
J. chem. Soc., 1957-1962

British Pharmacopoeia Commission (1973)   British Pharmacopoeia, London,
HMSO, p. 169

Chatten, L.G., Triggs, E.J. & Glowach, S.J. (1976)   Quantitative assay
of anti-fertility agents by i.r. spectroscopy.   J. Pharm. Belg.,
31, 63-79   [Chem. Abstr., 85, 155766n]

Chatten, L.G., Yadav, R.N., Binnington, S. & Moskalyk, R.E. (1977)
Polarographic study of certain progestogens and their determination
in oral contraceptive tablets by differential pulse polarography.
Analyst (Lond.), 102, 323-327

Hara, S. & Hayashi, S. (1977)   Correlation of retention behaviour of
steroidal pharmaceuticals in polar and bonded reversed-phase liquid
column chromatography.   J. Chromatogr., 142, 689-703

Harvey, S.C. (1975)   Hormones.   In: Osol, A. et al., eds, Remington's
Pharmaceutical Sciences, 15th ed., Easton, PA, Mack, pp. 921-922

IARC (1974)   IARC Monographs on the Evaluation of Carcinogenic Risk
of Chemicals to Man, 6, Sex Hormones, Lyon, pp. 167-171

Martin, J.L., Duncombe, R.E. & Shaw, W.H.C. (1975)   Thin-layer
chromatographic test for the identification of some drugs: its
application to steroids, tetracyclines, penicillins and cephalosporins.   Analyst (Lond.), 100, 243-248

National Formulary Board (1975)   National Formulary, 14th ed., Washington
DC, American Pharmaceutical Association, pp. 222-225

Stenchever, M.A., Jarvis, J.A. & Kreger, N.K. (1969)   Effect of
selected estrogens and progestins on human chromosomes in vitro.
Obstet. Gynecol., 34, 249-251

Stillwell, W.G., Horning, E.C., Horning, M.G., Stillwell, R.N. & Zlatkis,
A. (1972)   Characterization of metabolites of steroid contraceptives
by gas chromatography and mass spectrometry.   J. Steroid Biochem.,
3, 699-706

Tausk, H. & deVisser, J. (1972)   International Encyclopedia of Pharmacology
& Therapeutics, Vol. II, section 48, Elmsford, NY, Pergamon Press,
pp. 35-194

US Food & Drug Administration (1978)   Oral contraceptive drug products. Physician and patient labeling; extension of effective date for physician labeling.   Fed. Regist., 43, 9863-9864

Wade, A., ed. (1977)   Martindale, The Extra Pharmacopoeia, 27th ed., London, The Pharmaceutical Press, p. 1395

Weikel, J.H., Jr & Nelson, L.W. (1977)   Problems in evaluating chronic toxicity of contraceptive steroids in dogs.   J. Toxicol. environ. Health, 3, 167-177

Windholz, M., ed. (1976)   The Merck Index, 9th ed., Rahway, NJ, Merck & Co., p. 427

ETHYNODIOL DIACETATE

A monograph on this substance was published previously (IARC, 1974). Relevant data that have appeared since that time have been evaluated in the present monograph.

1.   Chemical and Physical Data

1.1 Synonyms and trade names

Chem. Abstr. Services Reg. No.:   297-76-7

Chem. Abstr. Name: $(3\beta,17\alpha)$-19-Norpregn-4-en-20-yne-3,17-diol diacetate

Synonyms: $3\beta,17\beta$-Diacetoxy-17α-ethynyl-4-estrene; $3\beta,17\beta$-diacetoxy-17α-ethynyl-4-oestrene; ethinodiol diacetate; ethynodiol acetate; β-ethynodiol diacetate; 19-nor-17α-pregn-4-en-20-yne-3β,17-diol diacetate

Trade names[1]: 8080 C.B.; CB 8080; Cervicundin; Demulen; Demulen 28; Demulen 50; Femulen; [FH 027]; [Lueolas]; [Luteonorm]; Lutométrodiol; Luto-Metrodiol; Metrodiol; Metrodiol diacetate; Metrulen; Metrulen 50; Metrulen M; Metrulene; Neovulen; Ovulen; [Ovulen 0.5]; [Ovulen 1.0]; [Ovulen 1/50]; Ovulen 21; Ovulen 50; [Ovulene 50]; [Ovulen Mite]; SC 11800

1.2 Structural and molecular formulae and molecular weight

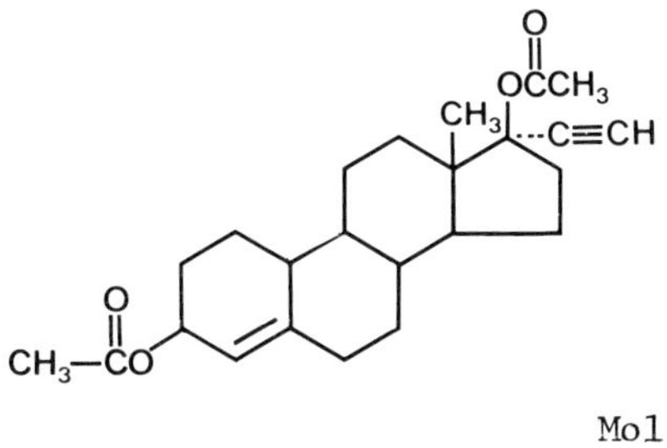

$C_{24}H_{32}O_4$ Mol. wt: 384.5

---

[1]Those in square brackets are preparations that are no longer produced commercially.

1.3 Chemical and physical properties

From Wade (1977) and Windholz (1976), unless otherwise specified

(<u>a</u>) <u>Description</u>: White crystals (from methanol and water)

(<u>b</u>) <u>Melting-point</u>: 126-127°C

(<u>c</u>) <u>Spectroscopy data</u>: λ_{max} 299, 236 and 244 nm after hydrolysis with methanolic hydrochloric acid; infra-red, nuclear magnetic resonance and mass spectral data have been tabulated (Lau & Sutter, 1974).

(<u>d</u>) <u>Optical rotation</u>: $[\alpha]_D$ -72.5° (in chloroform)

(<u>e</u>) <u>Solubility</u>: Practically insoluble in water; soluble in ethanol (1 in 15), chloroform (1 in 1), diethyl ether (1 in 3.5) and acetone; sparingly soluble in fixed oils

(<u>f</u>) <u>Stability</u>: Unstable to air and light

1.4 Technical products and impurities

Various national and international pharmacopoeias give specifications for the purity of ethynodiol diacetate in pharmaceutical products. For example, ethynodiol diacetate is available in the US as a USP grade containing 97-102% of the active ingredient. Tablets containing ethynodiol diacetate contain 93-107% of the labelled amount (US Pharmacopeial Convention Inc., 1975).

2. Production, Use, Occurrence and Analysis

2.1 Production and use

(<u>a</u>) Production

A method for the synthesis of ethynodiol diacetate was first patented in the US in 1965 (Klimstra, 1965): ethindrone is reduced to ethynodiol, which is acetylated with acetic anhydride in pyridine to produce ethynodiol diacetate. It is not known whether this is the process used for commercial production.

Ethynodiol diacetate is believed to be produced commercially in Italy and The Netherlands, but no information was available on the quantities produced.

It is not produced commercially in the US or Japan, and no data on imports were available.

(b) Use

Ethynodiol diacetate has applications similar to those of progesterone (see monograph, p. **491**). It is used in oral contraceptive tablets in a dose of 0.5-1 mg in combination with an oestrogen such as mestranol or ethinyloestradiol.   It is also used in the treatment of dysfunctional uterine bleeding and amenorrhoea in doses of 1-2 mg daily in combination with an oestrogen from day 5 to day 24 or 25 of the cycle (in severe cases the dose of ethynodiol diacetate may be increased to 4-6 mg).   In the treatment of endometriosis, the usual dose is 2-4 mg in combination with an oestrogen, for a minimum of 9 months (Wade, 1977).

In France, ethynodiol diacetate has been used in the treatment of advanced breast cancer at a dose of 50 mg per day (Cheix-Servonnat *et al.*, 1974).

No evidence was found that ethynodiol diacetate has been used in Japan in recent years.

The US Food & Drug Administration (1978) has ruled that with effect from 31 May 1978 all oral contraceptives for general use must carry patient and physician warning labels concerning use, risks and contraindications.

2.2 Occurrence

Ethynodiol diacetate is not known to occur naturally.

2.3 Analysis

Analytical procedures for the determination of ethynodiol diacetate as a bulk chemical and in pharmaceutical preparations have been reviewed (Lau & Sutter, 1974).   Typical analytical methods for its determination are summarized in Table 1.   Abbreviations used are: TLC, thin-layer chromatography; GC, gas chromatography; and UV, ultra-violet spectrometry. See also the section, 'General Remarks on Sex Hormones', p. 60.

TABLE 1

Analytical methods for ethynodiol diacetate

Sample matrix	Sample preparation	Assay procedure	Reference
Bulk chemical	—	GC	Feher & Bodrogi (1976)
Bulk chemical	Dissolve (chloroform-methanol)	Two-dimensional TLC (UV and acid spray)	Cavina et al. (1975)
Bulk chemical	Dissolve	TLC	Martin et al. (1975)
Bulk chemical	Dissolve (tetrahydrofuran); add silver nitrate	Titration (sodium hydroxide)	British Pharmacopoeia Commission (1973)
Tablets	Disintegrate (water, ethanol); add hydrochloric acid	UV (236 nm)	Görög (1977)
Tablets	Powder; triturate (aqueous methanol); filter; add hydrochloric acid; heat	UV (236 nm)	US Pharmacopeial Convention Inc. (1975)

3. Biological Data Relevant to the Evaluation

of Carcinogenic Risk to Humans

3.1 Carcinogenicity studies in animals

Oral administration

Mouse: Ethynodiol diacetate alone or in combination with oestrogens was incorporated into the diet of groups of 120 male and 120 female CF-LP mice (MTV[-])[1] for 80 weeks. The doses were identified only as low (2-5 times the human dose), medium (50-150 times) and high (200-400 times); the amounts were not specified. Administration of ethynodiol diacetate alone did not result in an increased incidence of tumours in any tissue of treated mice compared with controls, except in the liver where 32 benign tumours occurred in 120 treated males *versus* 18 and 19 in 2 control groups of 120 animals. When it was administered in combination with mestranol (1:1, 10:1 and 20:1), the numbers of pituitary tumours were 23-37 in treated groups and 2-8 in male and female controls. Administration of ethynodiol diacetate in combination with ethinyloestradiol (2:1 and 20:1) resulted in an increase in the incidence of pituitary tumours to 30-49 per group of 120 animals. Six malignant tumours of the connective tissue of the uterus (unspecified) were found in female mice fed ethynodiol di-acetate:ethinyloestradiol (20:1), compared with 0-1/120 in controls (Committee on Safety of Medicines, 1972).

Castrated male (C3H × RIII)F1 mice (MTV[+])[1] given   0.68 mg/kg bw per day ethynodiol diacetate had an increase in mammary tumour incidence from 10/61 to 11/26 but no change in the latent period (81 *versus* 82 weeks). In intact (C3H × RIII)F1 females administered 0.56-0.75 or 75-100 μg/kg bw per day, neither mammary tumour incidence nor latent period was altered (Rudali *et al.*, 1972).

Intact male (C3H × RIII)F1 mice (MTV+) given 3 mg/kg (ppm) Ovulen (90% ethynodiol diacetate and 10% mestranol) mixed into the diet (intake, 7.5-10 μg/mouse per day) showed an increased incidence of mammary tumours, from 0/76 to 14/25; in castrated males, the incidence was increased from 10/61 to 21/28. The high spontaneous incidence (161/167) and short latent period (30 weeks) in intact females were not altered in treated animals (37/38 within 33 weeks). In ovariectomized females, the tumour incidence was not altered by Ovulen (28/34 as compared with 20/26); but the latent period was reduced in both ovariectomized females (from 49 to 26 weeks) and castrated males (from 82 to 43 weeks) (Rudali, 1975).

---

[1]MTV[-]: mammary tumour virus not expressed; MTV[+]: mammary tumour virus expressed (see p. 62).

Rat: In groups of 105-180 rats fed ethynodiol diacetate alone or
with mestranol (10:1) at doses of 2-5 (low), 50-150 (medium) or 200-
400 (high) times the human dose, no increase in incidence of tumours was
observed.   Benign mammary tumours occurred in 10% of male rats treated
with ethynodiol diacetate alone, compared with 0 in controls; and malignant mammary tumours occurred in 5% of treated rats compared with 2.5%
in controls.   When it was given in combination with ethinyloestradiol
(2:1), malignant mammary tumours were observed in 10% of treated males
compared with 0 in controls and in 14% of treated female rats compared
with 5% in controls.   Administration of ethynodiol diacetate:mestranol
(20:1) resulted in an increased incidence of malignant mammary tumours
in groups of 120 females (from 0 to 15%) and 120 males (from 3 to 7%).
In a further group of 105 female rats that received ethynodiol diacetate:
mestranol (20:1), the incidence of malignant mammary tumours was not
increased (3% in controls, compared with 0 in treated rats) (Committee
on Safety of Medicines, 1972).

Monkey: In a preliminary report of a study in progress, a combination of ethynodiol diacetate:ethinyloestradiol (20:1) was administered
orally at 1, 10 and 50 times the human contraceptive dose (0.021, 0.21 and
1.05 mg/kg bw) cyclically (3 weeks on and 1 week off) to 3 groups of 16
mature (3-8-yr-old) female *Macaca mulatta* (rhesus) monkeys for 5 years.
Clinical examination during 65 cycles revealed the presence and subsequent disappearance of a nodule in one control animal and in one monkey in
the highest dose group (Drill & Golway, 1978).

3.2   Other relevant biological data

For a review of the biological activities of the progestin compounds,
see Tausk & deVisser (1972).   Ethynodiol diacetate has pronounced progestational effect when taken orally (Neumann, 1968; Tausk & deVisser,
1972).

(a)   Experimental systems

No data on the toxicity of this compound were available.

Embryotoxicity and teratogenicity

Oral or parenteral administration of 1 mg/kg bw ethynodiol diacetate
to CF-1 and CFW mice on days 7, 8 and 9 of gestation resulted in anomalies
in 30% of foetuses (retarded development, hydrocephalus, clubfoot, minor
skeletal anomalies) (Andrew *et al.*, 1972).

In rats injected subcutaneously with 0.1-1.0 mg/kg bw ethynodiol
diacetate 30 days before and 5 days after mating, pregnancy was inhibited
in a dose-dependent fashion, but no effects were seen in surviving foetuses.
S.c. doses of 2 or 5 mg/kg bw, or an oral dose of 5 mg administered during
days 2-4 of gestation or a s.c. dose of 5 mg/kg bw on day 1 also

terminated pregnancy.   In rabbits, a s.c. dose of 0.1-1 mg/kg bw or
2 mg/kg bw given orally from day of mating until day 28, or a s.c. dose
of 0.25 or 0.5 mg/kg bw or an oral dose of 2 mg/kg bw given on day 10 of
gestation until day 28, terminated pregnancy.   Doses that did not terminate pregnancy had no effect on litter size, weight of offspring or fertility
of adult progeny.   Treatment with ethynodiol diacetate on days 15-20 of
pregnancy had no androgenic effect on female progeny, as determined by ano-
genital distance (Saunders & Elton, 1967).

In rats given a combination of ethynodiol diacetate:mestranol (20:1)
orally, doses of 0.1-0.5 mg/kg bw ethynodiol diacetate administered 5
days before and 30 days after mating had no effect on conception.   Doses
of 2 or 5 mg/kg bw ethynodiol diacetate prevented conception totally.
When the combination was given during pregnancy from days 1-18 or 7-18
at doses of 0.2 or 0.4 mg/kg bw ethynodiol diacetate, respectively, no
effects were observed either on pregnancy or on the offspring.   Mixtures
containing 1 or 2 mg/kg bw ethynodiol diacetate administered orally on
days 1-21, or 0.1-2 mg/kg bw administered subcutaneously or 0.2-2 mg/kg
bw given orally on days 2-4 of gestation, terminated pregnancy in a dose-
and time-dependent fashion.   No malformations were seen in the 793 newborn
rats checked, and fertility in adult offspring was normal (Saunders &
Elton, 1967).

Metabolism

Ethynodiol diacetate is metabolized to the active progestin norethisterone (Tokuda *et al.*, 1967).

In rats, it is metabolized by deacetylation, ring A-saturation and
3-ketone formation.   A metabolite with a 6(7)-double bond probably arose
from dehydration of a 6-hydroxylated intermediate (Freudenthal *et al.*,
1971).

In baboons, both acetyl groups of ethynodiol diacetate, at C-3 and
C-17, were removed metabolically, but 3-deacetylation went much faster
than 17-deacetylation.   Enterohepatic circulation was considered to be
insignificant for this compound in this species;   it is excreted mostly
in bile and urine (Ishihara *et al.*, 1975).

Mutagenicity and other short-term tests

Female Holtzman rats treated orally for 5 days with 0.2 mg/kg bw
ethynodiol diacetate were sacrificed on day 6.   No damage to bone-marrow
chromosomes, as compared with corn-oil treated controls, was observed
(Edwards *et al.*, 1971).

The cyclic intake of oral contraceptives containing 1 mg ethynodiol
diacetate and 100 µg mestranol daily for at least 6 months did not significantly increase the frequency of chromosome aberrations in cultured
lymphocytes from 35 women (de Gutiérrez & Lisker, 1973).

(b) Humans

In humans, ethynodiol diacetate is deacetylated rapidly, and the ethynodiol is oxidized to norethisterone.   The metabolites produced also occur after metabolism of norethisterone itself (Cook *et al*., 1973; Kishimoto *et al*., 1972).

No significant difference in the frequency of abnormal karyotypes or in sex ratio was found in 124 abortuses of women who had taken oral contraceptives (including 13 who had taken 1 mg ethynodiol diacetate with 0.1 mg mestranol), in comparison with 122 abortuses of women who had never used oral contraceptives (Lauritsen, 1975).

3.3 Case reports and epidemiological studies

See the section, 'Oestrogens and Progestins in Relation to Human Cancer', p. 83 .

4. Summary of Data Reported and Evaluation[1]

4.1 Experimental data

Ethynodiol diacetate was tested in mice, rats and monkeys alone or in combination with oestrogens by oral administration.   In castrated male mice, it increased the incidence of mammary tumours, and in male rats it produced benign mammary tumours.   In combination with oestrogens, it increased the incidence of pituitary tumours in mice and of malignant mammary tumours in male and female rats.   The study in monkeys is still in progress.

Ethynodiol diacetate was reported to be embryolethal for pre- and postimplantation embryos and to have teratogenic effects in some species.

4.2 Human data

No case reports or epidemiological studies on ethynodiol diacetate alone were available to the Working Group.   Epidemiological studies on steroid hormones used in oestrogen-progestin contraceptive preparations have been summarized in the section, 'Oestrogens and Progestins in Relation to Human Cancer', p. 83.

---

[1]This section should be read in conjunction with pp. 62-64 in the 'General Remarks on Sex Hormones' and with the 'General Conclusions on Sex Hormones', p. 131.

4.3 Evaluation

There is *limited evidence* for the carcinogenicity of ethynodiol
diacetate in animals.   In humans, oral contraceptives containing oestrogens in combination with progestins have been related causally to an
increased incidence of benign liver adenomas and a decreased incidence
of benign breast disease.

5. References

Andrew, F.D., Williams, T.L., Gidley, J.T. & Wall, M.E. (1972)
Teratogenicity of contraceptive steroids in mice (Abstract).
Teratology, 5, 249

British Pharmacopoeia Commission (1973) British Pharmacopoeia, London,
HMSO, p. 199

Cavina, G., Moretti, G. & Petrella, M. (1975) A solvent system for the
separation of steroids with estrogenic and progestational activity
by two-dimensional thin-layer chromatography. J. Chromatogr., 103,
368-371

Cheix-Servonnat, F., Clavel, M., Bonnafous, N. & Pommatau, E. (1974)
Treatment of advanced breast cancer with ethynodiol diacetate (37
cases) (Fr.). Lyon Méd., 231, 715-724

Committee on Safety of Medicines (1972) Carcinogenicity Tests of Oral
Contraceptives, London, HMSO

Cook, C.E., Karim, A., Forth, J., Wall, M.E., Ranney, R.E. & Bressler,
R.C. (1973) Ethynodiol diacetate metabolites in human plasma.
J. Pharmacol. exp. Ther., 185, 696-702

Drill, V.A. & Golway, P.L. (1978) Effect of ethynodiol diacetate with
ethinyl estradiol on the mammary glands of rhesus monkeys: a preliminary report. J. natl Cancer Inst., 60, 1169-1170

Edwards, C.W., Calhoun, F.J. & Green, S. (1971) The effects of
mestranol and several progestins on chromosomes and fertility in the
rat (Abstract no. 157). Toxicol. appl. Pharmacol., 19, 421

Feher, T. & Bodrogi, L. (1976) Gas chromatographic determinations of
synthetic gestagen hormones. Acta pharm. Hung., 46, 73-77
[Chem. Abstr., 84, 147091y]

Freudenthal, R.I., Cook, C.E., Forth, J., Rosenfeld, R. & Wall, M.E.
(1971) The metabolism of ethynodiol diacetate by rat and human
liver. J. Pharmacol. exp. Ther., 177, 468-473

Görög, S. (1977) Analysis of steroids. XXIX. Single tablet assay
methods for the determination of progestins in oral contraceptives.
Zentralbl. Pharm., 116, 259-264

de Gutiérrez, A.C. & Lisker, R. (1973) Longitudinal study of the effects
of oral contraceptives on human chromosomes. Ann. Génét., 16, 259-
262

IARC (1974)   IARC Monographs on the Evaluation of Carcinogenic Risk of Chemicals to Man, 6, Sex Hormones, Lyon, pp. 173-178

Ishihara, M., Osawa, Y., Kirdani, R.Y. & Sandberg, A.A. (1975)   Metabolic fate of ethynodiol diacetate in the baboon. Steroids, 25, 829-847

Kishimoto, Y., Kraychy, S., Ranney, R.E. & Gantt, C.L. (1972)   Metabolism of oral contraceptives. I. Metabolism of ethynodiol diacetate in women. Xenobiotica, 2, 237-252

Klimstra, P.D. (1965)   19-Norandrostanes. US Patent, 3,176,013, 30 March to G.D. Searle & Co. [Chem. Abstr., 62, 14776h-14777e]

Lau, E.P.K. & Sutter, J.L. (1974)   Ethynodiol diacetate. In: Florey, K., ed., Analytical Profiles of Drug Substances, Vol. III, New York, Academic Press, pp. 254-279

Lauritsen, J.G. (1975)   The significance of oral contraceptives in causing chromosome anomalies in spontaneous abortions. Acta obstet. gynecol. scand., 54, 261-264

Martin, J.L., Duncombe, R.E. & Shaw, W.H.C. (1975)   Thin-layer chromato-graphic test for the identification of some drugs: its application to steroids, tetracyclines, penicillins and cephalosporins. Analyst (Lond.), 100, 243-248

Neumann, F. (1968)   Chemical constitution and pharmacologic action (Ger.). In: Langecker, H., ed., Handbuch der Experimenteller Pharmakologie, Vol. 22, Die Gestagene, Berlin, Springer, pp. 680-1025

Rudali, G. (1975)   Induction of tumors in mice with synthetic sex hormones. Gann Monogr., 17, 243-252

Rudali, G., Coezy, E. & Chemama, R. (1972)   Mammary carcinogenesis in female and male mice receiving contraceptives or gestagens. J. natl Cancer Inst., 49, 813-819

Saunders, F.J. & Elton, R.L. (1967)   Effects of ethynodiol diacetate and mestranol in rats and rabbits, on conception, on the outcome of preg-nancy and on the offspring. Toxicol. appl. Pharmacol., 11, 229-244

Tausk, M. & deVisser, J. (1972)   International Encyclopedia of Pharma-cology and Therapeutics, Vol. II, section 48, Elmsford, NY, Pergamon Press, pp. 35-194

Tokuda, G., Murakami, A., Higashiyama, S., Mizoguchi, S., Iwasaki, S. & Orino, K. (1967)   17α-Ethynyl-4-estrene-3β,17β-diol-diacetate (Jpn.). Folia Endocrinol. Jpn., 43, 905-914

US Food & Drug Administration (1978)   Oral contraceptive drug products.
    Physician and patient labeling; extension of effective date for
    physician labeling.   Fed. Regist., 43, 9863-9864

US Pharmacopeial Convention Inc. (1975)   The US Pharmacopeia, 19th rev.,
    Rockville, MD, pp. 191-193

Wade, A., ed. (1977)   Martindale, The Extra Pharmacopoeia, 27th ed.,
    London, The Pharmaceutical Press, pp. 1398-1399

Windholz, M., ed. (1976)   The Merck Index, 9th ed., Rahway, NJ, Merck
    & Co., p. 507

17α-HYDROXYPROGESTERONE CAPROATE

1. Chemical and Physical Data

1.1 Synonyms and trade names

Chem. Abstr. Services Reg. No.: 630-56-8

Chem. Abstr. Name: 17-[(1-Oxohexyl)oxy]pregn-4-ene-3,20-dione

Synonyms: 17α-Hexanoyloxypregn-4-ene-3,20-dione; HPC; 17-hydroxypregn-4-ene-3,20-dione hexanoate; 17α-hydroxyprogesterone *n*-caproate; 17α-hydroxyprogesterone hexanoate; progesterone caproate

Trade names: Capron; Corlutin L.A.; Delalutin; Depo-proluton; Duralutin; Estralutin; Gesterol L.A.; Hormofort; Hylutin; Hyproval-PA; Hyroxon; Idrogestene; Lutate; Luteocrin; Luteocrin Depot; Lutopron; Neolutin; Pharlon; Primolut Depot; Progestérone-Retard Pharlon; Proluton Depot; Relutin; Squibb; Syngynon; Teralutil

1.2 Structural and molecular formulae and molecular weight

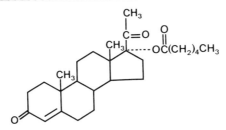

$C_{27}H_{40}O_4$ Mol. wt: 428.6

1.3 Chemical and physical properties

From Wade (1977) and Windholz (1976), unless otherwise specified

(a) Description: White needles

(b) Melting-point: 119-121°C

(c) Spectroscopy data: λ_{max} 241 nm (E_1^1 = 396.6) in ethanol; infra-red, nuclear magnetic resonance and mass spectral data have been tabulated (Florey, 1975).

(d) Optical rotation: $[\alpha]_D^{20}$ +61° (1% w/v chloroform)

(e) Solubility: Insoluble in water; soluble in ethanol (1 in 10), chloroform (1 in 0.4), diethyl ether (1 in 10), sesame oil (25-29 mg/ml) and butyl levulinate (350-400 mg/ml)

(f) Stability: Light-sensitive

1.4 Technical products and impurities

Various national and international pharmacopoeias give specifications for the purity of 17α-hydroxyprogesterone caproate in pharmaceutical products. For example, it is available in the US as a USP grade containing 97-103% active ingredient on an anhydrous basis and not more than 0.1% water and 0.6% free *n*-caproic acid. Injections in 125 and 250 mg/ml doses contain 90-110% of the stated amount of 17α-hydroxyprogesterone caproate in vegetable oil (US Pharmacopeial Convention Inc., 1975). Similar preparations are available in the UK (Wade, 1977). In Japan, 17α-hydroxyprogesterone caproate is available as injections.

In Austria, it is available as 125, 250 and 500 mg doses in oily solutions (Binder *et al.*, 1978). In France, it is available as 250 and 500 mg doses in oily solutions (Anon., 1978).

2. Production, Use, Occurrence and Analysis

2.1 Production and use

(a) Production

A method for synthesizing 17α-hydroxyprogesterone caproate was first patented by Kaspar *et al.* (1956) by the esterification of hydroxyprogesterone with caproic anhydride in the presence of *para*-toluenesulphonic acid. It is not known whether this method is used commercially.

No evidence was found that 17α-hydroxyprogesterone caproate has ever been produced commercially in the US. However, commercial production of 17α-hydroxyprogesterone in the US was first reported in 1963 (US Tariff Commission, 1964); only one US company reported production of an unspecified amount (see preamble, p. 20) in 1975 and 1976 (US International Trade Commission, 1977a,b). In 1975, US production of 13 oestrogen and progestin substances, including 17α-hydroxyprogesterone, amounted to 10.5

thousand kg (US International Trade Commission, 1977a). Data on US imports and exports of 17α-hydroxyprogesterone and its caproate ester are not available.

17α-Hydroxyprogesterone caproate is believed to be produced commercially in Italy, but no information was available on the quantity produced. It is produced in Austria and the Federal Republic of Germany (Binder *et al.*, 1978) and in France (Anon., 1978). Other esters of 17α-hydroxyprogesterone (e.g., the acetate) are believed to be produced commercially in the Federal Republic of Germany, France, The Netherlands and the UK, but no information was available on the quantities produced.

17α-Hydroxyprogesterone caproate was first marketed commercially in Japan in 1954-1955. It is not produced there, and imports amounted to approximately 200 kg in 1976 and 1977.

(b) Use

17α-Hydroxyprogesterone caproate, used in human medicine, is administered by i.m. injection for the treatment of menstrual disorders, including amenorrhoea and dysfunctional uterine bleeding, for the production of secretory endometrium and desquamation and for threatened abortion. For cyclic therapy, a 28-day cycle is used in which 20 mg oestradiol valerate or benzoate are given on day 1 of each cycle followed by a 125-250 mg injection of 17α-hydroxyprogesterone caproate and 5 mg oestradiol valerate or benzoate two weeks later. For continuous therapy, 250 mg 17α-hydroxyprogesterone caproate are administered once a week. It is also used for the treatment of advanced neoplasms of the uterus, in a dose of 1 g one or more times weekly (Harvey, 1975; Wade, 1977), and for the testing of endogenous oestrogen production, as a single dose of 250 mg. 17α-Hydroxyprogesterone caproate has also been proposed for use in the prevention of premature labour and birth (Johnson *et al.*, 1975).

In Japan, 17α-hydroxyprogesterone caproate is used (frequently in combination with progesterone or oestradiol derivatives) for the treatment of threatened abortion, menstrual disorders and sterility.

2.2 Occurrence

17α-Hydroxyprogesterone caproate is not known to occur naturally.

2.3 Analysis

Analytical methods for determing 17α-hydroxyprogesterone caproate in pharmaceutical preparations and as a bulk chemical have been reviewed (Florey, 1975). Typical analytical methods are summarized in Table 1. Abbreviations used are: TLC, thin-layer chromatography; HPLC, high-pressure liquid chromatography; and UV, ultra-violet spectrometry. See also the 'General Remarks on Sex Hormones', p. 60.

TABLE 1

Analytical methods for 17α-hydroxyprogesterone caproate

Sample matrix	Sample preparation	Assay procedure	Reference
Bulk chemical	Dissolve (ethanol)	UV (240 nm)	British Pharmacopoeia Commission (1973)
Bulk chemical	Dissolve (chloroform-methanol)	Two-dimensional TLC; acid spray and UV	Cavina et al. (1975)
Bulk chemical	Dissolve (dioxane)	UPLC (UV, 254 nm)	Hara & Hayashi (1977)
Bulk chemical	Spot; pyrolyse (110°C, 18 hrs)	TLC	Martin et al. (1975)
Bulk chemical	Dissolve (ethanol)	UV (240 nm)	US Pharmacopeial Convention Inc. (1975)
Injection formulation	Dissolve (chloroform); derivatize (isonicotinic acid hydrazide)	UV (380 nm)	British Pharmacopoeia Commission (1973)
Injection formulation	Dissolve (methanol); derivatize (isonicotinic acid hydrazide)	UV (380 nm)	US Pharmacopeial Convention Inc. (1975)

3. Biological Data Relevant to the Evaluation
of Carcinogenic Risk to Humans

3.1 Carcinogenicity studies in animals

Subcutaneous and/or intramuscular administration

Rat: Two groups of 15 female Wistar rats were given 3 mg/kg bw *N*-nitrosodiethylamine in the drinking-water for life, alone (mean survival time, 156 days) or in combination with weekly s.c. injections of 20 mg/kg bw 17α-hydroxyprogesterone caproate in sesame oil (mean survival time, 145 days). Liver carcinomas occurred in 100% of animals in the group given the nitrosamine and in 78% of those given the combination (Boquoi & Kreuzer, 1965).

Rabbit: Of 19 young, random-bred female rabbits injected intramuscularly with 13 mg 17α-hydroxyprogesterone caproate suspended in sesame oil on alternate weeks for up to 109 weeks, 14 developed numerous cysts of the endometrium during the first 267 days. In 7/8 animals still alive at 109 weeks, cysts were unilocular and lined with a single layer of cuboidal or columnar epithelium, which was often ciliated. In control rabbits, there were a few cysts of less than 0.3 mm in diameter; in 2, there were small non-neoplastic polyps with a fibrous core (Messner & Sommers, 1966) [The Working Group noted that this experiment was not designed to examine carcinogenesis].

3.2 Other relevant biological data

For a review of the biological activities of the progestin compounds, see Tausk & deVisser (1972) 17α-Hydroxyprogesterone caproate has approximately the same order of activity as progesterone, with 4-6 times its duration of action. For a comparison of its activity with that of other progestational compounds, see the 'General Remarks on Sex Hormones', p. 44.

No data on the toxicity, metabolism or mutagenicity of this compound were available.

No virilizing effects were observed in DBA mice given daily s.c. injections of 0.25 mg 17α-hydroxyprogesterone caproate on days 16-19 of gestation (Johnstone & Franklin, 1964) or in Sprague-Dawley rats given 5 mg daily from day 14-19 of gestation (Lerner *et al.*, 1962).

3.3 Case reports and epidemiological studies

No data were available to the Working Group.

4. Summary of Data Reported and Evaluation[1]

4.1 Experimental data

17α-Hydroxyprogesterone caproate was tested in rabbits by repeated subcutaneous injection. The data were insufficient to evaluate the carcinogenicity of this compound.

4.2 Human data

No case reports or epidemiological studies on 17α-hydroxyprogesterone caproate were available to the Working Group.

4.3 Evaluation

The available experimental and human data are inadequate to evaluate the carcinogenicity of 17α-hydroxyprogesterone caproate.

---

[1]This section should be read in conjunction with pp. 62-64 in the 'General Remarks on Sex Hormones' and with the 'General Conclusions on Sex Hormones', p. 131.

5. References

Anon. (1978)   Dictionnaire Vidal, 54th ed., Paris, Office de Vulgarisa-
tion Pharmaceutique, pp. 1652-1653

Binder, E., Breit, A., Zekert, F. & Zimmermann, G. (1978)   Austria-Codex
1978/79, Wien, Osterreichischer, Apotheker, p. 655

Boquoi, E. & Kreuzer, G. (1965)   Influence of oestrogenic and progestational hormones on liver changes and tumours produced by diethylnitros-
amine in the rat (Ger.).   Arch. Geschwulstforsch., 26, 223-233

British Pharmacopoeia Commission (1973)   British Pharmacopoeia, London,
HMSO, pp. 235-236

Cavina, G., Moretti, G. & Petrella, W. (1975)   A solvent system for the
separation of steroids with estrogenic and progestational activity
by two-dimensional thin-layer chromatography.   J. Chromatogr., 103,
368-371

Florey, K., ed. (1975)   Analytical Profiles of Drug Substances, Vol. 4,
New York, Academic Press, pp. 211-224

Hara, S. & Hayashi, S. (1977)   Correlation of retention behaviour of
steroidal pharmaceuticals in polar and bonded reversed-phase liquid
column chromatography.   J. Chromatogr., 142, 689-703

Harvey, S.C. (1975)   Hormones.   In: Osol, A. et al., eds, Remington's
Pharmaceutical Sciences, 15th ed., Easton, PA, Mack, pp. 922-923

Johnson, J.W.C., Austin, K.L., Jones, G.S., Davis, G.H. & King, T.M.
(1975)   Efficacy of 17α-hydroxyprogesterone caproate in the prevention of premature labor.   N. Engl. J. Med., 293, 675-680

Johnstone, E.E. & Franklin, R.R. (1964)   Assay of progestins for fetal
virilizing properties using the mouse.   Obstet. Gynecol., 23, 359-
362

Kaspar, E., Pawlowski, K.H., Junkmann, K. & Schenck, M. (1956)   17α-Acyl-
oxyprogesterones.   US Patent, 2,753,360, 3 July to Schering A.-G.
[Chem. Abstr., 51, 2076b,c]

Lerner, L.J., DePhillipo, M., Yiacas, E., Brennan, D. & Borman, A. (1962)
Comparison of the acetophenone derivative of 16α,17α-dihydroxy-
progesterone with other progestational steroids for masculinization
of the rat fetus.   Endocrinology, 71, 448-451

Martin, J.L., Duncombe, R.E. & Shaw, W.H.C. (1975)   A thin-layer chromatographic test for the identification of some drugs: its application to steroids, tetracyclines, penicillins and cephalosporins. Analyst (Lond.), 100, 243-248

Meissner, W.A. & Sommers, S.C. (1966)   Endometrial changes after prolonged progesterone and testosterone administration to rabbits.   Cancer Res., 26, 474-478

Tausk, M. & deVisser, J. (1972)   International Encyclopedia of Pharmacology and Therapeutics, Vol. II, section 48, Elmsford, NY, Pergamon Press, pp. 35-194

US International Trade Commission (1977a)   Synthetic Organic Chemicals, US Production and Sales, 1975, USITC Publication 804, Washington DC, US Government Printing Office, pp. 90, 102

US International Trade Commission (1977b)   Synthetic Organic Chemicals, US Production and Sales, 1976, USITC Publication 833, Washington DC, US Government Printing Office, p. 148

US Pharmacopeial Convention Inc. (1975)   The US Pharmacopeia, 19th rev., Rockville, MD, pp. 245-246

US Tariff Commission (1964)   Synthetic Organic Chemicals, US Production and Sales, 1963, TC Publication 143, Washington DC, US Government Printing Office, p. 134

Wade, A., ed. (1977)   Martindale, The Extra Pharmacopoeia, 27th ed., London, The Pharmaceutical Press, pp. 1400-1401

Windholz, M., ed. (1976)   The Merck Index, 9th ed., Rahway, NJ, Merck & Co., p. 643

LYNOESTRENOL

1. Chemical and Physical Data

1.1 Synonyms and trade names

Chem. Abstr. Services Reg. No.: 52-76-6

Chem. Abstr. Name: (17α)-19-Norpregn-4-en-20-yn-17-ol

Synonyms: 3-Desoxynorlutin; ethinylestrenol; Δ^4-17α-ethinylestren-17β-ol; 17α-ethinyl-17β-hydroxyestr-4-ene; ethinyloestrenol; Δ^4-17α-ethinyloestren-17β-ol; 17α-ethinyl-17β-hydroxyoestr-4-ene; ethynylestrenol; 17α-ethynylestrenol; 17α-ethynylestr-4-en-17β-ol; ethynyloestrenol; 17α-ethynyloestrenol; 17α-ethynyloestr-4-en-17β-ol; linestrenol; linoestrenol; lynenol; lynestrenol; 19-nor-17α-pregn-4-en-20-yn-17-ol

Trade names: Exluten; Exluton; Exlutona; Lyndiol; Minilyn; Noracycline; Orgametil; Orgametril; Orgametrol

1.2 Structural and molecular formulae and molecular weight

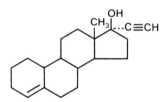

$C_{20}H_{28}O$ Mol. wt: 284.4

1.3 Chemical and physical properties

From Wade (1977) and Windholz (1976)

(a) Description: White, odourless, tasteless, crystalline powder

(h) Melting-point: 158-160°C

(c) <u>Optical rotation</u>: $[\alpha]_D$ -13° (chloroform)

(d) <u>Solubility</u>: Practically insoluble in water; soluble in 100%
    ethanol (1 in 15), acetone (1 in 12), chloroform (1 in 8) and
    diethyl ether (1 in 12)

(e) <u>Stability</u>: Unstable to air and light

1.4 Technical products and impurities

No specifications for the purity of lynoestrenol were found in
the available national pharmacopoeias or national formularies. In the
UK and Japan, it is available in combination tablets containing 2.5 mg
lynoestrenol and 0.075 mg mestranol; in the UK it is also available in
combination with 0.05 mg ethinyloestradiol (Wade, 1977).

2.   Production, Use, Occurrence and Analysis

2.1 Production and use

(a) Production

Synthesis of lynoestrenol was first reported in 1959 (de Winter *et
al.*, 1959), by treatment of 19-nortestosterone with ethane-1,2-dithiol
and boron trifluoride to give the 3-thioketal; treatment with sodium in
liquid ammonia gives 17β-hydroxyoestr-4-ene, which by oxidation with
chromic acid gives oestr-4-en-17-one. This can be converted to lynoestrenol
by treatment with lithium acetylide or Grignard reagent. Whether this
is the method used for commercial production is not known.

Lynoestrenol is believed to be produced in Italy and The Netherlands,
but no information was available on the quantities produced.

It is not produced in the US, and separate data on US imports are
not available.

It was first marketed in Japan in 1970; it is not produced there,
and imports amounted to about 75 kg in 1975, 55 kg in 1976 and 65 kg in
1977.

(b) Use

Lynoestrenol is used primarily as a component of contraceptive
tablets in a dose of 2.5 mg in conjunction with an oestrogen such as
ethinyloestradiol or mestranol. It is used in a cyclic regimen (22 days
on and 6 days off). It is also used (usually in combination with mestranol)
in the treatment of dysfunctional uterine bleeding and endometriosis at
a dose of 5 mg daily (Wade 1977).

The US Food & Drug Administration (1978) has ruled that with effect from 31 May 1978 all oral contraceptives for general use must carry patient and physician warning labels concerning use, risks and contra-indications.

2.2 Occurrence

Lynoestrenol is not known to occur naturally.

2.3 Analysis

Typical analytical methods for the determination of lynoestrenol are summarized in Table 1. Abbreviations used are: GC/FID, gas chromatography/flame-ionization detection; TLC, thin-layer chromatography; and IR, infra-red spectrometry. See also the section, 'General Remarks on Sex Hormones', p. 60.

TABLE 1

Analytical methods for lynoestrenol

Sample matrix	Sample preparation	Assay procedure	Reference
Bulk chemical	Dissolve (tetrahydrofuran); add silver nitrate	Titration (sodium hydroxide)	British Pharmacopoeia Commission (1973)
Bulk chemical	Dissolve (chloroform:methanol, 1:1)	Two-dimensional TLC (UV, acid spray)	Cavina *et al.* (1975)
Bulk chemical	Dissolve	TLC	Puech *et al.* (1975)
Tablets	Powder; extract (acetone); evaporate; dissolve (aqueous alkali); extract (carbon tetrachloride)	IR (1130 cm^{-1})	Bellomonte (1971)
Tablets	Extract	GC/FID	Moretti *et al.* (1974)
Tablets	Powder; wash (petroleum ether); extract (chloroform); evaporate; dissolve (ethanol); add silver nitrate & ammonium hydroxide; dilute (water); extract (diethyl ether); add acetic anhydride; evaporate	Titration (perchloric acid)	Roushdi *et al.* (1974)
Pharmaceutical preparations	Dissolve (ethanol); precipitate (silver nitrate); filter; derivatize excess silver ion (dithizonate)	Colorimetry (472 nm)	Rizk *et al.* (1973)

3. Biological Data Relevant to the Evaluation of Carcinogenic Risk to Humans

3.1 Carcinogenicity studies in animals

Oral administration

Mouse: Lynoestrenol alone or in combination with mestranol (33:1) was incorporated into the diet of groups of 114-123 male or female Swiss random-bred mice for 80 weeks at three levels, low (2-5 times the human contraceptive dose), medium (50-150 times) and high (200-400 times). The amounts were not specified. Benign liver-cell tumours occurred in 7% of male mice fed lynoestrenol alone, compared with 2% of controls. In females, malignant mammary tumours occurred in 4% of mice fed lynoestrenol, in 6% fed the combination and in 0/47 controls (Committee on Safety of Medicines, 1972).

Rat: Groups of 189 female rats were fed lynoestrenol or lynoestrenol: mestranol (33.3:1) at low (2-5 times the human contraceptive dose), medium (50-150 times) and high (200-400 times) doses. Malignant mammary tumours occurred in 3% of rats fed lynoestrenol and in 0/114 controls (Committee on Safety of Medicines, 1972).

Three groups of female Wistar rats received 40 mg/kg bw N-nitroso-methylurea (NMU) on 3 subsequent days. One group received an oral contraceptive (0.25 mg lynoestrenol + 0.075 mg mestranol) daily for 30 days before NMU treatment, whereas the other group received the contraceptive after the treatment. The third group served as controls. Tumour induction (especially of nephroblastomas) was changed only in the group that received the oral contraceptive before the carcinogen: a significant decrease was observed (Thomas et $al.$, 1972).

3.2 Other relevant biological data

For a review of the biological activities of the progestin compounds, see Tausk & deVisser (1972). Lynoestrenol has pronounced progestational effects when taken orally (Neumann, 1968; Tausk & deVisser, 1972). Its relative biological activity is indicated in the 'General Remarks on Sex Hormones', p. 44.

No data on its toxicity were available.

Embryotoxicity and teratogenicity

No effect was observed in the 7-day old embryos of rats that received s.c. injections of 0.1 mg lynoestrenol on days 2, 3, 4 and 5 of gestation; a dose of 1 mg terminated pregnancy (Castro-Vazquez et $al.$, 1971).

In female golden Syrian hamsters that received a contraceptive steroid containing 0.6 mg lynoestrenol and 18.7 µg mestranol (route unspecified) daily for 4.5-8 months, fertility was found to be normal; no effects were seen on the sexual behaviour or fecundity of offspring of the following two generations (Cottinet *et al.*, 1974).

No data on teratogenicity and embryotoxicity at later stages of development were available.

Metabolism

In rabbits, lynoestrenol is metabolized to norethisterone *via* ethynodiol (Okada *et al.*, 1964; Mazaheri *et al.*, 1970). The data of Murata (1968) infer that this pathway also occurs in humans.

Mutagenicity and other short-term tests

No significant difference in the frequency of abnormal karyotypes or in sex ratio was found in 124 abortuses of women who had taken oral contraceptives (including 15 who had taken 2.5 mg lynoestrenol with 0.075 mg mestranol), in comparison with 122 abortuses of women who had never used oral contraceptives (Lauritsen, 1975).

Dominant lethal mutations were observed in female mice treated for 3 days prior to mating with doses of 420 µg lynoestrenol and 12.5 µg/kg bw mestranol (Badr & Badr, 1974). [For a consideration of the possible mutagenicity of this compound, see 'General Remarks on Sex Hormones, p. 64].

3.3 Case reports and epidemiological studies

See the section, 'Oestrogens and Progestins in Relation to Human Cancer', p. 83.

4. Summary of Data Reported and Evaluation[1]

4.1 Experimental data

Lynoestrenol was tested by oral administration in mice and rats, alone or in combination with mestranol. It did not increase the incidence of tumours.

---

[1]This section should be read in conjunction with pp. 62-64 in the 'General Remarks on Sex Hormones' and with the 'General Conclusions on Sex Hormones', p. 131.

4.2 Human data

No case reports or epidemiological studies on lynoestrenol alone were available to the Working Group. Epidemiological studies on steroid hormones used in oestrogen-progestin oral contraceptive preparations have been summarized in the section, 'Oestrogens and Progestins in Relation to Human Cancer', p. 83.

4.3 Evaluation

No evaluation of the carcinogenicity of lynoestrenol could be made. In humans, oral contraceptives containing oestrogens in combination with progestins have been related causally to an increased incidence of benign liver adenomas and a decreased incidence of benign breast disease.

5. References

Badr, F.M. & Badr, R.S. (1974) Studies on the mutagenic effect of contraceptive drugs. I. Induction of dominant lethal mutations in female mice. Mutat. Res., 26, 529-534

Bellomonte, G. (1971) Infrared spectrophotometric determination of lynestrenol in the presence of mestranol in [pharmaceutical] tablets (Ital.). Ann. Ist. Super. Sanità, 7, 102-105 [Chem. Abstr., 76, 49999r]

British Pharmacopoeia Commission (1973) British Pharmacopoeia, London, HMSO, p. 273

Castro-Vazquez, A., Macome, J.C., De Carli, D.N. & Rosner, J.M. (1971) On the mechanism of action of oral contraceptives. I. Effect of lynestronol on ovum implantation and oviductal morphology in the rat. Fertil. Steril., 22, 741-744

Cavina, G, Moretti, G. & Petrella, M. (1975) A solvent system for the separation of steroids with estrogenic and progestational activity by two-dimensional thin-layer chromatography. J. Chromatogr., 103, 368-371

Committee on Safety of Medicines (1972) Carcinogenicity Tests of Oral Contraceptives, London, HMSO

Cottinet, D., Czyba, J.C., Dams, R. & Laurent, J.L. (1974) Effect of long-term administration of anti-ovulatory steroids on the fertility of female golden hamsters and their offspring (Fr.). C.R. Soc. Biol. (Paris), 168, 517-520

Lauritsen, J.G. (1975) The significance of oral contraceptives in causing chromosome anomalies in spontaneous abortions. Acta obstet. gynecol. scand., 54, 261-264

Mazaheri, A., Fotherby, K. & Chapman, J.R. (1970) Metabolism of lynestrenol to norethisterone by liver homogenate. J. Endocrinol., 47, 251-252

Moretti, G., Petrella, M., Taggi, F. & Cavina, G. (1974) Contribution to the standardization of a gas chromatographic method for the analysis of an oestrogenic and progestational combination. Ann. Ist. Super. Sanità, 10, 224-232

Murata, S. (1968) Study on the metabolism of estrane progestins in the human body (Jpn.). Folia endocrinol. Jpn., 43, 1083-1096

Neumann, F. (1968) Chemical constitution and pharmacologic action (Ger.).
    In: Langecker, H., ed., Handbuch der Experimenteller Pharmakologie,
    Vol. 22, Die Gestagene, Berlin, Springer, pp. 680-1025

Okada, H., Ota, S., Take, H. & Yamamoto, H. (1964) 17α-Ethinyl-4-estrene-
    17β-ol (Jpn.). Folia endocrinol. Jpn., 40, 1095-1098

Puech, A., Kister, G. & Chanal, J. (1975) Structure-mobility relation-
    ships in thin-layer chromatography. Applications to some
    progestogens (Fr.). J. Chromatogr., 108, 345-353

Rizk, M., Vallon, J.J. & Badinand, A. (1973) Colorimetric determination
    of acetylenic steroids by Ag^+ ions (Fr.). Anal. chim. acta., 65,
    220-222

Roushdi, I.M., El Sebai, A.I. & Belal, S. (1974) New methods for the
    estimation of acetylenic steroids (non-aqueous titrimetric method).
    Egypt. J. pharm. Sci., 15, 217-221

Tausk, M. & deVisser, J. (1972) International Encyclopedia of Pharma-
    cology and Therapeutics, Vol. II, section 48, Elmsford, NY,
    Pergamon Press, pp. 35-194

Thomas, C., Rogg, H. & Bücheler, J. (1972) Cancer inducing effect of
    N-nitrosomethylurea after administration of hormonal
    contraceptives (Ger.). Beitr. Pathol., 146, 332-338

US Food & Drug Administration (1978) Oral contraceptive drug products.
    Physician and patient labeling: extension of effective date for
    physician labeling. Fed. Regist., 43, 9863-9864

Wade, A., ed. (1977) Martindale, The Extra Pharmacopoeia, 27th ed.,
    London, The Pharmaceutical Press, pp. 1401-1402

Windholz, M., ed. (1976) The Merck Index, 9th ed., Rahway, NJ, Merck &
    Co., p. 732

de Winter, M.S., Siegmann, C.M. & Szpilfogel, S.A. (1959) 17-Alkylated
    3-deoxo-19-nortestosterones. Chemistry and Industry, 11 July, p. 905

MEDROXYPROGESTERONE ACETATE

A monograph on this substance was published previously (IARC, 1974). Relevant data that have appeared since that time have been evaluated in the present monograph.

1. Chemical and Physical Data

1.1 Synonyms and trade names

Chem. Abstr. Services Reg. No.: 71-58-9

Chem. Abstr. Name: (6α)-17-(Acetyloxy)-6-methylpregn-4-ene-3, 20-dione

Synonyms: 17α-Acetoxy-6α-methylprogesterone; depomedroxy-progesterone acetate; 17-hydroxy-6α-methylpregn-4-ene-3,20-dione acetate; 17α-hydroxy-6α-methylprogesterone acetate; 6α-methyl-17-acetoxyprogesterone; 6α-methyl-17α-hydroxy-progesterone acetate; metipregnone

Trade names[1]: Amen; Clinovir; Depcorlutin; Depo-Clinovir; Depo-Provera; [Depo Progevera]; Deporone; Farlutal; [Farlutal Depot]; Farlutin; Gesinal; [Gesinol]; Gestapuran; Gestapuron; [Gestovex]; Luteocrin; [Luteocrin Orale]; Lutopolar; Lutoral; Lutoral (Farmit); MAP; Metigestrona; Metilgestene; MPA; Nogest; Oragest; Perlutex; Prodasone; Progestalfa; Progevera; Promone-E; [Protex]; Provera; Proverone; Provest; Repromix; Sirprogen; Sodelut 'G'; U 8839; [Verafem]; Veramix; Veramix Plus V

---

[1]Those in square brackets are preparations that are no longer produced commercially.

1.2   Structural and molecular formulae and molecular weight

C₂₄H₃₄O₄   Mol. wt: 386.5

1.3   Chemical and physical properties

From Wade (1977) and Windholz (1976), unless otherwise specified

(a)   Description: White to off-white crystals (Hawley, 1977)

(b)   Melting-point: 207-209°C

(c)   Spectroscopy data: λ_{max} 240 nm (E_1^1 = 411) (in ethanol)

(d)   Optical rotation: $[\alpha]_D$ +61° (in chloroform)

(e)   Solubility: Insoluble in water; soluble in ethanol (1 in 800), acetone (1 in 50), chloroform (1 in 10) and dioxane (1 in 60); sparingly soluble in methanol; slightly soluble in diethyl ether

(f)   Stability: Unstable to air and light

1.4   Technical products and impurities

Various national and international pharmacopoeias give specifications for the purity of medroxyprogesterone acetate in pharmaceutical products. For example, it is available in the US as a USP grade containing 97-103% active ingredient on a dried basis. Sterile suspensions in 50, 100 and 400 mg/ml doses contain 90-110% of the stated amount of medroxyprogesterone acetate, and tablets in 2.5 and 10 mg doses contain 93-107% (US Pharmacopeial Convention Inc., 1975).

In the UK, medroxyprogesterone acetate is available in sterile suspensions of 50 mg/ml in 1, 3 and 5 ml vials and in 5 and 100 mg tablets (Wade, 1977).

In Japan, it is available in tablets.

2. Production, Use, Occurrence and Analysis

2.1 Production and use

(a) Production

A method for synthesizing medroxyprogesterone acetate was first reported in 1958, by (1) treating the bisethylene ketal of 17α-hydroxy-progesterone with peracetic acid to give a mixture of $5\alpha,6\alpha$-epoxy-17α-hydroxypregnane-3,20-dione bisethylene ketal and the corresponding $5\beta,6\beta$-epoxide; (2) the α-epoxide is separated from the mixture and refluxed with methylmagnesium bromide in tetrahydrofuran; (3) the resulting bisethylene ketal of $5\alpha,17\alpha$-dihydroxy-6β-methylpregnane-3,20-dione can be dehydrated to 6β-methyl-17α-hydroxyprogesterone and then epimerized to 6α-methyl-17α-hydroxyprogesterone; or it can be hydrolysed to $5\alpha,17\alpha$-dihydroxy-6β-methylpregnane-3,20-dione, which is dehydrated and epimerized to 6α-methyl-17α-hydroxyprogesterone; (4) acylation with acetic anhydride-acetic acid-*para*-toluenesulphonic acid produces medroxyprogesterone acetate (Babcock *et al.*, 1958). Several patents for synthesis routes have since been issued; in one method, the 3,17-ethylene ketal of 17α-hydroxyprogesterone is epoxidized at the 5,6-position with perbenzoic acid, and treatment of the epoxide with methyl-magnesium bromide followed by mild acid is used to open the epoxy ring and to methylate the 6-position. The resulting 5α-hydroxy-6β-methyl-3-one compound is dehydrated to introduce the 4,5-double bond, and the ketal group at the 17-position is removed with acid. Equilibration with a base converts the resulting diketone alcohol to the more stable 6α-methyl configuration, and acetylation produces medroxyprogesterone acetate (Klimstra, 1969). It is not known whether this method is used for commercial production.

Commercial production of medroxyprogesterone acetate in the US was first reported in 1964 (US Tariff Commission, 1965). In 1975 and 1976, only one US company reported production of an undisclosed amount (see preamble, p. 20) (US International Trade Commission, 1977a,b); in 1975, US production of 13 oestrogen and progestin substances, including medroxyprogesterone acetate, amounted to 10.5 thousand kg (US International Trade Commission, 1977a). Data on US imports and exports of this compound are not available.

Commercial production of medroxyprogesterone acetate in the UK was first reported in 1965. It is believed to be produced commercially in Italy, the UK and eastern European countries, but no information was available on the quantities produced. European imports in 1977 are estimated to have amounted to 200 thousand to 2 million kg.

Medroxyprogesterone acetate was first marketed commercially in Japan in 1967. It is not produced there, and imports amounted to 30 kg in 1976 and 1977.

(b) Use

In the US, medroxyprogesterone acetate is administered orally for the treatment of secondary amenorrhoea and dysfunctional uterine bleeding. The usual dose is 2.5-10 mg per day for 5-10 days, starting on the assumed 16th-21st day of the menstrual cycle, and continued for 2 cycles in the case of bleeding. It is also administered for the treatment of endometriosis, orally in doses of 2.5 mg daily for 2-3 weeks, followed by daily doses of 10-15 mg thereafter, or intramuscularly in doses of 50 mg per week or 100 mg every other week. An i.m. injection of medroxy-progesterone acetate is used in the treatment of recurrent or metastatic endometrial carcinoma (Harvey, 1975; Murad & Gilman, 1975).

Medroxyprogesterone acetate is used in countries other than the US as a contraceptive agent, when it is given intramuscularly as 150 mg doses at the beginning of a cycle; effectiveness lasts at least 3 months. It has also been used in the treatment of threatened or habitual abortion in oral doses of 10-40 mg daily or by i.m. administration of 50 mg daily until the signs disappear, then weekly. It is also given by i.m. injection for the treatment of endometriosis, in doses of 50 mg weekly or 100 mg every 2 weeks for 6 months or more (Wade, 1977).

Other uses for medroxyprogesterone acetate in human medicine include: (1) the treatment of dysmenorrhoea, premenstrual tension, and luteal infertility, in oral doses of 2.5-10 mg for 10-20 days, starting on the 6th-16th day of each cycle; (2) as an adjunct to cyclical therapy with oestrogen, at oral doses of 10-20 mg per day for the last 7-10 days of each cycle; and (3) for pregnancy testing as a single 50 mg dose or divided into 5 successive daily doses (Harvey, 1975). It has also been used in the treatment of carcinomas of the breast, testis, ovary and kidney (Wade, 1977).

In Japan, medroxyprogesterone acetate is used in the treatment of threatened abortion.

It has been used in veterinary medicine as follows: (1) in mares, for the treatment of follicular ovarian cysts with persistent oestrus, early habitual abortion, impending abortion, prevention of oestrus and during anoestrus; (2) in bitches, for prevention of oestrus, during anoestrus, abbreviation of oestrus and pseudopregnancy; and (3) in cats, for prevention of oestrus, during anoestrus and abbreviation of oestrus (Harvey, 1975).

2.2 Occurrence

Medroxyprogesterone acetate is not known to occur naturally.

2.3 Analysis

Typical analytical methods for the determination of medroxyprogesterone acetate are summarized in Table 1. Abbreviations used are: GC/ECD, gas chromatography/electron-capture detection; TLC, thin-layer chromatography; UV, ultra-violet spectrometry; and RIA, radioimmunoassay. See also the section, 'General Remarks on Sex Hormones', p. 60.

TABLE 1

Analytical methods for medroxyprogesterone acetate

Sample matrix	Sample preparation	Assay procedure	Sensitivity or limit of detection	Reference
Bulk chemical	Dissolve (chloroform:methanol, 1:1)	TLC (two-dimensional)	-	Cavina et al. (1975)
Bulk chemical	Dissolve	TLC	-	Puech et al. (1975)
Bulk chemical	Dissolve (chloroform); derivatize (isonicotinic acid hydrazide)	UV (380 nm)	-	US Pharmacopeial Convention Inc. (1975)
Suspensions	Extract (chloroform); derivatize (isonicotinic acid hydrazide)	UV (380 nm)	-	US Pharmacopeial Convention Inc. (1975)
Tablets	Powder; suspend (water); extract (chloroform); derivatize (isonicotinic acid hydrazide)	UV (380 nm)	-	US Pharmacopeial Convention Inc. (1975)
Parenteral preparations	Dissolve (ethanol)	Polarography	150 µg/ml	Chatten et al. (1976)
Plasma	Add labelled medroxyprogesterone acetate; extract (benzene:isooctane, 2:1); add antiserum	RIA	200 pg/ml (0.3 ml sample)	Hiroi et al. (1975)
Plasma	Extract (cyclohexane); derivatize (heptafluorobutyrate)	GC/ECD	1 ng/ml (5 ml sample)	Kaiser et al. (1974)

3. Biological Data Relevant to the Evaluation
of Carcinogenic Risk to Humans

3.1 Carcinogenicity studies in animals

Subcutaneous and/or intramuscular administration

Mouse: In a study reported in an abstract, 33 female Marsh mice, 3
months of age, were given an i.m. injection of 5 mg medroxyprogesterone
acetate (Depo-Provera, which contains 100 mg/ml) into the medial aspect
of the left thigh and the same dose 1 month later into the right thigh;
animals were followed for 20 months. Equal numbers of litter mates
received isotonic saline. No increase in the number of tumours was
observed (Bischoff & Bryson, 1977).

Dog: Four and 16 female beagle dogs were given an i.m. injection of
2.5 or 62.5 mg/kg bw medroxyprogesterone acetate every 3 months. Mammary
nodules developed in both groups, the first being detected after 20 and
15 months, respectively. Some mammary nodules also developed in 16
control dogs, the first being detected after 17 months. The difference
in the incidence of nodules was not significant; however, there were 10
times as many nodules per dog in the treated groups than in the controls,
and, in addition, 3/4 dogs in the higher dosage group had malignant
mammary tumours with metastases. All dogs given the higher dose had
died or had been killed by the end of the fourth year. No such malignant
tumours were found in dogs that died or were sacrificed prior to month
42 of administration or in any of the control dogs (Finkel & Berliner,
1973; WHO, 1973) [The Working Group noted that full details of the
study have not become available].

3.2 Other relevant biological data

For a review of the biological activities of the progestin compounds,
see Tausk & deVisser (1972). Medroxyprogesterone acetate displays high
parenteral and oral progestational activity in animals and humans
(Desaulles & Krähenbühl, 1959; Neumann, 1968). For the relative activity
of this compound compared with that of other progestins, see 'General
Remarks on Sex Hormones', p. 44.

No data on the toxicity of medroxyprogesterone acetate were available.

Embryotoxicity and teratogenicity

No significant dose-related malformations were seen in rats or mice
given s.c. injections of 3-3000 mg/kg bw medroxyprogesterone acetate
daily for 3, 6 or 9 days during days 7-15 of gestation (mice) or days 8-
16 (rats) (Andrew & Staples, 1977).

S.c. administration to rats of 0.3-1 mg/animal medroxyprogesterone acetate on days 17-20 of gestation had a virilizing effect on the external genitalia of offspring; doses of 3-30 mg induced the development of prostate glands in female progeny (Cupceancu & Neumann, 1969).

In rats, s.c. injection of 12.5 mg medroxyprogesterone acetate on the day of mating caused delayed implantation; when 1 μg oestrone was given additionally on day 4, delayed implantation was abolished. When the oestrone was administered on day 3, embryos were destroyed in the morula-blastula stage (Dickmann, 1973).

Daily s.c. injections to guinea-pigs of 1 mg medroxyprogesterone acetate/animal from day 18 after mating until day 60 led to masculinization of the external and internal genitalia of offspring (Foote et al., 1968).

Medroxyprogesterone acetate was injected subcutaneously to rabbits at doses of 0.1-30 mg/kg bw per day for 3, 6 or 9 days during days 7-15 of gestation. Toxic effects were seen with 10 and 30 mg/kg bw, and a significant dose-related increase in foetal mortality occurred. The incidence of cleft palate was also dose-related: it was observed in 6%, 28% and 43% of offspring of animals given the compound from day 13-15 of gestation in doses of 1, 3 and 10 mg/kg bw, respectively (Andrew & Staples, 1977).

Absorption, distribution, excretion and metabolism

I.m. injections of medroxyprogesterone acetate have a pronounced storage effect; for instance, in *Macaca mulatta* (rhesus) monkeys, peak concentrations were detected in plasma 2 weeks later, followed by a gradual decline (Zaki et al., 1978).

In baboons, the amount involved in enterohepatic circulation is small (Ishihara et al., 1976).

In dogs, medroxyprogesterone acetate is metabolized more slowly than progesterone (Runić et al., 1976). Glucuronide conjugates are excreted in urine and bile. Loss of the 17α-acetyl group, which varies in baboons from 30-70%, is greater than in the case of chlormadinone acetate (see monograph, p. 371), and appears to be similar in baboons and humans (Ishihara et al., 1976).

Mutagenicity and other short-term tests

No damage to bone-marrow cells was observed in female rats treated orally for 5 days with 10 mg/kg bw medroxyprogesterone acetate, as compared with controls treated with corn oil (Edwards et al., 1971).

3.3 Case reports and epidemiological studies

(a) Breast

One study carried out in Thailand showed no difference in the prevalence of palpable breast nodules in users and nonusers of medroxy-progesterone acetate, although limitations in the study design preclude firm conclusions (McDaniel & Pardthaisong, 1973).

(b) Cervix

There are two reports on the effect of injection of progestins on the development of cancer of the cervix. In the first (Powell & Seymour, 1971; Seymour & Powell, 1970), 1123 women in the US were given medroxy-progesterone acetate injections every 3 months for a total of 14,000 person-months. About half of the women received supplementary oestrogen. Dysplasia and carcinoma *in situ* were found in rates about twice as high as prevailing rates for women in a selected comparison population; however, the progestin-treated women were older, more parous and of lower socio-economic status.

Conflicting results were obtained by Dabancens *et al.* (1974) in Chile. They found no difference in the incidences of dysplasia and cancer *in situ* in women injected with medroxyprogesterone acetate or with chlormadinone acetate and in those with intrauterine devices. However, the progestin-treated women in this study were older and of higher parity than the women using intrauterine devices.

4. Summary of Data Reported and Evaluation[1]

4.1 Experimental data

Medroxyprogesterone acetate was tested in mice and dogs by intra-muscular administration. It produced mammary tumours in dogs.

Medroxyprogesterone acetate was reported to have teratogenic effects in some species.

4.2 Human data

One epidemiological study concerning the development of breast nodules and two studies concerning the development of dysplasias and carcinoma *in situ* of the uterine cervix have been reported. The results of these studies were conflicting and difficult to interpret because of

---

[1]This section should be read in conjunction with pp. 62-64 in the 'General Remarks on Sex Hormones' and with the 'General Conclusions on Sex Hormones', p. 131.

methodological problems. Epidemiological studies on steroid hormones used in contraceptive preparations have been summarized in the section, 'Oestrogens and Progestins in Relation to Human Cancer', p. 83 .

4.3 Evaluation

There is *limited evidence* for the carcinogenicity of medroxyprogesterone acetate in dogs. Epidemiological studies on medroxyprogesterone acetate are inadequate for an evaluation of the carcinogenicity of this compound in humans.

5. References

Andrew, F.D. & Staples, R.E. (1977) Prenatal toxicity of medroxy-progesterone acetate in rabbits, rats and mice. Teratology, 15, 25-32

Babcock, J.C., Gutsell, E.S., Herr, M.E., Hogg, J.A., Stucki, J.C., Barnes, L.E. & Dulin, W.E. (1958) 6α-Methyl-17α-hydroxy-progesterone 17-acylates; a new class of potent progestins. J. Am. chem. Soc., 80, 2904-2905

Bischoff, F. & Bryson, G. (1977) Medroxyprogesterone administration in female Marsh mice (Abstract no. 9). Proc. Am. Assoc. Cancer Res., 18, 3

Cavina, G., Moretti, G. & Petrella, M. (1975) A solvent system for the separation of steroids with estrogenic and progestational activity by two-dimensional thin-layer chromatography. J. Chromatogr., 103, 368-371

Chatten, L.G., Yadav, R.N. & Madan, D.K. (1976) The determination of certain Δ^4-3-ketosteroids in some parenteral formulations by differential pulse polarography. Pharm. acta helv., 51, 381-383

Cupceancu, B. & Neumann, F. (1969) Sensitivity differences of different genital tract structures of female rat fetuses due to the effect of medroxyprogesterone acetate or norethisterone acetate (Ger.). Endokrinologie, 54, 66-80

Dabancens, A., Prado, R., Larraguibel, R. & Zañartu, J. (1974) Intraepithelial cervical neoplasia in women using intrauterine devices and long-acting injectable progestogens as contraceptives. Am. J. Obstet. Gynecol., 119, 1052-1056

Desaulles, P.A., & Krähenbühl, C. (1959) Modern developments in the field of gestagen therapy (Ger.). In: Nowakowski, H., ed., Modern Development in the Field of Gestagen Therapy. Hormones Used in Veterinary Medicine, Berlin, Springer, pp. 1-10

Dickmann, Z. (1973) Postcoital contraceptive effects of medroxypro-gesterone acetate and oestrone in rats. J. Reprod. Fertil., 32, 65-69

Edwards, C.W., Calhoun, F.J. & Green, S. (1971) The effects of mestranol and several progestins on chromosomes and fertility in the rat (Abstract no. 157). Toxicol. appl. Pharmacol., 19, 421

Finkel, M.J. & Berliner, V.R. (1973) The extrapolation of experimental findings (animals to man): the dilemma of the systemically administered contraceptives. Bull. Soc. pharmacol. environ. Pathol., 4, 13-18

Foote, W.D., Foote, W.C. & Foote, L.H. (1968) Influence of certain natural and synthetic steroids on genital development in guinea-pigs. Fertil. Steril., 19, 606-615

Harvey, S.C. (1975) Hormones. In: Osol, A. *et al.* eds, Remington's Pharmaceutical Sciences, 15th ed., Easton, PA, Mack, p. 923

Hawley, G.G., ed. (1977) The Condensed Chemical Dictionary, 9th ed., New York, Van Nostrand-Reinhold, p. 542

Hiroi, M., Stanczyk, F.Z., Goebelsmann, U., Brenner, P.F., Lumkin, M.E. & Mishell, D.R., Jr (1975) Radioimmunoassay of serum medroxy-progesterone acetate (Provera®) in women following oral and intravaginal administration. Steroids, 26, 373-385

IARC (1974) IARC Monographs on the Evaluation of Carcinogenic Risk of Chemicals to Man, 6, Sex Hormones, Lyon, pp. 157-163

Ishihara, M., Kirdani, R.Y., Osawa, Y. & Sandberg, A.A. (1976) The metabolic fate of medroxyprogesterone acetate in the baboon. J. Steroid Biochem., 7, 65-70

Kaiser, D.G., Carlson, R.G. & Kirton, K.T. (1974) GLC determination of medroxyprogesterone acetate in plasma. J. pharm. Sci., 63 420-424

Klimstra, P.D. (1969) The role of progestin and estrogen in fertility control and maintenance. In: The Chemistry and Biochemistry of Steroids, Los Altos, CA, Geron-X, pp. 66-67

McDaniel, E.B. & Pardthaisong, T. (1973) Incidence of breast nodules in women receiving multiple doses of medroxyprogesterone acetate. J. biosoc. Sci., 5, 83-88

Murad, F. & Gilman, A.G. (1975) Estrogens and progestins. In: Goodman, L.S. & Gilman, A., eds, The Pharmacological Basis of Therapeutics, 5th ed., New York, Macmillan, pp. 1439-1445

Neumann, F. (1968) Chemical constitution and pharmacologic action (Ger.). In: Langecker, H., ed., Handbuch der Experimenteller Pharmakologie, Vol 22, Die Gestagene, Berlin, Springer, pp. 680-1025

Powell, L.C., Jr & Seymour, R.J. (1971) Effects of depo-medroxy-progesterone acetate as a contraceptive agent. Am. J. Obstet. Gynecol., 110, 36-41

Puech, A., Kister, G. & Chanal, J. (1975) Structural-mobility relationships in thin-layer chromatography. Applications to some progestogens (Fr.). J. Chromatogr., 108, 345-353

Runić, S., Miljković, M., Bogumil, R.J., Nahrwold, D. & Bardin, W. (1976) The in vivo metabolism of progestins. I. The metabolic clearance rates of progesterone and medroxyprogesterone acetate in the dog. Endocrinology, 99, 108-113

Seymour, R.J. & Powell, L.C., Jr (1970) Depo-medroxyprogesterone acetate as a contraceptive. Obstet. Gynecol., 36, 589-596

Tausk, M. & deVisser, J. (1972) International Encyclopedia of Pharmacology and Therapeutics, Vol. II, section 48, Elmsford, NY, Pergamon Press, pp. 35-194

US International Trade Commission (1977a) Synthetic Organic Chemicals, US Production and Sales, 1975, USITC Publication 804, Washington DC, US Government Printing Office, pp. 90, 102

US International Trade Commission (1977b) Synthetic Organic Chemicals, US Production and Sales, 1976, USITC Publication 833, Washington DC, US Government Printing Office, p. 148

US Pharmacopeial Convention Inc. (1975) The US Pharmacopeia, 19th rev., Rockville, MD, pp. 299-300

US Tariff Commission (1965) Synthetic Organic Chemicals, US Production and Sales, 1964, TC Publication 167, Washington DC, US Government Printing Office, p. 135

Wade, A., ed. (1977) Martindale, The Extra Pharmacopoeia, 27th ed., London, The Pharmaceutical Press, pp. 1402-1404

WHO (1973) Advances in methods of fertility regulation. Report of a WHO Scientific Group. World Health Org. tech. Rep. Ser., No. 527, pp. 13-14

Windholz, M., ed. (1976) The Merck Index, 9th ed., Rahway, NJ, Merck & Co., p. 751

Zaki, K., Atkinson, L.E. & Segal, S.J. (1978) Medroxyprogesterone acetate: peripheral serum levels and its effects on pituitary and ovarian functions in the rhesus monkey. Arzneim.-Forsch., 28, 1003-1008

MEGESTROL ACETATE

1. Chemical and Physical Data

1.1 Synonyms and trade names

Chem. Abstr. Services Reg. No.: 595-33-5

Chem. Abstr. Name: 17α-(Acetyloxy)-6-methylpregna-4,6-diene-3,-20-dione

Synonyms: 6-Dehydro-6-methyl-17α-acetoxyprogesterone; 17α-hydroxy-6-methylpregna-4,6-diene-3,20-dione acetate; megestryl acetate; 6-methyl-$\Delta^{4,6}$-pregnadien-17α-ol-3,20-dione acetate

Trade names: 5071; BDH 1298; Co-Ervonum; Delpregnin; DMAP; Kombiguens; Magestin; Megace; Megage; Megeron; Minigest; Niagestin; Nuvacon; Ovaban; Ovarid; Ovex; Planovin; SC-10363; Serial 28; Tri-Ervonum; Volidan; Volidan 21; Voplan; Weradys

1.2 Structural and molecular formulae and molecular weight

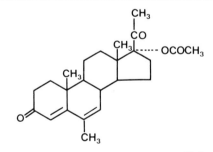

$C_{24}H_{32}O_4$ Mol. wt: 384.5

1.3 Chemical and physical properties

From Wade (1977) and Windholz (1976)

(a) Description: Crystals (from methanol)

(b) Melting-point: 214-216°C

(c) Optical rotation: $[\alpha]_D^{24}$ +5° (in chloroform)

(d) Spectroscopy data: λ_{max} 287 nm (E_1^1 = 653.3) (in ethanol)

(e) Solubility: Practically insoluble in water; soluble in ethanol (1 in 55), chloroform (1 in 0.8) and diethyl ether (1 in 130); soluble in acetone and benzyl alcohol; slightly soluble in fixed oils

(f) Stability: Unstable to light

1.4 Technical products and impurities

Megestrol acetate is available in the UK, containing 97-103% active ingredient on a dried basis (British Pharmacopoeia Commission, 1973). It is available in the US in tablets in 20 and 40 mg doses (Kastrup, 1977).

2. Production, Use, Occurrence and Analysis

2.1 Production and use

(a) Production

Megestrol acetate was first synthesized in 1959 by the dehydrogenation of medroxyprogesterone acetate with chloranil (Ringold *et al.*, 1959); however, it is not known if this is the method used for commercial production (Chinn *et al.*, 1969).

Commercial production of megestrol acetate in the US was first reported in 1976, when one company reported production of an undisclosed amount (see preamble, p. 20) (US International Trade Commission, 1977). Separate data on US imports and exports are not available.

It is believed to be produced commercially in Italy, but no information was available on the quantity produced.

Megestrol acetate is neither produced nor imported in Japan.

(b) Use

Megestrol acetate is used in human medicine in the US for the treatment of endometrial and breast carcinoma (Harvey, 1975; Wade, 1977). It has also been used for the treatment of acne, hirsutism and sexual infantilism in female patients (Wade, 1977). It has been used in some countries as an oral contraceptive, in combination with an

oestrogen such as ethinyloestradiol.   It is not employed for this
purpose in the US (Harvey, 1975), and such usage was discontinued in
the UK in 1975 (Wade, 1977).

Veterinary use of megestrol acetate as a progestational agent for
oestrus regulation has been reported (Windholz, 1976).

2.2 Occurrence

Megestrol acetate is not known to occur naturally.

2.3 Analysis

Typical analytical methods for the determination of megestrol
acetate are summarized in Table 1.   Abbreviations used are: UV, ultra-
violet spectrometry;   GC/MS, gas chromatography/mass spectrometry;
TLC, thin-layer chromatography;   CC, column chromatography;   and RIA,
radioimmunoassay.   See also the section, 'General Remarks on Sex
Hormones', p. 60.

TABLE 1

Analytical methods for megestrol acetate

Sample matrix	Sample preparation	Assay procedure	Sensitivity or limit of detection	Reference
Bulk chemical	Dissolve (ethanol)	UV (287 nm)	-	British Pharma-copoeia Commission (1973)
Bulk chemical	Dissolve (chloroform:methanol, 1:1) to 0.1% concentration	Two-dimensional TLC (UV, acid spray)	-	Cavina et al. (1975)
Tablets	Extract (acetone); centrifuge; decant; reduce volume	Two-dimensional TLC (UV, acid spray)	0.5 µg by UV; 1 µg using acid spray	Simard & Lodge (1970)
Blood plasma	Extract (diethyl ether:chloroform, 3:1); CC (silica gel); isolate; derivatize (monomethoxime)	GC/MS	200 pg/ml	Adlercreutz et al. (1974)
Blood plasma	Add to tracer solution; incubate; pre-cipitate; centrifuge; dissolve preci-pitate (water); extract (benzene:petroleum ether, 2:3); evaporate; dissolve (buffer)	RIA	30 pg/ml	Adlercreutz et al. (1975)
Urine	Multiple CC; TLC; isolate & derivatize (monomethoxime, trimethylsilyl ether)	GC/MS	-	Adlercreutz et al. (1975)

3. Biological Data Relevant to the Evaluation of Carcinogenic Risk to Humans

3.1 Carcinogenicity studies in animals

(a) Oral administration

Mouse: Megestrol acetate alone or in combination with ethinyl-oestradiol (5:1 and 80:1) was incorporated into the diet of groups of 78-97 male and female BDH-SPF mice daily for 80 weeks. The doses were identified only as low (2-5 times the human contraceptive dose), medium (50-150 times) or high (200-400 times); the amounts administered were not specified. The administration of the 80:1 combination resulted in an increased incidence of malignant mammary tumours in females (32% *versus* 3% in controls) and in males (17% *versus* 0 in controls) (Committee on Safety of Medicines, 1972).

Rat: Administration of megestrol acetate alone or in combination with ethinyloestradiol (5:1 and 80:1) for 104 weeks did not affect the incidence of tumours in groups of 73-81 male and female rats (Committee on Safety of Medicines, 1972).

Dog: In a long-term study, megestrol acetate was administered orally to groups of 20 pure-bred female beagles, 6-12 months of age at the start of the experiment. It was given as doses of 0.01, 0.10 and 0.25 mg/kg bw per day in coconut oil by capsule; these represented 1, 10 and 25 times the projected human dose on a mg/kg bw basis. Dogs were killed at 2, 4 and 7 years for histopathological examination. During the first 4 years of the study, the number of animals bearing palpable mammary nodules increased with time and with the dose admi-nistered; controls were free of nodules at the end of this period. Of 38 grossly detected nodules that were evaluated microscopically, 27 (71%) were classified as nodular hyperplasia and 5 (13%) as benign mixed mammary tumours; no adenocarcinomas were observed (Nelson *et al.*, 1973). The study was terminated at 7 years, and the final report (Weikel & Nelson, 1977) indicates an increase in the number of neoplasias from 5 at 4 years to 29 at 7 years (benign mammary tumours from 5 to 19; ductal papillomas from 0 to 1; mammary adenocarcinomas from 0 to 10). There was also a dose-response trend in tumour development: the numbers of neoplastic lesions were 0, 11 and 19 for animals treated with 0.01, 0.10 and 0.25 mg/kg bw per day, respectively [The Working Group noted the lack of information concerning the number of tumour-bearing animals].

(b) Subcutaneous and/or intramuscular administration

Rat: Groups of 10 female Wistar rats were given s.c. injections of 5, 10 or 15 mg/kg bw of a mixture of ethinyloestradiol:megestrol

acetate (1:8) in olive oil once every other day for 30 days.   Mammary
fibroadenomas occurred in 2/10, 4/8 and 2/9 survivors at between 29 and
59 weeks, compared with none in 10 surviving controls (Hisamatsu, 1972)
[The Working Group noted the small numbers in each group].

3.2 Other relevant biological data

For a review of the biological activity of the progestin compounds,
see Tausk & deVisser (1972).   Megestrol acetate displays high parenteral
and oral progestational activity in animals and humans (Neumann, 1968).
For the activity of this compound relative to that of other progestins,
see 'General Remarks on Sex Hormones', p. 44.

No data on the toxicity, embryotoxicity or teratogenicity of
megestrol acetate were available.

Megestrol acetate, like the related compounds chlormadinone acetate
(p. 371) and medroxyprogesterone acetate (p. 424), is metabolized much more
slowly than progesterone.   Metabolic studies *in vitro* and structural
considerations (Cooke & Vallance, 1965) showed that the 17α-acetoxy group
hinders metabolizing enzymes of rabbit liver, and the 6-methyl group those
of rat liver.   The 6(7)-double bond confers additional resistance to
metabolism by enzymes of rabbit liver.

No chromosomal effects were observed when 0.1-100 µg/ml megestrol
acetate were added to cultures of lymphocytes grown from the blood of
healthy women (Stenchever *et al.*, 1969).

No significant difference in the frequency of abnormal karyotypes or
in sex ratio was found in 124 abortuses of women who had taken oral
contraceptives (including 11 who had taken 4 mg megestrol acetate with
0.05 mg mestranol), in comparison with 122 abortuses of women who had
never used oral contraceptives (Lauritsen, 1975).

3.3 Case reports and epidemiological studies

See the section, 'Oestrogens and Progestins in Relation to Human
Cancer', p. 83.

4. Summary of Data Reported and Evaluation[1]

4.1 Experimental data

Megestrol acetate alone or with ethinyloestradiol was tested in mice, rats and dogs by oral administration and in rats by subcutaneous administration. It produced mammary tumours in dogs when tested alone and in mice when tested in combination with ethinyloestradiol. Experiments in which it was tested in rats in combination with ethinyloestradiol were negative or inadequate.

4.2 Human data

No case reports or epidemiological studies on megestrol acetate alone were available to the Working Group. Epidemiological studies on steroid hormones used in oestrogen-progestin contraceptive preparations have been summarized in the section, 'Oestrogens and Progestins in Relation to Human Cancer', p. 83.

4.3 Evaluation

There is *limited evidence* for the carcinogenicity of megestrol acetate in dogs. In humans, oral contraceptives containing oestrogens in combination with progestins have been related causally to an increased incidence of benign liver adenomas and a decreased incidence of benign breast disease.

---

[1]This section should be read in conjunction with pp. 62-64 in the 'General Remarks on Sex Hormones' and with the 'General Conclusions on Sex Hormones', p. 131.

5. References

Adlercreutz, H., Nieminen, U. & Ervast, H.-S. (1974)   A mass fragmento-
    graphic method for the determination of megestrol acetate in plasma
    and its application to studies on the plasma levels after administra-
    tion of the progestin to patients with carcinoma corporis uteri.
    J. Steroid Biochem., 5, 619-626

Adlercreutz, H., Martin, F., Wahlroos, Ö. & Soini, E. (1975)   Mass
    spectrometric and mass fragmentographic determination of natural
    and synthetic steroids in biological fluids.   J. Steroid Biochem.,
    6, 247-259

British Pharmacopoeia Commission (1973)   British Pharmacopoeia, London,
    HMSO, pp. 281-282

Cavina, G., Moretti, G. & Petrella, M. (1975)   A solvent system for
    the separation of steroids with estrogenic and progestational
    activity by two-dimensional thin-layer chromatography.   J. Chroma-
    togr., 103, 368-371

Chinn, L.J., Klimstra, P.D., Baran, J.S. & Pappo, R. (1969)   The
    Chemistry and Biochemistry of Steroids, Los Altos, CA, Geron-X,
    p. 67

Committee on Safety of Medicines (1972)   Carcinogenicity Tests of Oral
    Contraceptives, London, HMSO

Cooke, B.A. & Vallance, D.K. (1965)   Metabolism of megestrol acetate and
    related progesterone analogues by liver preparations in vitro.
    Biochem. J., 97, 672-677

Harvey, S.C. (1975)   Hormones.   In: Osol, A., et al., eds, Remington's
    Pharmaceutical Sciences, 15th ed., Easton, PA, Mack, p. 925

Hisamatsu, T. (1972)   Mammary tumorigenesis by subcutaneous administration
    of a mixture of megestrol acetate and ethynylestradiol in Wistar rats.
    Gann, 63, 483-485

Kastrup, E.K., ed. (1977)   Facts and Comparisons, St Louis, MO, Facts &
    Comparisons Inc., p. 665

Lauritsen, J.G. (1975)   The significance of oral contraceptives in
    causing chromosome anomalies in spontaneous abortions.   Acta
    obstet. gynecol. scand., 54, 261-264

Nelson, L.W., Weikel, J.H., Jr & Reno, F.E. (1973)   Mammary nodules in
    dogs during four years' treatment with megestrol acetate or chlorma-
    dinone acetate.   J. natl Cancer Inst., 51, 1303-1311

Neumann, F. (1968)   Chemical constitution and pharmacologic action
    (Ger.).   In: Langecker, H., ed., Handbuch der Experimenteller
    Pharmakologie, Vol. 22, Die Gestagene, Berlin, Springer, pp. 680-
    1025

Ringold, H.J., Ruelas, J.P., Batres, E. & Djerassi, C. (1959)   Steroids.
    CXVIII. 6-Methyl derivatives of 17α-hydroxyprogesterone and of
    Reichstein's substance 'S'.   J. Am. chem. Soc., 81, 3712-3716

Simard, M.B. & Lodge, B.A. (1970)   Thin-layer chromatographic identifi-
    cation of estrogens and progestogens in oral contraceptives.
    J. Chromatogr., 51, 517-524

Stenchever, M.A., Jarvis, J.A. & Kreger, N.K. (1969)   Effect of selected
    estrogens and progestins on human chromosomes in vitro.   Obstet.
    Gynecol., 34, 249-251

Tausk, M. & deVisser, J. (1972)   International Encyclopedia of Pharma-
    cology and Therapeutics, Vol. II, section 48, Elmsford, NY,
    Pergamon Press, pp. 35-194

US International Trade Commission (1977)   Synthetic Organic Chemicals,
    US Production and Sales, 1976, USITC Publication 833, Washington
    DC, US Government Printing Office, p. 149

Wade, A., ed. (1977)   Martindale, The Extra Pharmacopoeia, 27th ed.,
    London, The Pharmaceutical Press, pp. 1404-1405

Weikel, J.H., Jr & Nelson, L.W. (1977)   Problems in evaluating chronic
    toxicity of contraceptive steroids in dogs.   J. Toxicol. environ.
    Health, 3, 167-177

Windholz, M., ed. (1976)   The Merck Index, 9th ed., Rahway, NJ, Merck
    & Co., p. 752

NORETHISTERONE and NORETHISTERONE ACETATE

A monograph on these substances was published previously (IARC, 1974). Relevant data that have appeared since that time have been evaluated in the present monograph.

1. Chemical and Physical Data

Norethisterone

1.1 Synonyms and trade names

Chem. Abstr. Services Reg. No.: 68-22-4

Chem. Abstr. Name: (17α)-17-Hydroxy-19-norpregn-4-en-20-yn-3-one

Synonyms: Anhydroxynorprogesterone; ethinylnortestosterone; 17α-ethinyl-19-nortestosterone; ethynylnortestosterone; 17α-ethynyl-19-nortestosterone; 17-hydroxy-19-nor-17α-pregn-4-en-20-yn-3-one; norethindrone; norethisteron; 19-norethisterone; norethynodrone; 19-nor-17α-ethynyl-17β-hydroxy-4-androsten-3-one; 19-nor-17α-ethynyltestosterone; norpregneninolone

Trade names[1]: [Anovlar 21]; Anovule; [Anzolan]; Brevicon; Brevicon-28 Day; Conludaf; Conludag; [Conlumin]; [Conlunett]; [Conlunett 21]; [Conlutan]; [Conluten]; [Dianor]; Gestest; [Gynostat]; [Gynovlar]; Micronett; Micronor; Micronovum; Mini-Pe; Modicon; Modicon 28; [Nor 50]; Noralutin; Norfor; Norgestin; Noriday; [Noridei]; Norinyl; Norinyl-1/28; Norinyl-1; Norinyl-2; Norluten; Norlutin; Norluton; Nor-QD; [Norquentiel]; NSC-9564; [Orlestrin]; [Orthonovin]; [Ortho-Novin]; Ortho-Novin 1/50; Ortho-Novin 1/80; [Ortho-Novin 2]; [Ortho-Novin Mite]; [Ortho-Novin Sq.]; [Orthonovum]; [Orthonovum N]: Ortho-Novum;

---

[1]Those in square brackets are preparations that are no longer produced commercially.

[Ortho-Novum 1/50]; [Ortho-Novum 1/80]; [Ortho-Novum 2];
[Ortho-Novum Sq.]; Ovcon-35; Ovysmen; [Plan]; Primolutin;
Primolut N; [Primosiston]; [Progynon C]; Proluteasi; [Regovar];
SC 4640

1.2 Structural and molecular formulae and molecular weight

$C_{20}H_{26}O_2$ Mol. wt: 298.4

1.3 Chemical and physical properties

From Wade (1977) and Windholz (1976), unless otherwise specified

(a) Description: White crystalline powder with a slightly bitter
taste

(b) Melting-point: 203-204°C

(c) Spectroscopy data: λ_{max} 240 nm (E_1^1 = 575) in ethanol; infra-
red, nuclear magnetic resonance and mass spectral data have
been tabulated (Shroff & Moyer, 1975).

(d) Optical rotation: $[\alpha]_D^{20}$ -31.7° (in chloroform)

(e) Solubility: Practically insoluble in water and fixed oils;
soluble in ethanol (1 in 150), acetone (1 in 80), chloroform
(1 in 30) and pyridine (1 in 5); soluble in dioxane; slightly soluble in diethyl ether

(f) Stability: Unstable to air and light

1.4 Technical products and impurities

Various national and international pharmacopoeias give specifications
for the purity of norethisterone in pharmaceutical products. For example,
norethisterone is available in the US as a USP grade containing 97-102%

active ingredient on an anhydrous basis.   It is also available in doses
of 0.35-10 mg as tablets containing 90-110% of the stated amount of norethisterone, either by itself or in combination with mestranol or ethinyloestradiol (Kastrup, 1977, 1978; US Pharmacopeial Convention Inc., 1975).

In the UK, norethisterone is available in tablets containing 0.35,
0.5, 1, 2 and 5 mg and in combination with mestranol and ethinyloestradiol
(Wade, 1977).

In Japan, norethisterone is available in tablets containing 4 mg in
combination with ethinyloestradiol.

Norethisterone acetate

1.1 Synonyms and trade names

Chem. Abstr. Services Reg. No.:   51-98-9

Chem. Abstr. Name: (17α)-17-(Acetyloxy)-19-norpregn-4-en-20-yn-3-one

Synonyms: 17α-Ethinyl-19-nortestosterone acetate; 17α-ethinyl-19-
nortestosterone 17β-acetate; 17α-ethynyl-19-nortestosterone
acetate; 17-hydroxy-19-nor-17α-pregn-4-en-20-yn-3-one acetate;
norethindrone acetate; norethindrone 17-acetate; norethisteron
acetate; 19-norethisterone acetate; norethynyltestosterone
acetate; 19-norethynyltestosterone acetate; norethysterone acetate

Trade names: [Ablacton]; [Anovlar]; Anovlar 21; Controvlar;
[Duogynon Oral]; Etalontin; [Gestest]; [Gynovlane]; Gynovlar 21;
Loestrin; Loestrin-21; [Milli-Anovlar]; Minovlar; [N Gestakliman];
[Norinyl]; Norlestrin; Norlestrin 21; Norlestrin 28; Norlestrin
Fe; Norlutate; [Norlutate A]; Norlutin-A; Norlutin acetate;
Orlest 21; [Orlest 28]; Orlutate; Ovcon 50; Primodos; Primolut-
Nor; Primosiston; [Profinix]; Prolestrin; SH 420; Zorane

1.2 Structural and molecular formulae and molecular weight

$C_{22}H_{28}O_3$ Mol. wt: 340.5

1.3 Chemical and physical properties

From Wade (1977) and Windholz (1976), unless otherwise specified

(a) Description: White crystalline powder with a slightly bitter
taste

(b) Melting-point: 161-162°C

(c) Spectroscopy data: λ_{max} 240 nm (E_1^1 = 549).   Infra-red
spectral data have been tabulated (Grasselli & Ritchey, 1975).

(d) Optical rotation: $[\alpha]_D^{20}$ -32 to -38° (2% w/v in dioxane)
(US Pharmacopeial Convention Inc., 1975)

(e) Solubility: Practically insoluble in water; soluble in
ethanol (1 in 1.5), acetone (1 in 4), chloroform (1 in <1),
dioxane (1 in 2) and diethyl ether (1 in 18)

(f) Stability: Unstable to light

1.4 Technical products and impurities

Various national and international pharmacopoeias give specifications
for the purity of norethisterone acetate in pharmaceutical products.   For
example, norethisterone acetate is available in the US as a USP grade
containing 97-103% active ingredient on a dried basis.   It is also available in tablets containing 1-5 mg and which have 90-110% of the stated
amount of norethisterone acetate, either by itself or in combination with
ethinyloestradiol (Kastrup, 1977, 1978; US Pharmacopeial Convention Inc.,
1975).

In the UK, norethisterone acetate is available in tablets containing
1, 1.5, 2.5, 3, 4, 5 and 10 mg, by itself and in combination with mestranol
and ethinyloestradiol (Wade, 1977).

Norethisterone acetate is available in Japan in 4 mg doses as tablets in combination with ethinyloestradiol.

2. Production, Use, Occurrence and Analysis

2.1 Production and use

(a) Production

A method for synthesizing norethisterone was first reported in 1954 (Djerassi *et al.*, 1954) in which oestrone was converted to its methyl ether, which was reduced to oestradiol 3-methyl ether with lithium aluminium hydride; a Birch reduction gave the 1,4-dihydroaromatic compound, which by an Oppenauer oxidation produced the 17-ketone; this was ethinylated to produce the 17-ethinyl carbinol, and subsequent acid hydrolysis of the 3-methyl ether linkage using hydrochloric acid produced norethisterone. In a method for synthesizing norethisterone acetate, first patented in 1957 (Engelfried *et al.*, 1957), norethisterone is acetylated with acetic anhydride in pyridine. It is not known whether these processes are used for commercial production.

Norethisterone is believed to be produced commercially in the Federal Republic of Germany, France, Italy, The Netherlands and the UK. Norethisterone acetate is believed to be produced in the Federal Republic of Germany, France and Italy. No information was available on the quantities produced.

Norethisterone and its acetate were first marketed in Japan in 1969. They are not produced there, and imports of norethisterone amounted to approximately 35 kg in 1975, 45 kg in 1976 and 35 kg in 1977; imports of norethisterone acetate amounted to approximately 250 kg in 1975, 220 kg in 1976 and 180 kg in 1977.

Norethisterone and its acetate are not produced in the US, and separate data on imports are not available.

(b) Use

Small amounts of norethisterone, an orally-active progestin, have been used in human medicine since 1957. It is used for the treatment of conditions such as: (1) amenorrhoea (in doses of 10-20 mg daily from the 5th to the 24th day of the cycle), (2) dysfunctional uterine bleeding (at a level of 15 mg daily for 10 days) and (3) endometriosis (10 mg daily, increased to 20-30 mg for a maintenance dose and continued for 9-12 months). It is also used for the treatment of premenstrual tension and dysmenorrhoea. To delay or prevent menstruation, it is given in doses of 15-30 mg daily (Wade, 1977).

Since 1962 the most common use of norethisterone in the US has been as the progestin in progestin-oestrogen combination oral contraceptives. The usual dose is 0.5-2 mg daily in combination with mestranol or ethinylo-estradiol (given from the 5th to the 25th day of the cycle followed by 7 tablet-free days).   It is also used continuously at a daily dose of 0.35 mg in the so called contraceptive 'mini-pill' (Harvey, 1975;   Wade, 1977).

In Japan, norethisterone is used in doses of 5-10 mg 1-2 times daily for the treatment of endometriosis.

The medicinal use of norethisterone acetate is similar to that of norethisterone, as an orally-active progestin for the treatment of primary and secondary amenorrhoea and in the treatment of dysfunctional uterine bleeding in doses of 2.5-10 mg daily.   For the treatment of endometriosis, an initial daily dose of 5 mg is increased every 2 weeks by 2.5 mg to a maintenance dose of 15 mg daily.   Doses of 30-60 mg daily have been used in the treatment of inoperable malignant neoplasms of the breast or as an adjunct to surgery or radiotherapy.   The major use of norethisterone acetate is as a progestin in progestin-oestrogen combination oral contra-ceptives.   Doses of 1, 1.5, 2.5, 3 or 4 mg are given daily in conjunction with ethinyloestradiol from the 5th to the 25th day of the cycle with an interruption of 7 days between the cycles (Wade, 1977).

Less than 1000 kg norethisterone and norethisterone acetate are used in France annually.

The US Food & Drug Administration (1978) has ruled that with effect from 31 May 1978 oral contraceptives for general use must carry patient and physician warning labels concerning use, risks and contraindications.

2.2 Occurrence

Norethisterone and its acetate are not known to occur naturally.

In a study carried out in a factory producing oral contraceptives, norethisterone was found in various sectors of the working environment, at levels ranging from 0.30-59.56 $\mu g/m^3$, and in wipe samples at levels of 0.019-14.7 $\mu g/cm^2$ (Harrington et $al.$, 1978).

2.3 Analysis

Analytical procedures for the determination of norethisterone as a bulk chemical and in pharmaceutical preparations have been reviewed (Shroff & Moyer, 1975).   Typical analytical methods for norethisterone and norethisterone acetate are summarized in Tables 1 & 2.   Abbreviations used are: GC, gas chromatography; TLC, thin-layer chromatography; UV, ultra-violet spectrometry; GC/MS, gas chromatography/mass spectrometry; HPLC, high-pressure liquid chromatography; CC, column chromatography; RIA, radioimmunoassay; and IR, infra-red spectrometry.   See also the section, 'General Remarks on Sex Hormones', p. 60.

TABLE 1

Analytical methods for norethisterone

Sample matrix	Sample preparation	Assay procedure	Sensitivity or limit of detection	Reference
Bulk chemical	Dissolve (tetrahydrofuran); add silver nitrate	Titration (sodium hydroxide)	-	British Pharmacopoeia Commission (1973)
Bulk chemical	Dissolve (chloroform-methanol)	Two-dimensional TLC (UV, acid spray)	-	Cavina et al. (1975)
Bulk chemical	Dissolve	HPLC (UV)	-	Hara & Hayashi (1977)
Bulk chemical	Dissolve	TLC, HPLC	-	Hara & Mibe (1975)
Tablets	Disintegrate (water); dilute (aqueous methanol containing tetramethylammonium bromide)	Polarography	-	Opheim (1977)
Tablets	Powder; wash (petroleum ether); extract (chloroform); evaporate; dissolve (ethanol); add silver nitrate & ammonium hydroxide; dilute (water); extract (chloroform); add acetic anhydride	Titration (perchloric acid)	-	Roushdi et al. (1974)
Tablets	Extract (chloroform); derivatize (isonicotinic acid hydrazide)	UV (380 nm)	-	Wu (1977)
Ointments	Suspend (aqueous methanol); wash (cyclohexane); add potassium aluminium sulphate; extract (chloroform)	HPLC (UV)	-	Landgraf & Jennings (1973)

Table 1 (continued)

Sample matrix	Sample preparation	Assay procedure	Sensitivity or limit of detection	Reference
Air in pharma-ceutical manufacturing plants	Extract from glass-fibre filter (diethyl ether); evaporate; derivatize (trimethylsilyl ether)	GC	~ 2 ng	Harrington et al. (1978)
Plasma	Extract (diethyl ether); GC (Sephadex); evaporate; add labelled norethisterone & antiserum	RIA	7-15 pg	Verma et al. (1976)
Plasma	Extract (ethyl acetate: petroleum ether, 1:1); evaporate; add labelled norethisterone & antiserum	RIA	20 pg	Walls et al. (1977)
Urine and plasma	Isolate by a series of extractions, hydrolysis & chromatographic separations; derivatize (trimethylsilyl ether & methoxime)	GC/MS	–	Braselton et al. (1977)
Urine	–	GC	–	Feher & Bodrogi (1976)

TABLE 2

Analytical methods for norethisterone acetate

Sample matrix	Sample preparation	Assay procedure	Reference
Bulk chemical	Dissolve (tetrahydrofuran); add silver nitrate	Titration (sodium hydroxide)	British Pharmacopoeia Commission (1973)
Bulk chemical	Dissolve (chloroform:methanol, 1:1)	Two-dimensional TLC (UV, acid-spray)	Cavina *et al.* (1975)
Bulk chemical	—	IR	Chatten *et al.* (1976)
Tablets	Extract (95% ethanol); concentrate; add buffer	Polarography	Chatten *et al.* (1977)
Tablets	Powder; wash (petroleum ether); extract (chloroform); evaporate; dissolve (ethanol); add silver nitrate & ammonium hydroxide; dilute (water); extract (diethyl ether); add acetic anhydride; concentrate	Titration (perchloric acid)	Roushdi *et al.* (1974)

3. Biological Data Relevant to the Evaluation

of Carcinogenic Risk to Humans

3.1 Carcinogenicity studies in animals

(a) Oral administration

Mouse: Groups of 24 virgin female C57L mice received 7 or 70 µg
of a mixture of norethisterone:ethinyloestradiol (50:1) in oil by
gavage, 5 times per week, commencing when the animals were 13 weeks of
age.   Pituitary tumours were found at autopsy after 84-89 weeks in 5/8
surviving mice given the higher dose and in 7/15 given the lower dose,
compared with 2/15 controls.   Hepatomas were found in 10/96 mice treated
with norethisterone:ethinyloestradiol and in a concurrent experiment
with norethynodrel:mestranol, but there is no indication in which groups
they arose.   No hepatomas were found in 48 controls (Poel, 1966).

Norethisterone and its acetate alone or in combination with oestrogens
were incorporated into the diet of groups of 120 male and 120 female CF-LP
(MTV-)[1] mice.   The doses were identified only as low (2-5 times the human
contraceptive dose), medium (50-150 times) and high (200-400 times);   the
amounts were not specified.   An increased incidence of benign liver-cell
tumours occurred in groups of male mice treated with norethisterone and its
acetate (33/120 and 35/120, compared with 18/120 and 19/120 in the 2 groups
of controls);   female mice showed no increase in liver-cell tumour incidence.
Incidences of pituitary tumours were increased in female mice fed norethisterone alone (4-8/120 in controls, 23/120 in treated mice), and in male
and female mice given combinations of norethisterone acetate:ethinyloestra-
diol (50:1) (from 2/120 to 25/120 in males and from 4-8/120 to 32/120 in
females) or of norethisterone:mestranol (20:1) (2/120 to 15/120 in males
and 4-8/120 to 31/120 in females).   No increase in the incidence of
pituitary tumours was observed when norethisterone acetate was given alone
(Committee on Safety of Medicines, 1972).

Rat: Groups of 120 male and 120 female rats were fed norethisterone
or norethisterone:mestranol (20:1) at low (2-5 times the human contraceptive dose), medium (50-150 times) and high (200-400 times) doses.   The
numbers of benign liver-cell tumours were increased in males, to 23%
compared with 4% in controls.   The same treatments induced benign and
malignant mammary tumours in male rats (4% and 12%, compared with 0 in
controls);   and administration of norethisterone:mestranol resulted in
an increased incidence of malignant mammary tumours in females, from 5
to 30%.   Feeding of norethisterone acetate:ethinyloestradiol (50:1) was
associated with an increase in the incidence of benign mammary tumours in

---

[1]MTV-:   mammary tumour virus not expressed (see p. 62)

male rats from 2 to 28%, but there were no increases in the incidences of tumours of other tissues in either males or females with this regime (Committee on Safety of Medicines, 1972).

Groups of 50 male and 50 female Sprague-Dawley-derived albino rats were fed 75 mg/kg of diet (3-4 mg/kg bw per day) of a mixture of 98% norethisterone acetate and 2% ethinyloestradiol for 2 years [the effective number of animals was not given]; 100 males and 100 females were used as controls. An increase in the incidences of regenerative liver nodules (10% *versus* 2%) and of liver adenomas (4% *versus* 0) was observed. In females, the incidence of benign mammary tumours was unchanged, but the proportions of fibroepithelial tumours to adenomas varied from 57% and 5% in controls to 38% and 32% in the test groups. In males the proportions were 1% and 0 in controls and 36% and 2% in the test groups. With a dietary concentration of 7.5 mg/kg, the incidence of regenerative liver nodules was still increased (13% *versus* 2% in the controls), as was that of liver adenomas (3% *versus* 0); however, the incidence of benign mammary tumours was unchanged, and the proportions of fibroepithelial tumours to adenomas were similar in male and female controls and in test groups. The incidence of adenocarcinomas was increased slightly only in groups given 75 mg/kg (8% *versus* 2% in controls) (Schardein *et al.*, 1970).

Pretreatment of intact female Sprague-Dawley rats with 0.25 mg Norlestrin (norethisterone:ethinyloestradiol, 50:1) daily for 10 days resulted in an increase in the incidence of mammary tumours induced by a single oral administration of 8 mg 7,12-dimethylbenz[a]anthracene (DMBA) from 17/38 to 18/22 rats. Pretreatment with 1 mg Norlestrin for 10 days had no significant effect on the incidence of such tumours produced by DMBA (McCarthy, 1965).

Wistar rats of both sexes were fed 0.01% and 0.02% of the oral contraceptive Sophia (norethisterone:mestranol, 100:1) for 2 years and 1 year, respectively, in food pellets, resulting in daily doses of 1.53 mg norethisterone and 0.015 mg mestranol in the 0.01% group and 3.74 mg and 0.037 mg for females and 4.28 and 0.43 mg for males in the 0.02% group. In those fed 0.01%, 6 mammary tumours and 1 pituitary tumour developed in 39 effective females as compared with 0/6 female controls. No tumours were seen in 18 males treated with 0.01%, whereas 4/9 male controls developed mammary fibroadenomas. Considerable losses of animals occurred due to intercurrent deaths. Animals fed 0.02% lived for only one year. No tumours were observed within that time in animals of either group (Takahashi, 1974).

Dog: In a report of a study in progress, it was stated that groups of 16 female beagle dogs, 6-12 months of age at the start of the experiment, were given norethisterone in combination with ethinyloestradiol at dose levels of 1, 10 and 25 times the projected human dose for 54 months on 21/28 days per month: norethisterone, 20, 200 and 500 µg/kg bw, and ethinyloestradiol, 1, 10 and 25 µg/kg bw. Dose-related cystic

endometrial hyperplasia and pyometra were observed.   During the 5th
year, one mammary nodule was found by palpation in a dog receiving the
intermediate dose (Weikel & Nelson, 1977).

(b) Subcutaneous implantation

Mouse: In 25 BALB/c mice implanted subcutaneously with pellets
containing 40% norethisterone and 60% cholesterol for 76-77 weeks, absorption of norethisterone was estimated to be between 3.6 and 15.9 µg per
day (mean, 7.7 µg per day).   Granulosa-cell tumours of the ovary were
detected in 13 animals;   only 2 could be seen macroscopically (Lipschütz
et al., 1966, 1967).

3.2 Other relevant biological data

For a review of the biological activities of the progestin compounds,
see Tausk & deVisser (1972).

(a) Experimental systems

No data on the toxicity of norethisterone and norethisterone acetate
were available.

Embryotoxicity and teratogenicity

Norethisterone containing 1% mestranol was given at a concentration
of 10 mg/kg bw per day orally to mice on days 8-15 and 14-17 of gestation
and at doses of 1 and 3 mg/kg bw per day on days 8-17;   rabbits received
doses of 1, 3 or 10 mg/kg bw per day on days 8-20 of gestation.   Significant embryolethality was induced in both species only by administration
of the highest dose and only by administration from days 8-15 of gestation in mice.   No malformations were observed (Takano, 1964;   Takano et
al., 1966).

When mice were given single injections (route not specified) or oral
doses of 0.5 or 1 mg/kg bw norethisterone on days 8-16 of gestation,
anomalies were induced in 3-57% of foetuses;   these included retarded
development, hydrocephalus, clubfoot and minor skeletal anomalies
(Andrew et al., 1972).

S.c. injection of 1-10 mg norethisterone into rats from day 15-20
of gestation induced pseudohermaphrodism and an altered sex ratio (male
foetuses only) (Revesz et al., 1960).   S.c. injection of 0.3-30 mg per
day norethisterone acetate between day 17 and 20 of gestation into rats
had a virilizing effect on the external genitalia (Cupceancu & Neumann,
1969).

Injection (route not specified) of 1 or 2.5 mg from day 15-19 of
gestation into rats induced a dose-dependent genital virilization in

female foetuses; those exposed to the higher dose did not develop an
external vaginal opening.   Adult females that had been treated prenatally had a normal cycle (Whalen *et al.*, 1966).

I.m. administration of 25 mg norethisterone to *Macaca mulatta*
(rhesus) monkeys daily on 5 days/week, starting from day 27-35 of pregnancy
and continuing until delivery, terminated 8/10 pregnancies.   Female
foetuses showed virilization of the external genitalia and hypoplastic
ovaries; males showed cryptorchidism (Wharton & Scott, 1964).

Absorption, distribution, excretion and metabolism

Norethisterone has a similar plasma half-life in rhesus monkeys and
humans (Nygren *et al.*, 1974).

After incubation of norethisterone with dog liver microsomes the
$4\beta,5\beta$-epoxide of norethisterone and a 6-oxygenated norethisterone derivative were obtained as minor metabolites (Cook *et al.*, 1974).

Rabbit liver homogenates (Palmer *et al.*, 1969) catalyse the de-
ethinylation of norethisterone, giving rise to the metabolite oestr-4-
ene-3,17-dione.   Rabbits excrete norethisterone metabolites predominantly in the urine (Kamyab *et al.*, 1967), while rats excrete them to 80%
in bile (Hanasono & Fischer, 1974).   Similar figures have been reported
for the closely related norethynodrel (see monograph, p. 470).

Norethisterone is a common intermediate in the metabolism of the
19-nortestosterone progestins, because ethynodiol diacetate (see monograph, p. 387), lynoestrenol (see monograph, p. 407). and norethynodrel
(see monograph, p. 461) are partly converted to norethisterone (Breuer,
1977).

Mutagenicity and other short-term tests

No damage to bone-marrow chromosomes was observed in female rats
treated orally for 5 days with 4 mg/kg bw norethisterone and sacrificed
on day 6 (Edwards *et al.*, 1971).

Dominant lethal mutations were observed within 2 weeks in female
mice treated orally with 10 mg norethisterone acetate daily for 4 weeks
before mating (Röhrborn & Hansmann, 1974) [For a consideration of the
possible mutagenicity of this compound, see 'General Remarks on Sex
Hormones', p. 64].   No dominant lethal mutations were observed in
female mice treated for 3 days prior to mating with 170 µg/kg bw
norethisterone and 8.5 µg/kg bw ethinyloestradiol (Badr & Badr, 1974).

(b) Humans

When ^{3}H- or ^{14}C-norethisterone was given orally to men, about half
of the dose was excreted in the urine; 50-65% of the urinary radioactivity
was sulphate conjugates. The major sulphate conjugate was that of
5β-oestrane-3β,17β-diol; the major glucuronide conjugate was that of
5β-oestrane-3α,17β-diol. The other metabolites in the glucuronide and
sulphate fraction were produced by reduction of norethisterone at C-3 and
at the double-bond of ring A (Gerhards et al., 1971; Murata, 1968).
Norethisterone is transformed by reductive enzymes to four isomeric ring-A-
reduced (5α and 5β) 3α- or 3β-hydroxy metabolites (Breuer, 1977; Ranney,
1977).

No studies on the metabolism of norethisterone acetate were available;
however, by analogy to lynoestrenol acetate (Coert et al., 1975), it may
be inferred that the compound is transformed metabolically to free norethisterone.

No chromosomal effects were observed when various concentrations of
norethisterone or norethisterone acetate were added to cultures of human
lymphocytes (Singh & Carr, 1970; Stenchever et al., 1969) or in the
peripheral lymphocytes of women who had taken oestrogen-progestin oral
contraceptives containing norethisterone (Shapiro et al., 1972).

3.3 Case reports and epidemiological studies

See the section, 'Oestrogens and Progestins in Relation to Human
Cancer', p.83 .

4. Summary of Data Reported and Evaluation[1]

4.1 Experimental data

Norethisterone and its acetate alone or in combination with
oestrogens were tested in mice, rats and dogs by oral administration and
in mice by subcutaneous implantation. When administered alone to mice,
norethisterone increased the incidence of benign liver-cell tumours in
males and of pituitary tumours in females and produced granulosa-cell
tumours of the ovary in females. Administration of norethisterone acetate
alone increased the incidence of benign liver-cell tumours in male mice.
In male rats, administration of norethisterone alone increased the
incidence of benign liver-cell tumours.

---

[1]This section should be read in conjunction with pp. 62-64 in the
'General Remarks on Sex Hormones' and with the 'General Conclusions on
Sex Hormones', p. 131.

Norethisterone in combination with mestranol, or the acetate in combination with ethinyloestradiol, increased the incidence of pituitary tumours in mice of both sexes; norethisterone in combination with ethinyloestradiol increased the incidence of pituitary tumours in female mice. In combination with mestranol it increased the incidence of benign liver-cell tumours in male rats and of malignant mammary tumours in animals of both sexes. Norethisterone acetate in combination with ethinyloestradiol increased the incidence of benign mammary tumours in male rats in one study and increased the incidence of benign liver-cell and mammary tumours in rats of both sexes in a further study.

A study in dogs in which it was given in combination with ethinyloestradiol is still in progress.

Norethisterone is embryolethal in some species and produces virilization in female foetuses.

4.2 Human data

No case reports or epidemiological studies on norethisterone or norethisterone acetate alone were available to the Working Group. Epidemiological studies on steroid hormones used in oestrogen-progestin oral contraceptive preparations have been summarized in the section, 'Oestrogens and Progestins in Relation to Human Cancer', p. 83 .

4.3 Evaluation

There is *limited evidence* for the carcinogenicity of norethisterone and of its acetate in animals. In humans, oral contraceptives containing oestrogens in combination with progestins have been related causally to an increased incidence of benign liver adenomas and a decreased incidence of benign breast disease.

5. References

Andrew, F.D., Williams, T.L., Gidley, J.T. & Wall, M.E. (1972)   Terato-
    genicity of contraceptive steroids in mice (Abstract).   Teratology,
    5, 249

Badr, F.M. & Badr, R.S. (1974)   Studies on the mutagenic effect of contra-
    ceptive drugs.   I. Induction of dominant lethal mutations in female
    mice.   Mutat. Res., 26, 529-534

Braselton, W.E., Lin, T.J., Mills, T.M., Ellegood, J.O. & Mahesh, V.B.
    (1977)   Identification and measurement by gas chromatography-mass
    spectrometry of norethindrone and metabolites in human urine and
    blood.   J. Steroid Biochem., 8, 9-18

Breuer, H. (1977)   Metabolic pathways of steroid contraceptive drugs.
    In: Garattini, S. & Berendes, H.W., eds, Pharmacology of Steroid
    Contraceptive Drugs, New York, Raven Press, pp. 73-88

British Pharmacopoeia Commission (1973)   British Pharmacopoeia, London,
    HMSO, pp. 323-324

Cavina, G., Moretti, G. & Petrella, M. (1975)   A solvent system for the
    separation of steroids with estrogenic and progestational activity
    by two-dimensional thin-layer chromatography.   J. Chromatogr., 103,
    368-371

Chatten, L.G., Triggs, E.J. & Glowach, S.J. (1976)   Quantitative assay of
    antifertility agents by I.R. spectroscopy.   J. Pharm. Belg., 31,
    63-79 [Chem. Abstr., 84, 155766n]

Chatten, L.G., Yadav, R.N., Binnington, S. & Moskalyk, R.E. (1977)
    Polarographic study of certain progestogens and their determination
    in oral contraceptive tablets by differential pulse polarography.
    Analyst (Lond.), 102, 323-327

Coert, A., Geelen, J. & van der Vies, J. (1975)   Metabolites of lynestrenol
    acetate in the bile of rats after intravenous administration; a
    comparison with lynestrenol.   Acta endocrinol., 78, 791-800

Cook, C.E., Dickey, M.C. & Christensen, H.D. (1974)   Oxygenated norethin-
    drone derivatives from incubation with beagle liver.   Drug Metab.
    Disposition, 2, 58-64

Committee on Safety of Medicines (1972)   Carcinogenicity Tests of Oral
    Contraceptives, London, HMSO

Cupceancu, B. & Neumann, F. (1969)   Sensitivity differences of different genital tract structures of female rat fetuses due to the effect of medroxyprogesterone acetate or norethisterone acetate (Ger.). Endocrinology, 54, 66-80

Djerassi, C., Miramontes, L., Rosenkranz, G. & Sondheimer, F. (1954) Steroids.   LIV. Synthesis of 19-nor-17α-ethynylstestosterone and 19-nor-17α-methyltestosterone.   J. Am. chem. Soc., 76, 4092-4094

Edwards, C.W., Calhoun, F.J. & Green, S. (1971)   The effects of mestranol and several progestins on chromosomes and fertility in the rat (Abstract no. 157).   Toxicol appl. Pharmacol., 19, 421

Engelfried, O., Kaspar, E., Popper, A. & Schenck, M. (1957)   17-Alkyl-19-nortestosterone acylates.   German Patent, 1,017,166, 10 October to Schering Akt.-Ges. [Chem. Abstr., 53, 22096e]

Feher, T. & Bodrogi, L. (1976)   Gas chromatographic determination of synthetic gestagen hormones.   Acta pharm. hung., 46, 73-77 [Chem. Abstr., 84, 147091y]

Gerhards, E., Hecker, W., Hitze, H., Nieuweboer, B. & Bellmann, O. (1971) The metabolism of norethisterone (17α-ethinyl-4-oestren-17β-ol-3-one) and of dl- and d-norgestrel (13-ethyl-17α-ethinyl-4-oestren-17β-ol-3-one) in man (Ger.).   Acta endocrinol., 68, 219-248

Grasselli, J.G. & Ritchey, W.M., eds (1975)   CRC Atlas of Spectral Data and Physical Constants for Organic Compounds, 2nd ed., Vol. III, Cleveland, OH, Chemical Rubber Company, p. 234

Hanasono, G.K. & Fischer, L.J. (1974)   The excretion of tritium-labeled chlormadinone acetate, mestranol, norethindrone, and norethynodrel in rats and the enterohepatic circulation of metabolites.   Drug Metab. Disposition, 2, 159-168

Hara, S. & Hayashi, S. (1977)   Correlation of retention behaviour of steroidal pharmaceuticals in polar and bonded reversed-phase liquid column chromatography.   J. Chromatogr., 142, 689-703

Hara, S. & Mibe, K. (1975)   The solvent selectivity of the mobile phase in thin-layer chromatography in relation to the mobility and the structure of steroidal pharmaceuticals.   Chem. pharm. Bull., 23, 2850-2859

Harrington, J.M., Rivera, R.O. & Lowry, L.K. (1978)   Occupational exposure to synthetic estrogens - the need to establish safety standards.   Am. ind. Hyg. Assoc. J., 39, 139-143

Harvey, S.C. (1975)   Hormones.   In: Osol, A. *et al.*, eds, Remington's
    Pharmaceutical Sciences, 15th ed., Easton, PA, Mack, pp. 923-924

IARC (1974)   IARC Monographs on the Evaluation of Carcinogenic Risk of
    Chemicals to Man, 6, Sex Hormones, Lyon, pp. 179-189

Kamyab, S., Littleton, P. & Fotherby, K. (1967)   Metabolism and tissue
    distribution of norethisterone and norgestrel in rabbits.   J.
    Endocrinol., 39, 423-435

Kastrup, E.K., ed. (1977)   Facts and Comparisons, St Louis, MO, Facts
    & Comparisons Inc., pp. 107b, 108b-108e

Kastrup, E.K., ed. (1978)   Facts and Comparisons, St Louis, MO, Facts
    & Comparisons Inc., p. 106

Landgraf, W.C. & Jennings, E.C. (1973)   Steroid determination from
    complex mixtures by high pressure chromatographic techniques.
    J. pharm. Sci., 62, 278-281

Lipschütz, A., Iglesias, R., Salinas, S. & Panasevich, V.I. (1966)
    Experimental conditions under which contraceptive steroids may
    become toxic.   Nature, 212, 686-688

Lipschütz, A., Iglesias, R., Panesevich, V.I. & Salinas, S. (1967)
    Ovarian tumours and other ovarian changes induced in mice by two
    19-nor-contraceptives.   Br. J. Cancer, 21, 153-159

McCarthy, J.D. (1965)   Influence of two contraceptives on induction of
    mammary cancer in rats.   Am. J. Surg., 110, 720-723

Murata, S. (1968)   Study of the metabolism of estrane progestins in the
    human body (Jpn.).   Folia Endocrinol. Jpn., 43, 1083-1096

Nygren, K.-G., Lindberg, P., Martinsson, K., Bosu, W.T.K. & Johansson,
    E.D.B. (1974)   Radioimmunoassay of norethindrone: peripheral
    plasma levels after oral administration to humans and rhesus monkeys.
    Contraception, 9, 265-278

Opheim, L.-N. (1977)   Determination of norethisterone in tablets by
    differential pulse polarography.   Anal. chim. acta, 89, 225-229

Palmer, K.H., Feierabend, J.F., Baggett, B. & Wall, M.E. (1969)
    Metabolic removal of a 17α-ethynyl group from the antifertility
    steroid, norethindrone.   J. Pharmacol. exp. Ther., 167, 217-222

Poel, W.E. (1966)   Pituitary tumours in mice after prolonged feeding
    of synthetic progestins.   Science, 154, 402-403

Ranney, R.E. (1977)   Comparative metabolism of 17α-ethynyl steroids used in oral contraceptives.   J. Toxicol. environ. Health, 3, 139-166

Revesz, C., Chappel, C.I. & Gaudry, R. (1960)   Masculinization of female fetuses in the rat by progestational compounds.   Endocrinology, 66, 140-144

Röhrborn, G. & Hansmann, I. (1974)   Oral contraceptives and chromosome segregation in oocytes of mice.   Mutat. Res., 26, 535-544

Roushdi, I.M., El Sabai, A.I. & Belal, S. (1974)   New methods for the estimation of acetylenic steroids (non-aqueous titrimetric method).   Egypt. J. pharm. Sci., 15, 217-221

Schardein, J.L., Kaump, D.H., Woosley, E.T. & Jellema, M.M. (1970)   Long-term toxicologic and tumorigenesis studies on an oral contra-ceptive agent in albino rats.   Toxicol. appl. Pharmacol., 16, 10-23

Shapiro, L.R., Graves, Z.R. & Hirschhorn, K. (1972)   Oral contraceptives and *in vivo* cytogenic studies.   Obstet. Gynecol., 39, 190-192

Shroff, A.P. & Moyer, E.S. (1975)   Norethindrone.   In: Florey, K., ed., Analytical Profiles of Drug Substances, Vol. 4, New York, Academic Press, pp. 269-293

Singh, O.S. & Carr, D.H. (1970)   A study of the effects of certain hormones on human cells in culture.   Can. med. Assoc. J., 103, 349-350, 373

Stenchever, M.A., Jarvis, J.A. & Kreger, N.K. (1969)   Effect of selected estrogens and progestins on human chromosomes *in vitro*.   Obstet. Gynecol., 34, 249-251

Takahashi, A. (1974)   Chronic toxicity and effects of an oral contracep-tive (Sophia) on reproductive organs and blood coagulation in Wistar rats.   J. Nara med. Assoc., 25, 684-724

Takano, K. (1964)   The effect of several synthetic progestagens administered to pregnant animals upon their offspring.   Proc. Congenital Anomalies Res. Assoc. Jpn., 4, 3-4

Takano, K., Yamumura, H., Suzuki, M. & Nishimura, H. (1966)   Teratogenic effect of chlormadinone acetate in mice and rabbits.   Proc. Soc. exp. Biol. (N.Y.), 121, 455-457

Tausk, M. & deVisser, J. (1972)   International Encyclopedia of Pharmacology and Therapeutics, Vol. II, section 48, Elmsford, NY, Pergamon Press, pp. 35-194

US Food & Drug Administration (1978)   Oral contraceptive drug products.
    Physician and patient labeling; extension of effective date for
    physician labeling.   Fed. Regist., 43, 9863-986

US Pharmacopeial Convention Inc. (1975)   The US Pharmacopeia, 19th rev.,
    Rockville, MD, pp. 344-347

Verma, P., Curry, C. & Ahluwalia, B. (1976)   A radioimmunoassay for
    norethindrone.   II. Plasma levels in hypertensive and normotensive
    oral contraceptive users.   Anal. Lett., 9, 91-103

Wade, A., ed. (1977)   Martindale, The Extra Pharmacopoeia, 27th ed.,
    London, The Pharmaceutical Press, pp. 1410-1413

Walls, C., Vose, C.W., Horth, C.E. & Palmer, R.F. (1977)   Radioimmuno-
    assay of plasma norethisterone after ethynodiol diacetate administra-
    tion.   J. Steroid Biochem., 8, 167-171

Weikel, J.H., Jr & Nelson, L.W. (1977)   Problems in evaluating chronic
    toxicity of contraceptive steroids in dogs.   J. Toxicol. environ.
    Health, 3, 167-177

Whalen, R.E., Peck, C.K. & LoPiccolo, J. (1966)   Virilization of female
    rats by prenatally administered progestin.   Endocrinology, 78, 965-
    970

Wharton, L.R., Jr & Scott, R.B. (1964)   Experimental production of
    genital lesions with norethindrone.   Am. J. Obstet. Gynecol., 89,
    701-715

Windholz, M., ed. (1976)   The Merck Index, 9th ed., Rahway, NJ, Merck
    & Co., pp. 868-869

Wu, J.Y.P. (1977)   Collaborative study of an assay for progestational
    steroids in individual contraceptive tablets.   J. Assoc. off.
    anal. Chem., 60, 922-925

NORETHYNODREL

A monograph on this substance was published previously (IARC, 1974). Relevant data that have appeared since that time have been evaluated in the present monograph.

1. Chemical and Physical Data

1.1 Synonyms and trade names

Chem. Abstr. Services Reg. No.: 68-23-5

Chem. Abstr. Name: (17α)-17-Hydroxy-19-norpregn-5(10)-en-20-yn-3-one

Synonyms: 17α-Ethynyl-17-hydroxy-5(10)-estren-3-one; 17α-ethynyl-17-hydroxy-5(10)-oestren-3-one; 17-hydroxy-19-nor-17α-pregn-5(10)-en-20-yn-3-one; 13-methyl-17-ethynyl-17-hydroxy-1,2,3,4,6,7,8,9,11,12,13,14,16,17-tetradecahydro-15*H*-cyclopenta[*a*]phenanthren-3-one; norethinodrel

Trade names[1]: Conovid; Conovid E; Enavid; Enavid E; Enidrel; Enovid; Enovid-E; Enovid-E21; [Noretynodrel]; [Norolen]; Previson; SC-4642; [Singestrol]

1.2 Structural and molecular formulae and molecular weight

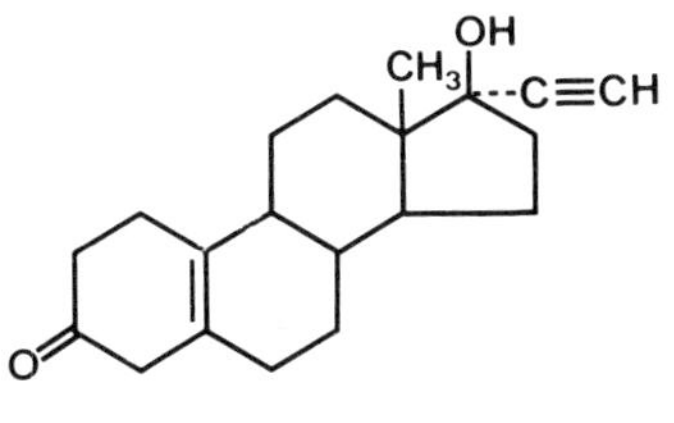

$C_{20}H_{26}O_2$ Mol. wt: 298.4

---

[1]Those in square brackets are preparations that are no longer produced commercially.

1.3 Chemical and physical properties of the pure substance

From Wade (1977) and Windholz (1976)

(a) Description: White, odourless, crystalline powder

(b) Melting-point: 169-170°C

(c) Optical rotation: $[\alpha]_D$ +108° (1% w/v chloroform)

(d) Solubility: Insoluble in water; soluble in ethanol (1 in 30),
chloroform (1 in 7) and diethyl ether (1 in 60); soluble in
acetone; very slightly soluble in light petroleum

(e) Stability: Unstable to air and light

1.4 Technical products and impurities

Various national and international pharmacopoeias give specifications for the purity of norethynodrel in pharmaceutical products. For
example, norethynodrel is available in the US as a NF grade containing
97-101% active ingredient (National Formulary Board, 1975). In the US
it is available in 2.5-10 mg doses as tablets in combination with mestranol.
In the UK it is also available in 2.5 and 5 mg doses as tablets in
combination with mestranol. Norethynodrel normally contains about 1%
mestranol (see monograph, p. 257) from the manufacturing process, and
the amount must be stated on the label (Wade, 1977).

2. Production, Use, Occurrence and Analysis

2.1 Production and use

(a) Production

Synthesis of norethynodrel was first reported in 1954, in which
oestradiol 3-methyl ether was reduced with lithium in liquid ammonia and
the intermediate oxidized; ethynolation produced the 3-methyl ether of
norethynodrel; treatment of this ether with acetic acid in methanol
gave norethynodrel (Colton, 1954, 1955). It is not known whether this
process is used for commercial production.

Commercial production of norethynodrel in the US was first reported
in 1962 (US Tariff Commission, 1963); however, it has not been reported
since 1965 (US Tariff Commission, 1967).

Commercial production of norethynodrel in the UK was first reported in 1957. Annual production of norethynodrel in western Europe is in the range of 100 thousand to 1 million kg; Italy, The Netherlands and the UK are believed to be the major producing countries. It is also made commercially in Hungary, but no information was available on the quantity produced. Imports into Austria, Belgium, the Federal Republic of Germany, Luxembourg, Switzerland and The Netherlands in 1977 were 10-100 thousand kg each.

Norethynodrel was first marketed commercially in Japan in 1962. It is not produced there, and imports amounted to about 1 kg in 1975-1977.

(b) Use

Norethynodrel is used primarily as a progestin in oral contraceptives, mostly in combination with an oestrogen such as mestranol. It is normally given daily from day 5-24 of the cycle in doses of 2.5-5 mg with 0.075-0.1 mg mestranol. In the treatment of dysfunctional uterine bleeding, it is given from day 5-24 of the cycle in doses of 5-10 mg daily. Higher doses (up to 20-30 mg daily) may be required initially to control bleeding. In the treatment of endometriosis, the usual dose is 2.5 mg initially; this is increased to 10-20 mg daily and maintained for at least 6-9 months (Wade, 1977).

From 200 thousand to 2 million kg norethynodrel are used annually in Europe.

The US Food & Drug Administration (1978) has ruled that with effect from 31 May 1978 oral contraceptives for general use must carry patient and physician warning labels concerning use, risks and contraindications.

2.2 Occurrence

Norethynodrel is not known to occur naturally.

2.3 Analysis

Typical analytical methods for the determination of norethynodrel are summarized in Table 1. Abbreviations used are: GC, gas chromatography; TLC, thin-layer chromatography; and UV, ultra-violet spectrometry. See also the section, 'General Remarks on Sex Hormones', p. 60 .

Table 1

Analytical methods for norethynodrel

Sample matrix	Sample preparation	Assay procedure	Reference
Bulk chemical	Dissolve (chloroform-methanol)	Two-dimensional TLC (acid spray, UV)	Cavina *et al*. (1975)
Bulk chemical	Dissolve	TLC	Martin *et al*. (1975)
Bulk chemical	Dissolve (methanol); add hydrochloric acid; dilute (methanol)	UV (240 nm)	National Formulary Board (1975)
Tablets	Disintegrate (water-ethanol); add base; reduce (sodium borohydride)	UV (240 nm)	Görög (1977)
Tablets	Powder, wash (petroleum ether); extract (chloroform); evaporate; dissolve (ethanol); add silver nitrate & ammonium hydroxide; dilute (water); extract (chloroform); add acetic anhydride; concentrate	Titration (perchloric acid)	Roushdi *et al*. (1974)
Tablets	Extract (chloroform); derivatize (isonicotinic acid hydrazide)	UV (380 nm)	Wu (1977)
Urine	–	GC	Feher & Bodrogi (1976)

3. Biological Data Relevant to the Evaluation
of Carcinogenic Risk to Humans

3.1 Carcinogenicity studies in animals

In some of the following investigations norethynodrel was administered as the commercial product 'Enovid', containing 98.5% norethynodrel and 1.5% mestranol. The experimental data have therefore been summarized both in this monograph and in that on mestranol (p. 257). It should be noted that effects reported may reflect the action of an individual constituent or of the combination.

(a) Oral administration

Mouse: Groups of 24 virgin female C57L mice [MTV⁻][1] received 7 or 70 μg of a mixture of norethynodrel:mestranol (50:1) in oil by gavage, 5 times per week, commencing when the animals were 13 weeks of age. Pituitary tumours were found at autopsy in 7/77 mice given the higher dose that lived 84 weeks and in 6/11 mice given the lower dose, compared with 2/15 controls that lived 90 weeks. Hepatomas were found in 10/96 treated mice in this and in a concurrent experiment with norethisterone: ethinyloestradiol (50:1), but no indication was given in which group they arose. No hepatomas were found in 48 control animals (Poel, 1966).

Female BALB/c mice [MTV⁻] were fed a liquid diet (Metrecal) containing Enovid such that each mouse consumed 10-12.5 μg each day. All of the 8 mice that survived more than 74 weeks of treatment had early or infil-trating carcinomas of the cervix. No carcinomas of the uterine corpus or cervix or of the vagina were found in 42 untreated females that lived 103-130 weeks nor in 8 females given Metrecal for 79-102 weeks (Dunn, 1969).

Castrated male (C3H x RIII)F1 mice (MTV⁺)[1] that received 15 mg/kg of diet Enovid (average intake, 30-40 μg/mouse per day) had an increased incidence of mammary tumours, from 10/61 to 20/23. The latent period for tumour development was decreased in both castrated males and ovariec-tomized females, but the incidence in ovariectomized females was not significantly increased. In intact female RIII mice, Enovid had no effect on incidence or on latent period. Administration of norethynodrel alone in the diet, at 13.5 mg/kg (intake, 25-35 μg/mouse per day), altered neither the incidence nor the latent period of mammary tumours in intact female RIII, C3H or (C3H x RIII)F1 (MTV⁺) mice nor in ovariec-tomized (C3H x RIII)F1 females. In castrated (C3H x RIII)F1 males, the mammary tumour incidence was increased from 10/61 to 29/29, and the latent period was reduced from an average of 82 to 37 weeks (Rudali, 1975).

----

[1]MTV⁻: = mammary tumour virus not expressed; MTV⁺: = mammary tumour virus expressed (see p. 62)

Twenty female BALB/c mice [MTV⁻] were fed a liquid diet (Metrecal) containing an estimated dose of 10-12.5 µg Enovid/mouse per day for an average period of 15 months. Of 16 mice that lived for 10 months or more, 3 developed precancerous lesions and 2, squamous-cell carcinomas of the cervix and/or vagina. Of a group of 40 mice treated with Enovid and with intravaginal inoculations of herpesvirus type 2, 31 survived 10 months or more; of these, 1 developed a precancerous lesion and 6, squamous-cell carcinomas of the cervix and/or vagina. In 15/20 control mice that lived for 10 months or more, 1 precancerous lesion of the cervix was detected (Muñoz, 1973).

Norethynodrel alone or in combination with mestranol (66:1 and 25:1) was incorporated into the diet of groups of 120 male and 120 female CF-LP mice for 80 weeks. The doses were identified only as low (2-5 times the human contraceptive dose), medium (50-150 times) and high (200-400 times); the amounts were not specified. Both norethynodrel alone and in the combinations resulted in an increased incidence of pituitary tumours in males and females, from a range of 2-8 tumours in control groups to incidences of 30-47 in the treated groups. Most of the increased incidences were related to the medium and high doses. Small numbers of benign adrenal tumours were found. Eight malignant mammary tumours were found, of which 5 occurred in female mice that received the high dose of norethynodrel alone, compared with 4/240 controls (Committee on Safety of Medicines, 1972).

Swiss-Webster random-bred mice received 1.25 mg/kg bw per day norethynodrel or a combination of norethynodrel with mestranol (25:1) (1.25 and 0.05 mg/kg/ bw per day) as a single daily oral administration in corn oil for 50-80 weeks. Benign hepatocellular tumours were observed in 0/50 and 2/50 mice administered norethynodrel and the combination, respectively. One of 50 controls also developed this tumour. In another series, CF-LP mice of both sexes were given low, intermediate and high doses corresponding to 2.5, 30 and 50 times the human dose of norethynodrel and of norethynodrel:mestranol combinations (25:1 and 66:1) in the diet. The dosages were: norethynodrel, 0.125 mg/kg bw per day (2.5x), 1.50 mg/kg bw per day (30x) and 5.0 mg/kg bw per day (100x); norethynodrel: mestranol (25:1), 0.13 mg/kg bw per day (2.5x), 1.56 mg/kg bw per day (30x) and 2.60 mg/kg per day (50x); norethynodrel:mestranol (66:1), 0.125 mg/kg bw per day (2.5x), 1.50 mg/kg bw per day (30x) and 5.0 mg/kg bw per day (100x). The incidences of liver tumours in control mice were 6/39 in males and 0/39 in females. When norethynodrel was given alone, liver tumours were observed in 7/40, 1/40 and 3/40 males and in 0/39, 0/40 and 2/39 females at low, intermediate and high dose levels, respectively. When given in combination with mestranol (25:1), the tumour incidences were 8/40, 7/40 and 1/39 in males and 1/39, 0/38 and 1/39 in females, respectively, for the above dose levels. When the ratio of norethynodrel:mestranol was increased (66:1), the tumour incidences were 4/40, 5/39 and 1/40 in males, and 1/40, 1/40 and 0/38 in females for the three dose levels (Barrows *et al.*, 1977).

Rat: Groups of 120 male and 120 female rats received norethynodrel alone or in combination with mestranol (66:1 and 25:1) at low (2-5 times the human contraceptive dose), medium (50-150 times) or high (200-400 times) doses. Administration of norethynodrel alone increased the incidence of benign liver-cell tumours in males from 3 to 24%, mostly at the medium and high dose levels; malignant hepatomas occurred in 8% of the males, mainly in animals receiving the medium and high doses. Administration of norethynodrel with mestranol (66:1) resulted in a similar increase in incidence of benign liver-cell tumours (29%) in males, but the increase in malignant tumours (2% compared with 0 in the controls) is of doubtful significance. Female rats given the same treatments had much lower incidences of benign liver-cell tumours (<5%) and no malignant liver-cell tumours. Norethynodrel alone induced pituitary tumours in 43% of male rats (compared with 6% in controls); 25:1 norethynodrel:mestranol increased the incidence in males to 15%; only 2% of animals receiving the 66:1 combination had such tumours. Female rats ingesting norethynodrel alone had no pituitary tumours, but these occurred in 20% of female rats fed 25:1 norethynodrel:mestranol, compared with 8% in controls. Both benign and malignant mammary tumours were seen in male rats given norethynodrel with or without mestranol (15-19%, compared with 0 in controls); but in female rats the incidence of malignant tumours was increased only in the groups fed 25:1 norethynodrel: mestranol (20%, compared with 7% in controls). It was stated, but not tabulated, that these increases occurred almost entirely in the high-dose group (Committee on Safety of Medicines, 1972).

In a group of 21 female Wistar rats given gastric instillations of 3 mg Enovid 6 times per week for 50 weeks, no mammary tumours were observed. The same treatment in 2 further groups of 47 and 24 rats neither increased nor decreased the induction of tumours by 3-methylcholanthrene (Gruenstein *et al*., 1964). Administration of Enovid in sesame oil by gavage to Sprague-Dawley rats resulted in a small inhibition of the induction of mammary tumours by 7,12-dimethylbenz[*a*]anthracene (DMBA) (Stern & Mickey, 1969; Weisburger *et al*., 1968). Daily administration of 0.25 mg Enovid by gavage in corn oil for 10 days prior to the administration of a single dose of 8 mg DMBA to 21 intact female Sprague-Dawley rats increased the incidence of breast cancer to 17/21, compared with 17/38 in controls that received DMBA only. Pretreatment for 10 days with 1 mg Enovid did not affect subsequent tumour incidence in 22 intact females (McCarthy, 1965).

Monkey: In a study still in progress at the time of reporting, an adenocarcinoma of the mammary gland arose after 18 months in 1/6 female *Macaca mulatta* (rhesus) monkeys administered 1 mg Enovid per day. Widespread metastases were associated with the tumour (Kirschstein *et al*., 1972) [The Working Group noted the incomplete reporting of this experiment].

In a preliminary report of a study in progress, oral administration of Enovid-E (2.5 mg norethynodrel and 0.1 mg mestranol per human dose) in dosages 1, 10 and 50 times the average human contraceptive dose to mature rhesus monkeys (16 per group) resulted in no clinical evidence of mammary gland lesions or tumours after 5 years (Drill et al., 1974).

(b) Subcutaneous and/or intramuscular administration

<u>Mouse</u>: Nulliparous C3H/HeJ female mice (MTV[+]) were given 0.1 mg Enovid by s.c. injection twice weekly from 1 month of age for 21 months. A significant increase (P<0.001) in the incidence of mammary tumours was observed in Enovid-treated mice as compared with controls (30/100, as compared with 14/100) (Welsch et al., 1977).

<u>Rat</u>: Repeated s.c. injections of 10 or 100 μg Enovid per day for 40 days into 2 groups of 25 female Sprague-Dawley rats for 40 days reduced the number of mammary tumours/rat produced by a single i.v. injection of 5 mg DMBA given on day 25 of treatment. The average numbers of tumours/rat were 10.9 in 37 controls given DMBA alone, compared with 7.6 and 3.9 in rats given 10 and 100 μg Enovid per day, respectively (Welsch & Meites, 1969).

<u>Hamster</u>: Thrice weekly s.c. injections of 34 mg/kg bw Enovid in sesame oil, reduced to 17 mg/kg bw at 94 weeks and to 8.5 mg/kg bw at 104 weeks, did not affect the incidence of any tumour type in 46 male Syrian golden hamsters (Sichuk et al., 1967) [The Working Group noted that the average age of the animals at the start of the experiment was 76 weeks and that 50% of the animals had died by 103 weeks].

(c)   Subcutaneous implantation

<u>Mouse</u>: In 24 female BALB/c mice implanted subcutaneously with pellets containing 40% norethynodrel and 60% cholesterol, absorption was estimated to be about 5.5 μg per day. Granulosa-cell tumours of the ovary were found in 2 animals (Lipschütz et al., 1966, 1967).

3.2 Other relevant biological data

For a review of the biological activity of the progestin compounds, see Tausk & deVisser (1972). The biological activity of norethynodrel is similar to that of norethisterone, but it has a weaker progestational activity; it also has an intrinsic oestrogenic activity.

(a) Experimental systems

No data on the toxicity of norethynodrel were available.

Embryotoxicity and teratogenicity

Mice given 10 mg/kg bw norethynodrel orally, daily from day 8-15 of gestation, had significant embryolethality (98.9%), but not when it was given on days 14-17 of gestation (Takano *et al.*, 1966).

Mice were given 0.2-2.4 mg/kg bw norethynodrel or its 3-hydroxy metabolites as an oral or parenteral dose, either singly or on 3 consecutive days, between days 6-16 of gestation; congenital anomalies occurred in offspring. A single dose of 1.2 mg/kg bw norethynodrel or its metabolite given between days 8-16 of gestation produced congenital abnormalities (retarded development, hydrocephalus, clubfoot and minor skeletal anomalies) in 10-30% of offspring (Andrew *et al.*, 1972).

Mice that received a single s.c. injection of 0.1 mg/kg bw norethynodrel in combination with mestranol (Enovid) on day 7, 10, 12, 15 or 17 of gestation had normal foetuses, with no external or internal genital anomalies; however, treatment on the 10th day of gestation led to a significant decrease in aggressive behaviour of male offspring later in life (Abbatiello & Scudder, 1970).

Oral administration of norethynodrel or its metabolites, 17α-ethynyl-estr-5(10)-ene-3α,17β-diol and 17α-ethynyl-estr-5(10)-ene-3β,17β-diol at daily doses of 0.15, 0.3 or 0.6 mg/kg bw on days 8, 9 and 10 or 11, 12 and 13 of gestation resulted in an increased number of resorptions and intrauterine deaths on days 11-13. Teratogenic effects included exencephaly, internal hydrocephalus and partial cryptorchidism. The most effective agent was the 3β,17β-diol (Gidley *et al.*, 1970).

S.c. administration of 0.5 and 1.0 mg/kg bw norethynodrel to pregnant rats on days 2, 3 and 4 of gestation terminated a significant number of pregnancies (Saunders, 1965). Administration of 0.083-2.5 mg/kg bw per day norethynodrel on days 10-17 of gestation to rats induced 100% foetal resorptions. A dose of 0.0083 mg/kg bw per day induced 42% resorptions; no virilizing effect was observed in females, and in males the weight of the testes was significantly lowered and the descent of testes was delayed in 35.5% of animals (Roy & Kar, 1967).

Sixty female rats were given 1 mg/kg bw Enidrel (9.2 mg norethynodrel, 0.075 mg mestranol) intragastrically daily for 2 months, at which time they were mated. In 30 animals in which treatment was continued for the 15 days of gestation, complete foetal resorption occurred rapidly; however, after 2 weeks without treatment, fertility rates and litter sizes were normal. In the 30 animals in which treatment was discontinued, fertility and pre- and postnatal development of the offspring were normal. No teratogenic effects were observed (Tuchmann-Duplessis & Mercier-Parot, 1972).

S.c. injection of 1 mg norethynodrel (Enovid) to guinea-pigs daily
from day 18-60 of gestation prevented pregnancy (Foote *et al.*, 1968).

Metabolism

The metabolism of norethynodrel has been reviewed (Ranney, 1977).
Major metabolites of norethynodrel in mice, rats, guinea-pigs and rabbits
are the 3α- and 3β-alcohols [17α-ethynyl-3α (or 3β),17β-dihydroxy-5(10)-
oestrene] and norethisterone (Freudenthal *et al.*, 1971a, 1973; Palmer
et al., 1969). However, marked species differences were observed in the
amount of the 3α-epimer formed from the 3β-compound (17α-ethynyl-3β,17β-
dihydroxy-5(10)-oestrene) in liver homogenates: the conversion ratios
varied from 90% in rats to less than 3% in guinea-pigs, hamsters and
mice (Freudenthal *et al.*, 1971b). In most species, polyhydroxylated
metabolites occur, which have not yet been characterized (Freudenthal,
1971a, 1973).

Norethynodrel undergoes an acid-catalysed, non-enzymic, partial
rearrangement to norethisterone, as demonstrated by incubation with rabbit
gastric juice (Arai *et al.*, 1962).

Mutagenicity and other short-term tests

Doses of 20-10,000 μg norethynodrel per plate did not induce mutations
in *Salmonella typhimurium* strains TA98, TA100, TA1535, TA1537 or TA1538,
with or without mouse or rat liver homogenate (Lang & Redmann, 1979).

No damage to bone-marrow chromosomes was observed in female Holtzman
rats treated orally for 5 days with 0.2 mg/kg bw norethynodrel and
sacrificed on day 6 (Edwards *et al.*, 1971).

Treatment with norethynodrel did not change the rate of polyploid
cells in human lymphocyte cultures *in vitro* (Singh & Carr, 1970).

(b) Humans

When women were given ^{3}H-norethynodrel, metabolites were isolated
that had retained the Δ-5(10)-ene structure, indicating that these
metabolites did not originate from norethisterone; other metabolites
contained the Δ-4-ene structure, which is characteristic of norethisterone.
Metabolites have also been isolated and identified that originate from
reductive processes at C-3 and by saturation of ring A (Cook *et al.*,
1972; Palmer *et al.*, 1969).

Part of norethynodrel must undergo oxidative metabolism, since
Layne *et al.* (1963) isolated and tentatively identified C-10-hydroxylated
metabolites.

A study has been made of the chromosome numbers and characteristics of cultured leucocytes from 77 mothers who had taken one or more types of oral contraceptives, including norethynodrel, and from their 108 babies, compared with similar numbers of controls. The number of abnormal cells was significantly higher in babies born to mothers who had been taking norethynodrel: 4.6% abnormal cells in test babies *versus* 2.0% in controls (Bishun *et al.*, 1975).

3.3 Case reports and epidemiological studies

See the section 'Oestrogens and Progestins in Relation to Human Cancer', p. 83 .

4. Summary of Data Reported and Evaluation[1]

4.1 Experimental data

Norethynodrel was tested in mice, rats and monkeys alone or in combination with mestranol by oral administration. It was also tested alone in mice by subcutaneous implantation, and in combination with mestranol in mice, rats and hamsters by subcutaneous injection.

When given alone, norethynodrel increased the incidence of pituitary tumours in mice of both sexes and of mammary tumours in castrated males of one strain; it also increased the incidence of liver-cell, pituitary and mammary tumours in male rats.

When given in combination with mestranol, it increased the incidence of pituitary, mammary, vaginal and cervical tumours in female mice, of pituitary tumours in male mice, of mammary tumours in castrated male mice, of benign liver-cell tumours in male rats and of malignant mammary tumours in rats of both sexes. The study in hamsters was of too short duration to be considered for evaluation.

Oral administration of norethynodrel in combination with mestranol to *Macaca mulatta* monkeys for 5 years did not increase the incidence of mammary tumours; the study is still in progress.

Norethynodrel was reported to be embryolethal in some species and to have teratogenic effects in mice.

---

[1]This section should be read in conjunction with pp. 62-64 in the 'General Remarks on Sex Hormones' and with the 'General Conclusions on Sex Hormones', p. 131.

4.2 Human data

No case reports or epidemiological studies on norethynodrel alone
were available to the Working Group. Epidemiological studies on steroid
hormones used in oestrogen-progestin contraceptive preparations have
been summarized in the section, 'Oestrogens and Progestins in Relation
to Human Cancer', p. 83.

4.3 Evaluation

There is *limited evidence* for the carcinogenicity of norethynodrel
alone and in combination with mestranol in experimental animals. In
humans, oral contraceptives containing oestrogens in combination with
progestins have been related causally to an increased incidence of
benign liver adenomas and a decreased incidence of benign breast disease.

5. References

Abbatiello, E. & Scudder, C.L. (1970) The effect of norethynodrel with mestranol treatment of pregnant mice on the isolation-induced aggression of their male offspring. Int. J. Fertil., 15, 182-189

Andrew, F.D., Williams, T.L., Gidley, J.T. & Wall, M.E. (1972) Teratogenicity of contraceptive steroids in mice (Abstract). Teratology, 5, 249

Arai, K., Golab, T., Layne, D.S. & Pincus, G. (1962) Metabolic fate of orally administered [H^3]-norethynodrel in rabbits. Endocrinology, 71, 639-648

Barrows, G.H., Christopherson, W.M. & Drill, V.A. (1977) Liver lesions and oral contraceptive steroids. J. Toxicol. environ. Health, 3, 219-230

Bishun, N., Mills, J., Parke, D.V. & Williams, D.C. (1975) A cytogenetic study in women who had used oral contraceptives and in their progeny. Mutat. Res., 33, 299-310

Cavina, G., Moretti, G. & Petrella, M. (1975) A solvent system for the separation of steroids with estrogenic and progestational activity by two-dimensional thin-layer chromatography. J. Chromatogr., 103, 368-371

Colton, F.B. (1954) Estradienes. US Patent, 2,691,028, 5 Oct. to G.D. Searle & Co. [Chem. Abstr., 49, 117291]

Colton, F.B. (1955) 13-Methyl-17-ethynyl-17-hydroxy-1,2,3,4,6,7,8,9, 11,12,13,14,16,17-tetradecahydro-15H-cyclopentaphenanthren-3-one. US Patent, 2,725,389, 29 Nov. to G.D. Searle & Co. [Chem. Abstr., 50, 9454f]

Committee on Safety of Medicines (1972) Carcinogenicity Tests of Oral Contraceptives, London, HMSO

Cook, C.E., Twine, M.E., Tallent, C.R., Wall, M.E. & Bresler, R.C. (1972) Norethynodrel metabolites in human plasma and urine. J. Pharmacol. exp. Ther., 183, 197-205

Drill, V.A., Martin, D.P., Hart, E.R. & McConnell, R.G. (1974) Effect of oral contraceptives on the mammary glands of rhesus monkeys: a preliminary report. J. natl Cancer Inst., 52, 1655-1657

Dunn, T.B. (1969) Cancer of the uterine cervix in mice fed a liquid
    diet containing an antifertility drug. J. natl Cancer Inst., 43,
    671-692

Edwards, C.W., Calhoun, F.J. & Green, S. (1971) The effects of mestranol
    and several progestins on chromosomes and fertility in the rat
    (Abstract no. 157). Toxicol. appl. Pharmacol., 19, 421

Feher, T. & Bodrogi, L. (1976) Gas chromatographic determination of
    synthetic gestagen hormones (Hung.). Acta pharm. hung., 46,
    73-77 [Chem. Abstr., 84, 147091y]

Foote, W.D., Foote, W.C. & Foote, L.H. (1968) Influence of certain
    natural and synthetic steroids on genital development in guinea
    pigs. Fertil. Steril., 19, 606-615

Freudenthal, R.I., Cook, C.E., Twine, M., Rosenfeld, R. & Wall, M.E.
    (1971a) Metabolism of norethynodrel by rat liver. Biochem.
    Pharmacol., 20, 1507-1512

Freudenthal, R.I., Rosenfeld, R. & Wall, M.E. (1971b) Species and
    strain differences in the epimerization of $3\beta,17\beta$-dihydroxy-17α-
    ethynyl-$\Delta^{5(10)}$-estrene to the 3α-epimer. Biochem. Pharmacol., 20,
    2930-2933

Freudenthal, R.I., Martin, J., Cook, C.E. & Wall, M.E. (1973) Metabolism
    and distribution of norethynodrel in pregnant and nonpregnant mice.
    Toxicol. appl. Pharmacol., 24, 125-132

Gidley, J.T., Christensen, H.D., Hall, I.H., Palmer, K.H. & Wall, M.E.
    (1970) Teratogenic and other effects produced in mice by
    norethynodrel and its 3-hydroxymetabolites. Teratology, 3, 339-
    344

Görög, S. (1977) Single tablet assay methods for the determination of
    progestins in oral contraceptives. Analysis of steroids. XXIX.
    Zentralbl. Pharm., 116, 259-264

Gruenstein, M., Shay, H. & Shimkin, M.B. (1964) Lack of effect of
    norethynodrel (Enovid) on methylcholanthrene-induced mammary
    carcinogenesis in female rats. Cancer Res., 24, 1656-1658

IARC (1974) IARC Monographs on the Evaluation of Carcinogenic Risk of
    Chemicals to Man, 6, Sex Hormones, Lyon, pp. 191-200

Kirschstein, R.L., Rabson, A.S. & Rusten, G.W. (1972) Infiltrating duct
    carcinoma of the mammary gland of a rhesus monkey after administration
    of an oral contraceptive: a preliminary report. J. natl Cancer
    Inst., 48, 551-556

Lang, R. & Redmann, U. (1979) Non-mutagenicity of some sex hormones in the Ames' *Salmonella*/microsome mutagenicity test. Arch. Toxicol. (in press)

Layne,, D.S., Golab, T., Arai, K. & Pincus, G. (1963) The metabolic fate of orally administered ^{3}H-norethynodrel and ^{3}H-norethindrone in humans. Biochem. Pharmacol., 12, 905-911

Lipschütz, A., Iglesias, R., Salinas, S. & Panesevich, V.I. (1966) Experimental conditions under which contraceptive steroids may become toxic. Nature, 212, 686-688

Lipschütz, A., Iglesias, R., Panasevich, V.I. & Salinas, S. (1967) Ovarian tumours and other ovarian changes induced in mice by two 19-nor-contraceptives. Br. J. Cancer, 21, 153-159

Martin, J.L., Duncombe, R.E. & Shaw, W.H.C. (1975) A thin-layer chromatographic test for the identification of some drugs: its application to steroids, tetracyclines, penicillins, and cephalosporins. Analyst (Lond.), 100, 243-248

McCarthy, J.D. (1965) Influence of two contraceptives on induction of mammary cancer in rats. Am. J. Surg., 110, 720-723

Muñoz, N. (1973) Effect of herpesvirus type 2 and hormonal imbalance on the uterine cervix of the mouse. Cancer Res., 33, 1504-1508

National Formulary Board (1975) National Formulary, 14th ed., Washington DC, American Pharmaceutical Association, pp. 493-494

Palmer, K.H., Ross, F.T., Rhodes, L.S., Baggett, B. & Wall, M.E. (1969) Metabolism of antifertility steroids. I. Norethynodrel. J. Pharmacol. exp. Ther., 167, 207-216

Poel, W.E. (1966) Pituitary tumors in mice after prolonged feeding of synthetic progestins. Science, 154, 402-403

Ranney, R.E. (1977) Comparative metabolism of 17α-ethynyl steroids used in oral contraceptives. J. Toxicol. environ. Health, 3, 139-166

Roushdi, I.M., El Sabai, A.I. & Belal, S. (1974) New methods for the estimation of acetylenic steroids (non-aqueous titrimetric method). Egypt. J. pharm. Sci., 15, 217-221

Roy, S.K. & Kar, A.B. (1967) Foetal effect of norethynodrel in rats. Indian J. exp. Biol., 5, 14-16

Rudali, G. (1975) Induction of tumors in mice with synthetic sex hormones. Gann Monogr., 17, 243-252

Saunders, F.J. (1965) Effects on the course of pregnancy of norethynodrel with mestranol (Enovid) administered to rats during early pregnancy. Endocrinology, 77, 873-878

Sichuk, G., Fortner, J.G. & Der, B.K. (1967) Evaluation of the influence of norethynodrel with mestranol (Enovid) in middle-aged male Syrian (golden) hamsters, with particular reference to spontaneous tumours. Acta endocrinol., 55, 97-107

Singh, O.S. & Carr, D.H. (1970) A study of the effects of certain hormones on human cells in culture. Can. med. Assoc. J., 103, 349-350, 373

Stern, E. & Mickey, M.R. (1969) Effects of a cyclic steroid contraceptive regimen on mammary gland tumor induction in rats. Br. J. Cancer., 23, 391-400

Takano, K., Yamamura, H., Suzuki, M. & Nishimura, H. (1966) Teratogenic effect of chlormadinone acetate in mice and rabbits. Proc. Soc. exp. Biol. (N.Y), 121, 455-457

Tausk, M. & deVisser, J. (1972) International Encyclopedia of Pharmacology and Therapeutics, Vol. II, section 48, Elmsford, NY, Pergamon Press, pp. 35-194

Tuchmann-Duplessis, H. & Mercier-Parot, L. (1972) Effect of a contraceptive steroid on progeny (Fr.). J. Gynecol. Obstet. biol. Reprod., 1, 141-159

US Food & Drug Administration (1978) Oral contraceptive drug products. Physician and patient labeling; extension of effective date for physician labeling. Fed. Regist., 43, 9863-9864

US Tariff Commission (1963) Synthetic Organic Chemicals, US Production and Sales, 1962, TC Publication 114, Washington DC, US Government Printing Office, p. 134

US Tariff Commission (1967) Synthetic Organic Chemicals, US Production and Sales, 1965, TC Publication 206, Washington DC, US Government Printing Office, p. 125

Wade, A., ed. (1977) Martindale, The Extra Pharmacopoeia, 27th ed., London, The Pharmaceutical Press, p. 1413

Weisburger, J.H., Weisburger, E.K., Griswold, D.P., Jr & Casey, A.E. (1968) Reduction of carcinogen-induced breast cancer in rats by an anti-fertility drug. Life Sci., 7, 259-266

Welsch, C.W. & Meites, J. (1969) Effects of a norethynodrel-mestranol
     combination (Enovid) on development and growth of carcinogen-induced
     mammary tumours in female rats. Cancer, 23, 601-607

Welsch, C.W., Adams, C., Lambrecht, L.K., Hassett, C.C. & Brookes, C.L.
     (1977) 17β-Oestradiol and Enovid mammary tumorigenesis in C3H/HeJ
     female mice: counteraction by concurrent 2-bromo-α-ergocryptine.
     Br. J. Cancer, 35, 322-328

Windholz, M., ed. (1976) The Merck Index, 9th ed., Rahway, NJ, Merck
     & Co., p. 869

Wu, J.Y.P. (1977) Collaborative study of an assay for progestational
     steroids in individual contraceptive tablets. J. Assoc. off.
     Anal. Chem., 60, 922-925

NORGESTREL

A monograph on this substance was published previously (IARC, 1974). Relevant data that have appeared since that time have been evaluated in the present monograph.

1. Chemical and Physical Data

In contrast to other synthetic sex steroids, norgestrel is obtained by total synthesis, which yields equal amounts of the d and l optical isomers.

1.1 Synonyms and trade names

(a) d-Norgestrel

Chem. Abstr. Services Reg. No.: 797-63-7

Chem. Abstr. Name: (17α)-13-Ethyl-17-hydroxy-18,19-dinorpregn-4-en-20-yn-3-one

Synonyms: Denorgestrel; D-norgestrel; 13β-ethyl-17α-ethynyl-17β-hydroxygon-4-en-3-one; 17α-ethynyl-18-homo-19-nortestosterone; 13-ethyl-17-hydroxy-18,19-dinor-17α-pregn-4-en-20-yn-3-one; 17-ethynyl-18-methyl-19-nortestosterone; levonorgestrel

Trade names: Adepal; Duoluton; Eugynon; FH 122-A; Follistrel; Lo/Ovral; Micro-30; Microgynon 30; Microlut; Microluton; Microval; Mikro-30; Minidril; Monovar; Neogest; Ovral; Ovran; Ovran 30; Ovranette; Ovrette; SH 850; SH 70850; Stediril; TSP-6; Wy 3707

(b) dl-Norgestrel

Chem. Abstr. Services Reg. No.: 6533-00-2

Chem. Abstr. Name: $(17\alpha)(\pm)$-13-Ethyl-17-hydroxy-18,19-dinorpregn-4-en-20-yn-3-one

Synonyms: 13β-Ethyl-17α-ethynyl-17β-hydroxygon-4-en-3-one;
(+)-13-ethyl-17-hydroxy-18,19-dinor-17α-pregn-4-en-20-yn-3-one;
17α-ethynyl-18-homo-19-nortestosterone; α-norgestrel; (+)-
norgestrel; dl-norgestrel

Trade names[1]: Duoluton; Eugynon; [Eugynon 21]; [Eugynon 28];
Eugynon 30; Eugynon 50; [Eugynon ED]; [Evanor]; FH 122-A;
[Folinett]; [Follinyl]; Lo/Ovral; Micro-30; Microlut;
Microval; Monovar; [Neogentrol]; Neogest; [Neogynon];
[Neogynon 21]; [Neogynon 28]; [Neogynon ED]; [Neovlar 21];
[Nordiol 28]; Orval; Ovran; Ovrette; [Primovlar 21];
[Primovlar 28]; SH 850; SH 70850; Stediril; [Stediril D];
Wy 3707

1.2 Structural and molecular formulae and molecular weight

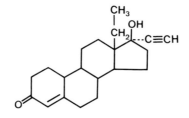

C$_{21}$H$_{28}$O$_2$ Mol. wt: 312.4

1.3 Chemical and physical properties

From Wade (1977) and Windholz (1976), unless otherwise specified

(a) Description: White crystals (from ethyl acetate or methanol)

(b) Melting-point: (+) form, 203-206°C; (-) form, 239-241°C

---

[1]Those in square brackets are preparations that are no longer
produced commercially.

(c) Spectroscopy data: λ_{max} 242 nm (E_1^1 = 541) in ethanol; infra-red, nuclear magnetic resonance and mass spectral data have been tabulated (Sopirak & Cullen, 1975).

(d) Optical rotation: $[\alpha]_D^{25}$ -42.5° (chloroform)

(e) Solubility: Insoluble in water; soluble in ethanol (1 in 120), chloroform (1 in 15), diethyl ether (1 in 400) and dioxane

(f) Stability: No decomposition observed after 5 years at room temperature, 1 year at 45°C, 1 month at 75°C and 1 month under direct ultra-violet light (Sopirak & Cullen, 1975)

1.4 Technical products and impurities

Various national and international pharmacopoeias give specifications for the purity of norgestrel in pharmaceutical products. For example, norgestrel is available in the US as a USP grade containing 98-102% active ingredient on a dried basis. Tablets in 0.5 mg doses in combination with 0.05 mg ethinyloestradiol contain 0.45-0.55 mg norgestrel (US Pharmacopeial Convention Inc., 1975). Tablets containing 0.075 mg norgestrel and tablets containing 0.3 mg norgestrel and 0.03 mg ethinyloestradiol are also available in the US (Kastrup, 1977).

In the UK, norgestrel is available in tablets in 0.075 mg doses and in various combinations with ethinyloestradiol: 0.5 mg norgestrel with 0.03 mg ethinyloestradiol, 0.5 mg norgestrel with 0.05 mg ethinyloestradiol, and 0.15 mg or 0.25 mg d-norgestrel with 0.03 mg ethinyloestradiol (Wade, 1977).

2. Production, Use, Occurrence and Analysis

2.1 Production and use

(a) Production

Several methods for the synthesis of norgestrel were reported in the early 1960s (Windholz, 1976). In a later method, 6-methoxy-1-tetralone is treated with vinylmagnesium bromide to form 6-methoxy-1-vinyl-1,2,3,4-tetrahydro-1-naphthol. This compound is condensed with 2-ethyl-1,3-cyclopentanedione to give 3-methoxy-8(14)-secooestra-1,3,5-(10),9(11)-tetraen-13-ethyl-18-nor-14,17-dione, which is made to undergo a ring closure to give the steroid skeleton. The 17-keto group is reduced with sodium borohydride, and the 14(15) double bond is reduced

with hydrogen over palladium on carbon. A Birch reduction is then used
to reduce the 8(9) double bond and the 1 and 4 positions of the A ring.
Oxidation of the alcohol is used to introduce a keto group at the 17
position. Treatment with acetylene gives the 17-ethynyl carbinol, and
hydrolysis of the 3-enol ether gives norgestrel (Klimstra, 1969). It is
not known whether this method is used for commercial production.

Commercial production of norgestrel in the US was first reported in
1969 (US Tariff Commission, 1971). In 1975 and 1976, only one US company
reported production of an undisclosed amount (see preamble, p. 20) (US
International Trade Commission, 1977a,b); however, in 1975, US production
of 13 oestrogen and progestin substances, including norgestrel, amounted
to 10.5 thousand kg (US International Trade Commission, 1977a). Data on
US imports and exports of norgestrel are not available.

Norgestrel is believed to be produced in western Europe by two
companies, one of which is located in France. Total western European
production is estimated to be less than 1000 kg.

Norgestrel is not produced or imported in Japan.

(b) Use

Norgestrel is used in human medicine primarily as a contraceptive
administered orally as a progestin-only tablet (commonly known as a
'minipill'), in a continuous daily dose of 0.075 mg. It is also used in
combination with ethinyloestradiol in doses of 0.3 or 0.5 mg norgestrel
with 0.03 or 0.05 mg ethinyloestradiol taken for 21 days starting on day
5 of the menstrual cycle (Harvey, 1975; Murad & Gilman, 1975). Norges-
trel:ethinyloestradiol combinations are also used to control menstrual
disorders and endometriosis (Wade, 1977).

2.2 Occurrence

Norgestrel is not known to occur naturally. Residues have been
detected in milk from nursing mothers taking oral contraceptives containing
norgestrel (Thomas *et al.*, 1977).

The US Food & Drug Administration (1978) has ruled that with effect
from 31 May 1978 all oral contraceptives for general use must carry
patient and physician warning labels concerning use, risks and contraindications.

2.3 Analysis

Analytical methods for the determination of norgestrel as a bulk
chemical have been reviewed (Sopirak & Cullen, 1975). Typical analytical
methods are summarized in Table 1. Abbreviations used are: UV, ultra-
violet spectrometry; CC, column chromatography; and RIA, radioimmunoassay.
See also the section, 'General Remarks on Sex Hormones', p. 60.

TABLE 1

Analytical methods for norgestrel

Sample matrix	Sample preparation	Assay procedure	Sensitivity or limit of detection	Reference
Bulk chemical	Dissolve (ethanol)	UV (241 nm)	-	US Pharmacopeial Convention Inc. (1975)
Tablets	Extract (dimethylformamide); reduce volume; add buffer	Polarography	-	Chatten et al. (1977)
Tablets	Extract (methanol:water, 15:2); reduce (sodium borohydride)	UV (241 nm)	-	GMrüg (1977)
Tablets	Powder; extract (chloroform); derivatize (isonicotinic acid hydrazide)	UV (∿ 380 nm)	-	Horwitz (1977)
Tablets	Powder; dissolve (aqueous ethanol)	UV (241 nm)	-	US Pharmacopeial Convention Inc. (1975)
Plasma	Dilute (water); extract (petroleum ether); evaporate; dissolve (ethanol); add labelled norgestrel and antiserum	RIA	30 pg/ml (0.1-1 ml sample)	Warren & Fotherby (1974)
Human milk	Add labelled norgestrel; extract (diethyl ether); CC (Sephadex LH/20); evaporate; dissolve (buffer); add antiserum	RIA	20 pg/ml (1 ml sample)	Thomas et al. (1977)

3. Biological Data Relevant to the Evaluation
of Carcinogenic Risk to Humans

3.1 Carcinogenicity studies in animals

Oral administration

Mouse: Norgestrel alone or in combination with ethinyloestradiol was incorporated into the diet of groups of 120 male and 120 female CF-LP mice (MTV$^-$)[1] for 80 weeks. The doses were identified only as low (2-5 times the human contraceptive dose), medium (50-150 times) and high (200-400 times); the amounts administered were not specified. Norgestrel administered alone or in combination with ethinyloestradiol (10:1) did not alter the incidence of tumours in any tissue compared with that in controls (Committee on Safety of Medicines, 1972).

Castrated (C3H x RIII)F1 mice (MTV$^+$) of both sexes were fed dl-norgestrel or d-norgestrel in the diet at levels of 1 or 0.5 mg/kg, respectively. Mammary carcinomas were observed in 22/31 dl-norgestrel-treated, 27/34 d-norgestrel-treated and 17/29 control female mice. In the corresponding males, the incidences were 9/32, 10/32 and 10/61. The increases in incidence were slightly raised, but the latencies of mammary tumours were unchanged (Rudali & Guggiari, 1974).

Rat: When norgestrel was administered alone or in combination with ethinyloestradiol (10:1) in the diet for 104 weeks to groups of 120 male and 120 female rats, there was no alteration in the incidence of tumours in any tissue compared with that in 80 male and 80 female controls (Committee on Safety of Medicines, 1972).

3.2 Other relevant biological data

Norgestrel is one of the most potent progestational compounds when taken orally. In contrast to other progestationally-active 19-nortestosterone derivatives, it can maintain pregnancy in subsequently castrated animals (Neumann, 1968). Only the d-enantiomer binds to the progestin receptor and is biologically active (Gerhards et al., 1971).

---

[1]MTV$^-$: mammary tumour virus not expressed; MTV$^+$: mammary tumour virus expressed (see p. 62)

Rats were given 0.5-30 µg norgestrel orally from day 1-7 of gestation or 2 µg on days 6-8, or in a single dose on day 6, 7 or 8. Administration of 2 µg continuously for 7 days terminated 100% of pregnancies; a single dose was effective only when given on day 6, terminating 57% of pregnancies; 2 µg given on days 6-8 terminated 50% of pregnancies (Dasgupta *et al.*, 1973).

No data on embryotoxicity at later stages of gestation or on teratogenicity were available.

The metabolism of *d*-, *l*- and *dl*-norgestrel has been reviewed by Ranney (1977). Norgestrel follows metabolic pathways similar to those of norethisterone (see monograph, p. 441). It has been suggested (Ranney, 1977) that the presence of an ethyl moiety at C-13 should slow down biotransformation; this may explain its very high progestational potency.

The *d*- and *l*-enantiomers of norgestrel are metabolized differently. The African green monkey metabolizes *d*-norgestrel *via* the same reductive pathways as are used in the metabolism of other progestational compounds, the major metabolite being 3α,5β-tetrahydro-*d*-norgestrel (13-ethyl-18, 19-dinor-5β,17α-pregn-20-yn-3α,17-diol). The biologically inactive *l*-norgestrel, however, is transformed mainly by hydroxylation at C-16. Metabolites of *l*-norgestrel are 16β-hydroxy-*l*-norgestrel, 16α-hydroxy-*l*-norgestrel, and a 16ξ-hydroxytetrahydro-*l*-norgestrel (Sisenwine *et al.*, 1974).

In women given oral doses of 1.5 mg *dl*-, *d*- or *l*-norgestrel, the main metabolites observed in the blood were: 3α,5β-tetrahydro-*d*-norgestrel following administration of *d*-norgestrel, and 16β-hydroxy-*l*-norgestrel following administration of *l*-norgestrel. Both metabolites occurred mainly as the glucuronide and sulphate conjugates, the glucuronide being derived predominantly from the *d*-enantiomer and the sulphate from the *l*-enantiomer (Sisenwine *et al.*, 1975). After administration of *dl*-norgestrel, the major metabolite in the urine was 16β-hydroxynorgestrel as the sulphate (Sisenwine *et al.*, 1973).

No data on the mutagenicity of norgestrel were available.

3.3 Case reports and epidemiological studies

See the section, 'Oestrogens and Progestins in Relation to Human Cancer', p. 83.

4. Summary of Data Reported and Evaluation[1]

4.1 Experimental data

Norgestrel was tested in mice and rats alone or in combination with ethinyloestradiol by oral administration. There was no increase in the incidence of tumours in either species.

Norgestrel is embryolethal for pre- and postimplantation embryos in rats.

4.2 Human data

No case reports or epidemiological studies on norgestrel alone were available to the Working Group. Epidemiological studies on steroid hormones used in oestrogen-progestin contraceptive preparations have been summarized in the section, 'Oestrogens and Progestins in Relation to Human Cancer', p. 83.

4.3 Evaluation

The available data in experimental animals and humans are insufficient to evaluate the carcinogenicity of norgestrel. In humans, oral contraceptives containing oestrogens in combination with progestins have been related causally to an increased incidence of benign liver adenomas and a decreased incidence of benign breast disease.

---

[1]This section should be read in conjunction with pp. 62-64 in the 'General Remarks on Sex Hormones' and with the 'General Conclusions on Sex Hormones', p. 131.

5. References

Chatten, L.G., Yadav, R.N., Binnington, S. & Moskalyk, R.E. (1977)
     Polarographic study of certain progestogens and their determination
     in oral contraceptive tablets by differential pulse polarography.
     Analyst (Lond.), 102, 323-327

Committee on Safety of Medicines (1972) Carcinogenicity Tests of
     Oral Contraceptives, London, HMSO, 1-23

Dasgupta, P.R., Srivastava, K. & Kar, A.B. (1973) Effect of
     d-norgestrel on early pregnancy in rats. Indian J. exp. Biol.,
     11, 321-322

Gerhards, E., Hecker, W., Hitze, H., Niewweboer, B. & Bellmann, O.
     (1971) Metabolism of norethisterone and dl- and d-norgestrel.
     Acta endocrinol., 68, 219-248

Görög, S. (1977) Analysis of steroids. XXIX. Single tablet assay
     methods for the determination of progestins in oral contraceptives.
     Zentralbl. Pharm., 116, 259-264

Harvey, S.C. (1975) Hormones. In: Osol, A. et al, eds, Remington's
     Pharmaceutical Sciences, 15th ed., Easton, PA, Mack, pp. 924,
     928

Horwitz, W. (1977) Official methods of analysis of the Association
     of Official Analytical Chemists. J. Assoc. off. anal. Chem., 60,
     483-484

IARC (1974) IARC Monographs on the Evaluation of Carcinogenic Risk
     of Chemicals to Man, 6, Sex Hormones, Lyon, pp. 201-205

Kastrup, E.K., ed. (1977) Facts and Comparisons, St Louis, MO, Facts
     & Comparisons Inc., pp. 108c-108e

Klimstra, P.D. (1969) The role of progestin and estrogen in fertility
     control and maintenance. In: Chinn, L.J., Klimstra, P.D.,
     Baran, J.S. & Pappo, R., eds, The Chemistry and Biochemistry of
     Steroids, Los Altos, CA, Geron-X, pp. 65-66

Murad, F. & Gilman, A.G. (1975) Estrogens and progestins. In: Goodman,
     L.S. & Gilman, A., eds, The Pharmacological Basis of Therapeutics,
     5th ed., New York, Macmillan, pp. 1441-1447

Neumann, F. (1968) Chemical constitution and pharmacologic action (Ger.).
    In: Langecker, H., ed., Handbuch der Experimenteller Pharmakologie,
    Vol. 22, Die Gestagene, Berlin, Springer, pp. 680-1025

Ranney, R.E. (1977) Comparative metabolism of 17α-ethynyl steroids
    used in oral contraceptives. J. Toxicol. environ. Health, 3,
    139-166

Rudali, G. & Guggiari, M. (1974) Studies on the carcinogenic effect
    of two norgestrels on the mammary gland of the mouse (Fr.).
    C.R. Soc. Biol. (Paris), 168, 1190-1194

Sisenwine, S.F., Kimmel, H.B., Liu, A.L. & Ruelius, H.W. (1973)
    Urinary metabolites of dl-norgestrel in women. Acta endocrinol.,
    73, 91-104

Sisenwine, S.F., Kimmel, H.B., Liu, A.L. & Ruelius, H.W. (1974)
    Stereoselective biotransformation of dl-norgestrel and its
    enantiomers in the African green monkey. Drug Metab. Disposition,
    2, 65-70

Sisenwine, S.F., Kimmel, H.B., Liu, A.L. & Ruelius, H.W. (1975) The
    presence of dl-, d- and l-norgestrel and their metabolites in
    the plasma of women. Contraception, 12, 339-353

Sopirak, A.M. & Cullen, L.F. (1975) Norgestrel. In: Florey, K.,
    ed., Analytical Profiles of Drug Substances, Vol. IV, New York,
    Academic Press, pp. 296-318

Thomas, M.J., Danutra, V., Read, G.F., Hillier, S.G. & Griffiths, K.
    (1977) The detection and measurement of D-norgestrel in human
    milk using Sephadex LH/20 chromatography and radioimmunoassay.
    Steroids, 30, 349-361

US Food & Drug Administration (1978) Oral contraceptive drug
    products. Physician and patient labeling; extension of effective
    date for physician labeling. Fed. Regist., 43, 9863-9864

US International Trade Commission (1977a) Synthetic Organic Chemicals,
    US Production and Sales, 1975, USITC Publication 804, Washington
    DC, US Government Printing Office, pp. 90, 102

US International Trade Commssion (1977b) Synthetic Organic Chemicals,
    US Production and Sales, 1976, USITC Publication 833,
    Washington DC, US Government Printing Office, p. 149

US Pharmacopeial Convention Inc. (1975) The US Pharmacopeia, 19th
    rev., Rockville, MD, pp. 347-348

US Tariff Commission (1971) Synthetic Organic Chemicals, US Production and Sales, 1969, TC Publication 412, Washington DC, US Government Printing Office, p. 118

Wade, A., ed. (1977) Martindale, The Extra Pharmacopoeia, 27th ed., London, The Pharmaceutical Press, pp. 1413-1414

Warren, R.J. & Fotherby, K. (1974) Radioimmunoassay of synthetic progestogens, norethisterone and norgestrel. J. Endocrinol., 62, 605-618

Windholz, M., ed. (1976) The Merck Index, 9th ed., Rahway, NJ, Merck & Co., p. 869

PROGESTERONE

A monograph on this substance was published previously (IARC, 1974). Relevant data that have appeared since that time have been evaluated in the present monograph.

1.   Chemical and Physical Data

1.1   Synonyms and trade names

Chem. Abstr. Services Reg. No.:   57-83-0

Chem. Abstr. Name: Pregn-4-ene-3,20-dione

Synonyms: Corpus luteum hormone; luteal hormone; luteine; luteohormone; Δ^4-pregnene-3,20-dione

Trade names[1]: Agolutin; Bio-luton; Colprosterone; Corlutin; Corlutina; Corlutone; Corluvite; Corporin; Corpormone; Cyclogesterin; [Cycloestrol]; [Duogynon]; [Emmenovis]; [Emonovister]; [Farlutal]; Flavolutan; [Foliluteina]; Fologenon; Gesterol; Gestin-E; Gestone; Gestormone; Gestron; Glanducorpin; Gynlutin; Gynolutone; Hormoflaveine; Hormoluton; Lipo-Lutin; Lucorteum; Lucorteum Sol; Luteinique; Luteinol; [Luteocrin]; Luteocrin normale; Luteodyn; [Luteo Folicular]; Luteogan; [Luteogyl]; Luteol; Luteopur; Luteosan; Luteosid; Luteostab; Luteosteron; Luteovis; [Lutestex]; [Lutestron]; Lutex; Lutex-Leo; Lutidon; Lutin; Lutociclina; Lutocor; Lutocyclin; Lutocyclin M; Lutocylin; Lutoform; Lutogyl; Lutogynon; [Lutovitamina E]; [Lut Ovociclina]; [Lut-ovocyclin]; Lutren; [Lutrogen]; Lutromone; [Lutrone]; Nalutron; Paragest; Paralut; Paralut Forte; [Percutacrine Lut.]; Percutacrine Luteinique; Piaponon; [Pre-cyclan-Leo]; Primolut; Primolut Depot; Profac-O; Progekan;

---

[1]Those in square brackets are preparations that are no longer produced commercially.

Progelan; Progestasert; Progeste; Progesterol; [Progesterone R];
Progestilin; [Progestilline Fort]; Progestin; Progestine;
Progestogel; Progestone; Progestron; Prolidon; Prolets;
Prolusteron; Proluton; [Proluton D]; [Proluton Dep.];
[Proluton-Oestradiol]; [Proluton Z]; [Protectona]; Protormone;
Sistociclina; [Stroluten]; [Synergon]; Syngesterone; Syngestrets;
[Synovex S]; Syntolutan; Syntolutin; [Syntoluton]; [Testo
Luteinica]; [Testoluton]; [Testoviron Prog.]; [Tocogestan];
[Trioestrine]; [Trioestrine R]; [Trioestrine Vitam.];
[Vit-E-Progesterone]

1.2   Structural and molecular formulae and molecular weight

$C_{21}H_{30}O_2$ Mol. wt: 314.5

1.3   Chemical and physical properties

From Weast (1977) & Windholz (1976) unless otherwise specified

(a) Description: Exists in two readily interconvertible forms:
     α-form – white orthorhombic prisms; β-form – white orthor-
     hombic needles

(b) Melting-point: α-form – 128.5–131°C; β-form – 121–122°C

(c) Density: α-form – d^{23} 1.166; β-form – d^{20} 1.171

(d) Spectroscopy data: λ_{max} 240 nm; infra-red, nuclear magnetic
     resonance and mass spectral data have been tabulated (Grasselli
     & Ritchey, 1975).

(e) <u>Optical rotation</u>: α-form - $[\alpha]_D$ +192°; β-form - $[\alpha]_D$ +172° to +182° (2% w/v in dioxane)

(f) <u>Solubility</u>: Practically insoluble in water; soluble in ethanol (1 in 8), arachis oil (1 in 60), chloroform (1 in <1), diethyl ether (1 in 16), ethyl oleate (1 in 60) and light petroleum (1 in 100) (Wade, 1977); soluble in acetone, dioxane and concentrated sulphuric acid; sparingly soluble in vegetable oils

1.4 Technical products and impurities

Various national and international pharmacopoeias give specifications for the purity of progesterone in pharmaceutical products. For example, progesterone is available in the US as a USP grade containing 98-102% active ingredient on a dried basis and not more than 3% foreign steroids and other impurities. Injections in a suitable solvent in 25, 50 and 100 mg/ml doses and tablets in 10 and 25 mg doses contain 90-110% of the stated amount of progesterone, and aqueous suspensions in 25, 50 and 100 mg/ml doses contain 93-107% of the stated amount (US Pharmacopeial Convention Inc., 1975). Progesterone is also available in the US in combination with oestrogenic substances in injections and tablets, as well as in a T-shaped intrauterine device containing a reservoir of 38 mg progesterone dispersed in medical-grade silicone oil (Kastrup, 1976, 1978).

In the UK, progesterone is available in injections in 10, 20, 25 and 50 mg/ml doses and in a 12 mg/ml dose in combination with 100 mg/ml α-tocopherol. It is also available in implants in 25, 50 and 100 mg doses and in an intrauterine device containing 38 mg progesterone (Wade, 1977).

In Japan, progesterone is available in injection form, and may be combined with oestradiol-17β or its esters.

2. Production, Use, Occurrence and Analysis

2.1 Production and use

(a) Production

Progesterone was isolated in 1929 from the corpora lutea of sows by Corner and Allen (Murad & Gilman, 1975) and was first synthesized by Butenandt and Schmidt in 1934 by heating 4β-bromo-5β-pregnane-3,20-dione with pyridine (Boit, 1969). Progesterone is produced commercially by (1) the degradation of diosgenin (obtained from the Mexican yam, *Dioscorea mexicana*) to pregnenolone, which is converted to progesterone by Oppenauer oxidation; or (2) the oxidation of stigmasterol (obtained from soya bean oil) to stigmastadienone, which undergoes further modifications to progesterone. Progesterone can also be produced using cholesterol as a starting material (Dorfman, 1966; Harvey, 1975).

Commercial production of progesterone in the US was first reported in 1939 (US Tariff Commission, 1940). In 1975 and 1976, only one US company reported production of an undisclosed amount (see preamble, p. 20) (US International Trade Commission, 1977a,b); in 1975, US production of 13 oestrogen and progestin substances, including progesterone, amounted to 10.5 thousand kg (US International Trade Commission, 1977a). Data on US imports and exports of progesterone are not available.

Commercial production of progesterone in the UK was first reported in 1950. It is produced commercially in France, The Netherlands and the UK and in eastern Europe, but no information was available on the quantities produced. In 1977, European imports are estimated to have amounted to over 2 million kg.

Progesterone was first marketed commercially in Japan in 1954-1955. It is not produced there, and imports amounted to 50 kg in 1976 and 40 kg in 1977.

(b) Use

Progesterone is used in human medicine for the treatment of secondary amenorrhoea and dysfunctional uterine bleeding, although progestational agents which are active orally are generally preferred to progesterone. Dosage regimens for the administration of progesterone as an i.m. injection vary, depending on whether it is administered as an aqueous suspension or as an oily solution. For dysfunctional uterine bleeding, aqueous suspensions are given in combination with oestrogen therapy in a dose of 5 mg per day or 10 mg every other day during the last 10 days of the cycle; oily solutions are given in a dose of 2-10 mg per day for 5 days, or until haemostasis occurs, or 50 mg followed by 10-20 mg per day for 4 days. Oily injections and tablets containing progesterone and oestrogenic substances are also used for the treatment of secondary amenorrhoea and dysfunctional uterine bleeding. Progesterone embedded in an intrauterine device is used for contraception (Harvey, 1975; Wade, 1977).

It has also been used in the treatment of female hypogonadism, dysmenorrhoea and premenstrual tension, habitual and threatened abortion, preeclampsia and toxaemia of pregnancy, mastodynia, uterine fibroma and neoplasms of the breast and endometrium (Harvey, 1975; Wade, 1977).

Human placental extracts (of which progesterone is believed to be the main constituent) have been used in preparations for cosmetic use (at levels of 0.1-1%), hair conditioners, shampoos and grooming aid tonics (<0.1%).

In Japan, progesterone is used for the treatment of menstrual disorders, in threatened abortion and in the treatment of sterility.

In veterinary medicine, progesterone is used to control habitual abortion and to delay oestrus and ovulation in cattle (50 mg per day), swine (50-100 mg per day) and dogs (50-75 mg of repository form) (Harvey, 1975).

About 100 thousand to 1 million kg progesterone each are used in Italy, Spain and the UK annually.

The US Food & Drug Administration (1977) requires that no residues of progesterone should be found in the uncooked edible tissues of lambs and steers.

2.2 Occurrence

Progesterone is a naturally occurring steroidal hormone found in a wide variety of tissues and biological fluids (see the section, 'General Remarks on Sex Hormones', pp. 42-56), including **cow**'s milk (Nuti *et al.*, 1975), where levels of 1-30 ng/ml have been found; and milk products, the highest level being found in butter (300 µg/kg) (Hoffman *et al.*, 1977). It has also been found to occur naturally in certain plant species (Weiler & Zenk, 1976).

2.3 Analysis

Analytical methods for determining progesterone in biological samples, based on radioimmunoassay and competitive protein binding techniques, have been reviewed (Abraham *et al.*, 1977; Johansson, 1975). Typical analytical methods are summarized in Table 1. Abbreviations used are: GC/ECD, gas chromatography/electron-capture detection; GC/FID, gas chromatography/ flame-ionization detection; GC/MS, gas chromatography/mass spectrometry; TLC, thin-layer chromatography; HPLC, high-pressure liquid chromatography; CC, column chromatography; MS, mass spectrometry; UV, ultra-violet spectrometry; RIA, radioimmunoassay; CPD, competitive protein binding. See also 'General Remarks on Sex Hormones', p. 60 .

TABLE 1

Analytical methods for progesterone

Sample matrix	Sample preparation	Assay procedure	Sensitivity or limit of detection	Reference
Bulk chemical	Dissolve (ethanol); evaporate; dissolve (98% sulphuric acid); let stand 2 hrs	UV (292 nm)	2 μg/ml	Hassan et al. (1976)
Bulk chemical	Dissolve (ethanol)	UV (230 nm)	1.25 μg/ml (1 ml cell)	Khayam-Bashi & Boroumand (1975)
Bulk chemical	Dissolve (methanol)	UV (241 nm)		US Pharmacopeial Convention Inc. (1975)
Injection	Dissolve (chloroform); derivatize (isonicotinic acid hydrazide)	UV (380 nm)		British Pharmacopoeia Commission (1973)
Injection	Extract (85% ethanol)	HPLC		King et al. (1974)
Injection	Derivatize (2,4-dinitrophenyl-hydrazine); isolate & weigh	Gravimetry		US Pharmacopeial Convention Inc. (1975)
Suspension	Filter & weigh	Gravimetry		US Pharmacopeial Convention Inc. (1975)
Tablets	Extract (acetone); evaporate; suspend (water); filter & weigh	Gravimetry		US Pharmacopeial Convention Inc. (1975)
Pharmaceutical preparations	Extract (diethyl ether); evaporate; dissolve residue (95% ethanol); make basic; add lead citrate	Back titration (ethylenediamine-tetraacetic acid)		Gajewska et al. (1975)
Plasma	Extract (diethyl ether); derivatize	GC/MS	0.2-0.25 μg/l	Dehennin et al. (1974)

Table 1 (continued)

Sample matrix	Sample preparation	Assay procedure	Sensitivity or limit of detection	Reference
Plasma	Dilute (sodium hydroxide); extract (diethyl ether ; evaporate; dilute (methanol: water, 7:3); wash (hexane); CC	GC/ECD GC/FID	1 µg/100 ml	Felér et al. (1975)
Plasma	Add labelled progesterone; extract (dichloromethane); evaporate; dissolve (50% methanol); extract (iso-octane); CC (Sephadex)	CPB	0.05 ng	Honda (1976)
Plasma	Isolate; reduce (enzyme); derivatize	GC/ECD	10 ng	Van der Molen & De Jong (1975)
Plasma	Add labelled progesterone; extract (dichloromethane); wash (water); evaporate; CC (Sephadex); dissolve (ethanol); add antiserum	RIA	5.7 pg	Sippell et al. (1978)
Plasma	Extract (acetone); isolate as Girard derivative; hydrolyse; extract (petroleum ether)	TLC	–	Weiss (1973)
Serum	Extract (hexane); TLC; isolate; derivatize (heptafluorobutyrate)	GC/MS	10 nM	Björkhem et al. (1975)
Serum	Dissolve (phosphate-gelatin buffer); extract (diethyl ether); evaporate; dissolve (70% ethanol); dilute (buffer); add labelled progesterone & antiserum in buffer	RIA	0.25 µg/l (0.2 ml sample)	Scott et al. (1978)

Table 1 (continued)

Sample matrix	Sample preparation	Assay procedure	Sensitivity or limit of detection	Reference
Urine	Derivatize (isopentyloxime-trimethylsilyl ether & benzyl-oxime-trimethylsilyl ether)	GC/MS	-	Baillie et al. (1974)
Ovarian tissue	Homogenize (sodium hydroxide); extract (diethyl ether-ethyl acetate-ethanol); wash (sodium hydroxide)	GC/FID	25 ng	Poteczin et al. (1975)
Ovarian tissue	Dry	MS	1 mg/kg (1.2 mg sample)	Snedden & Parker (1974)
Human myometrial tissue and rabbit uterus	Add labelled progesterone; digest (sodium hydroxide-sodium dodecyl sulphate); extract (ethyl acetate); CC (Sephadex); add antiserum	RIA	-	Batra & Bengtsson (1976)
Corpus luteum	Homogenize; extract (ethyl acetate); CC (silica gel); add antiserum	RIA	-	Shutt et al. (1975)
Tissue	Homogenize; extract (chloroform:methanol, 1:1); CC (Sephadex); isolate; derivatize (O-methyloxime trimethylsilyl ether)	GC/MS	-	Axelson et al. (1974)
Cultured adrenal & testicular cells	Extract (dichloromethane); wash (sodium hydroxide)	HPLC	2 ng	O'Hare et al. (1976)
Cow's milk	Extract (diethyl ether); evaporate; dissolve (diethyl ether:70% methanol, 1:4); chill; centrifuge; CC (Sephadex); TLC (Sephadex)	GC/FID RIA	-	Nuti et al. (1975)

3. Biological Data Relevant to the Evaluation
of Carcinogenic Risk to Humans

3.1 Carcinogenicity studies in animals

(a) Subcutaneous and/or intramuscular administration

Mouse: Thirteen CBA mice [MTV$^+$][1], 4-6 months of age, received 10 mg progesterone in arachis oil subcutaneously weekly until death. Mice were ovariectomized at the same time as they were given an intrauterine implantation of 0.1 mg 3-methylcholanthrene (MCA). At 20-29 weeks, 2 sarcomas of the uterine horn were found in 4 mice; 2 sarcomas were found in 4 other mice that died at 40-49 weeks. In 30 controls that received only MCA, 5 adenocarcinomas, 2 squamous carcinomas and 1 sarcoma were observed (Kaslaris & Jull, 1962).

In female C3H mice [MTV$^+$], 9-10 weeks of age, given 2.5 mg progesterone in peanut oil subcutaneously 5 times weekly for 19 weeks, the incidence of mammary tumours increased from 6/24 in vehicle controls to 21/24, and the latent period was reduced from 70 to 55 weeks. Progesterone did not result in tumours in 27 MTV$^-$[1] C3HeB mice observed for 42 weeks. It decreased the latent period for the induction of mammary tumours by MCA from 38 to 26 weeks in MTV$^+$ mice and from 40 to 25 weeks in MTV$^-$ mice (Poel, 1969).

A group of 16 ovariectomized C3H mice received weekly intravaginal applications of a 1% solution of 7,12-dimethylbenz[a]anthracene (DMBA) together with twice-weekly i.m. injections of 0.2 mg progesterone. The incidence of squamous-cell carcinomas increased from 5/15 to 9/16; no change was observed in the incidence of 'mixed carcinomas' (3/8 to 4/16) (Glucksmann & Cherry, 1962).

Rat: In rats, s.c. or i.m. injections of 3-4 mg progesterone per day resulted in a decreased latent period and/or increased incidence of mammary tumours induced by single doses of 20-30 mg DMBA or multiple oral doses of 10 mg MCA, but only when injections were commenced *after* administration of the carcinogen (Huggins & Yang, 1962; Huggins *et al*., 1959; Jabara *et al*., 1973). In experiments in which progesterone was injected for varying periods *before* administration of a carcinogen, the resulting incidence of mammary tumours was diminished significantly, from 13/20 to 6/16 (Jull, 1966) and from 29/29 to 20/25 (Welsch *et al*., 1968). Similar results were obtained by Briziarelli (1966) and Jabara *et al*. (1973). Experiments in which progesterone was injected together

---

[1]MTV$^+$: mammary tumour virus expressed; MTV$^-$: mammary tumour virus not expressed (see p. 62)

with an oestrogen after dosage with DMBA are difficult to interpret due to the known inhibitory effects of oestrogens on mammary carcinogenesis (McCormick & Moon, 1973). It has been shown that oestrogen treatment of ovariectomized rats is not sufficient to restore susceptibility to mammary carcinogenesis by MCA; however, s.c. treatment with a combination of progesterone and oestrogen is a sufficient replacement for the ovaries (Sydnor & Cockrell, 1963). Cantarow et al. (1948) reported an increased incidence (from 17/57 to 22/26) of mammary tumours in female rats fed 300 mg/kg of diet 2-acetylaminofluorene and injected intramuscularly with 0.5 mg progesterone 3 times weekly for life.

S.c. injection of 0.3 mg progesterone to female hooded rats 3 times weekly for 21 weeks increased the latent period of induction of mammary tumours by oestrone from 37 to 50 weeks but did not change their incidence (Cutts, 1964).

In intact rats, i.m. injections of 1 mg progesterone twice weekly retarded by approximately 4 weeks the induction of sarcomas of the cervix and vagina produced by local application of 1% DMBA in acetone weekly for life; but the induction of papillomas was promoted by 19 weeks. Progesterone alone did not increase the effects of the carcinogen in ovariectomized animals; however, when given with oestrogen, the incidence but not the latent period of tumour induction was restored to that of intact females (Glucksmann & Cherry, 1968).

Twice-weekly s.c. injections of 3 mg progesterone in 0.1 ml corn oil for 28 weeks to 65-day-old female Sprague-Dawley rats reduced the age at onset of mammary tumours induced by 30 mg DMBA given intragastrically at 50 days of age (52 versus 115 days; P<0.01) and increased the number of tumours per rat (4.8 versus 2.3) when compared with controls. Mammary tumour incidence at 28 weeks was not affected (19/20 versus 16/20). Progesterone counteracted only partially the inhibition of mammary tumorigenesis induced by hypothyroidism (Jabara & Maritz, 1973).

Daily s.c. injections of 4 mg progesterone for 20 days before and 20 days after a single i.v. injection of 5 mg DMBA into 20 60-day-old female Sprague-Dawley rats resulted in a lowered incidence (from 100% to 20%) and almost complete inhibition of the growth of tumours for 4 months after the DMBA injection. No mammary tumours appeared in rats treated with progesterone in combination with oestradiol benzoate (5 µg/day) during the same period (Kledzik et al., 1974).

In A x C rats hysterectomized and ovariectomized at 6 weeks of age, administration of progesterone by weekly s.c. injections (2 mg) or s.c. implantation (20 mg), beginning at 8 weeks of age, did not affect the incidence of mammary tumours induced by simultaneous administration of diethylstilboestrol by 82 weeks of age (18/39 or 17/33 versus 21/38). Latent period, number and histological type of mammary tumours were also unaltered by progesterone treatment (Segaloff, 1974).

Rabbit: S.c. injection of 10 mg progesterone twice weekly into 32 rabbits in which vaginal strings containing MCA had been inserted did not affect the incidence of vaginal tumours occurring within 20 months: the incidences were 4/31 in treated animals and 5/23 in controls (Alvizouri & Ramírez de Pita, 1964).

Dog: Long-term s.c. injections of progesterone for a total of 74 weeks, increasing in dosage from 0.08 to 22.5 mg daily, caused endometrial hyperplasia, inhibition of ovarian development and marked mammary hyperplasia in female beagle dogs. No tumours were reported in animals killed 24 hours after the last dose, but fibroadenomatous nodules occurred in 2/5 dogs given the highest doses of progesterone (Capel-Edwards *et al.*, 1973).

In a study reported as an abstract, mammary nodules were observed in female beagle dogs following weekly i.m. injections of progesterone at levels 1 and 24 times the human contraceptive dose of medroxyprogesterone acetate (Coleman *et al.*, 1976) [The Working Group noted that the results were preliminary and that the duration of treatment was not specified].

(b) Subcutaneous implantation

Mouse: Pellets containing 14 mg progesterone were implanted subcutaneously every 28 days for 104 weeks into 59 female C3H x A hybrid mice [MTV+]. Mammary carcinomas were found at a significantly earlier age and in a higher incidence (52/59 at 70 weeks) than among 58 untreated control mice (36/58 at 93 weeks). No mammary tumours appeared among 27 intact or 24 castrated, untreated male controls or among 27 intact, progesterone-treated males; however, 2/26 castrated males given progesterone developed mammary tumours (Trentin, 1954).

Absorption of 29 μg per day or more of progesterone from pellets implanted subcutaneously was necessary to suppress corpus luteum formation in the ovaries of mice. After 18 months' treatment with 59-900 μg per day progesterone, ovarian granulosa-cell tumours were found in 27/83 BALB/c mice. Only 3 of these tumours exceeded 5 mm in diameter, most of them measuring less than 0.5 mm. One microscopic tumour occurred among 33 control mice killed after 18 months (Lipschütz *et al.*, 1967a).

Following the absorption from s.c. pellets of 18-900 μg per day progesterone, sarcomas of the endometrial stroma were observed in 15/142 mice after a period of 18 months. No tumours were found in 33 controls (Lipschütz *et al.*, 1967a,b).

A group of 20 female BALB/c mice treated subcutaneously with 5 mg pellets of a progesterone-cholesterol mixture, replaced every 3-4 months, for an average of 17 months developed no precancerous or cancerous lesions of the cervix and/or vagina. However, when 39 mice were treated with intravaginal inoculations of herpes-virus type 2 in addition to the progesterone pellets, 1 precancerous lesion and 1 squamous-cell carcinoma of the cervix were observed. No tumours of the cervix or vagina were found in 15 untreated control mice; 1 precancerous lesion and 2 carcinomas were found in 19 mice treated with herpes-virus type 2 alone (Muñoz, 1973).

After local applications of MCA in 50 C57BL6 mice, s.c. implantations of 15 mg progesterone every 3 weeks for 9 weeks resulted in an increased incidence of vaginal-cervical invasive squamous-cell carcinomas, from 6/50 with MCA alone to 45/50 (Reboud & Pageaut, 1973).

Rat: Groups of A x C rats received s.c. implants of 25 mg pellets containing 200 mg/kg bw progesterone and were fed 0.025% N-2-fluorenyl-diacetamide; other groups were treated with N-2-fluorenyldiacetamide only; all animals were observed for 40 weeks. The incidences of liver-cell carcinomas in animals that received both compounds *versus* those in animals that received N-2-fluorenyldiacetamide alone were 11/11 *versus* 7/12 in intact males, 5/13 *versus* 1/9 in castrated males, 4/12 *versus* 0/14 in ovariectomized females and 0/9 *versus* 1/10 in intact females (Reuber & Firminger, 1962).

Female A x C rats were treated with diethylstilboestrol (DES) and/or progesterone (20 mg implanted intrascapularly) plus irradiation. The development of mammary tumours was inhibited by progesterone: from 12/21 with DES plus irradiation to 1/21 with DES plus progesterone plus irradiation; the incidence was 0/11 with progesterone plus irradiation (Segaloff, 1973).

(c) Neonatal exposure

Mouse: The long-term effects in female mice of neonatal exposure to steroid hormones, including progesterone, on the genital tract and mammary glands have been reviewed by Bern *et al*. (1975, 1976) and Takasugi (1976).

Neonatal female BALB/cfC3H mice [MTV$^+$] were given daily s.c. injections of 100 µg per day progesterone in sesame oil, alone or in combination with 5 or 20 µg per day oestradiol-17β for the first 5 days after birth; lesions of the genital tract and mammary glands were checked until they were 12 months of age. Persistent vaginal cornification was seen in all of 32 mice treated with progesterone alone; simultaneous administration of oestradiol-17β reduced the occurrence of vaginal cornification significantly [P<0.01]. Three of the 32 animals that received progesterone showed lesions of vaginal or cervical epithelia. Simultaneous administration of progesterone with oestradiol reduced the incidence of such lesions compared with that resulting from oestradiol alone, but increased their severity. Mammary tumour incidence was enhanced by progesterone alone (23/32) or in combination with oestradiol (5 µg, 20/32; 20 µg, 33/44), when compared with controls (5/17). Age at onset of mammary tumours was also significantly lower in mice given progesterone (P<0.01). No cervico-vaginal lesions or mammary tumours occurred in mice exposed neonatally to progesterone when they were ovariectomized at 40 days of age (Jones & Bern, 1977).

Daily s.c. injections of 100 µg progesterone in 0.02 ml sesame oil for 5 days beginning within 36 hrs after birth induced genital tract lesions in 15/24 BALB/cCrgl female mice (MTV⁻) at about 1.5-2 yrs of age. No such lesions were observed in 10 oil-treated or in 25 untreated control animals. Some lesions were transplantable, showing squamous-cell and/or adenocarcinomatous features. No mammary tumours were observed either in control or in progesterone-treated intact mice; however, 17/24 treated mice each had an average of 10 hyperplastic alveolar-like nodules and other dysplasias; 35 control mice had no such lesions (Jones *et al.*, 1977).

Rat: Of 30 Sprague-Dawley female rats that received single s.c. injections of 1.25 mg progesterone in 0.05 ml sesame oil at 5 days of age and an i.g. instillation of 20 mg DMBA at 55 days, 23 developed mammary tumours by 190 days of age. This incidence was similar to that in controls given DMBA only (20/33); however, the total number of adenocarcinomas was higher in progesterone-treated rats than in controls (44 *versus* 27) (Shellabarger & Soo, 1973).

3.2 Other relevant biological data

The biological activities of the progestin compounds have been reviewed (Tausk & deVisser, 1972) (see also 'General Remarks on Sex Hormones', p. 44).

No data on the toxicity of progesterone were available.

Embryotoxicity and teratogenicity

Injection of 3.5 mg progesterone on day 15 of gestation into the amniotic sacs of mouse embryos induced 61% mortality, compared with 13% in vehicle-injected controls. When this dose was injected subcutaneously on days 15, 16 and 17 of gestation, 65% mortality occurred (Petrelli & Forbes, 1964).

S.c. injection of 5-200 mg progesterone per day into rats on days 15-20 of gestation caused no abnormalities of external or internal genitalia in offspring (Revesz et al., 1960).

S.c. administration of 2.5-10 mg progesterone/rat per day between days 14-19 of gestation had no apparent virilizing effect on offspring (Lerner et al., 1962).

Injection of 1 mg progesterone per day to rabbits on days 1-4 of gestation had no discernible effect on 6.5-day-old blastocysts (Adams et al., 1961).

Daily injections of 30 mg/kg bw progesterone into 10 rabbits from day 8-16 of gestation caused virilization of the foetuses (increase in anourethral distance in both sexes) and an excess of males (F:M = 1.78:2.07) (Piotrowski, 1969).

Injection of 0.5, 1.0 and 1.0 mg progesterone into rabbits 2 and 1 days before mating and on day of mating, respectively, led to embryonic deaths by day 4 of gestation (McCarthy et al., 1977).

Daily s.c. injections of 1 mg progesterone per animal to 7 female guinea-pigs, from day 18 after mating until day 60, induced no masculinization (Foote et al., 1968).

I.m. injection of 25 μg progesterone combined with 12.5 μg oestrone into 183 multiparous sows during early gestation (day 14-23) increased litter size significantly. Higher concentrations (50 mg progesterone and 25 μg oestrone) had neither toxic nor teratogenic effects on the offspring (Wildt et al., 1976).

Single oral doses of 1.3-1.8 g progesterone given to ewes on day 14 after mating were neither toxic nor teratogenic to the offspring (Keeler & Binns, 1968).

Daily i.m. injections of 50 mg progesterone to Macaca mulatta (rhesus) monkeys on 5 days/week, from day 24-28 of gestation until term, induced no change in duration of pregnancy and no anomalies in the offspring (Wharton & Scott, 1964).

Metabolism

The metabolism of progesterone, especially in humans, has been reviewed by Zagorskaya (1975) and by Aufrère & Benson (1976).

In humans, progesterone is converted by reduction, hydroxylation, side-chain cleavage and conjugation. Qualitative (Aufrère & Benson, 1976) and quantitative (Little et al., 1975) species differences have been observed. In humans, most progesterone is metabolized by reductases, the main product being pregnanediol (5β-pregnane-3α,20α-diol), excreted as the glucuronide. In chimpanzees, progesterone is metabolized similarly, and pregnanediol is the major excretion product (YoungLai *et al.*, 1975); however, some non-human primates, such as baboons and rhesus monkeys, excrete androsterone as the major urinary product, implying that in these species side-chain cleavage predominates (Aufrère & Benson, 1976; Ishihara *et al.*, 1975).

Some species excrete acidic progesterone metabolites, i.e., metabolites that arise from hydroxylation at C-21 and further oxidation to the C-21-carboxyl derivative in the urine (Senciall & Dey, 1976). Rabbits excrete the largest amounts of this type of metabolite, followed by guinea-pigs, pigs and rats. Only negligible amounts are found in human urine (Senciall *et al.*, 1976).

Extrahepatic metabolism of progesterone also occurs to an appreciable extent. In rats, for instance, submaxillary gland tissue has been shown to contain 5α-reductase, 20α-reductase and 17α-hydroxylase (Coffey, 1973). Circulating progesterone can be utilized by the adrenals for the production of corticosteroids like aldosterone and corticosterone, as demonstrated by Vecsei & Kessler (1971) in rats.

Mutagenicity and other short-term tests

After i.m. injections of 1-25 mg progesterone per animal to male dogs every other day for 6 weeks, and s.c. injections of 1-100 mg per animal to female Chinese hamsters thrice weekly for 4 weeks, chromosomal abnormalities (stickiness, clumping, condensation), aneuploidy and polyploidy were observed in meiotic germ cells (Williams *et al.*, 1968, 1971, 1972).

Treatment of cultures of human embryonic fibroblasts and of renal epithelia with 1 µg/ml progesterone resulted in a two-fold increase in the number of chromosomal aberrations (Serova & Kerkis, 1974).

No chromosomal effects were observed when 0.1-100 µg/ml progesterone were added to cultures of lymphocytes grown from the blood of healthy women (Stenchever *et al.*, 1969).

3.3 Case reports and epidemiological studies

No data were available to the Working Group.

4. Summary of Data Reported and Evaluation[1]

4.1 Experimental data

Progesterone was tested by subcutaneous and intramuscular injection in mice, rats, rabbits and dogs and by subcutaneous implantation in mice and rats. It was tested alone in mice and dogs; in rats and rabbits it was always given in combination with other sex hormones.

When given alone, progesterone increased the incidence of ovarian, uterine and mammary tumours in mice; the data from dogs were insufficient to evaluate carcinogenicity.

Neonatal treatment with progesterone enhanced the occurrence of precancerous and cancerous lesions of the genital tract and resulted in increased mammary tumorigenesis in female mice.

4.2 Human data

No case reports or epidemiological studies on exogenous progesterone were available to the Working Group.

4.3 Evaluation

There is *limited evidence* for the carcinogenicity of progesterone in experimental animals. In the absence of epidemiological data, no evaluation of the carcinogenicity of progesterone to humans can be made.

---

[1]This section should be read in conjunction with pp. 62-64 in the 'General Remarks on Sex Hormones' and with the 'General Conclusions on Sex Hormones', p. 131.

5. <u>References</u>

Abraham, G.E., Manlimos, F.S. & Garza, R. (1977) <u>Radioimmunoassay</u>
<u>of steroids</u>. In: Abraham, G.E., ed., <u>Handbook of Radioimmunoassay</u>,
New York, Marcel Dekker, pp. 591-656

Adams, C.E., Hay, M.F. & Lutwak-Mann, C. (1961) The action of various
agents upon the rabbit embryo. <u>J. Embryol. exp. Morphol</u>., <u>9</u>,
468-491

Alvizouri, M. & Ramiréz de Pita, V. (1964) Experimental carcinoma of the
cervix. Hormonal influences. <u>Am. J. Obstet. Gynecol</u>., <u>89</u>, 940-945

Aufrère, M.B. & Benson, H. (1976) Progesterone: an overview and recent
advances. <u>J. pharm. Sci</u>., <u>65</u>, 783-800

Axelson, M., Schumacher, G. & Sjovall, J. (1974) Analysis of tissue
steroids by liquid-gel chromatography and computerized gas
chromatography-mass spectrometry. <u>J. chromatogr. Sci</u>., <u>12</u>, 535-540

Baillie, T.A., Brooks, C.J.W., Chambaz, E.M., Glass, R.C. & Madani, C.
(1974) <u>Comparison of isopentyloxime and benzyloxime trimethylsilyl</u>
<u>ethers in the characterization of urinary steroids of newborn infants</u>.
In: Frigerio, A. & Castagnoli, N., eds, <u>Mass Spectrometry in</u>
<u>Biochemistry and Medicine</u>, New York, Raven Press, pp. 335-348

Batra, S. & Bengtsson, L.P. (1976) A highly efficient procedure for the
extraction of progesterone from uterus and its compatibility with
subsequent radioimmunoassay. <u>J. Steroid Biochem</u>., <u>7</u>, 599-603

Bern, H.A., Jones, L.A., Mori, T. & Young, P.N. (1975) Exposure of
neonatal mice to steroids: longterm effects on the mammary gland
and other reproductive structures. <u>J. Steroid Biochem</u>., <u>6</u>, 673-676

Bern, H.A., Jones, L.A., Mills, K.T., Kohrman, A. & Mori, T. (1976)
Use of the neonatal mouse in studying longterm effects of early
exposure to hormones and other agents. <u>J. Toxicol. environ. Health</u>,
Suppl. <u>1</u>, 103-116

Björkhem, I., Blomstrand, R. & Lantto, O. (1975) Validation of routine
methods for serum progesterone determination using mass fragmentography.
<u>Clin. chim. acta</u>, <u>65</u>, 343-350

Boit, H.-G., ed. (1969) <u>Beilsteins Handbuch der Organischen Chemie</u>,
4th ed., Vol. 7, Syst. No. 673/H709, Berlin, Springer, p. 3649

British Pharmacopoeia Commission (1973) British Pharmacopoeia, London, HMSO, pp. 390-391

Briziarelli, G. (1966) Effects of hormonal pre-treatment against the induction of mammary tumors by 7,12-dimethylbenz(a)anthracene in rats. Z. Krebsforsch., 68, 217-223

Cantarow, A., Stasney, J. & Paschkis, K.E. (1948) The influence of sex hormones on mammary tumors induced by 2-acetaminofluorene. Cancer Res., 8, 412-417

Capel-Edwards, K., Hall, D.E., Fellowes, K.P., Vallance, D.K., Davies, M.J., Lamb, D. & Robertson, W.B. (1973) Long-term administration of progesterone to the female beagle dog. Toxicol. appl. Pharmacol., 24, 474-488

Coffey, J.C. (1973) In vitro progesterone metabolism in rat submaxillary gland: the formation of 20α-hydroxy-4-pregnen-3-one and other substances. Steroids, 22, 561-566

Coleman, M.E., Murchison, T.E. & Frank, D. (1976) Mammary nodules in dogs receiving Depo-provera and progesterone: an interim progress report. Toxicol. appl. Pharmacol., 37, 181

Cutts, J.H. (1964) Estrone-induced mammary tumors in the rat. II. Effect of alterations in the hormonal environment on tumor induction, behaviour and growth. Cancer Res., 24, 1124-1130

Dehennin, L., Reiffsteck, A. & Schüller, R. (1974) Simultaneous estimation of testosterone, progesterone and androstenedione by gas chromatography-mass spectrometry with a single ion detection correlation with radioimmunoassay. J. Steroid Biochem., 5, 767-768

Dorfman, R.I. (1966) Hormones (sex). In: Kirk, R.E. & Othmer, D.F., eds, Encyclopedia of Chemical Technology, 2nd ed., Vol. II, New York, John Wiley & Sons, pp. 122-124

Fehér, T., Fehér, K.G. & Bodrogi, L. (1975) A simple gas-liquid chromatographic method with electron capture detection for the determination of progesterone in the blood of humans and domestic animals. J. Chromatogr., 111, 125-132

Foote, W.D., Foote, W.C. & Foote, L.H. (1968) Influence of certain natural and synthetic steroids in genital development in guinea-pigs. Fertil. Steril., 19, 606-615

Gajewska, M., Lugowska, E. & Tomaszewska, E. (1975) Application of lead picrate to the determination of steroid hormones in pharmaceutical preparations (Pol.). Chem. Anal. (Warsaw), 20, 615-620 [Chem. Abstr., 84, 22139p]

Glucksmann, A. & Cherry, C.P. (1962) The effect of castration and of additional hormonal treatments on the induction of cervical and vulval tumours in mice. Br. J. Cancer, 16, 634-652

Glucksmann, A. & Cherry, C.P. (1968) The effect of oestrogens, testosterone and progesterone on the induction of cervico-vaginal tumours in intact and castrate rats. Br. J. Cancer, 22, 545-562

Grasselli, J.G. & Ritchey, W.M., eds (1975) CRC Atlas of Spectral Data and Physical Constants for Organic Compounds, 2nd ed., Vol. III, Cleveland, OH, Chemical Rubber Co., p. 193

Harvey, S.C. (1975) Hormones. In: Osol, A. et al., eds, Remington's Pharmaceutical Sciences, 15th ed., Easton, PA, Mack, pp. 924-925

Hassan, S.S.M., Abdel Fattah, M.M. & Zaki, M.T.M. (1976) Spectrophotometric determination of some steroid sex-hormones. Fresenius' Z. anal. Chem., 281, 371-377

Hoffman, B., Hamburger, R., Rattenberger, E. & Karg, H. (1977) Progesterone in milk and milk products and in fatty tissue of cattle. J. Toxicol. environ. Health, 3, 355-357

Honda, M. (1976) The simultaneous assay of progesterone, 17-hydroxy-progesterone and deoxycorticosterone in human plasma by competitive protein binding. Endocrinol. Jpn., 23, 259-264

Huggins, C. & Yang, N.C. (1962) Induction and extinction of mammary cancer. Science, 137, 257-262

Huggins, C., Briziarelli, G. & Sutton, H., Jr (1959) Rapid induction of mammary carcinoma in the rat and the influence of hormones on the tumors. J. exp. Med., 109, 25-42

IARC (1974) IARC Monographs on the Evaluation of Carcinogenic Risk of Chemicals to Man, 6, Sex Hormones, Lyon, pp. 135-146

Ishihara, M., Osawa, Y., Kirdani, R.Y. & Sandberg, A.A. (1975) Progesterone metabolism in the baboon. J. Steroid Biochem., 6, 1213-1218

Jabara, A.G. & Maritz, J.S. (1973) Effects of hypothyroidism and progesterone on mammary tumours induced by 7,12-dimethylbenz(a)-anthracene in Sprague-Dawley rats. Br. J. Cancer, 28, 161-172

Jabara, A.G., Toyne, P.H. & Harcout, A.G. (1973) Effects of time and duration of progesterone administration on mammary tumours induced by 7,12-dimethylbenz(a)anthracene in Sprague-Dawley rats. Br. J. Cancer, 27, 63-71

Johansson, E.D.B. (1975) Determination of progesterone in plasma by
    competitive protein binding (Ger.). In: Breuer, H., Hamel, D. &
    Krueskemper, H.L., eds, Methoden Hormonbestimmung, Stuttgart, Thieme,
    pp. 213-218 [Chem. Abstr., 83, 160067u]

Jones, L.A. & Bern, H.A. (1977) Long-term effects of neonatal treatment
    with progesterone, alone or in combination with estrogen, on the
    mammary gland and reproductive tract of female BALB/cfC3H mice.
    Cancer Res., 37, 67-75

Jones, L.A., Bern, H.A. & Wong, L.M. (1977) Cervicovaginal and mammary
    gland abnormalities in old BALB/cCrgl mice treated neonatally with
    progesterone. J. Toxicol. environ. Health, 3, 360-361

Jull, J.W. (1966) The effect of infection, hormonal environment and
    genetic constitution on mammary tumor induction in rats by 7,12-
    dimethylbenz(a)anthracene. Cancer Res., 26, 2368-2373

Kaslaris, E. & Jull, J.W. (1962) The induction of tumours following the
    direct implantation of four chemical carcinogens into the uterus of
    mice and the effect of strain and hormones thereon. Br. J. Cancer,
    16, 479-483

Kastrup, E.K., ed. (1976) Facts and Comparisons, St Louis, MO, Facts &
    Comparisons Inc., pp. 108g

Kastrup, E.K., ed. (1978) Facts and Comparisons, St Louis, MO, Facts &
    Comparisons Inc., pp. 104b, 107, 107a

Keeler, R.F. & Binns, W. (1968) Teratogenic compounds of Veratrum
    californicum (Durand). V. Comparison of cyclopian effects of
    steroidal alkaloids from the plant and structurally related compounds
    from other sources. Teratology, 1, 5-10

Khayam-Bashi, H. & Boroumand, M. (1975) Spectrophotometric estimation of
    estradiol-17β, progesterone, and testosterone. Biochem. Med., 14, 104-108

King, R.H., Grady, L.T. & Reamer, J.T. (1974) Progesterone injection assay
    by liquid chromatography. J. pharm. Sci., 63, 1491-1596

Kledzik, G.S., Bradley, C.J. & Meites, J. (1974) Reduction of carcinogen-
    induced mammary cancer incidence in rats by early treatment with hormones
    or drugs. Cancer Res., 34, 2953-2956

Lerner, L.J., DePhillipo, M., Yiacas, E., Brennan, D. & Borman, A. (1962)
    Comparison of the acetophenone derivative of 16α,17-α-dihydroxy-
    progesterone with other progestational steroids for masculinization
    of the rat fetus. Endocrinology, 71, 448-451

Lipschütz, A., Iglesias, R., Panasevich, V.I. & Salinas, S. (1967a) Granulosa-cell tumours induced in mice by progesterone. Br. J. Cancer, 21, 144-152

Lipschütz, A., Iglesias, R., Panasevich, V.I. & Salinas, S. (1967b) Pathological changes induced in the uterus of mice with the prolonged administration of progesterone and 19-nor-contraceptives. Br. J. Cancer, 21, 160-165

Little, B., Billiar, R.B., Rahman, S.S., Johnson, W.A., Takaoka, Y. & White, R.J. (1975) In vivo aspects of progesterone distribution and metabolism. Am. J. Obstet. Gynecol., 123, 527-534

McCarthy, S.M., Foote, R.H. & Maurer, R.R. (1977) Embryo mortality and altered uterine luminal proteins in progesterone-treated rabbits. Fertil. Steril., 28, 101-107

McCormick, G.M. & Moon, R.C. (1973) Effect of increasing doses of estrogen and progesterone on mammary carcinogenesis in the rat. Eur. J. Cancer, 9, 483-486

Muñoz, N. (1973) Effect of herpesvirus type 2 and hormonal imbalance on the uterine cervix of the mouse. Cancer Res., 33, 1504-1508

Murad, F. & Gilman, A.G. (1975) Estrogens and progestins. In: Goodman, L.S. & Gilman, A., eds, The Pharmacological Basis of Therapeutics, 5th ed., New York, Macmillan, p. 1436

Nuti, L.C., Wentworth, B.C., Karavolas, H.J., Tyler, W.J. & Ginther, O.J. (1975) Comparison of radioimmunoassay and gas-liquid chromatography analyses of progesterone concentrations in cow's milk. Proc. Soc. exp. Biol. (N.Y.), 149, 877-880

O'Hare, M.J., Nice, E.C., Magee-Brown, R. & Bullman, H. (1976) High-pressure liquid chromatography of steroids secreted by human adrenal and testis cells in monolayer culture. J. Chromatogr., 125, 357-367

Petrelli, E.A. & Forbes, T.R. (1964) Toxicity of progesterone to mouse fetuses. Endocrinology, 75, 145-146

Piotrowski, J. (1969) Experimental studies on the effect of some steroid hormones on the development of the rabbit fetus. II. (Pol.). Przegl. Lek., 25, 322-324

Poel, W.E. (1969) Bioassays with inbred mice: their relevance for the random-bred animal. Prog. exp. Tumor Res., 11, 440-460

Poteczin, E., Fehér, T., Kiss, C. & Györy, G. (1975) Gas chromatographic
    determination of unconjugated dehydroepiandrosterone, androstenedione,
    testosterone, pregnenolone and progesterone in human ovarian tissues.
    Endokrinologie, 64, 151-158

Reboud, S. & Pageaut, G. (1973) Co-carcinogenic effect of progesterone
    on 20-methylcholanthrene-induced cervical carcinoma in mice. Nature,
    241, 398-399

Reuber, M.D. & Firminger, H.I. (1962) Effect of progesterone and
    diethylstilbestrol on hepatic carcinogenesis and cirrhosis in AxC
    rats fed N-2-fluorenyldiacetamide. J. natl Cancer Inst., 29, 933-
    943

Revesz, C., Chappel, C.I. & Gaudry, R. (1960) Masculinization of female
    fetuses in the rat by progestational compounds. Endocrinology, 66,
    140-144

Scott, J.Z., Stanczyk, F.Z., Goebelsmann, U. & Mishell, D.R., Jr (1978)
    A double-antibody radioimmunoassay for serum progesterone using
    progesterone-3-(O-carboxymethyl)oximino[^{125}I]-iodohistamine as radio-
    ligand. Steroids, 31, 393-405

Segaloff, A. (1973) Inhibition by progesterone of radiation-estrogen
    induced mammary cancer in the rat. Cancer Res., 33, 1136-1137

Segaloff, A. (1974) The role of the ovary in estrogen production of
    mammary cancer in the rat. Cancer Res., 34, 2708-2710

Senciall, I.R. & Dey, A.C. (1976) Acidic steroid metabolites: evidence
    for the excretion of C-21-carboxylic acid metabolites of progesterone
    in rabbit urine. J. Steroid Biochem., 7, 125-129

Senciall, I.R., Harding, C.A. & Dey, A.C.((1976) Acidic steroid
    metabolites: species differences in the urinary excretion of acidic
    metabolites of progesterone. J. Endocrinol., 68, 169-170

Serova, I.A. & Kerkis, Y.J. (1974) Cytogenetic effect of some steroid
    hormones and change in activity of lysosomal enzymes in vitro (Russ.).
    Genetica, 10, 142-149

Shellabarger, C.J. & Soo, V.A. (1973) Effects of neonatally administered
    sex steroids on 7,12-dimethylbenz(a)anthracene-induced mammary
    neoplasia in rats. Cancer Res., 33, 1567-1569

Shutt, D.A., Shearman, R.P., Lyneham, R.C., Clarke, A.H., McMahon, G.R.
    & Goh, P. (1975) Radioimmunoassay of progesterone, 17-hydroxy-
    progesterone, estradiol-17β and prostaglandin F in human corpus
    luteum. Steroids, 26, 299-310

Sippell, W.G., Bidlingmaier, F., Becker, H., Brünig, T., Dürr, H., Hahn, H., Golder, W., Hollmann, G. & Knorr, D. (1978) Simultaneous radio-immunoassay of plasma aldosterone, corticosterone, 11-deoxycorticosterone, progesterone, 17-hydroxyprogesterone, 11-deoxycortisol, cortisol and cortisone. J. Steroid Biochem., 9, 63-74

Snedden, W. & Parker, R.B. (1976) The direct determination of estrogen and progesterone in human ovarian tissue by quantitative high resolution mass spectrometry. Biomed. Mass Spectrom., 3, 295-298

Stenchever, M.A., Jarvis, J.A. & Kreger, N.K. (1969) Effect of selected estrogens and progestins on human chromosomes in vitro. Obstet. Gynecol., 34, 249-251

Sydnor, K.L. & Cockrell, B. (1963) Influence of estradiol-17β, progesterone and hydrocortisone on 3-methylcholanthrene-induced mammary cancer in intact and ovariectomized Sprague-Dawley rats. Endocrinology, 73, 427-432

Takasugi, N. (1976) Cytological basis for permanent vaginal changes in mice treated neonatally with steroid hormones. Int. Rev. Cytol., 44, 193-224

Tausk, M. & deVisser, J. (1972) International Encyclopedia of Pharmacology and Therapeutics, Vol. II, section 48, Elmsford, NY, Pergamon Press, pp. 35-194

Trentin, J.J. (1954) Effect of long-term treatment with high levels of progesterone on the incidence of mammary tumors in mice. Proc. Am. Assoc. Cancer Res., 1, 50

US Food & Drug Administration (1977) Food and drugs. US Code Fed. Regul., Title 21, part 556.540, p. 364

US International Trade Commission (1977a) Synthetic Organic Chemicals, US Production and Sales, 1975, USITC Publication 804, Washington DC, US Government Printing Office, pp. 90, 102

US International Trade Commission (1977b) Synthetic Organic Chemicals, US Production and Sales, 1976, USITC Publication 833, Washington DC, US Government Printing Office, p. 149

US Pharmacopeial Convention Inc. (1975) The US Pharmacopeia, 19th rev., Rockville, MD, pp. 414-416

US Tariff Commission (1940) Synthetic Organic Chemicals, US Production and Sales, 1939, Report No. 140, Second Series, Washington DC, US Government Printing Office, p. 38

Van der Molen, H.J. & De Jong, F.H. (1975) Gas chromatographic determination of progesterone in plasma (Ger.). In: Breuer, H., Hamel, D. & Krueskemper, H.L., eds, Methoden Hormonbestimmung, Stuttgart, Thieme, pp. 219-229 [Chem. Abstr., 83, 160139u]

Vecsei, P. & Kessler, H. (1971) *In vivo* conversion of radioactive progesterone and corticosterone to adrenal cortical hormones in normal and ACTH-treated rats. Acta endocrinol., 68, 759-770

Wade, A., ed. (1977) Martindale, The Extra Pharmacopoeia, 27th ed., London, The Pharmaceutical Press, pp. 1422-1424

Weast, R.C., ed. (1977) CRC Handbook of Chemistry and Physics, 58th ed., Cleveland, OH, Chemical Rubber Co., p. C-444

Weiler, E.W. & Zenk, M.H. (1976) Radioimmunoassay for the determination of digoxin and related compounds in *Digitalis lanata*. Phytochemistry, 15, 1537-1545

Weiss, P.A.M. (1973) Progesterone determination in plasma from pregnant women by chromatogram-spectrophotometry (Ger.). Endokrinologie, 61, 1-8

Welsch, C.W., Clemens, J.A. & Meites, J. (1968) Effects of multiple pituitary homografts or progesterone on 7,12-dimethylbenz(a)anthracene-induced mammary tumors in rats. J. natl Cancer Inst., 41, 465-471

Wharton, L.R., Jr & Scott, R.B. (1964) Experimental production of genital lesions with norethindrone. Am. J. Obstet. Gynecol., 89, 701-715

Wildt, D.E., Culver, A.A., Morcom, C.B. & Dukelow, W.R. (1976) Effect of administration of progesterone and oestrogen on litter size in pigs. J. Reprod. Fertil., 48, 209-211

Williams, D.L., Runyan, J.W. & Hagen, A.A. (1968) Meiotic chromosome alterations produced by progesterone. Nature, 220, 1145-1147

Williams, D.L., Hagen, A.A. & Runyan, J.W., Jr (1971) Chromosome alterations produced in germ cells of dogs by progesterone. J. lab. clin. Med., 77, 417-429

Williams, D.L., Runyan, J.W., Jr & Hagen, A.A. (1972) Progesterone-induced alterations of oogenesis in the Chinese hamsters. J. lab. clin. Med., 79, 972-977

Windholz, M., ed. (1976) The Merck Index, 9th ed., Rahway, NJ, Merck
    & Co., p. 1007

YoungLai, E.V., Graham, C.E. & Collins, D.C. (1975) Metabolism of
    4-^{14}C-progesterone in the adult female chimpanzee. Steroids, 25,
    465-476

Zagorskaya, E.A. (1975) Metabolism of progesterone (Russ.). Probl.
    Endocrinol. (Moscow), 21, 102-110

ANDROGENS

TESTOSTERONE, TESTOSTERONE OENANTHATE and TESTOSTERONE PROPIONATE

A monograph on testosterone was published previously (IARC, 1974).
Relevant data that have appeared since that time have been evaluated in
the present monograph.

1. Chemical and Physical Data

Testosterone

1.1 Synonyms and trade names

Chem. Abstr. Services Reg. No.: 58-22-0

Chem. Abstr. Name: (17β)-17-Hydroxyandrost-4-en-3-one

Synonym: Δ^4-Androsten-17β-ol-3-one

Trade names[1]: [Ablacton]; Andrestraq; [Androfort]; Android-T;
Androlan; Androlin; Andronaq; [Andronoq]; [Androtest];
Andrusol; [Anertan]; [Aquaviron]; [Climanosid]; [Climaterine];
[Clivion]; [Combidurin]; Cormone; Cristerona T; [Cycladiene];
[Cycladiene M. Test.]; Depotest; Di-Met; Dura-Testrone;
[Estandron]; [Estandron-Prolong.]; [Foliteston]; [Foliteston
Retard]; Géno-cristaux Gremy; [Gineserpina]; [Heptylate de Test.];
Histerone; Homogene S; Homosteron; Homosterone; [Hormoduvadilan];
Hydrotest; [Klimanosid R]; [Lutestex]; Malestrone;
Mal-O-Fem; Malogen; Mertestate; Nendron; Neo-Hombreol; Neo-
Hombreol-F; Neotestis; Oreton; Oreton-F; Orquisteron;
Perandren; Percutacrine Androgénique; [Primodian D]; [Primodian
Depot]; Primotest; Primoteston; Rektandron; [Sterandryl];
Sterotate; Sustanon; Sustanone; [Synandrol]; Synandrol F;
Tesamone; Teslen; Tesone; Test 100; Testa denos; Testagen;

---

[1]Those in square brackets are preparations that are no longer
produced commercially.

Testalong; Testandrone; Testaqua; Test-Estrin; [Test.-Folliculline]; Testiculosterone; Testobase; Testodrin; [Test.-Oestr. R]; [Testo Folicular]; Testoject-50; Testolent; Testolin; [Testo Luteinica]; [Testoluton]; Testopropon; Testoral; [Testosid]; Testosteroid; Testosteron; [Testosterona]; Testoviron; [Testoviron Prog.]; Testoviron Schering; Testoviron T; Testro-Med; Testrone; Testryl; [Trioestrine]; [Trioestrine R]; [Trioestrine Vitam.]; Virormone; Virosterone

1.2 Structural and molecular formulae and molecular weight

$C_{19}H_{28}O_2$ Mol. wt: 288.4

1.3 Chemical and physical properties of the pure substance

From Wade (1977) and Windholz (1976), unless otherwise specified

(a) Description: White needles (from dilute acetone)

(b) Melting-point: 155°C

(c) Spectroscopy data: λ_{max} 283 nm; infra-red, nuclear magnetic resonance and mass spectral data have been tabulated (Grasselli & Ritchey, 1975).

(d) Optical rotation: $[\alpha]_D^{24}$ +109° (4% w/v in ethanol)

(e) Solubility: Practically insoluble in water; soluble in ethanol (1 in 5), chloroform (1 in 2), diethyl ether (1 in 100) and ethyl oleate (1 in 150); also soluble in acetone, dioxane and fixed oils

(f) Stability: Easily oxidized

1.4 Technical products and impurities

Various national and international pharmacopoeias give specifications for the purity of testosterone in pharmaceutical products. For example, testosterone is available in the US as a NF grade containing 97–103% active ingredient on a dried basis and not more than 3% foreign steroids and other impurities. Pellets in 75 mg doses contain 97–103% of the stated amount of testosterone, and sterile aqueous suspensions in 250 and 500 mg in 10 ml doses contain 90–110% of the stated amount (National Formulary Board, 1975). Testosterone is also available in the US in aqueous suspensions in 100 mg/ml doses and in combination (10 and 25 mg/ml) with oestrone (2 mg) or oestradiol (1 mg) (Kastrup, 1977).

In the UK, testosterone is **available** in implants in 25, 50, 100 and 200 mg doses and in sublingual tablets containing 10 mg in an inert, water-soluble, wax base (Wade, 1977).

In Japan, tablets containing 1 mg testosterone, 3 mg oestrogens and 7.5 mg thyroid hormones are available, as well as injections containing 4.76–23.8 mg testosterone and 0.24–1.2 mg oestradiol.

Testosterone oenanthate

1.1. Synonyms and trade names

Chem. Abstr. Services Reg. No.: 315-37-7

Chem. Abstr. Name: (17β)-17-[(1-Oxoheptyl)oxy]-androst-4-en-3-one

Synonyms: Testosterone enanthate; testosterone heptanoate; testosterone heptylate

Trade names: Androtardyl; Delatestryl; Orquisteron-E; Reposo-TMD; Testoenant

1.2 Structural and molecular formulae and molecular weight

$C_{26}H_{40}O_3$ Mol. wt: 400.6

1.3 Chemical and physical properties

    From Wade (1977) and Windholz (1976)

    (a) Description: Crystals

    (b) Melting-point: 36-37.5°C

    (c) Solubility: Practically insoluble in water; soluble in
         ethanol (1 in 0.3) and acetone (1 in 0.2); also soluble
         in chloroform, diethyl ether and fixed oils

1.4 Technical products and impurities

    Various national and international pharmacopoeias give specifications
for the purity of testosterone oenanthate in pharmaceutical products.
For example, it is available in the US as a USP grade containing
97-103% active ingredient. It is available as injections in doses of
100 and 200 mg in 1 ml, 0.5 and 1 g in 5 ml and 1 and 2 g in 10 ml
of a suitable vegetable oil containing 90-110% of the labelled amount
(Harvey, 1975; US Pharmacopoeial Convention Inc., 1975).

Testosterone propionate

1.1 Synonyms and trade names

    Chem. Abstr. Services Reg. No.: 57-85-2

    Chem. Abstr. Name: (17β)-17-(1-Oxopropoxy)-androst-4-en-3-one

    Synonyms: Δ^4-Androstene-17β-propionate-3-one; testosterone-17β-
propionate; testosterone-17-propionate; testosteron propionate

    Trade names: Agovirin; Androlon; Androsan; Androtest P;
Androteston; Anertan; Aguaviron; Bio-Testiculina; Enarmon;
Enarmon-oil; Homandren; Hormoteston; Malogen; Masenate;
Nasdol; Neo-Hombreol; NSC 9166; Okasa-Mascul; Orchiol;
Orchisteron P; Orchisterone P; Orchistin; Oreton; Oreton
Propionate; Pantestin; Paretest; Perandren; Propiokan;
Recthormone Testosterone; Solvotest; Stérandryl; Synerone;
Telipex; Testaform; Testex; Testine; Testodet; Testodrin;
Testogen; Testolets; Testonique; Testormol; Testosid;
Testoviron; Testoxyl; Testrex; Tostrin; TP; Uniteston

1.2 Structural and molecular formulae and molecular weight

$$C_{22}H_{32}O_3$$ Mol. wt: 344.5

1.3 Chemical and physical properties

From Wade (1977) and Windholz (1976)

(a) Description: Prisms (from ethanol and water)

(b) Melting-point: 118-122°C

(c) Optical rotation: $[\alpha]_D^{25}$ +83° to +90° (100 mg in 10 ml dioxane)

(d) Solubility: Practically insoluble in water; soluble in ethanol
     (1 in 6), acetone (1 in 4), arachis oil (1 in 35), ethyl
     oleate (1 in 20) and propylene glycol (1 in 30); also
     soluble in chloroform, dioxane, diethyl ether, fixed oils
     and methanol

1.4 Technical products and impurities

Testosterone propionate is available in the US as a USP grade
containing 97-103% active ingredient on a dried basis. It is available
as injections containing 10, 25, 50 and 100 mg per ml and as 100 mg, 250
mg, 500 mg and 1 g per 10 ml of solvent containing 88-112% of the stated
amount (Harvey, 1975; US Pharmacopeial Convention Inc., 1975).

2. Production, Use, Occurrence and Analysis

2.1 Production and use

(a) Production

Testosterone was first obtained in crystalline form in 1935 by David, who isolated it from bull testes. The first chemical synthesis of testosterone was reported by Butenandt and Hanisch in 1935, by heating 17β-acetoxyandrost-4-en-3-one (Boit, 1969). Testosterone can be prepared commercially from cholesterol or diosgenin (extracted from the Mexican yam, *Dioscorea mexicana*), by degradation to the key intermediate, dehydroepiandrosterone, which can be converted to testosterone by chemical (Oppenauer oxidation) or microbiological processes (Anon., 1977; Harvey, 1975). Recently, a new synthesis route has been reported to be in use, involving the removal of the saturated side chains from sitosterol using fermentation and subsequent build-up of the desired substituents (Anon., 1978).

Preparation of testosterone oenanthate was first described by Alter (1958). It can be prepared by the reaction of testosterone and oenanthic acid (Harvey, 1975). Testosterone propionate can be prepared by the reaction of testosterone with a propionyl halide, propionic acid, a propionic ester or propionic anhydride (Anon., 1939).

Commercial production of testosterone in the US was first reported in 1939 (US Tariff Commission, 1940) and was last reported in 1963 (US Tariff Commission, 1964). Data on US imports and exports of testosterone and its esters are not available.

No evidence was found that testosterone oenanthate has ever been produced commercially in the US. Commercial production of testosterone propionate in the US was first reported in 1937 (US Tariff Commission, 1938) and was last reported in 1960 (US Tariff Commission, 1961).

Testosterone and its esters are produced commercially in France, Italy, The Netherlands and the UK, but no information was available on the quantities produced.

Testosterone was first marketed commercially in Japan in 1953. It is not produced there, and imports amounted to 11-12 kg annually in 1975-1977.

(b) Use

Testosterone (the most active of the natural androgens) is used in human medicine for the treatment of a variety of conditions in both men and women. In men, it is used for the treatment of hypogonadism and eunuchoidism, for so-called 'male menopause' symptoms and for impotence due to androgen deficiency, in an i.m. dose of 25 mg 2-3 times per week, or (for hypogonadism) in a s.c. implant of 450 mg every 4-6 months.   In women, it is used for the treatment of metastatic breast cancer, in an i.m. dose of 25 mg 3 times per week for low-grade malignancies and up to 1 g per week for high-grade malignancies.   It has also been used for treatment of post-partum breast engorgement, in an i.m. dose of 50-100 mg 36-72 hrs after delivery.   It is also used for moderate to severe vasomotor symptoms of the climacteric, in an i.m. dose of 10-25 mg 1 or 2 times per week (Harvey, 1975;   Wade, 1977).

Testosterone has been used in the treatment of dysmenorrhoea and premenstrual tension, dysfunctional uterine bleeding, endometriosis, frigidity, for anabolic effects, hypopituitarism and Addison's disease (Harvey, 1975).

It is used in veterinary medicine, administered as an i.m. dose of 10-25 mg for dogs and 50-125 mg for horses (Harvey, 1975).

Testosterone oenanthate is used in human medicine for the treatment of the same conditions as testosterone.   It is administered intramuscularly as a solution in oil for slow release (the effect of a single i.m. injection may last 3 to 4 weeks).   It is used in the treatment of male hypogonadism, metastatic breast cancer in women, as an anabolic agent and in osteoporosis, in doses of 100 to 400 mg every 2-4 weeks (Harvey, 1975;   Murad & Gilman, 1975).

Testosterone propionate is used in human medicine for the treatment of the same conditions as testosterone.   Its initial action is faster than that of testosterone, but its duration of action is somewhat shorter. It is given intramuscularly for different male hypogonadal states at levels of 10-25 mg per day 2-4 times a week or orally at a dose of 5-20 mg per day;   for anabolic effects it is given intramuscularly at levels of 5-10 mg per day;   and to prevent post-partum breast engorgement it is given intramuscularly at levels of 25-50 mg per day for 3-4 days starting at delivery or orally at a dose of 40 mg per day in divided doses for 3-5 days.   It is given for metastatic breast cancer in women in i.m. doses of 50-100 mg 3 times a week or orally at a dose of 200 mg per day for as long as improvement is obtained (Harvey, 1975;   Murad & Gilman, 1975).

Testosterone propionate has been used in hormonal skin care preparations for cosmetic use at levels of less than 0.1%.   It has been used in veterinary medicine in horses, cattle, sheep and dogs for androgenic hormone deficiency (Harvey, 1975).

In Japan, testosterone is used in the treatment of so-called 'male menopause' symptoms. Testosterone oenanthate and propionate are also used for this and other purposes, such as Klinefelter's syndrome, dysmenorrhoea and control of lactation.

Less than 1000 kg of testosterone are used in France annually.

The US Food & Drug Administration (1977) requires that no residues of testosterone should be found in the uncooked edible tissues of beef cattle.

2.2 Occurrence

Testosterone is a widely occurring natural androgen (see 'General Remarks on Sex Hormones', pp. 42-56).

2.3 Analysis

Analytical methods for determining testosterone in biological samples, based on gas chromatography (Sommerville & Collins, 1975), gas chromatography-mass spectrometry (Björkhem et al., 1976), radioimmunoassay (Abraham et al., 1977) and competitive protein binding (Serio et al., 1973) have been reviewed.

Typical analytical methods are summarized in Table 1. Abbreviations used are: GC, gas chromatography; GC/ECD, gas chromatography/electron-capture detection; GC/FID, gas chromatography/flame-ionization detection; GC/MS, gas chromatography/mass spectrometry; TLC, thin-layer chromatography; HPLC, high-pressure liquid chromatography; CC-column chromatography; ORD, optical rotatory dispersion; UV, ultra-violet spectrometry; FL, fluorimetry; RIA, radioimmunoassay; and CPD, competitive protein binding. See also 'General Remarks on Sex Hormones', p. 60.

TABLE 1

Analytical methods for testosterone

Sample matrix	Sample preparation	Assay procedure	Sensitivity or limit of detection	Reference
Bulk chemical	Dissolve (ethanol)	UV (240 nm)	-	British Pharmacopoeia Commission (1973)
Bulk chemical	Dissolve	HPLC	-	Hara & Hayashi (1977)
Bulk chemical	Dissolve	ORD (250 nm)	15 μg/ml	Hassan (1974)
Bulk chemical	Dissolve (ethanol); evaporate; dissolve (98 sulphuric acid); let stand 2 hrs	UV (470 nm)	2 μg/ml	Hassan et al. (1976)
Bulk chemical	Dissolve (methanol containing aluminium perchlorate); derivatize (isonicotinic acide hydrazide)	FL (495 nm)	0.25 nmol	Horikawa et al. (1978)
Bulk chemical	Dissolve (ethanol)	UV (240 nm)	1.25 μg/ml	Khayam-Bashi & Boroumand (1975)
Bulk chemical	Dissolve	HPLC	5 μg	Satyaswaroop et al. (1977)
Suspension	Dissolve (ethanol)	Polarography	-	Chatten et al. (1976)
Suspension	Dissolve (50% ethanol); acidify (sulphuric acid); extract (chloroform); derivatize (isonicotinic acid (hydrazide)	UV (397 nm)	-	Myrick et al. (1972)
Plasma	Derivatize (heptafluoro-butyrate); TLC	GC/ECD	10 pg	Castellanos Llorens & Aranda Baro (1974)

Table 1 (continued)

Sample matrix	Sample preparation	Assay procedure	Sensitivity or limit of detection	Reference
Plasma	Extract (diethyl ether); derivatize (heptafluoro-butyrate)	GC/MS	0.21 ng/ml	Dehennin et al. (1974
Plasma	Extract (dichloromethane); wash (sodium hydroxide); CC (silica gel)	FL	10 ng (5 ml sample)	Eechaute et al. (1972
Plasma	Add labelled testosterone; extract (diethyl ether); CC (Lipidex 5000); add anti-serum	RIA	120 ng/l (0.1 ml sample)	Goldzieher et al. (1978)
Plasma	Extract (ethyl acetate); TLC	CPB	0.5 ng	Joshi et al. (1974)
Plasma	Extract (dichloromethane-ethyl acetate); wash (sodium hy-droxide); TLC	FL	5 ng (2-3 ml sample)	Obst (1972)
Plasma	Add labelled testosterone; extract (diethyl ether); de-rivatize (heptafluorobutyrate); TLC	GC	6 ng (100 ml sample)	Vermeulen (1975)
Avian plasma	Add labelled testosterone; dilute (water); extract (dichloromethane); CC (Celite); add antiserum	RIA	15.6 pg	Wingfield & Farner (1975)
Serum and urine	Adjust to pH 1 (sulphuric acid); saturate (with solid ammonium sulphate); extract (diethyl ether:methanol, 3:1); evaporate; TLC; dissolve (buffer); hydrolyse (sul-phuric acid, 20 hrs, 40°C); extract (diethyl ether); add antiserum	RIA	—	Puah et al (1978)

Table 1 (continued)

Sample matrix	Sample preparation	Assay procedure	Sensitivity or limit of detection	Reference
Urine	Adjust to pH 5 (acetic acid); add labelled testosterone; hydrolyse (enzyme); extract (dichloromethane); wash (sodium carbonate, water); evaporate; derivatize (Girard T reagent); adjust to pH 6.5 (sodium hydroxide); wash (diethyl ether); hydrolyse (hydrochloric acid); extract (diethyl ether); chromatograph (paper); TLC	GC/FID	0.02 µg	Charransol et al. (1972)
Urine	Adjust to pH 5; hydrolyse (enzyme); extract (chloroform); wash (sodium hydroxide & hydrochloric acid)	TLC	5 ng	Egg & Huck (1971)
Urine	Extract; TLC; derivatize (trimethylsilyl); spot on alumina plate; heat (170-180°)	FL (466 nm)	–	Huck (1975)
Urine	Add labelled testosterone; extract (diethyl ether); TLC; add antiserum	RIA	10 pg	Kjeld et al. (1977)
Urine	TLC; oxidize (chromium (III) oxide); derivatize (2,4-dinitro-phenylhydrazone); TLC	Colorimetry	0.5 µg	Korneev (1973)
Amniotic fluid	Add labelled testosterone; precipitate (ammonium sulphate); dissolve (water); extract (hexane:ethyl acetate, 9:1); evaporate; add antiserum	RIA	–	Pirani et al. (1977); Wong et al. (1975)

Table 1 (continued)

Sample matrix	Sample preparation	Assay procedure	Sensitivity or limit of detection	Reference
Breast tumour tissue	Homogenize (acetone); decant; evaporate; dissolve (80% aqueous methanol); wash (petroleum ether); evaporate dissolve (diethyl ether); wash (water); evaporate; derivatize (trimethylsilyl)	GC/MS	30 ng (1 μl sample)	Millington et al. (1974)
Ovarian tissue	Homogenize (sodium hydroxide); extract (diethyl ether-ethyl acetate-ethanol); wash (sodium hydroxide)	GC/FID	25 ng	Poteczin et al. (1976)
Prostate tissue	Add labelled testosterone; adsorb (silica gel); wash (hexane); elute (ethyl acetate); TLC; add antiserum	RIA	10 pg	Albert et al. (1976)
Cultured adrenal & testicular cells	Extract (dichloromethane); wash (sodium hydroxide)	HPLC	2 ng	O'Hare et al (1976)

3. Biological Data Relevant to the Evaluation

of Carcinogenic Risk to Humans

3.1 Carcinogenicity studies in animals

(a) Subcutaneous and/or intramuscular administration

Mouse: S.c. injection of 0.25-1.25 mg testosterone propionate in
sesame oil weekly for life or for 25 weeks resulted in the absence of
hepatomas in 24 male C3H mice (MTV[+])[1]. The incidence in 16 untreated
non-breeding males of this strain was 6% (Schenken & Burns, 1943).

A reduced incidence of mammary tumours (3/12) was found after 20
months in virgin female C3H mice injected subcutaneously with 1.0-1.5 mg
testosterone propionate in olive oil weekly, compared with 18/38 in
controls after 12 months (Jones, 1941). S.c. injection of testosterone
propionate in doses ranging from 0.625-2.5 µg weekly reduced the incidence
of mammary cancers in 88 male and 92 female C3H mice also given 3.3-33.3
µg oestradiol benzoate weekly. A total of 17 mice developed mammary
tumours, with an average latent period of 61 weeks, compared with 51/118
given the oestrogen alone with an average latent period of 45 weeks
(Gardner, 1946).

Hamster: Kirkman (1957) summarized the characteristics of three
types of tumours (numbers not given) induced in Syrian hamsters by a
combined treatment with s.c. injection or s.c. implantation of oestrogen
plus testosterone. One of three tumour types arose from the uterine
endometrium, the second from the vas deferens-epididymis, and the third
type was a basal-cell epithelioma arising in the flank. All these
tumours retained a dependence for growth on a combination of oestrogen
with testosterone. The first two tumour types do not occur in untreated
hamsters.

Rabbit: I.m. injection of 15 mg testosterone oenanthate in sesame
oil to random-bred female rabbits on alternate weeks produced 2 adenomatous
polyps of the endometrium at 763 days in 1/21 animals. No significant
alterations were seen in other tissues, including ovary, adrenal, thyroid
and pituitary gland (Meissner & Sommers, 1966).

---

[1]MTV[+]: mammary tumour virus expressed (see p. 62)

(b) Subcutaneous implantation

Mouse: The incidence of leukaemia in 36 ovariectomized female
Rockefeller Institute Leukemia mice implanted with 3 mg pellets of
testosterone propionate and observed up to 55 weeks was 21/36 compared
with 22 in 26 untreated, intact females and 28 in 31 untreated,
ovariectomized females (Murphy, 1944).

Cervical-uterine tumours were found in 26/42 (C57BL x dba)F1 mice
implanted with 1-2 mg pellets of testosterone propionate twice weekly
for lifespan. The tumours were infiltrating and metastasized to the
lungs in 10 mice (van Nie *et al*., 1961).

Rat: Nb strain male rats received s.c. implants of 1-3 10 mg
pellets containing testosterone propionate:cholesterol in a ratio of
9:1. The pellets were replaced at 6-8-week intervals for as long as 91
weeks. Only rats treated for 6 months or more and in which pellets were
replaced at least 4 times were included in the data. Incidences of
prostatic carcinoma were 0/13, 5/30 and 11/55 in rats receiving 1, 2
and 3 pellets, respectively. The incidence in untreated rats of this
strain is 0.48% (2/409). The ages at onset of tumours were 48-78 and
37-89 weeks in rats treated with 2 and 3 pellets, respectively. Although
simultaneous implantation of an oestrone:cholesterol pellet altered the
incidence only slightly (8/45), it shortened the age at onset (40-60
weeks). The incidences of metastases were 2/5, 4/11 and 4/8 in rats
receiving 2 pellets, 3 pellets and 3 pellets plus oestrogen, respectively
(Noble, 1977).

The incidence of urinary bladder tumours in female Wistar rats
given 0.05% N-butyl-N-(4-hydroxybutyl)nitrosamine in drinking-water for
6 weeks was not altered by ovariectomy, when compared with controls,
during 24 weeks of observation (3/10 *versus* 2/11). S.c. implantation of
50 mg testosterone mixed with cholesterol in a ratio of 1:1 enhanced the
incidence of bladder tumours in nitrosamine-treated, ovariectomized
animals to 8/11 (P<0.05). Testosterone treatment without nitrosamine
induced no tumours (Okajima *et al*., 1975).

Male A x C rats were castrated at 12 or 52 weeks of age and given
s.c. implants of pellets containing testosterone propionate:cholesterol
(1:3) to give a dose of 200 mg/kg bw testosterone. Two weeks later, all
were fed 0.025% N-2-fluorenyldiacetamide for 4 weeks followed by 1 week
on the basal diet, until the carcinogen had been administered for 16
weeks. Animals were killed after 48 weeks. In rats implanted when 12-
weeks old, testosterone propionate resulted in a significantly increased
incidence of liver carcinomas when compared with controls given N-2-
fluorenyldiacetamide alone (25/25 *versus* 10/26; P=0.001). A less marked
but still significant effect of testosterone propionate was observed in
rats 52-weeks-old at the start of treatment (7/25 *versus* 0/27; P=0.001)
(Reuber, 1976).

Hamster: Two s.c. implantations at a 5-month interval of pellets
containing 100 mg testosterone propionate and 25 mg diethylstilboestrol
dipropionate into hamsters resulted in the induction of leiomyomas and
leiomyosarcomas along the uterine horns in 18/20 females and of similar
tumours in the epididymis of 17/20 males. These tumours appeared after
the 11th month; 2 females and 3 males died without tumours before that
time. No concurrent controls were used (Rivière *et al.*, 1961). Similar
tumours were described by Kirkman & Algard (1965).

(c) Neonatal exposure

Mouse: The long-term effects in female mice of neonatal exposure
to steroid hormones, including testosterone, on the genital tract and
mammary glands have been reviewed by Bern *et al.* (1975, 1976) and Takasugi
(1976). Short-term effects leading to persistent vaginal cornification
have been reported by Iguchi & Takasugi (1976) and Ohta & Iguchi (1976)
(see section 3.2).

Of female BALB/cCrgl mice injected subcutaneously with 25 µg
testosterone in water daily for the first 5 days after birth, 7/9 developed
hyperplastic epithelial lesions, resembling epidermoid carcinomas (vaginal
squamous-cell tumours), at about 71 weeks of age (Kimura & Nandi, 1967).
Thus, neonatal injections of androgen appear to act similarly to injections
of oestradiol-17β (Takasugi *et al.*, 1970).

Daily s.c. injections to virgin female BALB/cfC3H mice (MTV[+]) of 5
or 20 µg testosterone in 0.02 ml sesame oil for the first 5 days of
postnatal life resulted in an increased mammary tumour incidence by 16
months of age (42/49 and 22/35), compared with mice treated with
oestradiol-17β (8/35 and 32/64) or with ovine prolactin, bovine growth
hormone or the vehicle (0/40 and 9/43). The mean age at onset of tumours
of testosterone-treated mice was lower than that of those treated with
oestradiol-17β (8.5 months *versus* 11.0 months) (Mori *et al.*, 1976).

All of a group of virgin female SHN mice (MTV[+]) given daily s.c.
injections of 200 µg 5β-dihydrotestosterone in 0.02 ml olive oil during
the first 5 days of postnatal life developed mammary tumours by 6.2
months of age; the incidence in controls was 8/38 (P<0.01) (Yanai *et
al.*, 1977).

Rat: Twenty female albino rats were given s.c. injections of 0.5
mg testosterone propionate in arachis oil weekly from the age of 3 days,
the doses being increased to 1 mg when they were 21 days old and to 2.5
mg when they were 6 months of age. Nine rats died during the first 6
months. Of 10 rats that survived 16 months or more of continuous treatment,
3 had theca-cell ovarian tumours. The pituitaries were not enlarged,
but there was marked epithelial hyperplasia in the uteri of 5/10 rats.
Neither ovarian nor uterine tumours occurred in untreated rats of that
colony (Horning, 1958).

The incidence of mammary tumours induced by 7,12-dimethylbenz[a]-anthracene (DMBA) was decreased in Sprague-Dawley female rats given single s.c. injections of 1.25 mg testosterone propionate in 0.05 ml olive oil on the day of birth (20/32 *versus* 28/30; P<0.01). Age at onset of mammary tumours was greater in testosterone-treated rats than in the controls (15 *versus* 11.3 weeks; P<0.001); however, the mean number of tumours per rat and the growth rate were similar. In the rats treated neonatally with testosterone, 7 of the mammary tumours were adenocarcinomas and 13 were fibroadenomas, while all of the tumours in the positive controls were diagnosed as adenocarcinomas (Christakos *et al.*, 1976).

Female Sprague-Dawley rats were given a single s.c. injection of 1.25 mg testosterone propionate on day 2 of life and 20 mg DMBA by gavage at day 50. The induction of mammary dysplasia in rats given testosterone propionate was significantly greater than that in the controls (26/29 *versus* 26/40), while mammary tumour incidence was completely suppressed (1/29 *versus* 34/40) at 300 days of age (Yoshida & Fukunishi, 1978).

In female Sprague-Dawley rats, a single s.c. injection of 1 mg testosterone propionate in 0.05 ml sesame oil at 2 days of age enhanced the incidence of auditory sebaceous gland tumours induced by DMBA administered intragastrically at 50 days of age. The incidences of tumours 250 days after DMBA treatment were 8/32 and 1/20 in the experimental and control groups, respectively (P<0.05) (Yoshida & Fukunishi, 1977).

Single s.c. injections of 1.25 mg testosterone propionate in 0.05 ml sesame oil to female Sprague-Dawley rats at 5 days of age had little effect on the incidence of DMBA-induced mammary tumours at 190 days of age (18/36 *versus* 20/33). On the other hand, neonatal treatment with testosterone propionate decreased the mammary adenocarcinoma response to DMBA (11/24 *versus* 27/30) and increased the fibroadenoma response to DMBA (13/24 *versus* 3/30; P=0.01). No tumours appeared in rats given only testosterone propionate neonatally (Shellabarger & Soo, 1973).

3.2 Other relevant biological data

Toxic effects

Cells from C3 and C4 mammary nodule lines originally induced in BALB/cCrgl female mice by 7,12-dimethylbenz[a]anthracene (DMBA) were transplanted into the cleared mammary fat pads of 3-week-old BALB/c mice. When, after 8 weeks, testosterone was administered subcutaneously as pellets (18 mg) and left in place, tumour transformation was significantly inhibited in both C3 (9/18 *versus* 16/20; P<0.05) and C4 (13/30 *versus* 21/23; P<0.05) lines (Medina, 1977).

In all of female C57BL/Tw mice given daily s.c. injections of 100 μg testosterone, 50 μg testosterone propionate, 100 μg 5α-dihydrotestosterone or 50 μg 5α-dihydrotestosterone propionate in 0.02 ml sesame oil for the first 10 days of postnatal life and ovariectomized at 60 days, the cranial part of the vagina was lined with stratified epithelium with either cornification, parakeratosis or mucification by 90 days of age. Stratification only or stratification with superficial squamous metaplasia or cornification occurred in the uterine epithelia of 2/11 of those treated with testosterone propionate, in 6/8 of those treated with 5α-dihydrotestosterone and in 5/10 of those treated with 5α-dihydrotestosterone propionate (Iguchi & Takasugi, 1976).

Five daily s.c. injections of 100 μg testosterone or 5α-dihydrotestosterone in 0.02 ml sesame oil to groups of 40 female C57BL/Tw mice from the day of birth and bilateral ovariectomy on day 10 induced oestrogen-independent, persistent proliferation of the vaginal epithelium in adulthood (Ohta & Iguchi, 1976).

Embryotoxicity and teratogenicity

Various reports are available on the masculinizing effect of testosterone and testosterone propionate on female mammalian foetuses (Buno et al., 1967; Foote et al., 1968; Forsberg et al., 1977; Goldman et al., 1976; Goy et al., 1964; Phoenix et al., 1959).

Daily s.c. injections for 4-8 days of total doses of 0.5-80 mg testosterone to rats between days 10-20 of gestation and of total doses of 1-55 mg testosterone propionate between days 12-19 of gestation resulted in resorptions, necrosis, lethality, post-partum mortality and various degrees of masculinization in female offspring; the effects were correlated directly with dosage and period of administration (Greene et al., 1939).

A single s.c. injection of 4 mg/kg bw testosterone to rats between days 5-8 of gestation prevented implantation in 11/16 animals; injections on days 9-11 produced foetal loss or delayed parturition in 9/13 rats. Injection of 20 mg/kg bw on days 1, 5 or 9 led to foetal loss in all animals treated (Dreisbach, 1959).

Injection of 100 mg testosterone propionate on day 14 of gestation into rats induced small or absent mammary glands in offspring of both sexes and absence of nipples in 100% of females only (Jean & Jean, 1969).

Oral administration of 1.3-1.8 g testosterone to crossbred ewes, given as a single dose on the 14th day of gestation, was neither toxic nor teratogenic (Keeler & Binns, 1968).

Metabolism

Testosterone is the naturally occurring male sex hormone secreted
by the mammalian testis. It is transformed to 5α-dehydrotestosterone in
target organs such as the prostate, sebaceous glands and seminal vesicles;
only the latter compound binds to the androgen-receptor site in these
target organs (Kochakian, 1976).

The metabolism of testosterone and related compounds in animal
tissues has been reviewed (Kochakian & Arimasa, 1976). Variations in
testosterone metabolism occur between species, strains and sexes.

When labelled testosterone is given intragastrically to male
rats, about $\frac{1}{4}$ of the radioactivity appears in biliary metabolites within
12 hrs; half of these metabolites are glucuronides and half are sulphates.
The major metabolic routes are reductive and lead to formation of 5α-
dihydrotestosterone, androsterone and isomers thereof (epiandrosterone
and 3α-hydroxy-5β-androstan-17-one) and to androstandiols (5α-androstan-
3α,17β-diol, 5β-androstan-3α,17β-diol, 5α-androstan-3β,17β-diol) (Hetzel
et al., 1974).

Testosterone metabolites are conjugated differently in rats with a
high and in those with a low biliary excretion. Hydroxylation in rats
occurs at positions 7α, 11β, 15α and 15β (Matsui & Kinuyama, 1977).

Large quantitative differences in testosterone metabolism are
evident between female and male rats (Matsui et al., 1974, 1978). The
reason for this phenomenon is that many steroid-metabolizing enzymes in
rats are either androgen- or oestrogen-dependent; the sex hormones thus
act in an inductive or a repressive manner (Ghraf et al., 1975).

In Macaca mulatta (rhesus) monkeys, testosterone is metabolized and
conjugated in a way similar to that in baboons and humans, although
the rate of excretion was different and resembled more closely that of
the baboon than of humans (Yamamoto et al., 1978).

Extensive reductive metabolism of testosterone occurs not only in
the liver, but also in a variety of extrahepatic tissues, especially in
target organs of the sex hormones; the ultimately effective physiological
androgen is formed in the target tissues. Testosterone metabolism
occurs not only in the prostate and seminal vesicles but also in rat
uterus (Hoffmann et al., 1975), rabbit placenta (Marchut, 1977), rodent
testis (Mizutani et al., 1977) and primate brain (Sholiton et al.,
1974). In rats, the small intestine is also capable of metabolizing
testosterone (Geelen et al., 1977).

Esters of testosterone, such as the propionate, the heptanoate, the cypionate, the valerate, the isovalerate, the oenanthate and the undecanoate, are partially cleaved *in vivo* to release the parent compound. This has been demonstrated by oral administration of testosterone undecanoate in oily solution to rats: most of the compound is converted within the intestinal wall, the first step being partial splitting off of the fatty acid moiety. The non-metabolized portion, however, and the metabolite 5α-dihydrotestosterone undecanoate, are absorbed *via* the lymphatic system and made available for androgenic action to the organism (Coert *et al*., 1975).

Human metabolism of testosterone has been reviewed by Kochakian & Arimasa (1976). The main urinary metabolites of administered testosterone are 17-ketosteroids (androsterone and its isomers). Part of the injected testosterone is converted to oestrogens (see 'General Remarks on Sex Hormones', p. 59).

The Working Group considered that no relevant mutagenicity data on testosterone were presently available.

3.3   Case reports and epidemiological studies

See the section 'Oestrogens and Progestins in Relation to Human Cancer', p. 83.

4.   Summary of Data Reported and Evaluation[1]

4.1   Experimental data

Testosterone and its esters were tested in mice, rats and hamsters, by subcutaneous injection and/or implantation, and in rabbits by intramuscular injection.

Testosterone propionate implanted subcutaneously in mice induced cervical-uterine tumours, which metastasized in some cases; in rats, metastasizing prostatic adenocarcinomas were induced in males.

Neonatal treatment of female mice by subcutaneous injection of testosterone induced lesions of the genital tract and increased the mammary tumour incidence when the animals were adult. 5β-Dihydrotestosterone, which is considered to be hormonally inactive in adults,

_____

[1]This section should be read in conjunction with pp. 62-64 in the 'General Remarks on Sex Hormones' and with the 'General Conclusions on Sex Hormones' p. 131.

also increased the incidence of mammary tumours in mice when given neonatally by subcutaneous injection.

Testosterone is embryolethal in pre- and postimplantation embryos and causes virilization in female offspring.

4.2 Human data

No case reports or epidemiological studies on testosterone alone were available to the Working Group. There are limited data concerning the possible long-term effects of androgenic-anabolic steroids (pp. 102-103), which are related to testosterone. An association between these synthetic androgenic steroids and the occurrence of hepatocellular carcinomas has been suggested, but the evidence is inconclusive.

4.3 Evaluation

There is *sufficient evidence* for the carcinogenicity of testosterone in experimental animals. In the absence of adequate data in humans, it is reasonable, for practical purposes, to regard testosterone as if it presented a carcinogenic risk to humans. The only related data in humans, although insufficient for an evaluation, concern the possible long-term effects of androgenic anabolic-steroids.

5. References

Abraham, G.E., Manlimos, F.S. & Garza, R. (1977) Radioimmunoassay
    of steroids. In: Abraham, G.E., ed., Handbook of Radioimmunoassay,
    New York, Marcel Dekker, pp. 591-656

Albert, J., Geller, J., Geller, S. & Lopez, D. (1976) Prostate
    concentrations of endogenous androgens by radioimmunoassay.
    J. Steroid Biochem., 7, 301-307

Alter, S.A. (1958) Esters of cortical hormones, androgens, or estrogens
    by transesterification and alcoholysis. Spanish Patent, 241,206,
    22 April [Chem. Abstr., 54, 3532b]

Anon. (1939) $\Delta^{4,5}$-Androsten-3-on-17-ol propionate. Swiss Patent, 205,119,
    16 October, to l'Industrie Chimique à Bâle [Chem. Abstr., 35, 3040-5]

Anon. (1977) New steroid sources uproot Barbasco. Chemical Week,
    29 June, pp. 49-50

Anon. (1978) New steroid pathway put into production. Chemical
    & Engineering News, 24 July, p. 19

Bern, H.A., Jones, L.A., Mori, T. & Young, P.N. (1975) Exposure of
    neonatal mice to steroids: longterm effects on the mammary
    gland and other reproductive structures. J. Steroid Biochem.,
    6, 673-676

Bern, H.A., Jones, L.A., Mills, K.T., Kohrman, A. & Mori, T. (1976)
    Use of the neonatal mouse in studying longterm effects of early
    exposure to hormones and other agents. J. Toxicol. environ.
    Health, Suppl. 1, 103-116

Björkhem, I., Blomstrand, R.,Lantto, O., Svensson, L. & Öhman, G.
    (1976) Toward absolute methods in clinical chemistry:
    application of mass fragmentography to high-accuracy analyses.
    Clin. Chem., 22, 1789-1801

Boit, H.-G., ed. (1969) Beilsteins Handbuch der Organischen Chemie,
    4th ed., 3rd suppl., Vol. 8, part 2, Berlin, Springer, p. 892

British Pharmacopoeia Commission (1973) British Pharmacopoeia, London,
    HMSO, p. 402

Buno, W., Dominguez, R. & Carlevaro, E. (1967) Effects of testosterone
    propionate on guinea-pig foetuses (Abstract). Anat. Rec., 157, 352

Castellanos Llorens, J.M. & Aranda Baro, M. (1974) Determination of
    'free' testosterone in plasma by GLC-^{63}N ECD. Ann. Biol. clin. (Paris),
    32, 221-226

Charransol, G., Bobas-Masson, F., Guillemant, S. & Mauvais-Jarvis, P.
    (1972) Determination of urinary androstanediol and testosterone
    in normal men by gas-liquid chromatography. J. Chromatogr., 66,
    55-61

Chatten, L.G., Yadav, R.N. & Madan, D.K. (1976) The determination of
    certain Δ^4-3-ketosteroids in some parenteral formulations by
    differential pulse polarography. Pharm. acta helv., 51, 381-383

Christakos, S., Sinha, D. & Dao, T.L. (1976) Neonatal modification
    of endocrine functions and mammary carcinogenesis in the rat.
    Br. J. Cancer, 34, 58-63

Coert, A., Geelen, J., de Visser, J. & van der Vies, J. (1975)
    The pharmacology and metabolism of testosterone undecanoate,
    a new biologically active androgen. Acta endocrinol., 79, 789-800

Dehennin, L., Reiffsteck, A. & Schöller, R. (1974) Simultaneous
    estimation of testosterone, progesterone and androstenedione
    by gas chromatography-mass spectrometry with a single ion
    detection correlation with radioimmunoassay. J. Steroid Biochem.,
    5, 767-768

Dreisbach, R.H. (1959) The effects of steroid sex hormones on
    pregnant rats. J. Endocrinol., 18, 271-277

Eechaute, W., Demeester, G. & Leusen, I. (1972) Method for the
    fluorimetric determination of testosterone in the plasma (Fr.).
    Ann. Endocrinol., 33, 201-204 [Chem. Abstr., 78, 133038a]

Egg, D. & Huck, H. (1971) New fluorimetric determination of urinary
    testosterone by thin-layer chromatographic direct evaluation
    (Ger.). J. Chromatogr., 63, 349-355

Foote, W.D., Foote, W.C. & Foote, L.H. (1968) Influence of certain
    natural and synthetic steroids on genital development in guinea
    pigs. Fertil. Steril., 19, 606-615

Forsberg, J.-G., Gustafsson, T. & Jacobsohn, D. (1977) Abnormal
    nipples in female offspring of rats given testosterone during
    pregnancy. Arch. Anat. Microsc., 66, 207-216

Gardner, W.U. (1946) The incidence of mammary tumors and the structure
    of mammary glands of estrogen-plus-testosterone-treated mice.
    Cancer Res., 6, 493

Geelen, J., Coert, A., Meijer, R. & van der Vies, J. (1977) Comparison of the matabolism of testosterone undecanoate and testosterone in the gastrointestinal wall of the rat *in vitro* and *in vivo*. Acta endocrinol., 86, 216-224

Ghraf, R., Lax, E.R. & Schriefers, H. (1975) The hypophysis in the regulation of androgen and oestrogen dependent enzyme activities of steroid hormone metabolism in rat liver cytosol. Hoppe-Seyler's Z. physiol. Chem., 356, 127-134

Goldman, A.S., Shapiro, B.H. & Neumann, F. (1976) Role of testosterone and its metabolites in the differentiation of the mammary gland in rats. Endocrinology, 99, 1490-1495

Goldzieher, J.W., de la Pena, A. & Aivaliotis, M.M. (1978) Radioimmunoassay of plasma androstenedione, testosterone and 11β-hydroxyandrostenedione after chromatography on Lipidex-5000 (hydroxyalkoxypropyl Sephadex). J. Steroid Biochem., 9, 169-173

Goy, R.W., Bridson, W.E. & Young, W.C. (1964) Period of maximal susceptibility of prenatal female guinea pig to masculinizing actions of testosterone propionate. J. comp. Physiol. Psychol., 57, 166-174

Grasselli, J.G. & Ritchey, W.M., eds (1975) CRC Atlas of Spectral Data and Physical Constants for Organic Compounds, 2nd ed., Vol. IV, Cleveland, OH, Chemical Rubber Co., p. 580

Greene, R.R., Burrill, M.W. & Ivy, A.C. (1939) Experimental intersexuality. The effect of antenatal androgens on sexual development of female rats. Am. J. Anat., 65, 415-469

Hara, S. & Hayashi, S. (1977) Correlation of retention behaviour of steroidal pharmaceuticals in polar and bonded reversed-phase liquid column chromatography. J. Chromatogr., 142, 689-703

Harvey, S.C. (1975) Hormones. In: Osol, A. *et al.*, eds, Remington's Pharmaceutical Sciences, 15th ed., Easton, PA, Mack, pp. 932-934

Hassan, S.S.M. (1974) Optical rotary dispersion in quantitative analysis. Microdetermination of some steroid sex hormones. Fresenius' Z. anal. Chem., 269, 363-367 [Chem. Abstr., 81, 101490n]

Hassan, S.S.M., Abdel Fattah, M.M. & Zaki, M.T.M. (1976) Spectrophotometric determination of some steroid sex-hormones. Z. anal. Chem., 281, 371-377

Hetzel, W.-D., Kiehnscherf, R. & Staib, W. (1974) Excretion of
    isotopically labeled metabolites of testosterone in the bile of
    male rats. Hoppe-Seyler's Z. physiol. Chem., 355, 1143-1151

Hoffmann, U., Maass, H. & Lisboa, B.P. (1975) Metabolism of [4-^{14}C]-
    testosterone in the rat uterus *in vitro*. Eur. J. Biochem., 59,
    305-312

Horikawa, R., Tanimura, T. & Tamura, Z. (1978) Fluorometric determination
    of Δ^4-3-ketosteroids using aluminum salts and isonicotinylhydrazine.
    Anal. Biochem., 85, 105-113

Horning, E.S. (1958) Carcinogenic action of androgens. Br. J. Cancer,
    12, 414-418

Huck, H. (1975) Fluorimetric determination of testosterone on Al$_2$O$_3$ by
    thin-layer chromatographic separation of the trimethylsilyl ether
    derivatives (Ger.). J. Chromatogr., 110, 125-131

IARC (1974) IARC Monographs on the Evaluation of Carcinogenic Risk
    of Chemicals to Man, 6, Sex Hormones, Lyon, pp. 209-217

Iguchi, T. & Takasugi, N. (1976) Occurrence of permanent changes in
    vaginal and uterine epithelia in mice treated neonatally with
    progestin, estrogen and aromatizable or non-aromatizable androgens.
    Endocrinol Jpn., 23, 327-332

Jean, C. & Jean, C. (1969) Action of androgens on the differentiation
    of nascent mammary glands in newborn rats (Fr.) C.R. Soc. Biol.
    (Paris), 163, 1754-1758

Jones, E.E. (1941) The effect of testosterone propionate on mammary
    tumors in mice of the C3H strain. Cancer Res., 1, 787-789

Joshi, U.M., Naik, V.K. & Rao, S.S. (1974) Competitive protein
    binding assay for testosterone. In: Rastogi, G.K., ed.,
    Proceedings of Asia Oceania Congress on Endocrinology, Chandigarh,
    India, Endocrinology Society of India, pp. 427-430 [Chem. Abstr.,
    83, 75008f]

Kastrup, E.K., ed. (1977) Facts and Comparisons, St Louis, MO,
    Facts & Comparisons Inc., pp. 110, 110a, 113

Keeler, R.F. & Binns, W. (1968) Teratogenic compounds of *Veratrum
    californicum* (Durand). V. Comparison of cyclopian effects of
    steroidal alkaloids from the plant and structurally related
    compounds from other sources. Teratology, 1, 5-10

Khayam-Bashi, H. & Boroumand, M. (1975) Spectrophotometric estimation
    of 17β-estradiol, progesterone and testosterone. Biochem. Med.,
    14, 104-108 [Chem. Abstr., 84, 101787b]

Kimura, T. & Nandi, S. (1967) Nature of induced persistent vaginal
    cornification in mice. IV. Changes in the vaginal epithelium
    of old mice treated neonatally with estradiol or testosterone.
    J. natl Cancer Inst., 39, 75-93

Kirkman, H. (1957) Steroid tumorigenesis. Cancer, 10, 757-764

Kirkman, H. & Algard, F.T. (1965) Characteristics of an androgen/
    estrogen induced dependent leiomyosarcoma of the ductus deferens
    of the Syrian hamster. Cancer Res., 25, 141-143

Kjeld, J.M., Puah, C.M. & Joplin, G.F. (1977) Measurement of unconjugated
    testosterone, 5α-dihydrotestosterone and oestradiol in human
    urine. Clin. chim. acta, 80, 271-284

Kochakian, C.D., ed. (1976) Handbook of Experimental Pharmacology, Vol. 43,
    Anabolic Steroids, Berlin, Springer

Kochakian, C.D. & Arimasa, N. (1976) The metabolism in vitro of
    anabolic androgenic steroids by mammalian tissues. In: Kochakian,
    C.D., ed., Handbook of Experimental Pharmacology, Vol. 43, Anabolic
    Steroids, Berlin, Springer, pp. 287-359

Korneev, G.Y. (1973) Testosterone and androstenedione determination
    in the urine (Russ.) Probl. Endokrinol., 19, 46-50 [Chem. Abstr.,
    80, 67989zX

Marchut, M. (1977) In vitro metabolism of [4-^{14}C]androstenedione and
    [4-^{14}C]testosterone by rabbit placenta. Endocrinol. exp., 11, 139-146

Matsui, M. & Kinuyama, Y. (1977) Comparative fate of testosterone and
    testosterone sulphate in female rats: $C_{19}O_2$ and $C_{19}O_3$ steroid
    metabolites in the bile. J. Steroid Biochem., 8, 323-328

Matsui, M., Kinuyama, Y. & Hakozaki, M. (1974) Biliary metabolites of
    testosterone and testosterone glucosiduronate in the rat. Steroids,
    24, 557-573

Matsui, M., Kinuyama, Y., Hakozaki, M., Abe, F., Kawase, M. & Okada,
    M. (1978) Metabolism of testosterone and its conjugates by female
    rat liver. Chem. pharm. Bull., 21, 2764-2768

Medina, D. (1977) Tumor formation in preneoplastic mammary nodule
    lines in mice treated with nafoxidine, testosterone and
    2-bromo-α-ergocryptine. J. natl Cancer Inst., 58, 1107-1110

Meissner, W.A. & Sommers, S.C. (1966) Endometrial changes after
    prolonged progesterone and testosterone administration to
    rabbits. Cancer Res., 26, 474-478

Millington, D., Jenner, D.A., Jones, T. & Griffiths, K. (1974)
    Endogenous steroid concentrations in human breast tumours
    determined by high-resolution mass fragmentography. Biochem.
    J., 139, 473-475

Mizutani, S., Tsujimura, T., Akashi, S. & Matsumoto, K. (1977) Lack
    of metabolism of progesterone, testosterone and pregnenolone
    to 5α-products in monkey and human testes compared with rodent
    testes. J. clin. Endocrinol. Metab., 44, 1023-1031

Mori, T., Bern, H.A., Mills, K.T. & Young, P.N. (1976) Long-term
    effects of neonatal steroid exposure on mammary gland development
    and tumorigenesis in mice. J. natl Cancer Inst., 57, 1057-1062

Murad, F. & Gilman, A.G. (1975) Estrogens and progestins. In:
    Goodman, L.S. & Gilman, A., eds, The Pharmacological Basis of
    Therapeutics, 5th ed., New York, Macmillan, p. 1460

Murphy, J.B. (1944) The effect of castration, theelin and testosterone
    on the incidence of leukemia in a Rockefeller Institute strain
    of mice. Cancer Res., 4, 622-624

Myrick, J.W., Page, D.P. & Pfabe, Y.H. (1972) Semiautomated method
    for the analysis of methyltestosterone tablets and testosterone
    suspension. J. Assoc. off. anal. Chem., 55, 1175-1179

National Formulary Board (1975) National Formulary, 14th ed.,
    Washington DC, American Pharmaceutical Association, pp. 685-687

van Nie, R., Benedetti, E.L. & Mühlbock, O. (1961) A carcinogenic
    action of testosterone, provoking uterine tumours in mice.
    Nature, 192, 1303

Noble, R.L. (1977) The development of prostatic adenocarcinoma in Nb
    rats following prolonged sex hormone administration. Cancer Res.,
    37, 1929-1933

Obut, T.A. (1972) Simple method for fluorometric determination of
    testosterone in blood plasma (Russ.) Deposited Publ., VINITI
    5409-5473, 13 pp. [Chem. Abstr., 85, 30248j]

O'Hare, M.J., Nice, E.C., Magee-Brown, R. & Bullman, H. (1976) High-
    pressure liquid chromatography of steroids secreted by human
    adrenal and testis cells in monolayer culture. J. Chromatogr.,
    125, 357-367

Ohta, Y. & Iguchi, T. (1976) Development of the vaginal epithelium
    showing estrogen-independent proliferation and cornification in
    neonatally androgenized mice. Endocrinol. Jpn., 23, 333-340

Okajima, E., Hiramatsu, T., Iriya, K., Ijuin, M., Matsushima, S.
    & Yamada, K. (1975) Effects of sex hormones on development of
    urinary bladder tumours in rats induced by N-butyl-N-(4-hydroxy-
    butyl)nitrosamine. Urol. Res., 3, 73-79

Phoenix, C.H., Goy, R.W., Gerall, A.A. & Young, W.C. (1959)
    Organizing action of prenatally administered testosterone
    propionate on the tissues mediating mating behavior in the
    female guinea pig. Endocrinology, 65, 369-382

Pirani, B.B.K., Pairaudeau, N., Doran, T.A., Wong, P.Y. & Gardner,
    H.A. (1977) Amniotic fluid testosterone in the prenatal
    determination of fetal sex. Am. J. Obstet. Gynecol., 129,
    518-520

Poteczin, E., Fehér, T., Kiss, C. & Gyßry, G. (1975) Gas chromatographic
    determination of unconjugated dehydroepiandrosterone, androstenedione,
    testosterone, pregnenolone and progesterone in human ovarian
    tissue. Endokrinologie, 64, 151-158

Puah, C.M., Kjeld, J.M. & Joplin, G.F. (1978) A radioimmuno-chromato-
    graphic scanning method for the analysis of testosterone
    conjugates in urine and serum. J. Chromatogr., 145, 247-255

Reuber, M.D. (1976) Effect of age and testosterone on the induction
    of hyperplastic nodules, carcinomas, and cirrhosis of the liver
    in rats ingesting N-2-fluorenyldiacetamide. Eur. J. Cancer,
    12, 137-141

Rivière, M.R., Chouroulinkov, I. & Guérin, M. (1961) Long-term
    experimental action of hormones in hamsters with regard to their
    carcinogenic effect. II. Study of testosterone associated with
    an oestrogen (Fr.). Bull. Cancer, 48, 499-524

Satyaswaroop, P.G., Lopez de la Osa, E. & Gurpide, E. (1977)
    High pressure liquid chromatographic separation of C_{18} and C_{19}
    steroids. Steroids, 30, 139-145

Schenken, J.R. & Burns, E.L. (1943) Spontaneous primary hepatomas in
    mice of strain C3H. III. The effect of estrogens and testosterone
    propionate on their incidence. Cancer Res., 3, 693-696

Serio, M., Forti, G., Fiorelli, G. & Pazzagli, M. (1973) Methodologic considerations on the measurement of plasma androgens by competitive protein binding methods and radio-assays. In: James, V.H.T., Serio, M. & Martini, L., eds, Endocrinology and Functioning of Human Testis, Proceedings of a Symposium, 1972, Vol. 1, New York, Academic Press, pp. 15-40

Shellabarger, C.J. & Soo, V.A. (1973) Effects of neonatally administered sex steroids on 7,12-dimethylbenz(a)anthracene-induced mammary neoplasia in rats. Cancer Res., 33, 1567-1569

Sholiton, L.J., Taylor, B.B. & Lewis, H.P. (1974) The uptake and metabolism of labelled testosterone by the brain and pituitary of the male rhesus monkey (*Macaca mulatta*). Steroids, 24, 537-547

Sommerville, I.F. & Collins, W.P. (1975) Gas chromatographic determination of dehydroepiandrosterone, androstenedione and testosterone in plasma. In: Breuer, H., Hamel, D. & Krueskemper, H.L., eds, Methoden Hormonbestimmung, Stuttgart, Thieme, pp. 319-327 [Chem. Abstr., 83, 160076w]

Takasugi, N. (1976) Cytological basis for permanent vaginal changes in mice treated neonatally with steroid hormones. Int. Rev. Cytol., 44, 193-224

Takasugi, N., Kimura, T. & Mori, T. (1970) Irreversible changes in mouse vaginal epithelium induced by early post-natal treatment with steroid hormones. In: Kazda, S. & Denenberg, V.H., eds, The Post-natal Development of Phenotype, Prague, Academia, pp. 229-251

US Food & Drug Administration (1977) Food and drugs. US Code Fed. Regul., Title 21, part 556.708, p. 366

US Pharmacopeial Convention Inc. (1975) The US Pharmacopeia, 19th rev., Rockville, MD, pp. 490-492

US Tariff Commission (1938) Dyes and other Synthetic Organic Chemicals in the US, 1937, Report No. 132, Second Series, Washington DC, US Government Printing Office, p. 38

US Tariff Commission (1940) Synthetic Organic Chemicals, US Production and Sales, 1939, Report No. 140, Second Series, Washington DC, US Government Printing Office, p. 38

US Tariff Commission (1961) Synthetic Organic Chemicals, US Production and Sales, 1960, TC Publication 34, Washington DC, US Government Printing Office, p. 128

US Tariff Commission (1964) Synthetic Organic Chemicals, US Production and Sales, 1963, TC Publication 143, Washington DC, US Government Printing Office, p. 134

Vermeulen, A. (1975) Gas chromatographic determination of testosterone in plasma (Ger.). In: Breuer, H., Hamel, D. & Krueskemper, H.L., eds, Methoden Hormonbestimmung, Stuttgart, Thieme, pp. 298-303 [Chem. Abstr., 83, 160140n]

Wade, A., ed. (1977) Martindale, The Extra Pharmacopoeia, 27th ed., London, The Pharmaceutical Press, pp. 1429-1433

Windholz, M., ed. (1976) The Merck Index, 9th ed., Rahway, NJ, Merck & Co., pp. 1181-1182

Wingfield, J.C. & Farner, D.S. (1975) The determination of five steroids in avian plasma by radioimmunoassay and competitive protein-binding. Steroids, 26, 311-327

Wong, P.-Y., Wood, D.E. & Johnson, T. (1975) Routine radioimmunoassay of plasma testosterone, and results of various endocrine disorders. Clin. Chem., 21, 206-210

Yamamoto, Y., Manyon, A., Kirdani, R.Y. & Sandberg, A.A. (1978) Androgen metabolism in the rhesus monkey. Steroids, 31, 711-729

Yanai, R., Mori, T. & Nagasawa, H. (1977) Long-term effects of prenatal and neonatal administration of 5β-dihydrotestosterone on normal and neoplastic mammary development in mice. Cancer Res., 37, 4456-4459

Yoshida, H. & Fukunishi, R. (1977) Effect of neonatal administration of sex steroids on 7,12-dimethylbenz(a)anthracene-induced auditory sebaceous gland tumor in female rats. Gann, 68, 851-852

Yoshida, H. & Fukunishi, R. (1978) Effect of neonatal administration of sex steroids on 7,12-dimethylbenz[a]anthracene-induced mammary carcinoma and dysplasia in female Sprague-Dawley rats. Gann, 69, 627-631

OTHER

CLOMIPHENE and CLOMIPHENE CITRATE

1. Chemical and Physical Data

Clomiphene

1.1 Synonyms and trade names

Chem. Abstr. Services Reg. No.: 911-45-5

Chem. Abstr. Name: 2-[4-(2-Chloro-1,2-diphenylethenyl)phenoxy]-
N,N-diethylethanamine

Synonyms: Chloramiphene; [2-*para*-(2-chloro-1,2-diphenylvinyl)-
phenoxy]triethylamine; 2-[*para*-(β-chloro-α-phenylstyryl)phenoxy]-
triethylamine; clomifene; clomiphene B; 1-*para*-(β-diethylaminoethoxy)-
phenyl]-1,2-diphenylchloroethylene

1.2 Structural and molecular formulae and molecular weight

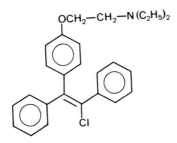

$C_{26}H_{28}ClNO$ Mol. wt: 406

1.3 Chemical and physical properties of the pure substance

No data were available in the standard pharmaceutical literature.

1.4 Technical products and impurities

No data were available.

Clomiphene citrate

1.1 Synonyms and trade names[1]

Chem. Abstr. Services Reg. No.: 50-41-9

Chem. Abstr. Name: 2-[4-(2-Chloro-1,2-diphenylethenyl)phenoxy]-*N*,*N*-diethylethanamine 2-hydroxy-1,2,3-propanetricarboxylate (1:1)

Synonyms: Clomifen citrate; clomiphene dihydrogen citrate; 2-[*para*-(2-chloro-1,2-diphenylvinyl)phenoxy]triethylamine citrate (1:1); racemic clomiphene citrate

Trade names: Clomid; Clomifeno; Clomivid; Clomphid; Chloramiphene; Dyneric; Genozym; Ikaclomin; Mer-41; MRL 41; MRL/41; NSC 35770; Omifin

1.2 Structural and molecular formulae and molecular weight

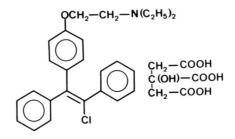

$C_{32}H_{36}ClNO_8$

Mol. wt: 598.1

1.3 Chemical and physical properties

From Wade (1977) and Windholz (1976) unless otherwise specified

(a) Description: White or pale-yellow, odourless powder

(b) Melting-point: 116.5-118°C; 117-119°C (Harvey, 1975)

---

[1]Clomiphene citrate can be separated into its *cis* and *trans* isomers, zuclomiphene and enclomiphene. In the US, zuclomiphene, the *cis* isomer, was previously called 'transclomiphene', and enclomiphene, the *trans* isomer, was previously called 'cisclomiphene' (Wade, 1977).

(c) Solubility: Slightly soluble in water (1 in 900), ethanol (1 in 40) and chloroform (1 in 800); freely soluble in methanol; practically insoluble in diethyl ether

(d) Stability: Unstable to air and light

1.4 Technical products and impurities

Various international pharmacopoeias specify the purity of clomiphene citrate used in pharmaceutical preparations. For example, in the US, it is available as a USP grade containing 98-101% (on the basis of the anhydrous material) of clomiphene citrate as a mixture of the *cis* and *trans* isomers, containing 1% max water, 0.002% max heavy metals and 30-50% of the *trans* isomer. It is also available in 50 mg tablets containing 93-107% of the stated amount of clomiphene citrate (US Pharmacopeial Convention Inc., 1975).

In the UK, the clomiphene citrate available contains 97-101% active ingredient (anhydrous basis) (British Pharmacopoeia Commission, 1973).

2. Production, Use, Occurrence and Analysis

2.1 Production and use

(a) Production

A method for the synthesis of clomiphene was first patented in 1959 (Allen *et al.*, 1959), by the reaction of 4-hydroxybenzophenone with 2-(diethylamino)ethyl chloride in toluene in the presence of alkali. The 4-[(2-diethylamino)ethoxy]benzophenone thus prepared is reacted with benzyl magnesium chloride, and the tertiary alcohol produced is dehydrated to give 2[*para*-(1,2-diphenylvinyl)phenoxy]triethylamine, chlorination of which yields clomiphene. The citrate can be made by reacting clomiphene with citric acid. It is not known whether this is the process used for commercial production.

No evidence was found that clomiphene or clomiphene citrate is produced in the US or Japan, and separate data are not available on US or Japanese imports.

Clomiphene citrate is believed to be produced commercially in France and in the UK, but no information was available on the quantities produced.

(b) Use

Clomiphene citrate is used in human medicine to induce ovulation in anovulatory and oligoovulatory women. The usual dose is 50 mg orally, daily for 5 days, starting on the fifth day of the menstrual cycle or at anytime in amenorrhoeic patients. If ovulation occurs, the same dosage is continued cyclically until conception is achieved. If ovulation does not occur, the cycle is repeated with 100 mg per day, and so on, providing that appropriate monitoring is effected (Harvey, 1975).

Clomiphene citrate has also been used in men to treat oligospermia, in doses of 50-200 mg daily, but the value of this treatment has not yet been established (Wade, 1977).

2.2 Occurrence

Clomiphene and clomiphene citrate are not known to occur naturally.

2.3 Analysis

No analytical procedures for the determination of clomiphene have been reported. Typical analytical procedures for the determination of clomiphene citrate are summarized in Table 1. Abbreviations used are: IR, infra-red spectrometry; UV, ultra-violet spectrometry. See also 'General Remarks on Sex Hormones', p. 60.

TABLE 1

Analytical methods for clomiphene citrate

Sample matrix	Sample preparation	Assay procedure	Reference
Bulk chemical	Add aqueous sodium hydroxide; extract (diethyl ether); evaporate; dissolve (carbon disulphide)	IR (13.16 & 13.51 μm)	British Pharmacopoeia Commission (1973)
Tablets	Powder; suspend (hydrochloric acid); filter	UV (292 nm)	British Pharmacopoeia Commission (1973)

3. Biological Data Relevant to the Evaluation
of Carcinogenic risk to Humans

3.1 Carcinogenicity studies in animals

Subcutaneous and/or intramuscular administration

Newborn rat: A single s.c. injection of 10-500 μg clomiphene
citrate (a mixture of *cis* and *trans* isomers) to one-day-old female
Sprague-Dawley rats resulted in multiple abnormalities of the reproductive
tract, including cystic ovaries, ovarian hypoplasia, hilus-cell tumours,
oviductal hyperplasia, pyometra, epithelial metaplasia, uterine cystic
hyperplasia and uterine tumours. The high dose (500 μg) produced some
forms of abnormality in 80-100% of animals, and intermediate and lower
doses in 10-50% (Clark & McCormack, 1977) [The Working Group noted the
incomplete reporting of the experiment].

3.2 Other relevant biological data

(a) Experimental systems

Clomiphene citrate is a mixture of two isomers: the *cis* form
possesses anti-oestrogenic activity while the *trans* form is oestrogenic.
It thus has slight oestrogenic and anti-oestrogenic effects, depending
on species and on numerous other factors such as treatment schedule and
the effect that is being considered (Murad & Gilman, 1975).

S.c. administration of daily doses of 20 mg/kg bw clomiphene
(unspecified) to female rats on days 7-10 of gestation was lethal to the
mothers (Marois & Marois, 1973).

Oral administration to mice of 1-3 mg/kg bw clomiphene citrate on
day 2 or on days 1-4 of gestation terminated pregnancy (Thomson, 1968).
Oral administration of 5-16 mg/kg bw caused inhibition of implantation
when given to mice in early gestation; it caused a dose-dependent
increase in the number of dead foetuses but had no effect on litter
size when given during the middle stages of gestation. A slight increase
in morphological abnormalities (clubfoot) was observed, and ossification
was accelerated in all groups (Suzuki, 1970a).

In rats, oral administration of 0.1 mg/kg bw clomiphene citrate
during early gestation induced 100% inhibition of implantation; administration of 5-10 mg/kg bw during the middle stage of pregnancy increased
foetal mortality by 14-20% (Suzuki, 1970b). Marois & Marois (1973)
observed a dose- and time-dependent effect of doses of 0.2-2 mg/kg bw
clomiphene (unspecified) on litter size and on foetal mortality. Oral
administration of 0.3 mg/kg bw per day on days 1-4 of gestation or of
0.9 mg/kg bw on any of the first 4 days prevented implantation in rats
(Nelson *et al.*, 1963).

Oral treatment of rats with 1-54 mg/kg bw per day clomiphene
(unspecified) starting 6.5 days after mating and continuing until day 20
of gestation induced mortality among the dams, decreased litter size,
inhibited skeletal ossification and caused various abnormalities in the
foetuses (hydronephrosis, hydroureter, deformed tails, exencephaly)
(Diener & Hsu, 1967).

S.c. injection of 0.2 mg/kg bw clomiphene (unspecified) to rats on
days 1 and 2 or 4-6 of gestation prevented implantation. Simultaneous
injection of 50 µg/animal oestradiol-17β or of 10 µg oestradiol-17β plus
5 mg progesterone during the clomiphene treatment on days 4-6 allowed
implantation, but embryo resorption occurred subsequently (Marois &
Marois, 1974).

A single daily s.c. injection of 2 mg/kg bw clomiphene citrate to
rats between days 6-14 of pregnancy resulted in hydramnios; doses of 50
mg/kg bw also induced cataracts in the foetuses. Daily administration
of 5 mg/rat progesterone from day 12 of pregnancy throughout gestation
inhibited these effects (Eneroth *et al*., 1971 [The Working Group noted
the inadequate reporting of the data].

When rabbits were fed 20 and 10 mg/animal clomiphene on days 1, 2 and
3 after artificial insemination, 22 and 34% of blastocysts found in the
uterus on day 6 were normal, compared with 89% in untreated animals
(Chang, 1964).

Oral administration of 1.5-4.5 mg/kg bw per day or i.m. administration
of 0.75-1.5 mg/kg bw per day clomiphene citrate for 1-4 days at various
stages between days 16 and 36 of gestation to 18 *Macaca mulatta* (rhesus)
monkeys resulted in 16 normal and 2 dead offspring (Courtney & Valerio,
1968).

Addition of 0.8 µg/ml clomiphene citrate to a culture medium prevented
development of mouse two-cell embryos in the blastocyst stage (Thomson,
1968).

No data on the metabolism of clomiphene and clomiphene citrate were
available.

(b) Humans

See 'General Remarks on Sex Hormones', p. 66.

It has been reported that treatment with human menopausal gonadotrophin
and clomiphene citrate increases the frequency of abnormal karyotypes
in spontaneous abortuses from 61% to over 80% (Boué & Boué, 1973).

3.3 Case reports and epidemiological studies

Schultze & Krause (1965) reported a case of granulosa-cell tumour of the ovary in a 28-year old female who had received clomiphene citrate therapy for two cycles (2 five-day courses of 100 mg per day). Two cases of bilateral breast cancer were reported in women aged 28 and 29 who had received such therapy (Bolton, 1977).

Molar pregnancies have been observed following induction of ovulation by clomiphene citrate (Burke, 1976; Schneiderman & Waxman, 1972; Wajntraub *et al.*, 1974); and rapid enlargement of uterine fibroids has also been reported (Felmingham & Corcoran, 1975; Frankel & Benjamin, 1973).

Moukhtar *et al.* (1977) reported the reversal of an endometrial carcinoma to a normal secretory endometrium following repetitive induction of ovulation with clomiphene citrate.

A 28-year old male who had received 1 mg 'cisclomiphene citrate' (enclomiphene, the *trans* isomer) daily for 10 weeks developed a germ-cell tumour with elements of seminoma and mature adult teratoma (Reyes & Faiman, 1973).

4. Summary of Data Reported and Evaluation[1]

4.1 Experimental data

Clomiphene citrate was inadequately tested in one experiment in newborn rats by subcutaneous injection; uterine and ovarian tumours were reported.

Clomiphene citrate is embryolethal for pre- and postimplantation embryos in several species and has various teratogenic effects in rats.

---

[1]This section should be read in conjunction with pp. 62-64 in the 'General Remarks on Sex Hormones' and with the 'General Conclusions on Sex Hormones', p. 131.

4.2 Human data

There are a few case reports of the occurrence of malignant and benign tumours at various sites in patients treated with clomiphene citrate, but there is no evidence of a causal relationship.

No definite association between clomiphene citrate administration and congenital defects in humans has been demonstrated.

4.3 Evaluation

The available experimental and human data are insufficient to evaluate the carcinogenicity of clomiphene citrate.

5. References

Allen, R.E., Palopoli, F.P., Schumann, E.L. & Van Campen, M.G., Jr
    (1959) Amine derivatives of triphenylethanol, triphenylethylene,
    and triphenylethane. US Patent, 2,914,561-4, 24 November, to
    Wm S. Merrell Co. [Chem. Abstr., 54, 5581e-5584e]

Bolton, P.M. (1977) Bilateral breast cancer associated with clomiphene.
    Lancet, ii, 1176

Boué, J.G. & Boué, A. (1973) Increased frequency of chromosomal
    anomalies in abortions after induced ovulation. Lancet, i, 679-
    680

British Pharmacopoeia Commission (1973) British Pharmacopoeia, London,
    HMSO, p. 116

Burke, M. (1976) Ectopic pregnancy, hydatidiform mole and clomiphene.
    Lancet, i, 41-42

Chang, M.C. (1964) Effects of certain antifertility agents on the
    development of rabbit ova. Fertil. Steril., 15, 97-106

Clark, J.H. & McCormack, S. (1977) Clomid or nafoxidine administered
    to neonatal rats causes reproductive tract abnormalities. Science,
    197, 164-165

Courtney, K.D. & Valerio, D.A. (1968) Teratology in Macaca mulatta.
    Teratology, 1, 163-172

Diener, R.M. & Hsu, B.Y.D. (1967) Effects of certain basic phenolic
    ethers on the rat fetus. Toxicol. appl. Pharmacol., 10, 565-576

Eneroth, G., Eneroth, P., Forsberg, U., Grant, C.A. & Gustafsson, J.-A.
    (1971) Clomiphene-induced hydramnios and fetal cataracts in rats
    inhibited by progesterone (Abstract). Teratology, 4, 487

Felmingham, J.E. & Corcoran, M. (1975) Letter. Br. J. Obstet. Gynaecol.,
    82, 431-432

Frankel, T. & Benjamin, F. (1973) Rapid enlargement of a uterine fibroid
    after clomiphene therapy. J. Obstet. Gynaecol. Br. Commonw., 80,
    764

Harvey, S.C. (1975) Hormones. In: Osol, A. et al., eds, Remington's
    Pharmaceutical Sciences, 15th ed., Easton, PA, Mack, pp. 920-921

Marois, M. & Marois, G. (1973) Effects of clomiphene on delivery in
    rats (Fr.). J. Gynecol. Obstet. Biol. Reprod., 2, 5-9

Marois, M. & Marois, G. (1974) Clomiphene, implantation and survival of foetuses (Fr.). C.R. Soc. Biol. (Paris), 168, 405-410

Moukhtar, M., Aleem, F.A., Hung, H.C., Sommers, S.C., Klinger, H.P. & Romney, S.L. (1977) The reversible behavior of locally invasive endometrial carcinoma in a chromosomally mosaic [45,X/46, Xr(X)] young woman treated with Clomid®. Cancer, 40, 2957-2966

Murad, F. & Gilman, A.G. (1975) Estrogens and progestins. Clomiphene. In: Goodman, L.S. & Gilman, A., eds, The Pharmacological Basis of Therapeutics, New York, Macmillan, p. 1435

Nelson, W.O., Davidson, O.W. & Wada, K. (1963) Studies on interference with zygote development and implantation. In: Enders, A.C., ed., Delayed Implantation, Chicago, University of Chicago Press, p. 183

Reyes, F.I. & Faiman, C. (1973) Development of a testicular tumour during cisclomiphene therapy. Can. med. Assoc. J., 109, 502-503, 506

Schneiderman, C.I. & Waxman, B. (1972) Clomid therapy and subsequent hydatidiform mole formation. A case report. Obstet. Gynecol., 39, 787-788

Schultze, K.W. & Krause, F.J. (1965) Clomiphene treatment and granulosa-cell tumour (Ger.). Geburtshilfe Frauenheilkd, 25, 918-923

Suzuki, M.R. (1970a) Effects of cyclofenil and clomiphene, ovulation inducing agents, on mouse fetuses (Jpn.). Oyo Yakuri, 4, 645-651

Suzuki, M.R. (1970b) Effects of oral cyclofenil and clomiphene, ovulation inducing agents, on pregnancy and fetuses in rats (Jpn.). Oyo Yakuri, 4, 635-644

Thomson, J.L. (1968) Effect of two non-steroidal antifertility agents on pregnancy in mice. I. Comparison of in-vitro and in-vivo effects on zygotes. J. Reprod. Fertil., 15, 223-231

US Pharmacopeial Convention Inc. (1975) The US Pharmacopeia, 19th rev., Rockville, MD, pp. 97-98

Wade, A., ed. (1977) Martindale, the Extra Pharmacopoeia, 27th ed., London, The Pharmaceutical Press, pp. 1392-1394

Wajntraub, G., Kamar, R. & Pardo, Y. (1974) Hydatidiform mole after treatment with clomiphene. Fertil. Steril., 25, 904-905

Windholz, M., ed. (1976) The Merck Index, 9th ed., Rahway, NJ, Merck & Co., p. 306

p. v	Table 1	*replace* Chemical *by* Chemicals
p. 9	3rd para. lines 5-6	*replace* age at *by* precocity of
p. 26	13	*replace* BIS(CHROMETHYL)ETHER *by* BIS(CHLOROMETHYL)ETHER
p. 33		*replace footnote 3 by* Pell, S. Mortality of workers exposed to dimethyl sulphate 1932-1974, submitted to the American Conference of Governmental and Industrial Hygienists, 1976
p. 37	37 line 2	*replace* lymphosarcomas, *by* lymphosarcomas and
p. 48	line 4	*replace* acrylonitride *by* acrylonitrile
p. 50	line 5	*delete*
p. 51	line 2	*replace* Azathioprine *by* Azothioprine
p. 67		*remove asterisk* (*) *after* Lead and certain lead compounds *replace* Peritoneum-mesothelioma (157) *by* Peritoneum-mesothelioma (158)
p. 70		*remove asterisk* (*) *after* Lead and certain lead compounds
p. 71	line 4	*replace* Anaesthetics, inhalational *by* Anaesthetics, volatile

CUMULATIVE INDEX TO IARC MONOGRAPHS ON THE EVALUATION

OF THE CARCINOGENIC RISK OF CHEMICALS TO HUMANS

Numbers underlined indicate volume, and numbers in italics indicate
page. References to corrigenda are given in parentheses. Compounds
marked with an asterisk (*) were considered by the Working Groups, but
monographs were not prepared because adequate data on their carcinogenicity
were not available.

2-Amino-4-nitrophenol*

2-Amino-5-nitrophenol*

Amitrole   *7*,*31*

Amobarbital sodium*

Anaesthetics, volatile   **11**,*285*

Anthranilic acid   **16**,*265*

Aniline   *4*,*27* (corr. *7*,*320*)

Apholate   *9*,*31*

Aramite®   *5*,*39*

Arsenic and inorganic arsenic compounds   *2*,*48*
  Arsenic pentoxide
  Arsenic trioxide
  Calcium arsenate
  Cascium arsenite
  Lead arsenate
  Potassium arsenate
  Potassium arsenite
  Sodium arsenate
  Sodium arsenite

Asbestos   *2*,*17* (corr. *7*,*319*)

                                                     14,   (corr. **15**,*341*)
                                                              (corr. **17**,*351*)

  Actinolite
  Amosite
  Anthophyllite
  Chrysotile
  Crocidolite
  Tremolite

Auramine   *1*,*69* (corr. *7*,*319*)

Aurothioglucose   **13**,*39*

Azaserine   **10**,*73* (corr. **12**,*271*)

Aziridine   *9*,*37*

2-(1-Aziridinyl)ethanol   *9*,*47*

Aziridyl benzoquinone   *9*,*51*

Azobenzene   *8*,*75*

Azothioprine*

B

Benz[*c*]acridine   *3*,*241*

J

Jacobine   10,*275*

L

Lasiocarpine   10,*281*

Lead salts   1,*40* (corr. 7,*319*)
                                                    (corr. 8,*349*)

    Lead acetate
    Lead arsenate
    Lead carbonate
    Lead phosphate
    Lead subacetate

Ledate   12,*131*

Light green SF   16,*209*

Lindane   5,*47*
                                            20,*195*

Luteoskyrin   10,*163*

Lynoestrenol   21,*407*

Lysergide*

M

Magenta   4,*57* (corr. 7,*320*)

Maleic hydrazide   4,*173* (corr. 18,*125*)

Maneb   12,*137*

Mannomustine and its dihydrochloride   9,*157*

Medphalan   9,*167*

Medroxyprogesterone acetate   6,*157*
                                            21,*417*

Megestrol acetate   21,*431*

Melphalan   9,*167*

Merphalan   9,*167*

Mestranol   6,*87*
                                            21,*257*

Methacrylic acid*

Methallenoestril*

Methoxychlor   5,*193*
                                            20,*259*

P

Parasorbic acid	10,*199* (corr. 12,*271*)
Patulin	10,*205*
Penicillic acid	10,*211*
Pentachlorophenol	20,*303*
Pentobarbital sodium*	
Phenacetin	13,*141*
Phenicarbazide	12,*177*
Phenobarbital	13,*157*
Phenobarbital sodium	13,*159*
Phenoxybenzamine and its hydrochloride	9,*223*
Phenylbutazone	13,*183*
ortho-Phenylenediamine*	
meta-Phenylenediamine and its hydrochloride	16,*111*
para-Phenylenediamine and its hydrochloride	16,*125*
N-Phenyl-2-naphthylamine	16,*325*
N-Phenyl-*para*-phenylenediamine*	
Phenytoin	13,*201*
Phenytoin sodium	13,*202*
Piperazine oestrone sulphate	21,*148*
Polyacrylic acid	19,*62*
Polybrominated biphenyls	18,*107*
Polychlorinated biphenyls	7,*261*
	18,*43*
Polychloroprene	19,*141*
Polyethylene (low-density and high-density)	19,*164*
Polyethylene terephthalate*	
Polyisoprene*	
Polymethylene polyphenyl isocyanate	19,*314*
Polymethyl methacrylate	19,*195*
Polyoestradiol phosphate	21,*286*
Polypropylene	19,*218*

R

Reserpine	10,*217*
Resorcinol	15,*155*
Retrorsine	10,*303*
Rhodamine B	16,*221*
Rhodamine 6G	16,*233*
Riddelliine	10,*313*
Rifampicin*	

S

Saccharated iron oxide	2,*161*
Safrole	1,*169* 10,*231*
Scarlet red	8,*217*
Selenium and selenium compounds	9,*245* (corr. 12,*271*)
Semicarbazide and its hydrochloride	12,*209* (corr. 16,*387*)
Seneciphylline	10,*319*
Senkirkine	10,*327*
Sodium diethyldithiocarbamate	12,*217*
Sodium equilin sulphate	21,*148*
Sodium oestrone sulphate	21,*147*
Soot, tars and shale oils	3,*22*
Spironolactone*	
Sterigmatocystin	1,*175* 10,*245*
Streptozotocin	4,*221* 17,*337*
Styrene	19,*231*
Styrene-acrylonitrile copolymers	19,*97*
Styrene-butadiene copolymers	19,*252*
Styrene oxide	11,*201* 19,*275*
Succinic anhydride	15,*265*
Sudan I	8,*225*

IARC MONOGRAPHS ON THE EVALUATION
OF THE CARCINOGENIC RISK OF CHEMICALS TO HUMANS

IARC Publications continued on inside back cover

LIVER CANCER	No. 1, 1971; 176 pages US$ 10.00; Sw. fr. 30.—
ONCOGENESIS AND HERPESVIRUSES	No. 2, 1972; 515 pages US$ 25.00; Sw. fr. 100.—
N-NITROSO COMPOUNDS ANALYSIS AND FORMATION	No. 3, 1972; 140 pages US$ 6.25; Sw. fr. 25.—
TRANSPLACENTAL CARCINOGENESIS	No. 4, 1973; 181 pages US$ 12.00; Sw. fr. 40.—
PATHOLOGY OF TUMOURS IN LABORATORY ANIMALS—VOLUME I— TUMOURS OF THE RAT PART 1	No. 5, 1973; 214 pages US$ 15.00; Sw. fr. 50.—
PATHOLOGY OF TUMOURS IN LABORATORY ANIMALS—VOLUME I— TUMOURS OF THE RAT PART 2	No. 6, 1976; 319 pages US$ 35.00; Sw. fr. 90.—
HOST ENVIRONMENT INTERACTIONS IN THE ETIOLOGY OF CANCER IN MAN	No. 7, 1973; 464 pages US$ 40.00; Sw. fr. 100.—
BIOLOGICAL EFFECTS OF ASBESTOS	No. 8, 1973; 346 pages US$ 32.00; Sw. fr. 80.—
N-NITROSO COMPOUNDS IN THE ENVIRONMENT	No. 9, 1974; 243 pages US$ 20.00; Sw. fr. 50.—
CHEMICAL CARCINOGENESIS ESSAYS	No. 10, 1974; 230 pages US$ 20.00; Sw. fr. 50.—
ONCOGENESIS AND HERPESVIRUSES II	No. 11, 1975; Part 1, 511 pages, US$ 38.00; Sw. fr. 100.— Part 2, 403 pages, US$ 30.00; Sw. fr. 80.—
SCREENING TESTS IN CHEMICAL CARCINOGENESIS	No. 12, 1976; 666 pages US$ 48.00; Sw. fr. 120.—
ENVIRONMENTAL POLLUTION AND CARCINOGENIC RISKS	No. 13, 1976; 454 pages US$ 20.00; Sw. fr. 50.—
ENVIRONMENTAL N-NITROSO COMPOUNDS—ANALYSIS AND FORMATION	No. 14, 1976; 512 pages US$ 45.00; Sw. fr. 110.—
CANCER INCIDENCE IN FIVE CONTINENTS—VOLUME III	No. 15, 1976; 584 pages US$ 40.00; Sw. fr. 100.—
AIR POLLUTION AND CANCER IN MAN	No. 16, 1977;; 331 pages US$ 35.00; Sw. fr. 90.—
DIRECTORY OF ON-GOING RESEARCH IN CANCER EPIDEMIOLOGY	No. 17, 1977; 599 pages US$ 10.00; Sw. fr. 25.—
ENVIRONMENTAL CARCINOGENS-SELECTED METHODS OF ANALYSIS VOL. 1: ANALYSIS OF VOLATILE NITROSAMINES IN FOOD	No. 18, 1978; 212 pages US$ 45.00; Sw. fr. 90.—
ENVIRONMENTAL ASPECTS OF N-NITROSO COMPOUNDS	No. 19, 1978; 566 pages US$ 50.00; Sw. fr. 100.—
NASOPHARYNGEAL CARCINOMA: ETIOLOGY AND CONTROL	No. 20, 1978; 610 pages US$ 60.00; Sw. fr. 100.—
CANCER REGISTRATION AND ITS TECHNIQUES	No. 21, 1978; 235 pages US$ 25.00; Sw. fr. 40.—
ENVIRONMENTAL CARCINOGENS—SELECTED METHODS OF ANALYSIS VOL. 2: VINYL CHLORIDE	No. 22, 1978; 142 pages US$ 45.00; Sw. fr. 75.—
PATHOLOGY OF TUMOURS IN LABORATORY ANIMALS—VOLUME II— TUMOURS OF THE MOUSE	No. 23, 1979; 669 pages US$ 60.00; Sw. fr. 60.—
ONCOGENESIS AND HERPESVIRUSES III	No. 24, 1978; Part 1, 580 pages, US$ 30.00; Sw. fr. 50.— Part 2, 519 pages, US$ 30.00; Sw. fr. 50.—
CARCINOGENIC RISKS—STRATEGIES FOR INTERVENTION	No. 25, 1979; 283 pages US$ 30.00; Sw. fr. 50.—
DIRECTORY OF ON-GOING RESEARCH IN CANCER EPIDEMIOLOGY 1978	No. 26, 1978; 550 pages Sw. fr. 30.—
DIRECTORY OF ON—GOING RESEARCH IN CANCER EPIDEMIOLOGY 1979	No. 28, 1979, 672 pages Sw. fr. 30.—
ENVIRONMENTAL CARCINOGENS— SELECTED METHODS OF ANALYSIS VOL. 3: POLYCYCLIC AROMATIC HYDROCARBONS	No. 29, 1979; 240 pages US$ 30.00; Sw. fr. 50.—

WHO/IARC publications may be obtained, direct or through booksellers, from:

ALGERIA : Société Nationale d'Edition et de Diffusion, 3 bd Zirout Youcef, ALGIERS

ARGENTINA : Carlos Hirsch SRL, Florida 165, Galerías Güemes, Escritorio 453/465, BUENOS AIRES

AUSTRALIA : *Mail Order Sales :* Australian Government Publishing Service Bookshops, P.O. Box 84, CANBERRA A.C.T. 2600 ; *or over the counter from* Australian Government Publications and Inquiry Centres *at :* 113–115 London Circuit, CANBERRA CITY A.C.T. 2600 ; Shop 42, The Valley Centre, BRISBANE, Queensland 4000 ; 347 Swanston Street, MELBOURNE VIC 3000 ; 309 Pitt Street, SYDNEY N.S.W. 2000 ; Mt Newman House, 200 St. George's Terrace, PERTH WA 6000 ; Industry House, 12 Pirie Street, ADELAIDE SA 5000 ; 156–162 Macquarie Street, HOBART TAS 7000 — Hunter Publications, 58A Gipps Street, COLLINGWOOD VIC 3066

AUSTRIA : Gerold & Co., Graben 31, 1011 VIENNA I

BANGLADESH : The WHO Programme Coordinator, G.P.O. Box 250, DACCA 5 — The Association of Voluntary Agencies, P.O. Box 5045, DACCA 5

BELGIUM : Office international de Librairie, 30 avenue Marnix, 1050 BRUSSELS — *Subscriptions to World Health only :* Jean de Lannoy, 202 avenue du Roi, 1060 BRUSSELS

BRAZIL : Biblioteca Regional de Medicina OMS/OPS, Unidade de Venda de Publicações, Caixa Postal 20.381, Vila Clementino, 04023 SÃO PAULO, S.P.

BURMA : *see* India, WHO Regional Office

CANADA : *Single and bulk copies of individual publications (not subscriptions) :* Canadian Public Health Association, 1335 Carling Avenue, Suite 210, OTTAWA, Ont. K1Z 8N8. *Subscriptions : Subscription orders, accompanied by cheque made out to the* Royal Bank of Canada, OTTAWA, Account World Health Organization, *should be sent to the* World Health Organization, P.O. Box 1800, Postal Station B, OTTAWA, Ont. K1P 5R5. *Correspondence concerning subscriptions should be addressed to the* World Health Organization, Distribution and Sales, 1211 GENEVA 27, Switzerland

CHINA : China National Publications Import Corporation, P.O. Box 88, PEKING

COLOMBIA : Distrilibros Ltd, Pío Alfonso García, Carrera 4a, Nos 36–119, CARTAGENA

CZECHOSLOVAKIA : Artia, Ve Smeckach 30, 111 27 PRAGUE 1

DENMARK : Ejnar Munksgaard, Ltd, Nørregade 6, 1164 COPENHAGEN K

ECUADOR : Librería Científica S.A., P.O. Box 362, Luque 223, GUAYAQUIL

EGYPT : Nabaa El Fikr Bookshop, 55 Saad Zaghloul Street, ALEXANDRIA

EL SALVADOR : Librería Estudiantil, Edificio Comercial B No 3, Avenida Libertad, SAN SALVADOR

FIJI : The WHO Programme Coordinator, P.O. Box 113, SUVA

FINLAND : Akateeminen Kirjakauppa, Keskuskatu 2, 00101 HELSINKI 10

FRANCE : Librairie Arnette, 2 rue Casimir-Delavigne, 75006 PARIS

GERMAN DEMOCRATIC REPUBLIC : Buchhaus Leipzig, Postfach 140, 701 LEIPZIG

GERMANY, FEDERAL REPUBLIC OF : Govi-Verlag GmbH, Ginnheimerstrasse 20, Postfach 5360, 6236 ESCHBORN — W. E. Saarbach, Postfach 101610, Follerstrasse 2, 5 COLOGNE 1 — Alex. Horn, Spiegelgasse 9, Postfach 3340, 6200 WIESBADEN

GREECE : G. C. Eleftheroudakis S.A., Librairie internationale, rue Nikis 4, ATHENS (T. 126)

HAITI : Max Bouchereau, Librairie "A la Caravelle", Boîte postale 111-B, PORT-AU-PRINCE

HONG KONG : Hong Kong Government Information Services, Beaconsfield House, 6th Floor, Queen's Road, Central, VICTORIA

HUNGARY : Kultura, P.O.B. 149, BUDAPEST 62 — Akadémiai Könyvesbolt, Váci utca 22, BUDAPEST V

ICELAND : Snaebjörn Jonsson & Co., P.O. Box 1131, Hafnarstraeti 9, REYKJAVIK

INDIA : WHO Regional Office for South-East Asia, World Health House, Indraprastha Estate, Ring Road, NEW DELHI 110002 — Oxford Book & Stationery Co., Scindia House, NEW DELHI 110000 ; 17 Park Street, CALCUTTA 700016 (*Sub-Agent*)

INDONESIA : M/s Kalman Book Service Ltd, Jln. Cikini Raya No. 63, P.O. Box 3105/Jkt., JAKARTA

IRAN : Iranian Amalgamated Distribution Agency, 151 Khiaban Soraya, TEHERAN

IRAQ : Ministry of Information, National House for Publishing, Distributing and Advertising, BAGHDAD

IRELAND : The Stationery Office, DUBLIN 4

ISRAEL : Heiliger & Co., 3 Nathan Strauss Street, JERUSALEM

ITALY : Edizioni Minerva Medica, Corso Bramante 83–85, 10126 TURIN ; Via Lamarmora 3, 20100 MILAN

JAPAN : Maruzen Co. Ltd, P.O. Box 5050, TOKYO International 100–31

KOREA, REPUBLIC OF : The WHO Programme Coordinator, Central P.O. Box 540, SEOUL

KUWAIT : The Kuwait Bookshops Co. Ltd, Thunayan Al-Ghanem Bldg, P.O. Box 2942, KUWAIT

LAO PEOPLE'S DEMOCRATIC REPUBLIC : The WHO Programme Coordinator, P.O. Box 343, VIENTIANE

LEBANON : The Levant Distributors Co. S.A.R.L., Box 1181, Makdassi Street, Hanna Bldg, BEIRUT

LUXEMBOURG : Librairie du Centre, 49 bd Royal, LUXEMBOURG

MALAYSIA : The WHO Programme Coordinator, Room 1004, Fitzpatrick Building, Jalan Raja Chulan, KUALA LUMPUR 05–02 — Jubilee (Book) Store Ltd, 97 Jalan Tuanku Abdul Rahman, P.O. Box 629, KUALA LUMPUR 01–08 — Parry's Book Center, K. L. Hilton Hotel, Jln. Treacher, P.O. Box 960, KUALA LUMPUR

MEXICO : La Prensa Médica Mexicana, Ediciones Científicas, Paseo de las Facultades 26, Apt. Postal 20–413, MEXICO CITY 20, D.F.

MONGOLIA : *see* India, WHO Regional Office

MOROCCO : Editions La Porte, 281 avenue Mohammed V, RABAT

MOZAMBIQUE : INLD, Caixa Postal 4030, MAPUTO

NEPAL : *see* India, WHO Regional Office

NETHERLANDS : N. V. Martinus Nijhoff's Boekhandel en Uitgevers Maatschappij, Lange Voorhout 9, THE HAGUE 2000

NEW ZEALAND : Government Printing Office, Mulgrave Street, Private Bag, WELLINGTON 1, *Government Bookshops at :* Rutland Street, P.O. Box 5344, AUCKLAND ; 130 Oxford Terrace, P.O. Box 1721, CHRISTCHURCH ; Alma Street, P.O. Box 857, HAMILTON ; Princes Street, P.O. Box 1104, DUNEDIN — R. Hill & Son, Ltd, Ideal House, Cnr Gillies Avenue & Eden St., Newmarket, AUCKLAND 1

NIGERIA : University Bookshop Nigeria Ltd, University of Ibadan, IBADAN — G. O. Odatuwa Publishers & Booksellers Co., 9 Hausa Road, SAPELE, BENDEL STATE

NORWAY : Johan Grundt Tanum Bokhandel, Karl Johansgt. 43, 1010 OSLO 1

PAKISTAN : Mirza Book Agency, 65 Shahrah–E–Quaid–E–Azam, P.O. Box 729, LAHORE 3

PAPUA NEW GUINEA : WHO Programme Coordinator, P.O. Box 5896, BOROKO

PHILIPPINES : World Health Organization, Regional Office for the Western Pacific, P.O. Box 2932, MANILA — The Modern Book Company Inc., P.O. Box 632, 926 Rizal Avenue, MANILA

POLAND : Składnica Księgarska, ul Mazowiecka 9, 00052 WARSAW (*except periodicals*) — BKWZ Ruch, ul Wronia 23, 00840 WARSAW (*periodicals only*)

PORTUGAL : Livraria Rodrigues, 186 Rua do Ouro, LISBON 2

SIERRA LEONE : Njala University College Bookshop (University of Sierra Leone), Private Mail Bag, FREETOWN

SINGAPORE : The WHO Programme Coordinator, 144 Moulmein Road, G.P.O. Box 3457, SINGAPORE 1 — Select Books (Pte) Ltd, 215 Tanglin Shopping Centre, 2/F, 19 Tanglin Road, SINGAPORE 10

SOUTH AFRICA : Van Schaik's Bookstore (Pty) Ltd, P.O. Box 724, 268 Church Street, PRETORIA 0001

SPAIN : Comercial Atheneum S.A., Consejo de Ciento 130–136, BARCELONA 15 ; General Moscardó 29, MADRID 20 — Librería Díaz de Santos, Lagasca 95, MADRID 6 ; Balmes 417 y 419, BARCELONA 6

SRI LANKA : *see* India, WHO Regional Office

SWEDEN : Aktiebolaget C. E. Fritzes Kungl. Hovbokhandel, Regeringsgatan 12, 103 27 STOCKHOLM

SWITZERLAND : Medizinischer Verlag Hans Huber, Länggass Strasse 76, 3012 BERNE 9

SYRIAN ARAB REPUBLIC : M. Farras Kekhia, P.O. Box No. 5221, ALEPPO

THAILAND : *see* India, WHO Regional Office

TUNISIA : Société Tunisienne de Diffusion, 5 avenue de Carthage, TUNIS

TURKEY : Haset Kitapevi, 469 Istiklal Caddesi, Beyoglu, ISTANBUL

UNITED KINGDOM : H. M. Stationery Office : 49 High Holborn, LONDON WC1V 6HB ; 13a Castle Street, EDINBURGH EH2 3AR ; 41 The Hayes, CARDIFF CF1 1JW ; 80 Chichester Street, BELFAST BT1 4JY ; Brazennose Street, MANCHESTER M60 8AS ; 258 Broad Street, BIRMINGHAM B1 2HE ; Southey House, Wine Street, BRISTOL BS1 2BQ. *All mail orders should be sent to* P.O. Box 569, LONDON SE1 9NH

UNITED STATES OF AMERICA : *Single and bulk copies of individual publications (not subscriptions) :* WHO Publications Centre USA, 49 Sheridan Avenue, ALBANY, NY 12210. *Subscriptions : Subscription orders, accompanied by check made out to the* Chemical Bank, New York, Account World Health Organization, *should be sent to the* World Health Organization, P.O. Box 5284, Church Street Station, NEW YORK, NY 10249. *Correspondence concerning subscriptions should be addressed to the* World Health Organization, Distribution and Sales, 1211 GENEVA 27, Switzerland. *Publications are also available from the* United Nations Bookshop, NEW YORK, NY 10017 (*retail only*), *and single and bulk copies of individual* International Agency for Research on Cancer *publications (not subscriptions) may also be ordered from the* Franklin Institute Press, Benjamin Franklin Parkway, Philadelphia, PA 19103

USSR : *For readers in the USSR requiring Russian editions :* Komsomolskij prospekt 18, Medicinskaja Kniga, Moscow — *For readers outside the USSR requiring Russian editions :* Kuzneckij most 18, Meždunarodnaja Kniga, Moscow G-200

VENEZUELA : Editorial Interamericana de Venezuela C.A., Apartado 50785, CARACAS 105 — Librería del Este, Apartado 60337, CARACAS 106

YUGOSLAVIA : Jugoslovenska Knjiga, Terazije 27/II, 11000 BELGRADE

ZAIRE : Librairie universitaire, avenue de la Paix Nº 167, B.P. 1682, KINSHASA I

Special terms for developing countries are obtainable on application to the WHO Programme Coordinators or WHO Regional Offices listed above or to the World Health Organization, Distribution and Sales Service, 1211 Geneva 27, Switzerland. Orders from countries where sales agents have not yet been appointed may also be sent to the Geneva address, but must be paid for in pounds sterling, US dollars, or Swiss francs.

Price: Sw. fr. 60.— US$ 35.00   Prices are subject to change without notice.   IARC/2/78